NAVIGATING DENTAL EDUCATION TRENDS AND TRANSFORMIN

This volume offers a comprehensive examination of contemporary trends, pioneering innovations, and [illegible] challenges in dental education, spanning undergraduate and postgraduate curricula. It examines how training evolves to address the dynamic exigencies of clinical practice, technological convergence, and learner-centric paradigms.

Key themes include:

- Curriculum design and outcome-based, competency-based, and choice-based education.
- Assessment strategies, mentorship, and interprofessional collaboration.
- Digital tools like simulation, gaming, and advanced diagnostics.
- Student, educator, and examiner perspectives on teaching, evaluation, and competencies.
- Clinical training, communication, professionalism, ethics, and care for special needs patients.

Together, these chapters illustrate emerging best practices and practical solutions aimed at improving the quality, effectiveness, and relevance of dental education.

This book is intended for dental educators, academic administrators, curriculum planners, postgraduate students, and researchers in health professions education. It will also be valuable to policymakers and clinicians interested in educational reform and evidence-informed teaching practices in dentistry.

Taylor & Francis Proceedings in Healthcare and Pharmaceutical Sciences

This series is a compilation of peer-reviewed conference proceedings in healthcare and pharmaceutical sciences. This prestigious series captures groundbreaking advances across the full spectrum of healthcare sciences, from basic biomedical research to clinical applications and pharmaceutical innovation.

Navigating Dental Education Trends and Transforming Dental Pedagogy
Edited by Adinegara Lutfi Abas and Srikant N

For more information about this series, please visit: www.routledge.com/Taylor–Francis-Proceedings-in-Healthcare-and-Pharmaceutical-Sciences/book-series/TFPHPS

Navigating Dental Education Trends and Transforming Dental Pedagogy

Edited by

Adinegara Lutfi Abas
Manipal University College (MUCM) Malaysia's Faculty of Allied Health

Srikant N
Manipal College of Dental Sciences Mangalore, Manipal Academy of Higher Education, Manipal, India

PROCEEDINGS OF THE INTERNATIONAL CONFERENCE ON DENTAL EDUCATION AND CURRICULUM CONCLAVE 6.0 (ICDECC2024), MANGALORE, INDIA, 27TH TO 29TH SEPTEMBER 2024

CRC Press
Taylor & Francis Group
Boca Raton London New York

CRC Press is an imprint of the
Taylor & Francis Group, an **informa** business

First edition published 2027
by CRC Press
4 Park Square, Milton Park, Abingdon, Oxon, OX14 4RN

and by CRC Press
2385 NW Executive Center Drive, Suite 320, Boca Raton FL 33431

CRC Press is an imprint of informa UK Limited

British Library Cataloguing-in-Publication Data
A catalogue record for this book is available from the British Library

ISBN: 978-1-041-32674-8 (hbk)
ISBN: 978-1-041-39036-7 (pbk)
ISBN: 978-1-042-01607-5 (ebk)

DOI: 10.1201/9781042016075

Typeset in Times New Roman
by MPS Limited, Chennai, India

Navigating Dental Education Trends and Transforming Dental Pedagogy – Abas and Srikant N (Eds)
© 2027 The Editor(s), ISBN: 978-1-041-32674-8

Contents

Preface

Contemporary dental education increasingly calls for rigorous, evidence-informed approaches to teaching, learning, and assessment. As institutions move toward competency-based frameworks and outcome-oriented curricula, the need for systematic scholarly evaluation of educational practices has become more pressing. This volume responds to that imperative by bringing together carefully designed studies and analytically grounded discussions that explore critical dimensions of dental education.

The chapters presented here draw on a wide range of research methodologies, including cross-sectional surveys, observational studies, mixed methods approaches, and structured educational interventions. Collectively, they examine curriculum design, assessment strategies, learner and faculty perspectives, mentoring systems, and the integration of digital technologies and simulation-based learning. Several contributions critically address the validity, reliability, and feasibility of assessment tools, while others evaluate innovative pedagogical approaches and their measurable impact on learning outcomes. Together, these works offer a robust body of empirical evidence to inform curriculum development, institutional policy, and instructional practice.

This book is intended for dental educators, health professions education researchers, and academic leaders seeking methodologically sound insights to support informed decision-making. It also serves as a valuable resource for postgraduate students and emerging scholars engaged in educational research design and implementation. By foregrounding systematic inquiry and critical evaluation, this volume aspires to contribute meaningfully to the advancement of dental education and to support the pursuit of sustained academic excellence.

 ISBN: 978-1-041-32674-8

Foreword

Education transcends the mere transmission of knowledge; it is the development of professionals who serve society with competence, compassion, and integrity. In dentistry, where scientific knowledge, technical skills, and patient interaction converge, the role of education is particularly significant. This book arises from a shared commitment to enhance dental education by preparing reflective practitioners for the challenges of contemporary oral healthcare.

The chapters are derived from the expertise of educators in the field of dentistry dedicated to effective teaching and substantive learning. They address innovations such as digital tools, simulation training, mentorship, and learner-centered approaches, while emphasizing ethical standards and patient-centered care. In addition to instructional methods and evaluation techniques, the book underscores essential qualities of excellence in education: curiosity, accountability, empathy, and commitment to lifelong learning. Each contribution prompts educators to adapt classrooms, clinics, and curricula to promote critical thinking and professional development.

This volume is designed for educators, academic administrators, and students who regard education as a dynamic process. It aims to reinforce dedication to teaching, encourage constructive discussion, and support the training of dental professionals who demonstrate skill, purpose, and compassion.

Dr. Dilip G Naik
Pro-Vice Chancellor, Manipal Academy of Higher Education,
Manipal, India

About the Editors

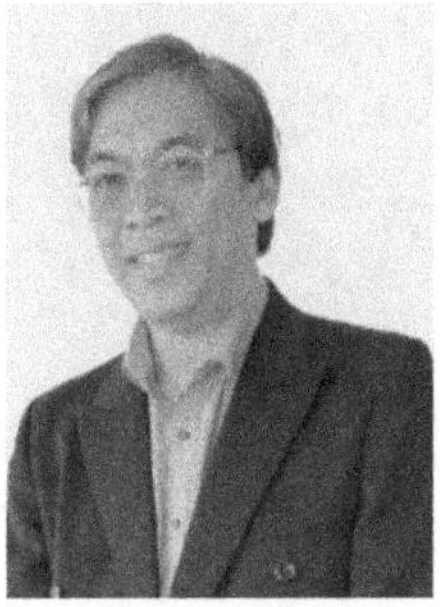

Adinegara Lutfi Abas currently serves as the Pro Vice Chancellor at Manipal University College Malaysia. He is a distinguished member of the Faculty of Allied Health & Psychology, where his contributions have significantly enriched both academic and research endeavors. He has around 49 scopus index publications in reputed scopus indexed journals to his credit. These publications have garnered a commendable 547 citations, a testament to the caliber and impact of his research. Furthermore, his h-index of 14 underscores the significance and influence of his scholarly output. A distinguishing feature of his work is its international collaboration, with approximately 10.5% of his publications being co-authored with researchers from other countries and regions.

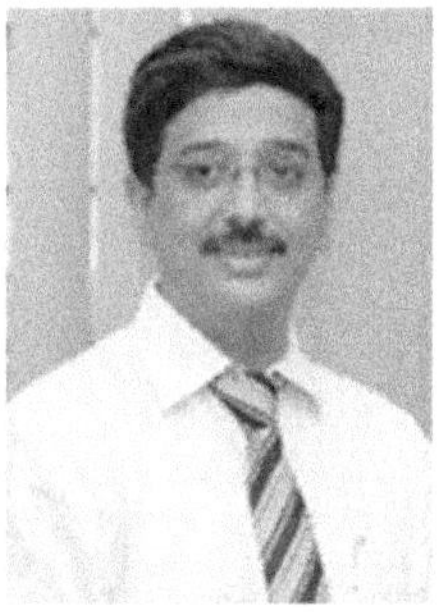

Srikant N serves as the professor and Head of the Department of Oral Pathology and Microbiology and the Coordinator for the Center for Forensic Odontology, Manipal College of Dental Sciences, Mangalore, MAHE. He is currently pursuing his PhD under the Manipal Academy of Higher Education, Manipal. He has authored and co-authored seven textbooks covering a wide range of oral and maxillofacial pathology and dental anatomy and histology. He has over 230 scientific publications with around 500 citations. He has many highly indexed research publications with a H index of 16 and an i10-index of 32, research grants, best research awards, best presentation awards, best teacher award, and technology innovation awards to his credit. His motto is to continue learning and disperse knowledge through the gained experience.

Navigating Dental Education Trends and Transforming Dental Pedagogy – Abas and Srikant N (Eds)
© 2027 The Editor(s), ISBN: 978-1-041-32674-8

Organizing Committee

Organising committee	
CHAIRPERSON	Dr. Junaid Ahmed, Professor & Associate Dean, Department of Oral Medicine and Radiology, MCODS, Mangalore
ORGANISING SECRETARY	Dr. Supriya Nambiar, Professor and Head, Department of Orthodontics and Dentofacial Orthopedics, MCODS, Mangalore
SCIENTIFIC COMMITTEE	
EDITORS	Dr. Srikant N., Professor & Associate Dean, Department of Oral Pathology and Microbiology, MCODS, Mangalore
	Dr. Adinegara Lutfi Abas, Pro Vice Chancellor, Manipal University College Malaysia (MUCM)
	Prof Dr. Soumendra Sahoo, Director, Center for Transformative Learning and HoD Ophthalmology, Manipal University College Malaysia
EDITORIAL TEAM	Dr Karuna Y M, Associate Professor, Department of Pediatric and Preventive Dentistry, MCODS, Mangalore
	Dr. Supriya Nambiar, Professor and Head, Department of Orthodontics and Dentofacial Orthopedics, MCODS, Mangalore
	Dr. Asavari Desai, Associate Professor, Department of Orthodontics and Dentofacial Orthopaedics, MCODS, Mangalore
	Dr. Prashanthi S. Madhyastha, Associate Professor and Incharge Head, Department of Dental Materials, MCODS, Mangalore
	Dr Bhagyalakshmi, Reader, Department of Orthodontics and Dentofacial Orthopedics, JSS Dental College and Hospital, Mysore
	Dr. Laxmish Mallya, Associate Professor, Department of Conservative Dentistry, MCODS, Mangalore
	Dr. Pushpanjali Krishnappa, Professor and Head, Department of Public Health Dentistry, Faculty of Dental Sciences, M.S.Ramaiah University of Applied Sciences, Bangalore
	Dr. Gulam Saidunnisa Begum, Professor & Head, Department of Biochemistry, College of Medicine and Health Sciences, National University of Science and Technology, Oman
	Dr. Shahista, Assistant Professor, Department of Orthodontics, RAK College of Dental Sciences, Ras Al-Khaimah, UAE
FOOD COMMITTEE	Dr. Sharon J.R. Saldanha, Associate Professor, Department of Prosthodontics and Crown and Bridge MCODS, Mangalore
	Dr. Sandipan Mukherjee, Senior Lecturer, Department of Prosthodontics and Crown & Bridge, MCODS, Mangalore
	Dr. David Kadakampally, Associate Professor, Department of Periodontology, MCODS, Mangalore
HOSPITALITY COMMITTEE	Dr. Nandita Shenoy, Associate Professor, Department of Oral Medicine and Radiology, MCODS, Mangalore
	Dr. Nandita K.P., Professor Head, Department of Oral Pathology & Microbiology, MCODS, Mangalore
	Dr. Avinash B.R., Senior Lecturer, Department of Public Heath Dentistry, MCODS, Mangalore
	Dr. Sandipan Mukherjee, Senior Lecturer, Department of Prosthodontics and Crown & Bridge, MCODS, Mangalore
	Dr. Mithun Pai B.H., Associate Professor, Department of Public Health Dentistry, MCODS, Mangalore
RECEPTION COMMITTEE	Dr. Shreya Hegde, Associate Professor, Department of Conservative Dentistry and Endodontics, MCODS, Mangalore
	Dr Arvind R, Professor & I/C Head, Department of Oral and Maxillofacial Surgery, MCODS, Mangalore
	Dr. Amoli Singh, Senior Lecturer, Department of Orthodontics and Dentofacial Orthopedics, MCODS, Mangalore
TREASURY	Dr. Junaid Ahmed, Professor & Associate Dean, Department of Oral Medicine and Radiology, MCODS, Mangalore
	Dr. Asavari Desai, Associate Professor, Department of Orthodontics and Dentofacial Orthopaedics, MCODS, Mangalore
	Dr. Nandita Shenoy, Associate Professor, Department of Oral Medicine and Radiology, MCODS, Mangalore

(*continued*)

Continued

Organising committee	
PRE CONFERENCE COMMITTEE	Dr. Nanditha Sujir, Associate Professor, Department of Oral Medicine and Radiology, MCODS, Mangalore Dr. Nandita Shenoy, Associate Professor, Department of Oral Medicine and Radiology, MCODS, Mangalore Dr Arvind R, Professor & I/C Head, Department of Oral and Maxillofacial Surgery, MCODS, Mangalore Dr. Shivangi Vats, Senior Lecturer, Department of conservative Dentistry and Endodontics, MCODS, Mangalore Dr. Vignesh Kamath, Assistant Professor, Department of Prosthodontics and Crown and Bridge MCODS, Mangalore Dr. Sandeep K M, Senior Lecturer, Department of Oral and Maxillofacial Surgery, MCODS, Mangalore Dr. David Kadakampally, Associate Professor, Department of Periodontology, MCODS, Mangalore

 ISBN: 978-1-041-32674-8

Scientific Committee

1. Prof. Dr Adinegara Lutfi Abas, Pro Vice Chancellor, Manipal University College Malaysia (MUCM), Faculty of Allied Health.
2. Dr. Srikant N, Professor, Department of Oral Pathology and Microbiology, Manipal College of Dental Sciences Mangalore, Manipal Academy of Higher Education, Manipal, India.
3. Dr. Vineet Dhar, Chair, Faculty of Pedodontics and Orthodontics, University of Maryland, USA.
4. Prof Dr. Soumendra Sahoo, Director, Center for Transformative Learning and HoD Ophthalmology, Manipal University College Malaysia.
5. Dr. Shashidhar Acharya, Professor, Department of Public Health Dentistry, Manipal College of Dental Sciences Manipal, Manipal Academy of Higher Education, Manipal, India.
6. Dr. Supriya Nambiar, Professor and Head, Department of Orthodontics and Dentofacial Orthopedics, Manipal College of Dental Sciences Mangalore, Manipal Academy of Higher Education, Manipal, India.
7. Dr. Karuna YM, Associate Professor, Department of Pediatric and Preventive Dentistry, Manipal College of Dental Sciences Mangalore, Manipal Academy of Higher Education, Manipal, India.
8. Dr. Asavari Desai, Associate Professor, Department of Orthodontics and Dentofacial Orthopedics, Manipal College of Dental Sciences Mangalore, Manipal Academy of Higher Education, Manipal, India.
9. Dr. Laxmish Malya, Associate Professor, Department of Conservative Dentistry, Manipal College of Dental Sciences Mangalore, Manipal Academy of Higher Education, Manipal, India.
10. Dr. Violet D'souza, Assistant Professor, Faculty of Dentistry, Dalhousie University.
11. Dr. Kalyan Chakravarthy, Associate professor, Department of Public Health Dentistry, Manipal College of Dental Sciences Manipal, Manipal Academy of Higher Education, Manipal, India.
12. Dr. Bhagyalakshmi Avinash, Professor in Orthodontics, Consultant Orthodontist, Faculty Advisor, M-FILIPE Manipal Academy of Higher Education, Manipal, India.
13. Dr. Gulam Saidunnisa Begum, Professor & Head, Department of Biochemistry, College of Medicine and Health Sciences, National University of Science and Technology, Oman.
14. Dr. Shashistha Parveen Dasnadi, Assistant Professor of Orthodontics, RAK college of dental Sciences, Ras Al Khaimah Medical and Health Sciences, University.
15. Dr. Puspanjali, Professor and Head, Department of Public Health Dentistry, Faculty of Dental Sciences, M.S. Ramaiah University of Applied Sciences, Bengaluru.
16. Dr. Samarika Dahal, Associate Professor and Head, Department of Oral Pathology, Institute of Medicine Marajgunj Medical Campus, Kathmandu.
17. Dr. Shivangi Vats, Senior Lecturer, Department of Conservative Dentistry and Endodontics, Manipal College of Dental Sciences, Mangalore.
18. Dr. Janina Loren D'Souza, Senior Lecturer, Department of Conservative Dentistry and Endodontics, Manipal College of Dental Sciences Mangalore, Manipal Academy of Higher Education, Manipal, India.
19. Dr. Vignesh Kamath, Senior Lecturer, Department of Prosthodontics, Manipal College of Dental Sciences, Mangalore.

Navigating Dental Education Trends and Transforming Dental Pedagogy – Abas and Srikant N (Eds)
 ISBN: 978-1-041-32674-8

A Module on Interprofessional Communication Skills for Health Care Undergraduate Students

Nandita Shenoy
Associate Professor, Department of Oral Medicine and Radiology, Manipal College of Dental Sciences Mangalore, Manipal Academy of Higher Education, Manipal, India

Gagan Bajaj
Department of Audiology and Speech-Language Pathology, Kasturba Medical College, Mangalore, Manipal Academy of Higher Education, Manipal, Karnataka, India

A M Ciraj
Department of Microbiology, Manipal Academy of Higher Education, Manipal, Karnataka, India

ABSTRACT: **Introduction:** In addition to professional skills, healthcare workers need good communication skills for good clinical practice. It is a backbone over which many areas of patient care rest, such as first-contact patient interviews, probing for associated and additional problems, counselling the patient, explaining treatment options and complications, and advising follow-up and rest.

Methods: An interprofessional group of 100 students belonging to various streams, mainly medical, dental, physiotherapy, and audiology, was chosen for this module. The assessment of students' preexisting knowledge of communication skills was carried out before the initiation of the course via the Communication Skill Attitude Scale (CSAS), which Rees and Sheard originally developed. A hybrid module was used wherein ten lectures were delivered online via Microsoft Teams, and feedback was obtained after each session via Microsoft Forms validated by my mentor. Onsite sessions were conducted for 5 hours, including small group discussions, roleplaying, and sessions with simulated patients. The training module for teaching communication skills included topics related to communication, leadership, teamwork, and professionalism, which were delivered by an interprofessional team of instructors. Posttest assessment was performed via the CSAS at the end of the module, and the values were compared with the pretest scores.

Results: Student's t test was used to compare the pretest and posttest scores, and a P value < 0.05 was considered to indicate statistical significance.

Discussion: Student Perceptions and Attitudes: Students perceived communication skills training positively. They highlighted the importance of integrating communication skills training longitudinally throughout the curriculum. There was significant statistical variation in attitudes, behaviours, and satisfaction among the students and between the groups at the end of the module, indicating the need for such a module in the health care curriculum.

Keywords: Communication, Empathy, Medical education, Physician—patient relations, Questionnaire

1 INTRODUCTION

Professional education has not kept pace with recent challenges largely because of fragmented, outdated, and static curricula that produce ill-equipped graduates with competencies mismatched with patient and population needs and a lack of teamwork. The development of empathy and a broader outlook toward patient care should be introduced early in their student life to prevent the loss of trust in the physician—patient relationship [1].

With the rise in consumerism in health care, patients look for a more patient-centered and person-focused doctor rather than a doctor who is characterized by high physician control [2]. The person-focused style mandates teaching the next generation good communication and empathy skills. Good communication is shown to increase the positive patient perception that is required for better recovery and better emotional health. This approach also benefits doctors by increasing work satisfaction and decreasing frustration in daily work [3].

1.1 *Aim*

This study aimed to identify the importance and perceptions of communication skill training via a validated communication training module among an interprofessional group of undergraduate students at a university in India.

DOI: 10.1201/9781042016075-1

The specific objectives were as follows:

- Identifying the perceptions and experiences of interprofessional undergraduate students with respect to communication skills

To assess the efficacy of the developed module and the knowledge, attitudes, and practices of the dental, medical, and allied health students

2 METHODOLOGY

An interprofessional group of 100 students belonging to various streams, mainly medical, dental, physiotherapy, and audiology, were chosen for this module. The module was well structured and validated by the medical education unit of the institution. Our study was conducted on an interprofessional group of students comprising medical, dental, physiotherapy, and audiology backgrounds, for a total of 100 students. The blended model of training was developed by the faculty of various specialties and trainers of medical education who are trained in skills training, e-learning, and telemedicine at the institute. Each module has online content with recorded lectures, including standard operating procedures (SOPs), videos demonstrating skills, and live sessions and simulation classes. The pre- and posttest CSAS questionnaires[4] were sent through Google Forms to these students, and the questionnaires consisted of dichotomous, open, and closed questions; Likert-type scale questions; and multiple-choice questions.

The assessment of students' preexisting knowledge of communication skills was carried out before the initiation of the program via the Communication Skill Attitude Scale (CSAS), which was originally developed by Rees and Sheard[5]. The training module was planned following Millers' pyramid for teaching communication skills, including topics related to communication, leadership, teamwork, and professionalism, which were covered through didactic lectures, small group discussions, roleplaying, and simulated patients. Posttest assessment was performed at the end of the module via the CSAS, and the values were compared with the pretest scores.

with the sequence of activity shown in Table 1.

3 RESULTS

The pretest and posttest CSAS scores were assessed, and statistical analysis was performed via paired t tests.

Table 1. Pre- and posttest differences among the study participants (n=100).

		(Audiology+ Physiotherapy) N=28		(Medical+Dental) N=72	
Pair	Variables	Mean difference ± SD*	P Value	Mean difference ± SD*	P Value
Pair 1	To be a good practitioner, I must have good communication skills.	−0.14±1.3	0.565	0.16±1.18	0.504
Pair 2	I can't see the point in learning communication skills.	−0.04±0.96	0.846	1.54±1.55	<**0.001*****
Pair 3	Nobody is going to fail to have poor communication skills.	0.36±1.25	0.143	0.46±1.33	<**0.001*****
Pair 4	Developing my communication skills is just as important as developing my knowledge of my specialty	0.39±1.42	0.156	0.96±1.54	**0.005*****
Pair 5	Learning communication skills has helped me or will help me respect patients.	0.29±1.24	0.234	0.50±1.17	**0.040*****
Pair 6	I haven't got time to learn communication skills.	−0.07±0.94	0.691	1.04±1.11	<**0.001*****
Pair 7	Learning communication skills is interesting.	0.25±1.08	0.229	0.08±1.09	0.72
Pair 8	I can't be bothered to turn up to sessions on communication skills.	−0.57±1.35	**0.033*****	−0.04±1.31	0.88
Pair 9	Learning communication skills has helped or will facilitate my team working skills.	0±1.28	1	0.58±1.09	**0.029*****
Pair 10	Learning communication skills has improved my ability to communicate with patients.	0.07±1.27	0.769	0.69±1.32	**0.013*****
Pair 11	Communication skills teaches the obvious and then complicates it.	0±1.31	1	−0.35±1.52	0.26
Pair 12	Learning communication skills is fun.	0.29±1.18	0.212	0.15±0.92	0.40
Pair 13	Learning communication skills is too easy.	−0.43±1.14	0.056	0.31±1.05	0.15
Pair 14	Learning communication skills has helped or will help	0.11±1.26	0.656	0.38±1.20	0.12

(continued)

Table 1. Continued

Pair	Variables	(Audiology+ Physiotherapy) N=28		(Medical+Dental) N=72	
		Mean difference ± SD*	P Value	Mean difference ± SD*	P Value
	me respect my colleagues.				
Pair 15	I feel confident after the training session communication skills given to me by nonclinical lecturers.	−1.61±1.17	**<0.001****	0.00±165	1.00
Pair 16	Learning communication skills has helped or will help me recognize patients' rights regarding confidentiality and informed consent.	−0.04±1.14	0.869	1.12±161	**0.002*****
Pair 17	Communication skills teaching would have a better image if it sounded more like a science subject.	−0.11±1.45	0.699	0.2±1.55	0.53
Pair 18	When applying for I thought it was a truly good idea to learn communication skills.	−0.43±1.07	**0.043*****	0.91±1.41	**0.006*****
Pair 19	I don't need good communication skills to be a doctor	−0.21±1.34	0.406	1.44±1.16	**<0.001*****
Pair 20	I find it hard to admit to having some problems with my communication skills.	0.57±1.14	**0.013*****	0.52±1.45	0.08
Pair 21	I think it's truly useful learning communication skills for my specialty.	−0.54±0.96	**0.007*****	0.00±1.54	1.00
Pair 22	My ability to pass exams will get me through l rather than my ability to communicate.	0.25±1.35	0.336	1.04±1.49	**0.003*****
Pair 23	I find it difficult to take communication skills learning seriously.	−0.14±1.15	0.515	0.72±1.21	**0.007*****
Pair 24	Learning communication skills is important because my ability to communicate is a lifelong skill.	0±1.12	1	0.56±1.00	**0.01*****
Pair 25	Communication skills learning should be left to psychology students, not dental students.	0.11±1.17	0.631	0.68±1.11	**0.005*****

*SD-Standard deviation **Paired t test applied *** p<0.05=statistically significant

4 DISCUSSION

The National Medical Commission of India introduced the Competency-Based Curriculum in Medical Education for undergraduate medical students in 2019 with a new module named Attitude, Ethics and Communication (AETCOM) [6]. To explore the need for such a module for dental and allied health students, a survey was designed through online Microsoft forms and was shared among faculty of various specialties to determine their experiences and attitudes towards teaching and evaluating their communication skills. The responses strongly supported the need for communication training involving components of leadership and professionalism.

4.1 *Phase I:—Quantitative part*

We compared the effectiveness of communication skills training as reported on a postintervention scale in which skills, attitudes, and satisfaction outcomes were assessed. There was a statistically significant difference in the value of being asked if they felt confident after the training session on the communication skills given to them. For better practices, learning communication skills was important, and there was a statistically significant difference between the values at postintervention (SD=−0.43±1.07 and p value=0.043). Many participants found it difficult to confess that they have issues admitting that they lack good communication skills, as was the case in our group; similar findings were also reported in studies by Clever *et al.* [7]

There were no statistically significant differences in many other parameters that were assessed, such as "my ability to pass exams will get me through my course rather than my ability to communicate".

Our experience with our study group showed that onsite sessions make enormous differences in communication skill training. Onsite sessions on role play, simulated patients, and active interactive sessions with trainers in communication have had great impacts on these students [8-10]. The pre- and posttest analysis results of this group revealed the importance of skill training that focused on practical matters such as learning interview techniques, consultation, simulations, or roleplay with peers. This study investigated undergraduate students' attitudes toward communication skills and revealed that the students held a significantly positive attitude toward subjects that imparted "soft skills" (e.g., communication skills) after the completion of the module.

Our findings revealed that these students had high levels of positive attitudes and low levels of negative views. A positive reaction to the onsite sessions suggested that these students were generally more interested in communication, as the study required voluntary participation. While a comparison of mean scores indicated the value of practicing communication skills, many people have concluded that poor communication skills are not a reason for failure in professional degree programs.

Our research participants believed that developing their communication skills improved their ability to collaborate with others, respect patients, and interact with them. Studies have demonstrated a statistically significant positive correlation between the acquisition of communication skills and the recognition of patients' rights to informed consent and confidentiality [11]. They found it difficult to take communication skills seriously, and they believed that psychology students, not healthcare personnel, should be in charge of teaching people these abilities. This led to a considerable decrease in values, according to the posttest survey. Owing to time constraints and hard workdays, the students believed that gaining communication skills would be useful; however, they also believed that developing communication skills is vital since they are lifetime skills. [12].

4.2 *Phase II: Qualitative part*

Following the phase I study, a small number of participants were selected for semistructured interviews on the basis of their answers to the questionnaire to obtain their opinions and a credible explanation for their distinct perceptions as study subjects of the hybrid module. They were chosen on the basis of factors that included their availability, willingness to engage, and capacity for thoughtful and eloquent communication of experiences and ideas. The positive feedback from the students regarding their level of satisfaction with the curriculum was evident in the results. They believed that a great deal of the information improved their understanding and made it possible for them to communicate with me in both personal and professional capacity. Some pupils expressed humility and gratitude to the resource people for their hard work and knowledge, which gave them excellent opportunities to study. The module was deemed interesting, highly instructive, and beautifully presented by the students. Additionally, they have begun putting some of the techniques and resources they were taught to use, and they report that it is doing extraordinarily well. Although many students wanted to bring their friends along, after a few sessions, we did not want any more participants. This thoughtful criticism is noted and subjected to a thematic examination.

5 CONCLUSIONS

We have provided an adequate opportunity for students to master the effective communication techniques necessary to manage their patients and develop best practices in this module. The novelty of our study is that communication modules were formally introduced to a group of interprofessional students for the first time, and feedback was obtained.

REFERENCES

[1] Haskard KB, Williams SL, DiMatteo MR, Rosenthal R, White MK, Goldstein MG. (2008). Physician and patient communication training in primary care: effects on participation and satisfaction. *Health Psychol.* 27:513–22.

[2] Pehrson C, Banerjee SC, Manna R, Shen MJ, Hammonds S, Coyle N, *et al.* (2016). Responding empathically to patients: development, implementation, and evaluation of a communication skills training module for oncology nurses. *Patient Educ Couns.* 99:610–6.

[3] Moore PM, Rivera S, Bravo-Soto GA, Olivares C, Lawrie TA. (2018). Communication skills training for healthcare professionals working with people who have cancer. *Cochrane Database Syst Rev.* 7:CD003751.

[4] C Rees, C Sheard, S Davies. (2002). The development of a scale to measure medical students' attitudes towards communication skills learning: The Communication Skills Attitude Scale (CSAS). *Med Educ*, 36, pp. 141–147

[5] Maguire P, Pitceathly C. (2002). Key communication skills and how to acquire them. *BMJ.* 325: 697–700. 10.1136/bmj.325.7366.697.

[6] C Rees, C Sheard. (2002). The relationship between medical students' attitudes towards communication skills learning and their demographic and education-related characteristics. *Med Educ*, 36, p. 1017

[7] Chandra Shaw S, Datta K, Lall M, Jaipurkar R, Shakya AK, Kanitkar M. (2024). Development of a hybrid undergraduate portfolio for the AETCOM module. *Med J Armed Forces India.* 80(2):192–198.

[8] Clever SL, Jin L, Levinson W, Meltzer DO. (2008). Does doctor™patient communication affect patient satisfaction with hospital care? Results of an analysis with a novel instrumental variable. *Health Serv Res.* 43: 1505–519

[9] Roter DL, Hall JA, Kern DE, Barker LR, Cole KA, Roca RP (1995). Improving physicians' interviewing skills and reducing patients' emotional distress. *Arch Intern Med.* 155: 1877–1884. 10.1001/archinte.1995.00430170071009.

[10] Hausberg, M.C., Hergert, A., Kröger, C. *et al.* (2012). Enhancing medical students' communication skills: development and evaluation of an undergraduate training program. *BMC Med Educ* 12, 16. https://doi.org/10.1186/1472-6920-12-16

[11] Hulsman RL, Ros WJ, Winnubst JA, Bensing JM. (1999). Teaching clinically experienced physician's communication skills. A review of evaluation studies. *Med Educ*; 33: 655–68.

[12] Windy Levinson, Cara S. Lesser, Ronald M. Epstain. (2010). Developing physician communication skills for patients centered care. *Health Affairs* 29 (7): 1310–1317.

[13] Rider EA. (2010). Interpersonal and communication skills. In: Rider EA, Nawotniak RH. *A Practical Guide to Teaching and Assessing the ACGME Core Competencies*, 2nd edition. Marblehead, MA: HCPro, Inc., pp 1–137.

Navigating Dental Education Trends and Transforming Dental Pedagogy – Abas and Srikant N (Eds)
 ISBN: 978-1-041-32674-8

Undergraduate Dental Education in Prosthodontics: Current Scenario and Future Trends

Shobha J Rodrigues, Thilak Shetty, Umesh Y Pai, Sharon Saldanha, and M Mahesh
Department of Prosthodontics, Manipal College of Dental Sciences Mangalore, Manipal Academy of Higher Education, Manipal, Karnataka, India

Sandipan Mukherjee, Ann Sales, Vignesh Kamath, and Prashant Bajantri
Department of Prosthodontics and Crown and Bridge, Manipal College of Dental Sciences Mangalore, Manipal Academy of Higher Education, Manipal, Karnataka, India

ABSTRACT: Dentistry in India is currently being challenged to maintain its professionalism. We produce 25000-30000 dental graduates annually. The challenges any dental university faces is to optimize education to its students, prioritize clinical service to its patients and still enforce mandatory regulations and codes of ethics. All this needs to be done in the face of changes in dentistry which is massively influenced by Artificial intelligence. The need of the hour is to make budding dentist a competent professional with skills required for utilizing the ever-changing and improving restorative materials and technology, while also being an accomplished diagnostician and critical thinker.This article is a narrative review of the current scenario in undergraduate teaching in the speciality of prosthodontics and the future trends that are influenced by the introduction of artificial intelligence in prosthodontics

1 INTRODUCTION

Dentistry in India is currently facing challenges in maintaining professionalism. Annually, we produce 25,000 to 30,000 dental graduates [1].

Dental universities must manage the complexities of optimizing student education, prioritizing clinical services for patients, and adhering to mandatory regulations and ethical standards. To address these issues, a dynamic and robust curriculum with effective feedback mechanisms is essential. This approach will keep stakeholders—students, faculty, and alumni—informed about the latest advancements in educational technology and help produce graduates who meet the current demands of healthcare delivery.

To facilitate this positive change, four key components are necessary: the Dental Council of India should recognize and mandate a dynamic curriculum that aligns with contemporary healthcare needs; the institution's administration must enforce it; faculty members should implement it; and students should adhere to it. This paper will examine the current landscape and trends in predoctoral prosthodontics, highlighting the role of educators in developing a responsive and effective curriculum to prepare future dentists for a digital world.

2 ROLE OF FACULTY IN PROSTHODONTICS

The predoctoral dental training program leading to the B.D.S. degree in India lasts a minimum of five years. Throughout this period, the Dental Council of India (DCI) required students to engage in full-time study at a DCI-recognized or DCI-approved dental college. During the five-year undergraduate program, instruction in clinical subjects must span at least three years. In prosthodontics, students receive training in preclinical complete denture prosthodontics during their first and second years.

Faculty in prosthodontics play a crucial role by providing information, supervising and supporting student learning, and facilitating the development of essential knowledge and skills.

3 IIND BDS

The assessment of the highest order, focusing on "what learners can do," must be designed to reflect the critical competencies required in the specialty of prosthodontics. Aligning outcomes and competencies with teaching and assessment in both clinical and preclinical training is essential. The preclinical curriculum for second-year BDS students in prosthodontics primarily emphasizes tooth arrangement and laboratory procedures related to complete denture prosthodontics [2].

DOI: 10.1201/9781042016075-2

Currently, the complete denture prosthodontics curriculum, as prescribed by the DCI and implemented at our institution, requires students to complete five-tooth arrangements and laboratory procedures [2]. Additionally, our school requires students to execute at least one laboratory investing and processing procedure for complete dentures. While these exercises are precursors of clinical requirements, students ultimately complete only five tooth arrangements and fabricate a single set of dentures in their preclinical training. Consequently, they have limited skills and experience in executing good complete dentures, sometimes resulting in suboptimal prostheses for patients.

As educators, we should prioritize what dental students should learn and make appropriate modifications in the curricula. For example, students need to grasp the principles of appropriate tooth arrangement and learn how to alter teeth positions in trial dentures to aesthetically and functionally satisfy patient requirements. Technology has transformed dentistry, and digital workflows are now standard in many practices. However, we must ask whether future practitioners are adequately prepared for this increasingly digitized landscape.

Digital technologies, including augmented reality (AR) and virtual reality (VR), offer invaluable interactive learning experiences that are accessible 24/7, along with objective evaluation methods [3].

Unfortunately, the insertion of CAD/CAM technology into predoctoral dental curricula is not common. If future practitioners are to be prepared to function in a digitized landscape, the inclusion of complete digital dentures in contemporary dental education is paramount. In addition, there is an increasing volume of research and clinical publications in this arena, and many companies offer digital complete dentures and increasing clinical application by practitioners because of their various advantages [3]. These prostheses present significant advantages that students should experience before graduation, ensuring that they are equipped for a career influenced by digital technology. Therefore, integrating digitization and e-learning into dental curricula is crucial for preparing future dentists.

Moreover, there is a relative lack of well-trained faculty members and available CAD/CAM units for students. It is imperative that our dental schools place greater emphasis on the use of digital workflows to prepare future practitioners for modern prosthodontics.

This need presents an excellent opportunity for students to learn tooth arrangements via computerized programs employed for fabricating digital dentures. Such programs enable students to understand tooth positioning for optimal aesthetics and functionality. Furthermore, faculty and students can play with the program to enhance learning and critique and identify various tooth positions. They can also provide partial arrangements on the basis of desired aesthetic or occlusal schemes, try various occlusal schemes allowing students to complete the arrangements and learn how to achieve specific outcomes. Thus, leveraging digital technology can significantly increase students' learning potential, allowing them to master much more than the DCI's mandatory curriculum in the same or even a shorter time frame.

4 III BDS

At the III BDS level, the DCI mandates a focus on predominant clinical training and didactic lectures in removable partial prosthodontics (RPD) [2]. While definitive prostheses typically consist of cast partial dentures, their cost often precludes their use in predoctoral training. As a result, students primarily work on creating transitional dentures for various Kennedy classifications. Currently, the traditional method for fabricating RPDs involves the use of irreversible hydrocolloids, and in cases of distal extensions, dual impressions are taken. The remaining steps align with those used in conventional complete denture prosthodontics.

Although students are introduced to all components of a cast partial framework and denture, they do not receive exposure to mouth preparations or the clinical application of a surveyor within their predoctoral program. While there is continuity in the learning process as students advance each year—building on knowledge from the second- to third-year students, it is crucial that third-year clinical students develop positive and responsible relationships with their patients. This relationship building can be fostered by observing the approaches of their educators in the clinic. Students cultivate professional behaviors and attitudes through role modeling and the hidden curriculum, making role modeling and supervision essential components of teaching in a clinical setting.

The traditional process for RPD fabrication can be summarized as follows: after an initial impression is taken via an irreversible hydrocolloid (alginate), all necessary mouth preparations are completed. This is followed by a final impression, which is made with elastomeric impression material or alginate via a custom tray. Additionally, border molding is required to capture detailed impressions of the distal extension edentulous areas [4,5].

Digital technology may be utilized here in a similar manner as explained for II BDS. Students may enjoy learning all the parts of the cast partial denture, including major connectors, minor connectors, rests, and direct and indirect retainers [4]. In addition, the justification for different designs in different Kennedy's classifications may be effectively understood.

5 FINAL BDS

At the final BDS level, the DCI mandates a focus on predominantly clinical training in removable prosthodontics and didactic lectures in fixed dental prosthodontics (FDP) [2]. Preclinical work involves demonstration and practical training in full veneer crowns for both anterior and posteriors. Wax patterns and castings are not part of their training.

Improved student performance in crown digitization and framework design was observed when computer-aided design/computer-aided manufacturing (CAD/CAM) courses were introduced in dental education [6].

The Department conducted an unpublished study where tooth preparations performed by the students were scanned by a laboratory scanner and constructive criticism was offered to improve their preparations. The students were then asked to repeat the preparations, and invariably, all performed better. In addition, students enjoyed designing a full crown via CAD rather than traditional waxing. Viewing their scanned crown preparations magnified on the screen improved students' understanding of the finishing line. The application of the IOS in simulation training showed that even inexperienced dental students could acquire the skills needed to use digital tools, and students preferred the IOS over conventional impressions [7–9]. Furthermore, work time was shorter with IOS than with conventional impressions [10]; [11] although more teaching time was required for digital scanning than for conventional impression techniques.

6 CURRENT ISSUES FACING THE DEPARTMENT

There is a paucity of well-trained faculty members, and the number of CAD/CAM units available to students limits its use. Faculty must be prepared for progressive training.

Some initial training was provided by the vendor at the institution. Additional training for faculty can take place through continuing education programmes. Additionally, faculty in the Department who use technology within their practices may also be a resource to support the integration of digital dentistry into the existing curriculum.

7 CONCLUSION

While undergraduate students today must be prepared for digital dentistry, they still need to acquire knowledge of conventional treatment strategies and processes. When they grow in the digital world, they easily adapt to digital features. Digital dentistry offers several options for an objective standardized evaluation of students' performance, which should be used for quality enhancement. It is currently a "teaching transition time", and new standards must be defined for dental education in general. Open questions remain, such as (i) in which phase of the dental curricula should digital technologies be introduced as routine tools; (ii) which analog techniques can be omitted; and (iii) which digital content should be taught in which disciplines?

No conflicts of interest

No funds were received.

REFERENCES

[1] Sharma S, Vijayaraghavan V, Tandon P, Kumar DR, Sharma H, Rao Y. (2012). Dental education: current scenario and future trends. *J Contemp Dent Pract.* 2012;13:107–10.

[2] BDS Course regulations. *Dental council of India.* Available online. https://dciindia.gov.in .Accessed 15th Oct 2024.

[3] Spielman AI. (2024). Dental education and practice: past, present, and future trends. Front Oral Health. :1368121.

[4] Phoenix RD, Cagna DR, Defreest CF. (2003). *Stewart's Clinical Removable Partial Prosthodontics.* 3rd ed. Chicago: Quintessence.

[5] Craig RG, Powers JM. (2002). *Restorative Dental Materials.* 11th ed. St. Louis: Mosby.

[6] Schwindling, F.S.; Deisenhofer, U.K.; Porsche, M.; Rammelsberg, P.; Kappel, S.; Stober, T. (2015). Establishing CAD/CAM in preclinical dental education: evaluation of a hands-on module. *J. Dent. Educ.* 79:1215–1221.

[7] Douglas, R.D.; Hopp, C.D.; Augustin, M.A. (2014). Dental students' preferences and performance in crown design: Conventional wax-added versus CAD. *J. Dent. Educ.* 78:1663–1672.

[8] Wegner, K.; Michel, K.; Seelbach, P.H.; Wostmann, B. (2017). A questionnaire on the use of digital denture impressions in a preclinical setting. *Int. J. Comput. Dent.* 20: 177–192.

[9] Schott, T.C.; Arsalan, R.; Weimer, K. (2019). Students' perspectives on the use of digital versus conventional dental impression techniques in orthodontics. *BMC Med. Educ.* 19:81.

[10] Zitzmann, N.U.; Kovaltschuk, I.; Lenherr, P.; Dedem, P.; Joda, T. (2017). Dental students' perceptions of digital and conventional impression techniques: A randomized controlled trial. *J. Dent. Educ.* 1:1227–1232.

[11] Lee, S.J.; Gallucci, G.O. (2013). Digital vs. conventional implant impressions: Efficiency outcomes. *Clin. Oral Implant. Res.* 24: 111–115.

[12] Marti, A.M.; Harris, B.T.; Metz, M.J.; Morton, D.; Scarfe,W.C.; Metz, C.J.; Lin,W.S. (2017). Comparison of digital scanning and polyvinyl siloxane impression techniques by dental students: Instructional efficiency and attitudes toward technology. *Eur. J. Dent. Educ.* 21: 200–205.

 ISBN: 978-1-041-32674-8

Essential Responses: Dental Education on Managing Medical Emergencies in the Dental Office

Shreya Hegde
Department of Conservative Dentistry and Endodontics, Manipal College of Dental Sciences Mangalore, Manipal Academy of Higher Education, Manipal, India

Deepak Hegde
Department of Orthopedics, K S Hegde Medical Academy, Deralakatte, Mangalore, Karnataka, India

M Roma
Department of Conservative Dentistry and Endodontics, Manipal College of Dental Sciences Mangalore, Manipal Academy of Higher Education, Manipal, India

1 INTRODUCTION

Medical crises can occur in dental practices, although catastrophic medical situations are providentially rare. More than half of oral health practitioners will have to handle some kind of medical emergency throughout their professional lives [1]. In the event of an emergency, waiting too long to provide care might have preventable repercussions. Ensuring that the dental team is properly educated in basic life support techniques and that basic emergency supplies and drugs are available will help lower the chance of death or major morbidity [2].

The kinds of medical crises that are most likely to occur at certain dental offices depend on the patient groups they serve and the procedures that are performed most frequently. When a clinician encounters such circumstances, the entire team should be competent, self-assured, and equipped with the most recent information to provide superior treatment during emergencies [3]. The significance of medical emergency management training requirements, including simulation training, and the necessity for medical crisis prevention, guidance and procedures. The regular implementation of simulation training is necessary to ensure that oral health practitioners are equipped to handle various medical problems. In the dental environment, prevention is the greatest means of being ready for medical crises hence, oral health practitioners need to stay up -to -date on medical emergency protocols [4].

Dentists worldwide still find it difficult to manage these kinds of situations in the dental clinic, even after finishing a qualified formal medical emergency training program for their undergraduate and graduate degrees [5]. In the past several years, a range of medical emergency training courses have been integrated into educational offerings via simulation model techniques and flipped classrooms. Both undergraduate and graduate management outcomes have significantly improved as a result of this extreme change in the more current instructional methodologies [6]. The requirement for clinicians to receive training in medical crises through several workshops persists although dentistry curricula differ around the sphere [7]. An overview of medical emergencies and effective management techniques is provided in this review, as this overview is crucial to the effectiveness of treatment outcomes.

2 METHODS

A comprehensive literature search was conducted across four databases (Medline through PubMed, Scopus, and Science Direct) using keywords such as dental education and its equivalents, dentistry, oral health, dental clinic, dental practice, and medical emergencies. Articles addressing the Dental Office's Medical Emergencies were screened and reviewed.

3 RESULTS

Medical crises that have occurred at dental offices include - vasovagal syncope, angina, hypoglycemia, epileptic seizures, asthma, anaphylaxis, and cardiac arrest [Table 1]. A medical emergency is predicted to occur for a general dentist practitioner (GDP) at least once every two years on average [8]. Emergency cases with vasovagal syncope are the most common. The incidence of vasovagal syncope seems to decline with expert knowledge, according to an investigation that revealed that 4.8% of GDPs witnessed 22% of all syncope [9].

 DOI: 10.1201/9781042016075-3

Table 1. Common medical emergencies encountered in dental practices in India [8].

Medical Emergency	Signs & Symptoms	Management
Syncope	– Feels faint/dizzy – Collapse & loss of consciousness – Pallor, sweating, slow pulse, low BP – Nausea	– Check for Airway, Breathing, Circulation, Disability, Exposure (ABCD) – Lie flat, elevate legs, and loosen tight clothing – Once consciousness returns, offer glucose in water – Slow recovery: consider alternative diagnosis – If unresponsive, check signs of life
Hypoglycemia	– Shaking/trembling – Slurred speech – Sweating & blurred vision – Tiredness – Confusion – Unconsciousness	– Check for ABCD – Offer 15-20g of a quick-acting carbohydrate (e.g., 4-5 Glucotabs tablets) – Once consciousness returns, offer oral carbohydrates
Epileptic Seizures	– Sudden collapse & loss of consciousness – Rigidity & cyanosis – Jerking movements of limbs – Noisy breathing – Tongue may be bitten – Frothing at the mouth	– Check for ABCD – Maintain a safe environment to prevent injury – Administer oxygen (15 liters/min) – Note the timing of the seizure – Once jerking movements cease, place in the recovery position – For prolonged convulsive seizures (5+ minutes), administer 10 mg of Midazolam oromucosal solution via the buccal route
Asthma	– Breathlessness & expiratory wheeze – Severe: inability to complete sentences in one breath, respiratory rate >25/min, pulse >110/min – Life-threatening: cyanosis, respiratory rate <8/min, pulse <50/min, exhaustion, confusion, decreased level of consciousness	– Check for ABCD – Sit upright and follow the patient's personalized asthma action plan (PAAP) – Administer 2 puffs (100 micrograms/puff) of a $\beta 2$ bronchodilator inhaler (e.g., Salbutamol); repeat as necessary – If unsatisfactory response or severe, administer oxygen (15 liters/min) and $\beta 2$ bronchodilator via a spacer, one puff at a time with tidal breathing, up to a maximum of 10 puffs
Anaphylaxis	– Sudden onset – Urticaria and/or angioedema, flushing, pallor – Respiratory distress (stridor, wheeze, or hoarseness) – Hypotension & tachycardia – Rapid progression of symptoms; skin and/or mucosal changes	– Check for ABCD – Lie flat and elevate legs (if breathing not impaired); administer oxygen (15 liters/min) – Administer 500 micrograms of adrenaline intramuscularly (0.5 ml of 1:1000 solution) – Repeat adrenaline at 5-minute intervals until adequate response
Cardiac Emergencies	– Chest pain or discomfort that suddenly occurs and does not go away, often feeling like pressure, squeezing, or heaviness – Pain may spread to left/right arm, neck, jaw, back, or stomach – Nausea, sweating, light-headedness, shortness of breath	– Check for ABCD – Call ambulance – Position the patient comfortably (typically sitting up) – Administer 400-800mcg of glyceryl trinitrate spray (typically 1-2 activations) sublingually – Chew dispersible aspirin (300 mg) unless there is a clear allergy

4 DISCUSSION

Numerous studies on knowledge, and proficiency have focused on the receptiveness of dentists to basic life support (BLS), advanced cardiovascular life support (ACLS), and cardiopulmonary resuscitation (CPR). They are life-saving techniques which dental professionals should be trained and certified to treat patients in emergencies [10]. A person's degree of competence is always based on their undergraduate and postgraduate education, as well as their experience and ongoing skill development. Postgraduate programs offer more advanced training and coursework.

List of training programs for BDS and MDS students focusing on medical emergency management: [10]

- Basic Life Support (BLS) Certification
- Advanced Cardiovascular Life Support (ACLS) Certification
- First Aid and Emergency Response Training
- Anaphylaxis and Allergic Reaction Management

- Myocardial Infarction Recognition and Management
- Seizure Management Training
- Respiratory Emergencies Management
- Airway Management Training
- Shock Management Training
- Emergency Pharmacology
- Syncope and Hypoglycemia Management
- Emergency Communication Skills Training
- Simulation-Based Emergency Drills
- Psychological First Aid and Stress Management
- Ethics and Legal Considerations in Medical Emergencies

When managing emergency circumstances in the clinic, the dentist should live up to the patient's expectations. However, occasionally, a dentist's lack of experience and confidence causes them to fail to handle such circumstances [11]. Patients anticipate that dentists will stock up on the necessary supplies to handle medical emergencies. While first aid knowledge and skills are ingrained and do not fade quickly after training, this is a well-known truth. In actuality, dental professionals frequently need to update their knowledge and attend skill training [12].

Implementing activities and assessment techniques to evaluate readiness for medical emergencies is essential to ensure that healthcare professionals are well-prepared to respond effectively. Here are some activities and assessment techniques that can be integrated into an institute to evaluate readiness: simulation-based training, role-playing with patient actors, full-scale emergency response drills, case-based discussion and debriefing, paper-based or digital assessment tools, skills stations, tabletop exercises, interdisciplinary training workshops, regular review and continuous education [8].

To improve the preparedness of handling the medical emergency in dental clinic there should be [13]

- Emergency Action Plans: Developing and implementing a comprehensive emergency action plan for the dental clinic.
- Use of Emergency Drugs and Equipment: Acquainting with the emergency drugs and equipment available in the clinic, such as epinephrine, oxygen, and emergency kits.
- Management of Specific Emergencies: Detailed protocols for managing specific emergencies like allergic reactions, hypoglycemia, and seizures.
- Mock Drills and Simulations: Conducting regular mock drills and simulations to ensure preparedness and improve response times.
- Legal and Ethical Considerations: Includes liability, medical emergency management, ethical principles, professional duties and billing practices.

All undergraduate and postgraduate students should be required to complete skill-based seminars and ongoing education program training to manage medical crises in dental clinics. However, it is clear that dentistry students need more than just basic skill training; they also need to take specialized courses to keep up with the latest developments in the field [14].

5 CONCLUSION

Different countries have different rates of medical emergencies at dentistry clinics. Many dentists are not confident enough to manage medical emergencies. Even while dentistry schools provide medical emergency training, it is insufficient; additional specialized courses must be taken. In the dentist office, a thorough understanding of emergency medical equipment should be obtained and supplied. Every dentist office is responsible for ensuring that patients receive safe and efficient care.

REFERENCES

[1] Anwar MA, Rehman IU, Khalil F, Saeed T, Shakeel S, Arif K, Kushef H. (2024). Knowledge, skills, and perceived competency in handling medical emergencies among dental house officers and general dentists: Knowledge, skills, and perceived competency in handling medical emergencies. *Pakistan Journal of Health Sciences*. 158-63.

[2] Mukherji A, Singh MP, Nahar P, Bhuvaneshwari S, Goel S, Mathur H. (2019). Competence of handling medical emergencies among dental graduates and post-graduate students—a cross-sectional questionnaire study. *J Indian Acad Oral Med Radiol*. 31:107–16.

[3] Singh N, Kachwaha P, Singhal D. (2018). Preparedness of dental students to manage medical emergencies in clinical dental set-up: a cross-sectional questionnaire survey. *Indian J Public Health Res Dev*. 9:289.

[4] Vaughan M, Park A, Sholapurkar A, *et al.* (2018). Medical emergencies in dental practice management requirements and international practitioner proficiency. A scoping review. *Aust Dent J*. 63(4):455–66.

[5] Clark MS, Wall BE, Tholström TC, *et al.* (2006). A twenty-year follow-up survey of medical emergency education in U.S. dental schools. *J Dent Educ*. 70(12):1316–9.

[6] Tanzawa T, Futaki K, Kurabayashi H, *et al.* (2013). Medical emergency education using a robot patient in a dental setting. *Eur J Dent Educ*. 17:e114–9.

[7] Sangamesh NC, Vidya KC, Pathi J, Singh A. (2017). Awareness, attitude, and knowledge of basic life support among medical, dental, and nursing faculties and students in the university hospital. *J Int Soc Prev Community Dent*. 7:161–7.

[8] Jevon P. (2020). Medical emergencies in the dental practice poster: Revised and updated. *British Dental Journal*. 229(2):97–104.

[9] Collange O, Bildstein A, Samin J *et al.* (2010). Prevalence of medical emergencies in the dental practice. *Resuscitation* 81: 915–916.

[10] Bernardi S, Fulgenzi MB, Rovera A, Rinaldi F, Trichilo S, Bianchi S. (2023). Dentistry and gender gap: an overview of the Italian situation. *Healthcare*. 11(6):828.

[11] Al-Turki O, Al-Hussyeen A, Al-Hammad N, Alhowaish L, Almaflehi N. (2017). Medical emergencies in dental practice. *J Dent Med Sci* 16: 1–9.

[12] Sutton RM, Nadkarni V, Abella BS. (2012). "Putting it all together" to improve resuscitation quality. *Emerg Med Clin North Am*. 30(1):105–22.

[13] Morales Romero JT, Herrera-Barraza VA, Ferrer-Valdivia NF. (2024). Initial Management of Medical Emergencies in Dental Practice: A Literature Review. *Odontoestomatología*. 26(44).

[14] Laurent F, Augustin P, Nabet C, *et al.* (2009). Managing a cardiac arrest: evaluation of final-year predoctoral dental students. *J Dent Educ*. 73:211–7.

 ISBN: 978-1-041-32674-8

Perception of Examinees and Examiners on Conventional vs Objectively Structured Viva-voce for Final BDS in the Subject of Prosthodontics

Deviprasad Nooji
Academics & Administration, Prosthodontics and Crown & Bridge, KVG Dental College and Hospital, Sullia, DK, Karnataka, India

Suhasini J Nagda
Former Dean, Nair Hospital Dental College, Mumbai, Maharashtra

Chinmay Shah
Professor and Head, Department of Physiology, Government Medical College, Bhavnagar, Gujarat

ABSTRACT: **Introduction** The viva-voce is intended to focus on the assessment of communication skills and convincing powers of the examinees, along with the knowledge. The conventional viva-voce (CVV) methods might vary in time allotted for each examinee, the number of questions asked to each examinee and also the difficulty levels of questions asked. Incorporation of objectively structured viva-voce (OSVV) might enhance the system of assessment by making it transparent and objective. Hence, this study was designed and conducted.

Objectives To evaluate the perception of examinees and examiners on CVV vs OSVV examination in prosthodontics.

Methods Forty selected examinees were subjected to conventional as well as objectively structured viva-voce by four different examiners. Separate responses were obtained through questionnaire from all the 40 examinees as well as 4 examiners participated in the study.

Results Both the examiners and examinees agreed that the conduction, transparency, coverage of syllabus, variations in questions, time dedicated for every examinee were better in OSVV than CVV. The **examiners** were more satisfied and felt it was easier to categorize the students as low performers of advanced Learners in OSVV. All the examiners and most of the examinees preferred OSVV over CVV as a better assessment tool.

Conclusion All the examiners and most of the examinees preferred OSVV over CVV for all assessments. Sensitization of students would be required to clarify the basic concepts of conducting viva-voce and the role of OSVV in achieving the same.

Keywords: Oral Assessment, Conventional Viva-voce, Traditional Viva-voce, Objectively Structured Viva-voce, Prosthodontics

1 INTRODUCTION

Examination is an integral part of assessment of knowledge in cognitive domain and skill in psychomotor domain, during the learning process [1,2]. The viva-voce is a tool mainly focusing on the levels of knowledge, communication skills and convincing powers of the student during the learning process [1,2]. It elicits the comprehensive application of basic knowledge and concepts along with the logical implications [1]. It can be used to evaluate the higher levels of cognition such as analysis, evaluation, and creation along with attitude, communication and convincing powers of examinee [1,3,4]. Even though the assessment of viva-voce is subjective, it has got a high face value and if used thoughtfully, rationally, objectively, and relevantly, it can assess the student beyond the written examinations [1].

The conventional viva-voce methods might vary in time allotted for each student, the number of questions asked to each student and also the difficulty levels of questions asked [5]. It has a poor content validity, low inter-rater and inter-case reliability, inconsistency in marking, and lack of standardization [5]. It is common that the traditional viva-voce is usually conducted towards the end of practical examination [6]. The students might be tiered and more apprehensive at that stage [6]. Also, the examiners might be restricted to the areas of their interest, with fixed whims and fancies, along with numerous environmental factors affecting the moment [6]. There could be multiple advantages of using objectively structured viva-voce such as better coverage of syllabus, better learner expression, reduced anxiety and shyness of the students [5].

The objectively structured viva-voce is used for assessment of students at few Dental Institutions around the world [3]. It is thought to be more transparent and unbiased [5]. All the students undergoing will be offered equal

 DOI: 10.1201/9781042016075-4

time, number as well as type of questions [5]. However, most of the institutions in India have not incorporated it [3]. Most of the dental teachers are following the traditional technique of conducting viva-voce and they must be educated about the objectively structured viva-voce [3].

Presently, most of the Dental Colleges in India are following the traditional Viva-voce during the University Exams as well as Internal Assessments [3]. However, following the objectively structured viva-voce in all the Dental Colleges across India, might enhance the system of assessment [3]. Hence, this study is designed for using objectively structured viva-voce in the subject of Prosthodontic and to compare its effect on the scores of the students along with the perceptions of both examinees and examiners.

This study was conducted with the aim to evaluate the perception of examinees and examiners on conventional vs objectively structured viva-voce for final BDS in the subject of prosthodontics. The Objective of the study was to evaluate the perception of IV BDS examinees and examiners on conventional vs objectively structured viva-voce examination in prosthodontics.

2 MATERIALS AND METHODS

This study was conducted in the Department of Prosthodontics at a Dental College affiliated to Rajiv Gandhi University of Health Sciences, Karnataka. The first forty students who were studying in IV BDS at Dental Colleges affiliated to Rajiv Gandhi University of Health Sciences, Karnataka, voluntarily filled the open registration form with informed consent, were selected to participate in the study.

2.1 *Selection of the examinees*

A registration form created on Google Forms with the information about the study was made available to all the students of IV BDS to go through it. Forty students who responded first were selected for this study. Those 40 students were further divided into 4 groups, namely Group-1, Group-2, Group-3, and Group-4, having 10 students each. All the 40 students were sensitized to participate in objectively structured viva-voce (OSVV) examination.

2.2 *Appointing the examiners*

Four Professors (A, B, C, and D) from the Department of Prosthodontics were appointed as examiners for the viva-voce examinations. All the 4 appointed examiners were trained to conduct objectively structured viva-voce (OSVV) examination.

2.3 *Categorising the viva questions*

Around 100 viva questions each in Complete Denture, Removable Partial Denture, Fixed Partial Denture, and Miscellaneous Topics (Maxillofacial, implants, Overdentures Immediate Denture etc.) of Prosthodontics, asked commonly for IV BDS in Prosthodontics Examinations were gathered. All the 400 questions were categorised as "Must Know - Easy", "Must Know - Difficult", "Desirable to Know - Easy", "Desirable to Know - Difficult" and "Nice to Know" as per the recommendation in BDS Regulations of Rajiv Gandhi University of Health Sciences, Karnataka [7]. Every question was printed separately on different coloured cards such as blue, green, yellow, pink and red corresponding to their category.

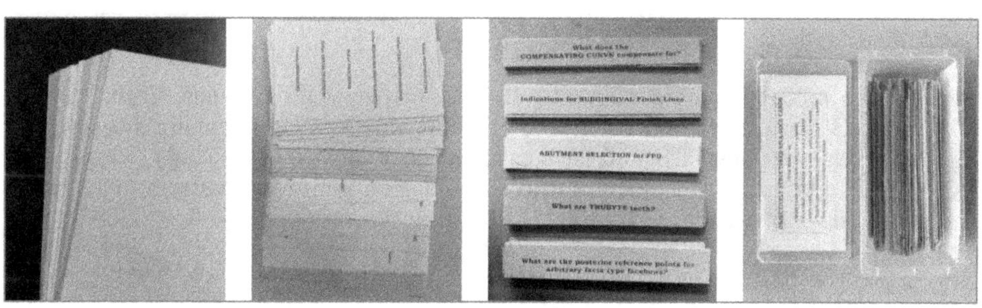

Figure 1. Preparation of viva-voce cards for objectively structured viva-voce (OSVV).

These cards were used to conduct objectively structured viva-voce (OSVV) by picking up 10 question cards randomly, in the proportions 4:2:2:1:1, carrying 2 marks each (Total 20 Marks) [7]. The marks were entered for each answer, onto the mark sheet created on Google Forms.

The Marks were allotted for Objectively Structured Viva-Voce as below.

Total Score: 20 Marks
Total Items: 10 Questions
Each question carries: 2 Marks
Marking rubric for each answer:

- No attempt made to answer: 0.0 Mark
- Attempts to answer without confidence: 0.5 Marks
- Answers partially with confidence: 1.0 Marks
- Answers correctly with confidence: 1.5 Marks
- Answers correctly and convincingly: 2.0 Marks.

The conventional viva-voce (CVV) were carried out by each examiner, by randomly asking few questions to each student for 20 Marks. The total marks obtained by each student was entered onto the mark sheet.

Viva-voce Evaluation:

Table 1. Conduction of Viva-voce Examinations by different Examiners for different groups of Examinees.

Evaluator	Evaluation – 1	Evaluation - 2	Evaluation – 1	Evaluation - 2
Evaluator - A	Group – 1 CVV	Group – 3 OSVV	Group – 2 CVV	Group – 4 OSVV
Evaluator – B	Group – 2 OSVV	Group – 4 CVV	Group – 1 OSVV	Group – 3 CVV
Evaluator - C	Group – 3 CVV	Group – 1 OSVV	Group – 4 CVV	Group – 2 OSVV
Evaluator - D	Group – 4 OSVV	Group – 2 CVV	Group – 3 OSVV	Group – 1 CVV

A cross-over study design was used to subject every examinee to both conventional viva-voce as well as objectively structured viva-voce by four different examiners. The questions from Complete Denture section of prosthodontics were used during Evaluation – 1, the questions from Removable Partial Denture section of prosthodontics are used during Evaluation – 2, the questions from Fixed Partial Denture section of prosthodontics are used during Evaluation – 3, and Miscellaneous Topics (Maxillofacial, implants, Overdentures Immediate Denture etc.) from prosthodontics are used during Evaluation – 4. All the examinees were also subjected to all the sets of questions either in conventional viva-voce (CVV) or objectively structured viva-voce (OSVV).

Table 2. Marksheet of OSVV.

S. No	P.N.	Q.1	Q.2	Q.3	Q.4	Q.5	Q.6	Q.7	Q.8	Q.9	Q.10	Total Marks	Time taken
1	1	0.5	0.5	0	1	0	0	1.5	0	0	0	3.5	5.56
2	5	1	1	1.5	1	1.5	1	2	0.5	0.5	1.5	12.5	5.07
3	9	0.5	0.5	0.5	0.5	0.5	0	0	0.5	0.5	0	3	4.36
4	13	0.5	1	1	1	1	0	0.5	1	1	0	5.5	7.01
5	17	0.5	0	0.5	0.5	0	0.5	0	0	0	0.5	2.5	5.41
6	21	1	1	1	1	0.5	1	1	0.5	1	1	6	6.55
7	25	1	1.5	0.5	0.5	1	0.5	1.5	2	0.5	0.5	8	3.53
8	29	0.5	1	0.5	1	0.5	0.5	2	0.5	0.5	0	5.5	4.1
9	33	1	0.5	1	0.5	1	1	0.5	1	0.5	0.5	4	5.5
10	37	0.5	1	0.5	0.5	0.5	0.5	1	0.5	0.5	0	3.5	2.42

Questionnaires: A pre-validated questionnaire was designed and created on Google Forms to obtain responses from all the 40 examinees participated in the study. Another pre-validated questionnaire was designed and created on Google Forms to obtain responses from all the 4 examiners participated in the study.

Data Collection: The responses for the questionnaires on Google Forms received from to all the examinees and examiners were extracted on M S Excel and subjected to statistical analysis.

3 RESULTS

All the Examiners of Prosthodontics preferred OSVV over CVV for all assessments. Most of the Examinees also preferred OSVV for their assessments. However, few students preferred CVV as the examiners were asking questions on the topics that they prepared for and also trying to get answers by giving clues.

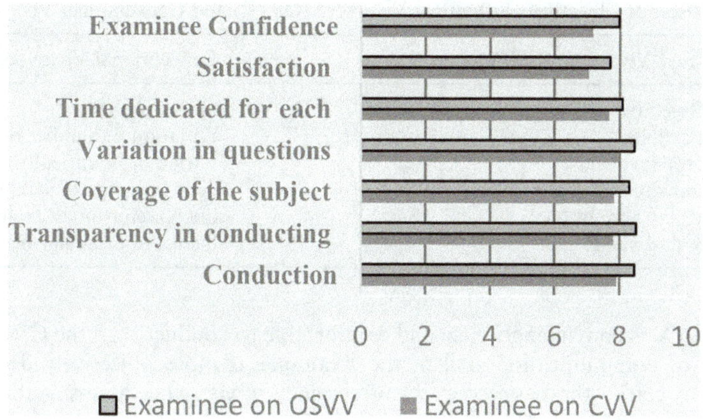

Figure 2A. Responses of Examinees on OSVV and CVV.

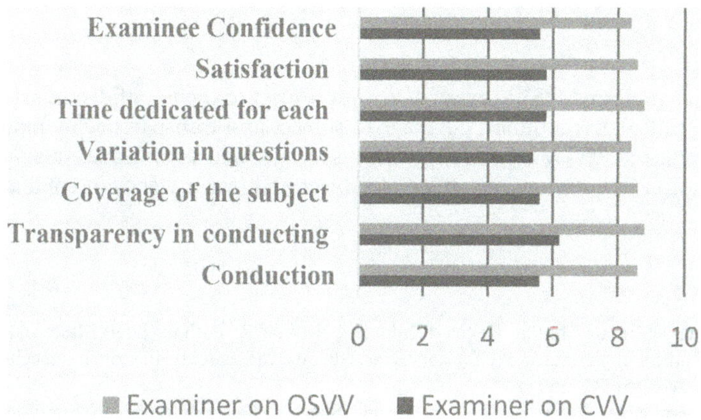

Figure 2B. Responses of Examiners on OSVV and CVV.

Both the examiners as well as examinees agreed that the confidence levels of examinees. Time dedicated for each examinee, variety of questions asked, coverage of the subjects, transparency in conduction of viva and ease of conduction were better in OSVV than CVV. However, the examinees were not in agreement that OSVV was more satisfying than CVV. This might be due to their regular exposure to CVV as routine assessment method and OSVV being a new method.

4 DISCUSSION

In the present study, the viva-voce questions were divided into five categories, namely, must know easy, must know difficult, desirable to know easy, desirable to know difficult and nice to know. This categorization was carried out based on the syllabus allocated by Rajiv Gandhi University of Health Sciences, Karnataka. Based on the categorization, the questions were printed on five different coloured cards, namely, blue, green, yellow, pink and red. These cards were used to conduct viva-voce in the ratio 4:2:2:1:1 respectively. Even the average time taken to conduct both traditional as well as objectively structured viva-voce were noted and compared in the study.

Minal C Patel et. al., (2021) found that the performances of students were better in OSVV than CVV. Also, the feedback from students and examiners agreed that OSVV was better than CVV [8]. However, set of four questions might not be adequate to cover the whole syllabus with different difficulty levels [8]. Pradnya Nikhade et. al., (2020) found no difference in the mean scores of two methods, those students scored better with modified OSVV were easily categorized as advanced learners [3].

The results of this study are in line with the studies reported in literature. The majority of the examinees and examiners felt that the viva questions were uniform, time given to think and to answer the given questions in front of examiner was adequate, stress faced due to sudden facing of the questions and examiner was less, there was equal time given to all the students for viva, examiner's personal bias was less, and they would prefer viva examination in future. [5,9] Majority of examinees also agreed that OSVV as more objective and unbiased. [5] Examinees preferred OSVV over CVV as it minimized the luck factor and reduced bias and it is a better assessment tool in regards to consistency, reliability, and validity. [10] (Table 3)

Table 3. Comparison of Objectively Structured Viva-voce (OSVV) and Conventional Viva-voce (CVV).

Objectively Structured Viva-voce (OSVV)	Conventional Viva-voce (CVV)
Transparent and Objective	More subjective
Better coverage of syllabus	Variation in number of questions
Minimum luck factor involved	Variation in difficulty levels of questions
Reduces anxiety and shyness of examinee	Poor coverage of syllabus
Reduced examiner bias and fatigue	Luck factor might be involved
Consistent, reliable and valid	Increased examiner bias

The conduction of OSVV is convincingly easy and comfortable to conduct than the CVV. Also, the coverage of subject and assessment of communication skill of the Examinee is more objectively done through OSVV. An attempt must be made to clarify the basic concepts of conducting viva-voce assessment, particularly objectively structured viva-voce to every student. All the examiners need to be trained in both preparation of viva questions and viva cards along with conduction of OSVV.

5 CONCLUSION

(1) Most of the examinees preferred OSVV over CVV, with respect to their confidence, satisfaction, time dedicated to each examinee, variation in questions, coverage of subject and transparency in conduction.
(2) All the examiners preferred OSVV over CVV, with respect to their confidence, satisfaction, time dedicated to each examinee, variation in questions, coverage of subject and transparency in conduction.

REFERENCES

[1] Ajeet Kumar Khilnani, Jaykaran Charan, Rekha Thaddanee, Rakesh R. Pathak, Sohil Makwana, Gurudas Khilnani. (2015). Structured oral examination in pharmacology for undergraduate medical students: Factors influencing its implementation. *Indian Journal of Pharmacology* 47(5):546–550

[2] D.C. Dhasmana, Suman Bala, Rajendra Sharma, Taruna Sharma, Saurabh Kohli, Neeraj Aggarwal, Juhi Kalra. (2016). Introducing structured viva voce examination in medical undergraduate pharmacology: A pilot study. *Indian Journal of Pharmacology* Vol 48(Supplement):S54–S56

[3] Pradnya Nikhade, Shweta Sedani, Nikhil Mankar, Abhilasha Das, Sindhu P, Shruti Mishra. (2020). Comparison of objectively structured viva voce and modified objectively structured viva voce as assessment tool during formative and summative examination in dentistry. *J Evolution Med Dent Sci* 9(40):2987–2991

[4] Sufia Naseem, Mehjbeen Javed, Ummul Baneen. (2019). Developing and implementing structured viva voce examination as a valid and reliable assessment tool in biochemistry for first year BDS students. *Journal of Clinical and Diagnostic Research* 13(7):05–08

[5] Poorva A. Sule, Milind R. Ubale, Sundaram Kartikeyan, Deepali D. Belurkar, Vrushali V. Kulkarni. (2017). comparative study of objectively structured versus traditional viva-voce in microbiology amongst second-year MBBS students. *IOSR Journal of Research & Method in Education* 7(3):15–18

[6] Tejas M. Khakhkhar, Neelesh Khuteta, Gurudas Khilnani. (2019). A comparative evaluation of structured and unstructured forms of viva voce for internal assessment of undergraduate students in Pharmacology. *International Journal of Basic & Clinical Pharmacology* 8(4):616–621

[7] Revised BDS Ordinance. http://www.rguhs.ac.in/courses_rguhs/dental_ordinances/dental_BDS%20CURRICULUM%20_rguhs.pdf

[8] Minal C Patel, Hasmukh D Shah, Archana S Nimbalkar, Tejas T Prajapati, Nilesh H Patel. (2021). Comparing the effectiveness of systematic recall time-based viva examination versus traditional viva examination of the 1st year medical undergraduates. *National Journal of Physiology, Pharmacy and Pharmacology* 11 (10): 1085–1089.

[9] Priti V Puppalwar, Alka Rawekar, Anita Chalak, Archana Dhok, Meenakshi Khapre. (2014). Introduction of objectively structured viva-voce in formative assessment of medical and dental undergraduates in biochemistry. *Journal of Research in Medical Education & Ethics* 4(3):321–325

[10] Shobha Kini. (2016). Student and faculty perception of objective structured Viva Voce (OSVV) as a reliable, objective and valid method of oral assessment. *Global Journal for Research Analysis* 5(5):376–377

 ISBN: 978-1-041-32674-8

Knowledge, Attitude and Practice of Mentorship among Dental Students in a University Teaching Hospital

Arjun Hari Rijal
Department of Periodontology and Oral Implantology, Kathmandu University School of Medical Sciences, Dhulikhel, Kavrepalanchok, Nepal

Laxman Gnawali
Kathmandu University School of Education, Hattiwan, Lalitpur, Nepal

Manoj Humagain
Department of Periodontology and Oral Implantology, Kathmandu University School of Medical Sciences, Dhulikhel, Kavrepalanchok, Nepal

Pratistha Ghimire
Consultant Prosthodontist, Methinkot Hospital, Bhakundebesi, Kavrepalanchok, Nepal

ABSTRACT: **Background:** Mentorship programme are focused on the mutual benefits of both the mentor and mentees. Any of the following components can be considered as a mentorship: emotional and psychological support, assistance with career development and role-modeling. Though there are numerous benefits to mentor and mentee, there is lack of organized or structured mentorship programme in the dental schools.

Aim: This study aims to find out the knowledge, attitude and practice of mentorship among the undergraduate dental students of a dental college.

Methodology: This qualitative cross-sectional study was conducted among undergraduate dental students of Kathmandu University School of Medical Sciences-Dhulikhel Hospital. The ten self-administered questionnaires were prepared in the google form and google link was sent to the second, third and fourth year undergraduate dental students. Basic introduction about mentorship was included in the beginning to minimize the confusion regarding the mentorship. Data were coded and analyzed using descriptive statistics.

Results: One hundred thirteen (113) students responded to the online questionnaire. 81.4 % students believed mentorship is very important in undergraduate level, 57.5% students were very satisfied with the current status of the provided mentorship, 52.2% students were given proper career advice and planning, 69.9% believed mentorship had improved their clinical skill and 67.3 % students believed mentorship programme is mandatory in undergraduate level.

Conclusion: Based on the findings of the current study, mentorship plays important role in development of the undergraduate students and should develop organized structured mentorship programme in undergraduate curriculum.

Keywords: dentistry, undergraduate students, mentorship

1 INTRODUCTION

The concept of mentorship has been used in practice for many years. In ancient mythological books, the terms "guru" as mentor and "shishya" as mentee have been used to represent the theme of mentorship. Mentorship is defined as "the advice and help provided by a mentor to a less experienced person over a period of time, especially as part of a formal programme in a company, university, etc." [1]. There is no universal definition of mentorship. The following components can be considered mentorship: "emotional and psychological support, assistance with career development and role modeling" [2]. The main basis of mentorship is the mutual benefit of both parties, i.e., mentors and mentees.

There are numerous advantages of mentorship available in the literature [3–5]. Mentorship can help mentees grow, improve their skills, and boost their chances of achieving their goals. This connection can have a positive effect on their education and career, leading to less burnout and depression, greater job satisfaction, and progress in

DOI: 10.1201/9781042016075-5

both personal and professional areas [4,5]. In dental colleges, there are more advantages of mentorship in improving clinical skills, academic progress and personal development.

Although there are numerous benefits to mentors and mentees, there is a lack of organized or structured mentorship programs in dental schools. There are numerous barriers in the development of mentorship programs. Some of them lack knowledge about mentorship among students and academicians, a very limited number of qualified mentors, limited training opportunities for mentors, improper matching of the mentor mentee, infrequent visits/lack adequate time provided by the mentor, etc [6]. To overcome these types of problems, the following strategies are suggested in the literature: (a) creating and setting up a formal mentorship program for students and faculty; (b) creating ways to track and measure the progress of the mentorship program; and (c) conducting long-term studies on mentees to assess the lasting effects of mentorship. [6]

Undergraduates that students are the future to be mentors. The knowledge, attitudes and practices of mentorship affect the future directions of these kinds of programs. Therefore, this study aims to determine the knowledge, attitudes and practices of mentorship among undergraduate dental students at a dental college.

2 METHODS

A descriptive cross-sectional study was conducted among undergraduate dental students at the Kathmandu University School of Medical Sciences, Dhulikhel Hospital, for a period of one month (May 10 to June 10, 2024). Institutional ethics committee approval was taken from the institutional review committee of Kathmandu University School of Medical Sciences (IRC-KUSMS, Ref No: 122/24). Informed consent was obtained before the questionnaire was completed in Google form. Introduction and informed consent were incorporated into the first page of the questionnaire. All the undergraduate dental students, from second- to fourth-year students, were included in the study. Students from other streams, such as the MBBS, nursing, and Bachelor in Physiotherapy, were excluded from the study.

The online survey questionnaire was prepared in Google form. Ten questions were included to assess the knowledge, attitudes and practices of mentorship. Out of the ten questions, eight were answered via a Likert scale, and the remaining two were multiple-choice questions. The self-administered questionnaire was first piloted with ten fourth-year students for content and face validity. Modifications of the questions were done according to the response of the students. Then question ions were distributed among 20 students in the one-week interval to find out the reliability of the same. The Cohen Kappa value was calculated which was 0.87. Then link of an online questionnaire was sent to all the students via different social media platforms, such as Vibers and Facebook Messages. Responses were collected and coded. Further analysis was performed via descriptive statistics.

3 RESULTS

This web-based questionnaire was administered to undergraduate dental students at Kathmandu University School of Medical Sciences. One hundred fifteen students (81.56%) responded to the questionnaire survey. The distribution of the students is as follows: second year, 34 (29.6%); third year, 44 (38.3%); and fourth year, 37 (32.2%). Out of the 115 participants, 19 (16.5%) were males, and the remaining were females. The ages of the participants ranged from 21–24 years, and the majority (50; 43.5%) were 22 years of age.

In terms of the importance of having a mentor at the undergraduate level, 94 (81.7%) participants believed that it was very important. Similarly, participants were asked how frequently they met their mentor, and the majority of them met weekly for mentorship purposes. The majority of the participants (67, 58.3%) were satisfied, while fewer than one percentage of the participants were dissatisfied with their mentor. With respect to achieving academic goals, 34 (29.6%) mentors always, 49 (42.6%) often, and 29 (25.2%) sometimes help to set and achieve academic goals (Table 1). Approximately 33% of the participants always/sometimes felt comfortable with their mentor regarding any issues. The majority of the participants (61, 53%) considered the advice provided by the mentor regarding their career to be effective. Almost 80 (70%) participants reported that the mentorship provided was effective in enhancing their clinical skills. The majority of the participants (78; 67.8%) agreed that mentorship is mandatory at the undergraduate level. According to the participants, the benefits of mentorship were as follows: clinical skill improvement 97 (84.3%), academic guidance 80 (69.6%), personal development 55 (47.8%), career advice 53 (46.1%) and research opportunities 41 (35.7%). In terms of how mentorship can be improved in dental schools, participants responded as follows: better matching of the mentor and mentee (66, 57.4%), increased frequency of meetings (57, 49.6%), more group mentoring sessions (48, 41.7%) and more training for mentors (36, 31.3%) (Table 1).

Table 1. Response of undergraduate students to the mentorship questionnaire.

SN	Questions	Response n (%)				
1.	**How would you rate the importance of having a mentor during your dental studies?**	**Very important**	**Important**	**Neutral**	**Not important**	**Not at all important**
		94 (81.7)	20 (17.4)	1 (0.9)	-	-
2.	**How often do you meet with your mentor?**	**Weekly**	**Biweekly**	**Monthly**	**Rarely**	**Never**
		64 (55.7)	7 (6.1)	12 (10.4)	29 (25.2)	3(2.6)
3.	**How satisfied are you with the guidance provided by your mentor?**	**Very satisfied**	**Satisfied**	**Neutral**	**Dissatisfied**	**Very dissatisfied**
		16 (13.9)	67 (58.3)	30 (26.1)	1 (0.9)	1 (0.9)
4.	**Does your mentor help you set and achieve your academic goals?**	**Always**	**Often**	**Sometimes**	**Rarely**	**Never**
		34 (29.6)	49 (42.6)	29 (25.2)	1 (0.9)	2 (1.7)
5.	**Do you feel comfortable discussing your academic challenges with your mentor?**	**Always**	**Often**	**Sometimes**	**Rarely**	**Never**
		21 (18.3)	38 (33)	39 (33.9)	13 (11.3)	4 (3.5)
6.	**How effective is your mentor in providing career advice and planning?**	**Very effective**	**Effective**	**Neutral**	**Ineffective**	**Very ineffective**
		15 (13)	61 (53)	36 (31.3)	3 (2.6)	
7.	**How has mentorship impacted your confidence in clinical skills?**	**Greatly improved**	**Improved**	**Neutral**	**Not improved**	**Declined**
		15 (13)	80 (69.6)	16 (13.9)	3 (2.6)	1 (0.9)
8.	**Do you think mentorship should be mandatory for all dental students?**	**Strongly agree**	**Agree**	**Neutral**	**Disagree**	**Strongly disagree**
		78 (68.6)	32 (27.8)	5 (4.3)	-	-
9.	**What aspect of mentorship do you find most beneficial? (Select all that apply, multiple selection possible)**	**Academic Guidance**	**Clinical Skills Improvement**	**Career Advice**	**Personal Development**	**Research Opportunities**
		80 (69.6)	97 (84.3)	53 (46.1)	55 (47.8)	41 (35.7)
10.	**How would you improve the mentorship program in your dental school?**	**Increase Frequency of Meetings**	**More Training for Mentors**	**Better Matching of Mentors and Mentees**	**More Group Mentoring Sessions**	**Other (Please specify)**
		57 (49.6)	36 (31.3)	66 (57.4)	48 (41.7)	1 (0.9)

4 DISCUSSION

A long history of mentorship practices exists in the literature. The concept of mentorship started in the United States of America in the 1970s to increase the status of junior staff by senior staff. Since then, unstructured forms of mentorship have been developed in the medical sector [3]. Although there was a lack of structured, formal forms of mentorship programs for medical doctors until the 1970s, there was proper implementation of mentorship in nursing programs. However, no universal definition of mentorship exists in the literature. Various terminologies have been used to mean the process of mentorship, such as "teaching", "guiding", "mentoring", "tutoring", and "coaching". The Standing Committee on Postgraduate Medical and Dental Education has defined mentorship as "*A process whereby an experienced, highly regarded, empathetic person (the mentor) guides another (usually younger) individual (the mentee) in the development and re-examination of their own ideas, learning, and personal and professional development. The mentor, who often (but not necessarily) works in the same organization or field as the mentee, achieves this by listening or talking in confidence to the mentee.* " [7] Similarly, Garmel (2004) explained the process of mentorship as "an insightful process in which the mentor's wisdom is acquired and modified as needed, as well as a process that is supportive and often protective. The successful mentor™mentee relationship therefore requires the active participation of both parties. The mentoring relationship can be structured or loose. It can be a relatively short process or an ongoing process. There can be breaks in the relationship, with its reestablishment occurring at some future time. The mentoring relationship is dynamic and evolves over time, during which both parties continually define and redefine their roles. It should be considered a process, not an end result, and the relationship must remain noncompetitive." [8]

Annette (2018) described the advantages of the mentorship program to mentors, mentees and organizations [4]. Benefits for the mentor include personal satisfaction from helping others, support on projects, improvement in leadership and coaching abilities, greater recognition, renewed interest in their own career, potential financial rewards, and career growth. Mentees also gain various benefits, such as higher job satisfaction, a sense of empowerment, more opportunities for research grants, improved productivity, more time for academic activities like publishing, greater confidence in their abilities, better networking opportunities, and career growth. The organization also gains from a mentorship program through better work performance, improved strategic planning, enhanced communication and workplace culture, employee development, retention and sharing of knowledge, lower staff turnover, faster training, and cost efficiency

Although there is a lack of uniformity in the process of mentoring, it provides numerous benefits for medical and dental undergraduate students [9]. In dentistry, it provides proper guidance in career selection, improves job satisfaction, and increases interest in research activities as well as research productivity [8,10]. Mentoring undergraduate students improves their academic success, increases interest in the specialty of medicine/dentistry and emotionally and mentally supports their well-being [3]. The literature suggests that mentees who receive proper mentorship have two advantages in their career path selection and development [11].

In the present study, participants were asked about the importance of mentorship at the undergraduate level; the majority of them responded very importantly, few responded importantly, and very few (<1%) responded neutrally. The response of the students may be due to the nature of the course, i.e., the requirement of theoretical as well as practical knowledge for success in their academic and clinical life. Similarly, the duration of active participation in mentorship activities or the availability of the mentor plays an important role in the success of the mentorship. In the present study, the majority of the participants met their mentor at one-week intervals. The amount of time needed from both the mentor and mentee was seen as the biggest obstacle to mentorship. [12] The unavailability of mentors up to one-week intervals may be due to the limited number of course hours provided to mentors by departments or institutions. Additionally, students are not available and are interested in being a part of the mentorship programme.

In this study, most of the participants (67, 58.3%) were satisfied with their mentor/mentorship activities, and a few (16, 13.9%) were very satisfied. However, 30 (26.1%) participants remained neutral to the current mentor and mentorship practice. The relationship between the mentor and mentee determines the level of satisfaction [12]. The relationship between the mentor and mentee relies on factors like seniority, being approachable, accessible, caring, understanding, patient, and honest. It also requires mutual respect, open communication, and the mentee's commitment to making the mentorship successful.

In the present study, 49 (42.6%), 34 (29.6%), and 25 (29.2%) participants often, always and sometimes, received help from the mentor to set and achieve their academic goals, respectively. This process is dependent on the characteristics of both the mentor and mentee. The characteristics of mentors include "personal attributes, generous, enthusiastic and motivating, patient and honest, responsive and excel at active listening", whereas the characteristics of mentees include "understanding, responsive, open to feedback, excels at active listening, honest and patient and nonjudgmental" [4].

Similarly, 39 (39.3%), 38 (33%) and 21 (18.3%) participants sometimes and always felt comfortable discussing their academic challenges with their mentor. This type of confidence depends on the personal characteristics of the mentor. A good mentor should have certain qualities, including a willingness to share personal and professional experiences, the ability to teach knowledge, skills, and values, and a readiness to create networking opportunities for the mentee [13]. Ideally, mentors should follow the principles listed below: [14] "provide a comfortable and safe learning environment, allow the mentee to be a part of planning future projects, provide opportunities for mentees to assess their own needs, encourage the joint formulation of learning objectives, identify resources needed to achieve personal and work goals, support mentees' attempts to achieve their goals and complete a joint evaluation of the mentees' goal achievement."

The majority of the participants believed that mentorship was beneficial to them. According to them, mentorship offers the following benefits to them: academic guidance, clinical skill improvement, career advice, personal development, and research opportunities. This relationship can be improved with various inputs. The participants suggested that the following measures can be implemented to nurture effective mentorship: increased frequency of meetings, more training for mentors, better matching of mentors and mentees, more group mentoring sessions, etc.

Implementing mentorship in a dental college is crucial for fostering student development and enhancing academic success. Firstly, the institution should establish a structured mentorship program that pairs experienced faculty members with students based on their interests and career goals. Regular one-on-one meetings should be scheduled to provide personalized guidance, support, and feedback on academic performance and clinical skills. Additionally, mentorship should extend beyond academics; mentors can help students navigate challenges such as stress management and work-life balance in the demanding field of dentistry.

To encourage collaboration, mentorship programs could include group workshops and seminars where mentors share their experiences and insights. Creating a platform for peer mentorship can also be beneficial, allowing senior students to guide juniors. Furthermore, continuous evaluation of the mentorship program is essential to ensure its effectiveness, adapting strategies based on student feedback to foster a supportive learning environment that nurtures future dental professionals.

5 CONCLUSION

In dental schools, the development of academics as well as clinical skills is mandatory. For this purpose, an effective mentorship relationship is needed. In the context of the present study, the participants were aware of the concepts of mentorship. They were aware of the importance of mentorship to set their academic goals, to increase their confidence, to develop clinical skills to treat patients with dental problems, and to obtain proper guidance to choose a proper career path. Similarly, mentorship offers numerous benefits, such as academic guidance, clinical skill improvement, career advice, personal development, and research opportunities. Accordingly, an increased frequency of meetings, more training for mentors, better matching of mentors and mentees, and more group mentoring sessions are needed to improve effective mentor™mentee relationships.

Conflict of interest

None.

ACKNOWLEDGEMENTS

The author would like to acknowledge all the second-year, third-year and fourth-year students of the Kathmandu University School of Medical Sciences for their active participation in this study.

REFERENCES

[1] Manser MH, Turton ND. (1998). *Advanced Learner's Dictionary*. Wordsworth Editions.

[2] Jacobi M. (1991). *Advanced* Mentoring and undergraduate academic success: A literature review. *Rev Educ Res*. 61(4):505–32.

[3] Frei E, Stamm M, Buddeberg-Fischer B. (2010). Mentoring programs for medical students-a review of the PubMed literature 2000–2008. *BMC Med Educ*. 10:1–4.

[4] Burgess A, van Diggele C, Mellis C. (2018). Mentorship in the health professions: a review. *Clin Teach.* 15(3):197–202.

[5] Arnesson K, Albinsson G. (2017). Mentorship–a pedagogical method for integration of theory and practice in higher education. *Nord J Stud Educ Policy*. 3(3):202–17.

[6] Tamale E, Atuhairwe I, Ssemwogerere A, Muhimbura B, Atimango L, Malinga PD, *et al.* (2024). Knowledge, attitudes, and practices of health professions students on mentorship: A cross-sectional study at a sub-Saharan African medical school. *Discover Education.* 3(1):27.

[7] Oxley J. (1998). Standing committee on postgraduate medical and dental education, *An Enquiry Into Mentoring*. SCOPME.

[8] Garmel GM. (2004). Mentoring medical students in academic emergency medicine. *Acad Emerg Med.* 11(12):1351–7.

[9] Jackson VA, Palepu A, Szalacha L, Caswell C, Carr PL, Inui T. "Having the right chemistry": A qualitative study of mentoring in academic medicine. *Acad Med.* 2003 Mar 1; 78(3):328–34.

[10] Sambunjak D, Straus SE, Marušić A. (2006). Mentoring in academic medicine: a systematic review. *Jama.* 296(9):1103–15.

[11] Dehon E, Cruse MH, Dawson B, Jackson-Williams L. (2015). Mentoring during medical school and match outcome among emergency medicine residents. *West J Emerg Med.* 16(6):927–930.

[12] Straus SE, Chatur F, Taylor M. (2009). Issues in the mentor–mentee relationship in academic medicine: A qualitative study. *Acad Med.* 84(1):135–9.

[13] Sangole AP, Abreu BC, Stein F. (2006). Mentoring review and reflections. *Occupational Therapy in Health Care.* 20(1):1–6.

[14] Kilgallon K, Thompson J. (2012). *Mentoring in Nursing and Healthcare: A Practical Approach.* John Wiley & Sons.

Navigating Dental Education Trends and Transforming Dental Pedagogy – Abas and Srikant N (Eds)
© 2027 The Author(s), ISBN: 978-1-041-32674-8

Assessment of Knowledge, Attitudes, and Practices Regarding Dentinal Hypersensitivity Management: Implications for Dental Curriculum Development

Diya Giridhar Kamath
Department of Conservative Dentistry and Endodontics, Manipal College of Dental Sciences, Manipal Academy of Higher Education, Manipal, India

Deepa Sai Giridhar Kamath
Department of Periodontology, Manipal College of Dental Sciences Mangalore, Manipal Academy of Higher Education, Manipal, India

Ramya Shenoy
Department of Public Health Dentistry Manipal College of Dental Sciences Mangalore, Manipal Academy of Higher Education, Manipal, India

ABSTRACT: INTRODUCTION: Dentinal hypersensitivity (DH) is defined as "a distinctive short sharp pain arising from exposed dentine, characteristically in response to an array of stimuli including thermal, tactile, evaporative, osmotic or chemical, which cannot be attributed to any other form of dental defect, disease or pathology." It is a prevalent condition in the dental field, yet there is discrepancy in the reported cases.The main causes have been reported to be under or overestimation of the condition, and poor management of the condition .This leads to long-term discomfort and significantly impacts on the quality of life (QoL) of sufferers. Multiple studies regarding DH have been conducted to address similar concerns, however there is still uncertainty regarding the cause, diagnostic techniques and treatment of DH. AIM OF THE STUDY: To describe the knowledge, attitudes, and practices of the management of Dentinal Hypersensitivity (DH) as perceived by a convenient (non-probability) selected sample of dentists in Mangalore. MATERIALS AND METHODS: A validated structured questionnaire was designed while considering the aims and objectives of the study. A Google survey form was created on the basis of queries on worldwide reports about DH including important predisposing factors, major triggers, mechanisms, differential diagnoses and patient management. The form was mailed to willing participants who fulfilled the inclusion criteria. RESULTS: Findings from 336 dentists revealed that dentinal hypersensitivity is a common problem either reported by patients or diagnosed by dentists. A considerable impact on the patients' quality of life was determined. It has a multifactorial etiology. A detailed diagnosis was revealed to be necessary for adequate treatment. However, it was revealed that there was a gap in patient awareness and a need to fulfil the same. The treatment options also varied. CONCLUSION: This study highlights that dentinal hypersensitivity is a common yet often underdiagnosed condition, primarily due to insufficient patient awareness and unclear treatment protocols. This underscores the need for improved education within dental training programs. Emphasizing both the identification of underlying etiological factors and the development of clear treatment guidelines could significantly increase diagnostic accuracy and patient care. Integrating comprehensive information about dentinal hypersensitivity into the dental curriculum will help bridge knowledge gaps, promote better clinical practices, and ultimately improve decision-making among future practitioners.

Keywords: Dentine hypersensitivity, Questionnaire, Diagnosis, Management

1 INTRODUCTION

Dentinal hypersensitivity (DH) is defined as "a distinctive short sharp pain arising from exposed dentine, characteristically in response to an array of stimuli including thermal, tactile, evaporative, osmotic or chemical, which cannot be attributed to any other form of dental defect, disease or pathology" [1]. DH is considered one of the most common conditions in the current dental scenario. However, there are discrepancies reported in the diagnosis and prevalence ranging from 1.1- 98% depending on the methodology of the tests (Self-reported/ Diagnosed by the dentist) and location (worldwide) of assessment. The main causes have been reported to be under or overestimation of the condition, and poor management of the condition [2].This has revealed to cause long-term discomfort and impacts on the quality of life (QoL) of sufferers. Multiple studies regarding DH have been conducted to address similar concerns; however there is still uncertainty regarding the cause, diagnostic techniques and treatment of DH [3,4]. This shows a clear gap in education at dental schools regarding diagnosis, treatment and long-term management of Dentinal hypersensitivity, as well as inadequate communication required for patient awareness. This study aimed to evaluate the knowledge and understanding of dental hypersensitivity (DH) among dental professionals in Mangalore.

 DOI: 10.1201/9781042016075-6

2 MATERIALS AND METHODS

This study was conducted through an email-based system. The dentists in Mangalore who fulfilled the eligibility criteria were invited. A validated questionnaire was sent through Google Forms. To ensure that the questions were relevant, the most common queries regarding dentinal hypersensitivity were gathered. These queries were used to frame appropriate questions, while ensuring that each one yielded a better insight into the subject response. The questions were then grouped into categories such as common causes, methods of diagnoses and treatment plan so as to have maintain good order and flow. The questionnaire was then compared to the standard format from similar studies. It was then reviewed by three subject experts to ensure that the questions adhered to the subject matter and could be used to thoroughly assess the current understanding regarding the same. Any redundant or irrelevant questions were removed. The questions were then tested by a small group of participants, similar to the target population, to ensure adequate comprehension and to check for any ambiguity that may ensue. The response pattern and the feedback from the same was then used to revise any discrepancies noted. It was once again reviewed by the experts, following the changed made, to ensure that the questionnaire was reliable. The final questionnaire included questions based on common concerns about Dentinal Hypersensitivity including major causative factors, diagnostic methods, management, patient compliance and need for patient education. (Table 1)

It was accompanied by a request to participate in the study, and a set of rules to follow. Anonymity was maintained throughout. Initially, the questionnaire included demographic details, years of experience, and their primary approach in such conditions. After that, the questions relied more on the ability of the dentist to diagnose and formulate a treatment plan. The last section included the need for patient awareness and education regarding the condition to ensure better diagnosis. It also revealed the compliance of the patient with the prescribed treatment.

Table 1. Common queries about dentinal hypersensitivity among dental professionals.

CAUSES	DIET AND BRUSHING HABITS
	RESTORATIVE FACTORS- CARIES, POST RESTORATIVE SENSITIVITY, AND BLEACHING
	PERIODONTAL FACTORS- PLAQUE, POCKETS, SCALING, PERIODONTAL SURGERY
	PSYCHOSOMATIC- BRUXISM, STRESS
	GENERAL HEALTH- ANATOMIC, SYSTEMIC/ HORMONAL
DIAGNOSIS	SELF-REPORTED BY THE PATIENT
	DENTAL EXAMINATION- AIRBLASTING/ THERMAL
	PERIODONTAL ASSESSMENT- MEASUREMENT OF RECESSION/ PROBING DEPTH
MANAGEMENT	DIET AND COUNSELLING
	THERAPEUTIC PASTES/ OTC AT HOME USE PRODUCTS
	FLUORIDE VARNISH
	SEALANTS
	PERIODONTAL THERAPY
	RESTORATION
	ENDODONTIC TREATMENT
PATIENT COMPLIANCE AND NEED FOR EDUCATION	COMPLIANCE OF TREATMENT PROVIDED
	PATIENT LEAFLET FOR EDUCATION

3 RESULTS

Among the 337 dentists 41.2% (139) dentists had been practicing dentistry for 5-10 years. 47.2% were practicing general dentistry whereas 52.8% who were dental specialists. 82.5% (278) dentists reported that the patients complained of hypersensitivity which lasted longer than 4 weeks. According to 64.1% (216) dentists the primary cause of DH can be periodontal disease, dental caries or psychosomatic factors.A total of 69.4% (234) of dentists reported that that the patients self-reported their condition and 70.6% (238) of dentists diagnosed it by air blasting and thermal tests. 65.9% (222) of dentists agreed that DH has a considerable impact on the quality of life for the patients.69.4 %(234) recommended diet counseling and improved brushing habits . 68.5 % prescribed therapeutic desensitizing agents in the management of DH. 70.3% of dentists in this study advocated sealants and fluoride varnishes in the treatment of DH.70.3 % (224) reported patient compliance with the treatment provided.70.9% (239) of the participants reported that pamphlets would be useful to educate them further regarding DH.

4 DISCUSSION

Dentin hypersensitivity is an extremely uncomfortable condition. This can often lead patients to become neglectful with respect to their oral health. Bacterial plaque that builds up on the tooth surface can worsen demineralization of the tooth and worsen any pre-existing gingival recession. This study aimed to determine the dentists' knowledge, attitudes and practices in the diagnosis and management of DH. In our study 82.8% of the participants reported that patients frequently complained of hypersensitivity which lasted longer than 4 weeks. DH is a common condition which can be routinely observed in dental practice. This is in accordance with the study performed by Zeola *et al.* (2020) [5] who reported that nearly 80% of dentists reported DH as routine condition in dental practice. In the study, 64.1% of dentists considered periodontal disease, dental caries, diet and psychosomatic factors as the etiologic agent. This is in accordance with the study by Gillian *et al.* (2019) [6] where they reported that 66% of dentists considered these etiologic factors. 70.6% of dentists in this study considered air blasting and thermal tests as suitable diagnostic methods for DH. This is in accordance with studies performed by Kopycka *et al.* (2017) [7] where he reported air blast and cold water tests as routine methods for diagnosing DH.

It was seen that 65.9% of dentists agreed that DH has a considerable effect on the quality of life (QoL) of the patients. This is in accordance with studies performed by Exarchou *et al.* (2019) [8] who conducted a study on Greece based dentists and reported that 76.4% of the studies reported the same. 68.5% prescribed therapeutic desensitizing toothpastes in the management of DH. Additional 70.3% of dentists in this study recommended sealants and fluoride varnish in the treatment of DH. This is similar to the findings of Pereira *et al.* (2018) [9] who reported majority of the dentists recommended this had a positive effect on the treatment of DH.70.9% of participants perceived the need to make patient leaflets to provide information about the condition. This is in accordance with study performed by Gilliam *et al.* (2019) [6] who reported that there is need for patient folders in terms of prevention and awareness of DH. A total of 43.9% of dentists reported patient compliance with their treatment strategies. This is in accordance with study conducted by Saif *et al.* (2019) [10] on Moroccan dentists in which 50% of dentists reported that patients were not compliant with treatment given by them

The limitations of this study include the relatively small and conveniently selected sample size in a small, limited region. The data were mostly self-reported which could lead to overestimation of knowledge and subjective rather than objective results. Following improved patient education, follow-up data were not assessed. Numerous treatment options are available, leading to wide variation in the management strategies.

When a patient presents symptoms indicative of DH, performing a thorough clinical assessment is vital. This ensures that other conditions are ruled out. It also helps to make an accurate diagnosis and a tailor-made treatment plan. An effective management strategy may require a personalized oral hygiene recommendations, desensitizing products and targeted treatments based on other related causes. Continuous professional development and updates regarding the latest research and protocols are necessary to maintain current knowledge about the subject.

Depending on the cause identified, a combination of customized oral hygiene instructions, the use of desensitizing agents and specialized treatment may be required to manage the condition. It is recommended that professionals regularly proceed to continue training to update their knowledge with new scientific data on the subject.

The majority of the dentists also reported poor patient compliance with prescribed treatment. This is mostly attributed to inadequate patient education and communication. The majority of the participants acknowledged the need for leaflets and other informative resources, and recognized the crucial role of patient awareness. This could also be improved by stressing the ill-effects of the same and introducing them to effective treatment options. This could improve patient adherence, leading to better outcomes.

This study stresses the necessity of integrating comprehensive, uniform and standardized information about DH into the dental curriculum. The various causes, diagnostic criteria and definitive treatments of DH to ensure that future dental professionals are more prepared to address this extremely common condition effectively. This would not only ensure better uniformity and efficient management of the condition, but also ensure better long term patient care. It also highlights the involvement of the different subjects in the dental curriculum for the effective management of DH (Table 2)

Table 2. Role of different dental specialties in the management of dentinal hypersensitivity.

Department	Managementof DH
Oral Pathology	Educating about the mechanism and causes of DH
Conservative Dentistry	Restoration techniques, application of desensitizing agents, fluoride varnishes. Educate students on appropriate materials for restoration.
Periodontics	Scaling and root planing, periodontal therapy. Focus on the relationship between gum health and DH, emphasizing non-invasive approaches.
Prosthodontics	Fabrication of crowns, bridges, and dentures. Teach students how to design restorations that minimize DH and provide comfort.
Orthodontics	Treatment planning involving tooth movement. Discuss how misalignment can contribute to DH and the importance of retention.
Oral Surgery	Extractions and surgical interventions. Highlight post-operative care and pain management strategies to address potential DH.

5 CONCLUSION

This study provides valuable insight into the current understanding of Dentinal Hypersensitivity. Although the majority of dentists are aware of its prevalence and impact , considerable variability is found in the diagnosis and treatment . A majority reported DHs lasting longer than four weeks indicating that the condition is persistent in the clinical scenario, but the treatment methods range from scaling and periodontal treatments to fluoride application, restorations or even endodontic treatment. This underscores the clear inconsistency, pointing towards the broader issue, a lack of effective treatment protocols.

In conclusion, this study reveals that while dental practitioners have a foundational understanding of the condition (DH), there is an urgent need to refine both diagnostic and treatment practices. The incorporation of improved educational content on DH in the dental curriculum, coupled with the development of standardized treatment protocols and improved patient education, can address these gaps. This will not only help improve the accuracy of the diagnosis and effectiveness of the treatment, but also enhance the patient outcomes and ultimately quality of life. Continued research, professional education and adherence to evidence-based practice will help improve the advancement of dental care with respect to Dentinal Hypersensitivity.

ACKNOWLEDGEMENT

NIL

REFERENCES

[1] Canadian Advisory Board on Dentin Hypersensitivity. (2003). Consensus-based recommendations for the diagnosis and management of dentin hypersensitivity. *J Can Dent Assoc* 69:221–226

[2] Bekes K, John MT, Schaller HG, Hirsch C. (2009). Oral health-related quality of life in patients seeking care for dentin hypersensitivity. *J Oral Rehabil* 36(1):45–51

[3] Gibson B, Boiko OV, Baker SR, *et al.* (2010). The everyday impact of dentine sensitivity: personal and functional aspects. *Soc Sci Dent* 1:11–21

[4] Cunha-Cruz J, Wataha JC, (2014). The burden of dentine hypersensitivity. In: Robinson PG, ed. *Dentine Hypersensitivity: Developing a Person-Centered Approach to Oral Health.* Oxford: Elsevier, 34–44

[5] Zeola LF, Teixeira DNR, Galvão ADM, Souza PG, Soares PV. (2020). Brazilian dentists' perception of dentin hypersensitivity management. *Braz Oral Res.* 33:e115. doi: 10.1590/1807-3107bor-2019.vol33.0115. PMID: 31939497.

[6] Gillam DG, Naser Dashti and Chatzopoulou D. (2019). A survey of the professional opinions of kuwaiti dentists for the treatment and management of dentine hypersensitivity: A questionnaire-based study. *Jacobs J Dentistry Res* 5(2): 046.

[7] Kopycka-Kedzierawski T, Meyerowitz C, Litaker M, Chonowski S. (2017). Management of Dentin Hypersensitivity by National Dental Practice-Based Research Network practitioners: results from a questionnaire administered prior to initiation of a clinical study on this topic. *BMC Oral Health* 17:41

[8] Exarchou C, Betsani I, Sakellari D. (2019). A survey of dentists in the management of dentine hypersensitivity: A questionnaire-based study. *Eur J Dent* 13:383–390

[9] Pereira R, Gillam DG, Bapatla S, Satyamurthy P (2018) Awareness of dentine hypersensitivity among general dental practitioners in Mumbai, India. *J Odontol* 2: 103.

[10] S Saif, M, Hamza, S Dhaimy. (2018). Moroccan dentist's perception and management of dentin hypersensitivity *International Journal of Dentistry Research* 3(1): 17–24

 ISBN: 978-1-041-32674-8

Digital Evaluation of Crown Preparations Done by Final Year Undergraduates

Prasanna Vadhani, Sivaranjani Gali, and SK Gayathri Devi
Department of Prosthodontics and Crown & Bridge, Faculty of Dental Sciences, Ramaiah University of Applied Sciences, New BEL Road, MSR Nagar, Bengaluru

ABSTRACT: Objective and reliable assessment of dental students is critical for psychomotor skill development in preclinical fixed prosthodontics. An objective method for evaluating crown preparations using an intraoral scanner and software is proposed in this study. Students were asked to perform a full veneer preparation for porcelain-fused-to-metal crowns on the upper left central incisor on a patient simulator. A total of 20 preparations were evaluated digitally using intraoral scanner based on pre-established criteria. Of these, only 12 preparations (60%) were deemed acceptable. Almost 55% of the preparations required improvement in terms of marginal integrity and structural durability. Assessment using intraoral scanning softwares (IOS) can address the limitations of subjectivity and provide immediate feedback to students, enhancing their understanding of tooth preparation in preclinical fixed prosthodontics. The goal is to leverage cutting-edge technologies to improve the assessment process, enhance learning outcomes, and better prepare students for clinical practice.

Keywords: Preclinical Prosthodontics, Fixed Prosthodontics, Tooth Preparation, Assessment, Intraoral scanners

1 INTRODUCTION

Preclinical fixed prosthodontics is included in the final year curriculum for dental students. They must perform full veneer preparations for porcelain-fused-to-metal crowns on anterior and posterior teeth [1]. Typically, the psychomotor skill assessment is conducted subjectively, lacking pre-established evaluation criteria. An objective and reliable evaluation of dental students in the preclinical setting is essential to ensure effective development of their psychomotor skills [2].

Learning to achieve an ideal crown preparation can be challenging due to the subjective assessments of clinical supervisors [3]. Grades in the record book are typically assigned without any objective criteria. This approach has limitations, such as a lack of complex real-world scenarios, shortage of professional supervision, and the subjective nature of skill assessments [4].

With the emergence of novel educational strategies and their implementation, dental education will inevitably undergo further evolution and transformation [5]. With the continuous advancement of digital dental technology, digital technologies have increasingly been incorporated into dental education, especially in preclinical training [6]. With the help of computer-assisted learning (CAL) or computer-assisted simulation (CAS), it is now possible to aim for a more objective assessment [7].

Digital tools such as intraoral scanners, computer-aided design (CAD) software, and artificial intelligence (AI) have the potential to revolutionize the way tooth preparation is assessed. These technologies offer increased accuracy in measuring preparation dimensions, improved consistency in evaluations, and the ability to provide immediate, detailed feedback. By integrating these digital solutions, dental education can address current challenges and better support students in mastering preclinical fixed prosthodontics [8].

Reduced errors in tooth preparation might lead to higher-quality restorations, leading to increased patient satisfaction. As students become proficient through standardized digital assessments, they are better prepared to deliver high-quality care in their professional practice.

We propose an objective method for evaluating crown preparations using intraoral scanner and software (IOS) through this study. It also serves as immediate feedback, helping students gain a better understanding of preclinical fixed prosthodontics.

2 MATERIALS AND METHODS

As part of the year-end assessment, students must complete full veneer preparations for porcelain-fused-to-metal crowns on either anterior or posterior teeth. Students are allotted 45 minutes to complete the preparation. We conducted a pilot study in which Trios 5 (3Shape) intraoral scanner and software was used to evaluate these preparations based on pre-established criteria. The criteria established by Sadid-Zadeh *et al.* in their 2019 study

 DOI: 10.1201/9781042016075-7

were utilized here based on the principles of tooth preparation [9]. Retention and resistance were evaluated by examining the taper and adjusting the path of insertion using the software. Structural durability was assessed by examining the amount of clearance and the extent of axial reduction. Marginal integrity was assessed by evaluating the configuration of the finish line.

The upper and lower jaws from the phantom models were scanned separately and together to obtain the bite scan (Figure 1A). This approach is crucial for assessing the amount of clearance provided. Lack of clearance, undercuts, and taper are visualized through color coding, which indicates the measurements (Figure 1B-D). An experienced single evaluator assessed the scans and graded each preparation as S (Standard met) or N (Needs Improvement) [9]. The grades were tabulated and analyzed for each criterion as well as overall as shown in Table 1.

Table 1. Grades for tooth preparation based on the rubrics.

S. No.	Retention & Resistance	Marginal Integrity	Structural Durability	Overall Acceptance
1	S	S	N	Yes
2	S	N	N	No
3	S	N	N	No
4	S	N	N	No
5	S	N	S	Yes
6	S	N	N	No
7	S	S	N	Yes
8	S	S	S	Yes
9	N	N	N	No
10	N	N	N	No
11	S	S	S	Yes
12	S	N	S	Yes
13	S	N	S	Yes
14	S	S	S	Yes
15	S	S	S	Yes
16	N	S	S	Yes
17	S	N	N	No
18	S	N	S	Yes
19	S	S	N	Yes
20	N	S	N	No

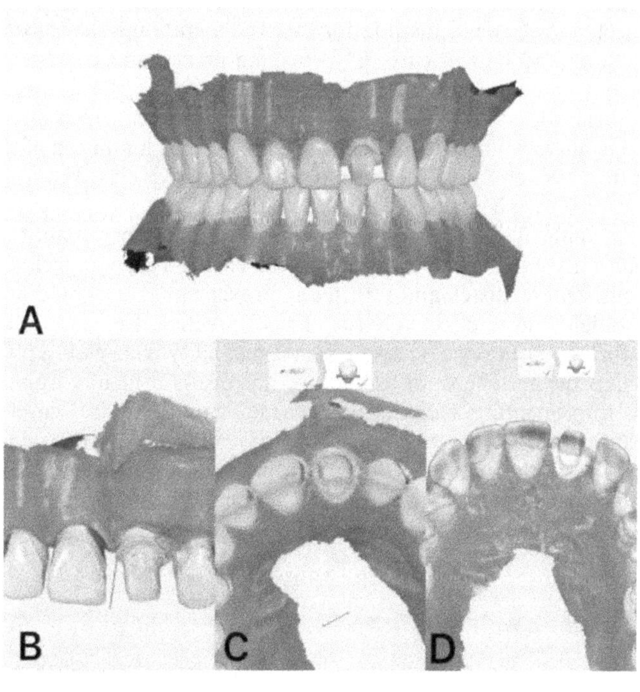

Figure 1. A- Upper and Lower Jaw Scanned with Bite B-D Lack of clearance, undercuts, and taper visualized through color coding.

3 RESULTS

A total of 20 preparations were evaluated digitally based on pre-established criteria [9]. Out of these, only 12 preparations (60%) were deemed acceptable. When assessed for resistance and retention form, 80% of the preparations met the standard criteria of performance. However, 55% of the preparations required improvement in terms of marginal integrity and structural durability.

4 DISCUSSION

Integrating digital dentistry courses into dental curriculum is essential for effectively training dental students and ensuring they can deliver high-quality patient care [10]. This study's aim was to propose an objective assessment method using an intraoral scanner and software. Digital assessments reduce the variability in evaluations by providing objective measurements, thus ensuring that all students are assessed according to the same criteria. Furthermore, the efficiency of digital tools allows for quicker feedback, which can accelerate the learning process and improve student outcomes.

Conventional methods in preclinical dental training provide advantages such as affordability, improved hand-eye coordination, and development of manual dexterity, making them a popular, time-tested option. However, they also have significant drawbacks, including non-calibrated evaluations, heavy dependence on subjective instructor judgments, and inconsistent student assessments. To overcome these issues, computerized dental teaching and assessment systems are proposed as alternatives, aiming to provide consistent feedback and enhance student learning and self-assessment [8].

Schubert *et al.* (2020) found that digitizing preparations with intraoral scanning improves the quality of all-ceramic single crown preparations, including marginal substance reduction, design, finish line homogeneity, and frequency of undercuts. This suggests that intraoral scanning enhances preparation quality by providing immediate visual feedback [11].

3Shape is the most widely used intraoral scanner because of its accuracy and precision [12,13]. The software offers various features for clinicians, including easy viewing, editing, and rescanning. Dentists can edit scans and rescan specific areas without starting over. The built-in occlusal clearance tool measures the space between the preparation and antagonist, using color codes to indicate if there is sufficient space for the restoration and allowing for adjustments before sending the impression to the lab. The Insertion Direction tool helps control convergence and divergence of prepared teeth and ensures optimal insertion direction before submitting the digital impression.

These features are extensively utilized by clinicians to enhance treatment outcomes. We suggest adopting them as an educational tool, allowing students to identify and correct their mistakes through self-assessment. Color coding facilitates easy visualization and provides immediate feedback for the students.

The proposed digital objective assessment method for tooth preparation holds substantial clinical significance, impacting both dental education and patient care. By providing precise and consistent evaluations, digital tools enhance the skill development of dental students, ensuring they acquire the necessary proficiency for clinical practice. This precision is crucial for achieving accurate tooth preparations, which directly affect the fit and functionality of dental restorations, thereby improving treatment outcomes. A limitation of this pilot study is the lack of operator training or calibration, which raises the potential for subjective bias. Future research with more established criteria and a larger sample size is necessary to address these issues.

A standardized rubric that outlines specific performance indicators for psychomotor skills should be incorporated into the BDS curriculum. By utilizing this method, we can ensure a more objective and reliable assessment of students' skills, fostering consistent feedback and targeted improvement. This would not only enhance skill development but also prepare students more effectively for clinical practice. Regular training for evaluators on the rubric's application would further ensure its effectiveness and reliability in assessing psychomotor skills.

However, challenges such as the initial cost of technology, the need for faculty training, and potential technical issues must be considered. Implementing a digital assessment method requires careful planning, including the integration of these tools into the existing curriculum and providing necessary training for both students and faculty. The success of this integration will depend on the institution's ability to support the adoption of new technologies and adapt to the changes in assessment practices. Future research should investigate low-cost scanners for educational purposes and evaluate the effectiveness of these assessment methods in comparison to traditional approaches.

5 CONCLUSION

Assessment using intraoral scanners (IOS) can address the limitations of subjectivity and provide immediate feedback to students, enhancing their understanding of tooth preparation in preclinical fixed prosthodontics. The goal is to leverage cutting-edge technologies to improve the assessment process, enhance learning outcomes, and better prepare students for clinical practice. While the transition to digital objective assessments presents challenges, the potential benefits for accuracy, consistency, and educational impact make it a compelling option for modernizing dental education.

ACKNOWLEDGMENTS

I am grateful to the Faculty of Dental Sciences, Ramaiah University of Applied Sciences for its invaluable support and resources throughout this study.

REFERENCES

[1] Dental Council of India. BDS Course regulations. (2007). Available from: https://dciindia.gov.in/Rule_Regulation/Revised_BDS_Course_Regulation_2007.pdf

[2] Sadid-Zadeh R, D'Angelo EH, Gambacorta J. (2018). Comparing feedback from faculty interactions and virtual assessment software in the development of psychomotor skills in preclinical fixed prosthodontics. *Clinical and Experimental Dental Research.* 4 (5):189–95.

[3] Seet RH, Soo PR, Leong KJ, Pang JJ, Lee FK, Tan MY. (2020). Crown preparations by undergraduate dental students: A comparison of conventional versus digital assessment via an intraoral scanner. *Journal of Dental Education.* 84(11):1303–13.

[4] Arora O, Sivaswamy V, Ahmed N, Ganapathy D. (2023). Effectiveness of digital visualization in teaching crown preparation to predoctoral dental students – A Pilot study. *Journal of Population Therapeutics and Clinical Pharmacology.* 30(12): 168–173.

[5] Wong ML, Lee TWO, Allen PF, Foong K. (2020). Dental education in Singapore: A journey of 90 years and beyond. *The Asia Pacific Scholar* 5:3–7.

[6] Liu L, Li J, Yuan S, *et al.* (2018). Evaluating the effectiveness of a preclinical practice of tooth preparation using digital training system: A randomised controlled trial. *Eur J Dent Educ.* 22(4): e679–e686.

[7] Maximilian N *et al.* (2024) Assessment of crown preparations with 'prepCheck' – A pilot study. *Romanian Journal of Medical and Dental Education.* 13(1): 102–110.

[8] Velioğlu N, Çabuk GG, Abdulai D, Geduk G, Cengiz S. (2023). Comparison of digital and traditional assessment methods in crown preparation: Pilot study. *International Journal of Applied Dental Sciences.* 9(4):17–22.

[9] Sadid-Zadeh R, DeLuca JT, Arany H, Li R. (2020). Assessment of teeth prepared by senior dental students for CAD/CAM restorations. *Journal of Dental Education.* 84(3):358–66.

[10] Cooper LF, Campbell SD, Garcia LT, Lefebvre CA. (2019). *The Current Impact of Digital Technology in Prosthodontics.* American College of Prosthodontists: Chicago, IL, USA. Available from: https://www.prosthodontics.org/assets/1/7/Digital_White_Paper_r1.pdf

[11] Schubert O, Erdelt KJ, Tittenhofer R, Hajtó J, Bergmann A, Güth JF. (2020). Influence of intraoral scanning on the quality of preparations for all-ceramic single crowns. *Clinical oral investigations.* 4511–18.

[12] Winkler J, Gkantidis N. (2020). Trueness and precision of intraoral scanners in the maxillary dental arch: an in vivo analysis. *Scientific Reports.* 2020 Jan 24;10(1):1172.

[13] Pellitteri F, Albertini P, Vogrig A, Spedicato GA, Siciliani G, Lombardo L. (2022). Comparative analysis of intraoral scanners accuracy using 3D software: an in vivo study. *Progress in Orthodontics.* 23(1):21.

Navigating Dental Education Trends and Transforming Dental Pedagogy – Abas and Srikant N (Eds)
 ISBN: 978-1-041-32674-8

A Narrative Review of Problem-Based Learning: A Learner-Based Approach in Dental Education

Urmila Paudel, Ashish Shrestha, Tarakant Bhagat, Santosh Kumari Agrawal, and Ujwal Gautam
Department of Public Health Dentistry, College of Dental Surgery, B. P. Koirala Institute of Health Sciences, Dharan, Nepal

Ramya Shenoy
Department of Public Health Dentistry, Manipal College of Dental Sciences Mangalore, Manipal Academy of Higher Education, Manipal, Karnataka, India

ABSTRACT: The objective of this review is to explore the applicability of problem-based learning (PBL) methods in dental education. Problem-based learning (PBL) is an active student-centered learning methodology that has been increasingly used worldwide in various medical education systems. It inspires students to actively learn, develop habits of critical thinking, and search for new ideas and factors related to a real-world problem. The concept of PBL in dental education started in the 1990s. The inclusion of PBL in dental education helps in identifying various clinical problems on the basis of various factors responsible for its causation. It provides a broad view regarding the utilization of physiological, pathological and anatomical concepts in solving a problem. The dental students can later independently use such knowledge in future dental careers. This PBL methodology has been implemented in basic and clinical subjects' dental curricula since 2014 at the B.P. Koirala Institute of Health Sciences. The literatures suggests that the inclusion of problem-based learning (PBL) in curricula is an effective teaching/ learning strategy compared with traditional learning methods. This strategy could help dental students to deal with various problems throughout their course of learning.

Keywords: Problem-based learning, dental education, curriculum

1 INTRODUCTION

Problem-based learning (PBL) is a student-centered learning approach carried out among small groups of students under the supervision of a tutor. Students may think critically, analyze, and solve real-world problems with this learning approach. In problem-based learning, the problem is assigned to students, and they are actively involved in finding solutions to the problem whereas in traditional learning, students receive information about the utilization of existing problems [1–3].

The PBL has been included in the dental curriculum for a few decades. It was first developed at the Faculty of Odontology in Malmo, Sweden, in 1990. The integration of PBL into the dental curriculum has helped students identify clinical problems more accurately and effectively with evidence-based solutions. It acts as a mainstay for an integrated core curriculum. PBL enables students to apply their knowledge of anatomy, pathology and physiology to understand the underlying causes of dental problems [4–6].

Since then, PBL has been followed in different countries throughout the world. In PBL, the problem to be included is given to the students on the basis of certain facts. The students need to define the problem, gather information, generate hypotheses and know the factors responsible for its causation [7,8].

Our main objective is to review the literature on how the integration of PBL in dental education can help develop new learning skill in solving a defined problem, increase communication skills and strengthen teamwork among the dental students.

2 METHODS

Various databases such as PubMed, Hinari, Google Scholar and cross-references were searched for this narrative review. The relevant articles from these databases were searched. The keywords used for searching articles were as follows:

Problem-based learning OR team-based learning OR traditional based learning or AND Dental Education OR Dental curriculum OR Medical education OR Clinical studies/ studies/ Research/ review Fifteen articles from 2014 – 2024 A.D were selected for the review.

 DOI: 10.1201/9781042016075-8

Inclusion criteria:

(1) Qualitative, observational and experimental studies and systematic reviews/ reviews including problem-based learning as a learning method in dental education.
(2) Studies including PBL and dental education, and their comparison with traditional methods of learning.

Exclusion criteria:

(1) Studies available in languages other than the English language.
(2) Papers whose full text was not available in the online database.

3 RESULTS

According to this report, problem-based learning has been adopted by a number of academic fields worldwide. Problem based learning has been widely used in dental curricula throughout countries such as the USA, Canada, the UK, Spain, Australia and Southeast China. The involvement of students in PBL has shown that they formulate innovative ideas and concepts. In PBL, students are always motivated and stimulated to solve problems given to them. The PBL fosters the growth of communication, problem-solving, and critical thinking skills [9]. The studies revealed a positive response favoring problem-based learning in dental education [2,5,10]. The pre and posttest comparisons following the PBL sessions revealed that the dental students were interactive, collaborative, goal and research oriented [1].

The study conducted among students with five focus group discussions revealed that PBL was the most effective model to support self-regulation among dental students. This illustrated the need for all incoming students to be formally introduced to PBL settings [11].

Most of the studies have conducted PBL among a small group of students under the supervision of facilitators. They reported that students found it more stimulating and practical to solve real world problems [10]. This study suggests that the inclusion of PBL in the dental curriculum requires instructors to have adequate knowledge and skills to facilitate student learning [12]. The curriculum focuses on problems, and integrated learning is prioritized instead of separating basic and clinical science components [13]. Most of the studies have compared PBL with traditional methods of learning. These studies showed that that PBL is more effective among dental students than teacher-based lectures are [14,15]. Most of the review studies suggest that the PBL curriculum is more effective than the traditional curriculum in dental education [2,15]. The use of PBL via radiography has a beneficial effect on radiological education. Effective guidance by tutors in small groups helps them learn new skills [16].

4 DISCUSSION

Problem-based learning is an effective learning approach for enhancing students' competency and broadening their horizons of knowledge. Various studies have reported the effectiveness of including PBL in dental education. In contrast to the positive findings, one study that applied the concept of PBL among dental students in the first, third and fifth years did not show the expected improvement in the learning approach [17]. When it came to handling fixed prostheses and removable partial dentures, the students who were taught using traditional methods showed noticeably more proficiency than those who were taught using PBL. This could be because PBL students believe their manual skills are at a lower level [18].

The implementation of PBL in the curriculum increases the workload among students since they must actively be involved in collecting resources. The barriers to its implementation include inadequate resources and limited faculty members. In addition, barriers to the implementation of PBL in the course could be a lack of faculty dedication, inadequate motivation among students [19]. There might be a lack of information obtained directly from teachers on various subjects which might cause problems during exams. The costs, resources and time allocated to train facilitators does create issues with PBL in crowds.

Accreditation standards for the BDS in Nepal suggest that dental colleges should implement innovative teaching methodologies that are limited to self-directed learning, PBL and structured interactive sessions (SIS). In Nepal, out of 19 medical colleges, only 11 have included PBL in their course [20]. The dental curriculum of BPKIHS has included PBL since 2014 for second- and third-year BDS students and planning to implement this program for fourth- and fifth-year students. This has helped students correlate basic and clinical knowledge in dentistry to solve this problem. The students involved in PBL themselves identify the gap in their knowledge and work on the part to solve the problem.

5 CONCLUSION

Problem-based learning (PBL) enhances networking skills, team work and appreciation of interdisciplinary approaches. Problem-based learning can help dental students develop problem-solving abilities. This promotes their communication and collaboration with team members which help them prepare to face real world challenges as dental professionals.

The implementation of PBL in the dental curriculum necessitates a rational increase in training for facilitators and resources for students. Medical/ dental colleges can make the provision of various workshops, seminars to help faculty members to effectively conduct this type of teaching methodology.

REFERENCES

[1] Ali SS. (2019). Problem based learning: a student-centered approach. *Canadian Center of Science and Education*. 12(5):73.

[2] Bassir SH, Sadr-Eshkevari P, Amirikhorheh S, Karimbux NY. (2014). Problem–based learning in dental education: A systematic review of the literature. *Journal of Dental Education*. 78(1):98–109.

[3] Wood DF. (2003). ABC of learning and teaching in medicine: Problem based learning. *British Medical Journal*. 326(7384):328–30.

[4] Rohlin M, Petersson K, Svensäter G. (1989). The Malmö model: A problem-based learning curriculum in undergraduate dental education. *European Journal of Dental Education*. 2(3):103–14.

[5] Tayyeb R. (2013). Effectiveness of problem based learning as an instructional tool for acquisition of content knowledge and promotion of critical thinking among medical students. *Journal of the College of Physicians and Surgeons Pakistan* 23.

[6] Joshi T, Budhathoki P, Adhikari A, Poudel A, Raut S, Shrestha DB. (2021). *Improving Medical Education: A Narrative Review. Cureus [Internet]*. [cited 2024 Aug 26]; Available from: https://www.cureus.com/articles/74079-improving-medical-education-a-narrative-review

[7] Dolmans DHJM, Schmidt HG. (1949). What drives the student in problem-based learning? *Medical Education*, 28(5):372–80.

[8] Jones RW. (2006). Problem-based learning: description, advantages, disadvantages, scenarios and facilitation. *Anaesth Intensive Care*. 34(4):485–8.

[9] Ali. (2023). 2022 Does problem-based learning facilitate enactment of learner agency in undergraduate. *European Journal of Dental Education*. 27:823–832.

[10] Rimal J, Paudel B, Shrestha A. (2015). Introduction of problem-based learning in undergraduate dentistry program in Nepal. *International Journal of Applied Basic Medical Research*. 5(4):45.

[11] Ali K, Daud A, Ba Hattab R, Philip N, Matoug-Elwerfelli M, Anweigi L, *et al.* (2023). Development of self-regulation amongst dental students in problem-based learning curricula: A qualitative study. *European Journal of Dental Education*. 27(2):388–95.

[12] Von Bergmann H, Walker J, Dalrymple KR, Shuler CF. (2017). Dental faculty members' pedagogic beliefs and curriculum aims in problem-based learning: An exploratory study. *Journal of Dental Education*. 81(8):937–47.

[13] Alrahlah A. (2016). How effective the problem-based learning (PBL) in dental education. A critical review. *The Saudi Dental Journal*. 28(4):155–61.

[14] Quratulain Javaid, Ambreen Usmani. (2024). Effectiveness of problem-based learning strategies compared to conventional anatomy teaching approaches. *Journal of Pakistan Medical Association*. 74(2):264–71.

[15] Oderinu OH, Adegbulugbe IC, Orenuga Omolola O, Butali A. (2020). Comparison of students' perception of problem-based learning and traditional teaching method in a Nigerian dental school. *Eur J Dental Education*. 24(2):207–12.

[16] Lawal O, Ramlaul A, Murphy F. (2021). Problem based learning in radiography education: A narrative review. *Radiography. Radiography*. 27(2):727–32.

[17] Haghparast H, Ghorbani A, Rohlin M. (2017). Dental students' perception of their approaches to learning in a PBL programme. *European Journal of Dental Education*. 21(3):159–65.

[18] Montero J, Dib A, Guadilla Y, Flores J, Santos JA, Aguilar RA, *et al.* (2018). Dental students' perceived clinical competence in prosthodontics: Comparison of traditional and problem-based learning methodologies. *Journal of Dental Education*. 82(2):152–62.

[19] Farrukh K, Ambreen Usmani, Syed Bilal Yousuf. (2023). Assessment of problem-based learning in dental education and exploring barriers to its implementation: theory to reality. *Journal of Pakistan Medical association*. 73(11):2247–50.

[20] Nepal Medical Council. (2017). Accreditation standards for the BDS.

Integrating Outreach Activities in the Undergraduate Curriculum for Dental Education: A Narrative Review

Suveksha Pandey, Ashish Shrestha, Tarakant Bhagat, Santosh Kumari Agrawal, and Ujwal Gautam
Department of Public Health Dentistry, College of Dental Surgery, B.P. Koirala Institute of Health Sciences, Dharan, Nepal

Ramya Shenoy
Department of Public Health Dentistry, Manipal College of Dental Sciences Manglore, Manipal College of Higher Education, Manipal, Karnataka, India

ABSTRACT: The objective of this review is to explore possibilities for integrating dental outreach activities as a mandatory training requirement for dental undergraduate students. As a part of training, outreach programs are not adapted by many dental colleges. This review provides evidence highlighting the necessity, usefulness and challenges of adopting outreach programs for students. Dental outreach programs can be effective approaches for the prevention of oral diseases and the promotion of oral health. School health programs are ideal programs because they cover large groups of people, including students, parents, teachers and staff. Students are the trained manpower required for the implementation of these programs in communities. It will contribute to the future preparedness of students by helping them build confidence and can enable them to implement their learning in practice. Moreover, students will be introduced to several dimensions of health and illness, as this platform allows them to interact with people from diverse backgrounds. These programs have challenges and limitations on their own. These factors should be addressed to make the program more acceptable and sustainable. Proper training, supervision and support for dental students in outreach programs can significantly contribute to improving the oral health of a community. The focus should be on developing a curriculum involving outreach programs for undergraduate students.

Keywords: Outreach activities, dental students, community

1 BACKGROUND

Oral health is a vital component of overall health, maintaining self-esteem and having a proper quality of life. Despite the wide importance of oral health, they are neglected [1]. Oral diseases are largely preventable. Initiation of oral diseases can be avoided if proper oral care habits are practiced. If the disease has already started, its progression into a serious condition can be interrupted if it is diagnosed and treated at early stages [2]. They can be prevented through an effective public health approach [3].

One among such program can be the dental outreach program where the first approach to diagnosis and prevention of oral problems can be possible. It has the capacity to engage the community with health institutions or organizations [4]. There is sufficient evidence showing the effectiveness of outreach programs in improving the oral health of participants [4–8]. However, the implementation of effective outreach programs often faces challenges such as time constraints, high workloads, limited resources, inadequate funding and a shortage of qualified human resources [9]. One solution to address the lack of human resources can be the integration of undergraduate dental students into outreach programs.

A dental student, after graduating from the dental college is expected to practice the principles of prevention and health promotion in his professional career. He must understand the social, cultural and environmental dimensions of health and disease. Apart from these a dental surgeon should be able to showcase his proficiency on research, communication skills and group activities. All these abilities is intended to prepare him/her to efficiently handle the challenges that might come along the way in future.Hh [10]

The incorporation of outreach programs in the academic curriculum of oral health professionals can be a useful approach for developing the academic skills and social responsibilities among undergraduate students. These programs are mutually beneficial to both students and community and also strengthens the bond between communities and institutions [11].

The objective of this review is to explore possibilities for integrating dental outreach activities as a mandatory training requirement for dental undergraduate students.

DOI: 10.1201/9781042016075-9

2 METHODS

Electronic databases (PubMed, Hinari, Google Scholar) and reference lists from key papers were used to identify articles relevant to this narrative review. Literature from the past 10 years, i.e., from 2014–2024, was used. The articles were searched via keywords such as the following:

Undergraduate dental students OR dental students OR dental curriculum AND Community service OR Dental Outreach Program OR Outreach program OR Community engagement OR Community inclusion OR Community involvement OR Outreach program OR School Oral Health Program OR Community-based education OR Community dental clinics OR Clinical studies/Studies/Research/Review The titles and abstracts were also screened for inclusion using the following inclusion and exclusion criteria:

Inclusion criteria:

(1) Papers that included the involvement of undergraduate dental students in various types of outreach activities.
(2) All types of studies, including case reports, reviews, cross-sectional studies and reviews, were included in the study.

Exclusion criteria:

(1) Papers that included research related to outreach activities but did not involve undergraduate dental students.
(2) Papers in languages other than English.
(3) Papers for which the full text was not available in online databases.

3 RESULTS

A total of 200 articles were screened for review, out of which only 15 articles were included. The findings suggest that the practice of incorporating outreach activities in undergraduate dental education is prevalent in many dental colleges across the globe [11–15]. Dental students are involved in community activities either in their third [13], fourth or final year of dentistry [11,13,15–17] or even during their internship period [18]. Students are seen to participate for a day, two, or even weeks or months depending upon the curriculum of their universities [11,13–15,17,18]. The programs are planned in the form of community-based dental education, service-learning programs or extramural programs. Programs were conducted in community clinics, public health clinics, peripheral satellite centers, oral outreach treatment camps, residential homes, indigenous clinics or hospital clinics [11,12,15–19]. The services provided included oral screening, extraction, restoration, scaling and polishing, sealant application, atraumatic restorative treatment and oral health education [11,12,14,18]. Students had the opportunity to diagnose, treat, interact with the patient and educate them [18].

In most of the studies, outreach programs for students were assessed by gathering information from the students through questionnaires, [11,12,18] surveys [13,17,19] or written assignments [14,15]. The studies were conducted with various designs, including experimental [11,16,18], cross-sectional [12,13,20–24] or qualitative [14,15,19] and case reports [17]. A scoping review was also conducted that assessed various outreach programs [25].

The benefits from outreach programs evaluated from these studies can be grouped into four major entities:

(1) Academic development: Three studies [11–13] concluded that outreach programs were beneficial in terms of the academic aspects of students.
(2) Personal development: Seven studies [11–15,18,21] reported that outreach programs enhanced the personality of dental students in terms of various aspects.
(3) Social responsibility: Seven studies [11,13,14,17,19,21,22] reported improved social responsibility among dental students after their involvement in outreach activities.
(4) Interprofessional learning: One study [13] showed that outreach programs were beneficial in terms of interprofessional learning.

The long-term impact of community-based developmental education was assessed in one of the studies, where dentists who participated in such activities during their student life were assessed for their involvement in charitable care even after years of graduation [23].

One study evaluated the perceptions of dentists who supervise dental students at outreach clinics [24]. Three studies appraised the limitations of performing dental procedures in outreach activities by dental students [12,17,18].

4 DISCUSSION

The studies revealed that the outreach program provided an exciting opportunity to face a real-world scenario. It was beneficial to them, as it helped them build confidence, develop communication skills, increase clinical confidence, gain momentum in their clinical work, develop patient management skills, enhance their leadership skills and help them understand their strengths and weaknesses [11–14,18]. A qualitative study performed by Major *et al.* revealed that students initially felt anxious about treating large numbers and different types of populations. They thought patient management would be a challenge and that the clinic would consist of outdated instruments. They were also apprehensive about working independently in the clinic. The perceptions of these students changed after they participated in a outreach program [15].

Students were allowed to handle patients independently during the postings, which also reinforced their academic knowledge and broadened their clinical experience [11–13]. The supportive learning environment in such centers allows them to concentrate on learning [13].

Such programs strengthen the social ties between society and the profession. They were beneficial to communities in terms of developing oral hygiene status, oral health knowledge and attitudes. The students also had a positive impact on the community in terms of healthy oral practices [7,8]. A study performed by Behar-Horenstein *et al.* [14] revealed that students became more aware of disparities after becoming involved in such activities. They understood the difficulties of the underserved population and improved their connectedness with them [17,21,22] They realized their professional responsibilities to serve the oral health needs of people with low income and sought their willingness to volunteer in such communities in the future [19]. They became familiar with the primary healthcare system and understood the social determinants of oral disease more broadly [13].

The students worked as teams with dental hygienists and dental nurses, which gave them new insights into the profession of dentistry [13].

Supervisors also believed that exposing students to real- world earlier during the training phase helped students develop the necessary skills such as communication, interprofessional interaction, critical analysis of a situation and provided wide clinical exposure. Students could be benefited from the guidance and suggestions provided by the supervisors regarding practice and time management [24].

The Institute of Medicine and the Commission on Dental Accreditation have recommended that dental programs incorporate Community-Based Dental Education as a part of the student training program in the U.S [23,26]. The Association for Dental Education in Europe (ADEE) highlights the necessity of the involvement of dental students in health promotion and preventive programs [27]. The dental council of India has also directed compulsory participation in satellite clinics in remote areas to complete their internship programs during the Bachelor of Dental Surgery (BDS) course [18]. Accreditation standard for the BDS program in Nepal encourages students to know about the health system in hospital and community, understand various determinants of health existing in the society and practice preventive strategies for the community as well as individual level [10]. However, no such periphery programs that helps students to develop understanding of the community by being in the community is considered mandatory.

Studies from Australia [17], India [18], Saudi Arabia [12], and the United States [14,23] indicate that outreach programs are practiced throughout the world and are tailored according to the circumstances suited for their universities. In the context of Nepal, a dental outreach program is conducted on a regular basis by the Department of Public Health Dentistry at the B.P. Koirala Institute of Health Sciences, Dharan, Nepal. Students in their fourth year, final year and internship period regularly visit different outreach centers where they provide oral health education, perform screening, perform needful treatment, such as extractions, atraumatic restorative treatment and the application of pit and fissure sealants. Referral is performed for cases that are not possible to treat in the outreach center. These activities in the community have helped students increase their confidence, make them more oriented toward preventive activities and make them more socially accountable. Such changes in students' behavior are evident in clinical practice as well. No evidence regarding the involvement of dental students in periphery posts is available at other universities in Nepal. Curriculum of BDS in Nepal requires reformation for preparing students to compete in a global as well as local scenario. The postings can start from third year where they can take surveys of small community and develop the basic understanding of community. In the fourth year and final year they can be utilized to provide health education, perform oral examination in schools or primary health centers and provide simple treatments such as extraction and Atraumatic Restorative Treatments which can be performed without much resources. In the internship period, students can be posted in remote community hospitals along with the supervisors where they can examine, diagnose, treat or refer the cases. Initial phase of the program would require coordination with the community hospitals, public health dentists and the local people.

Several limitations in performing dental procedures have been identified in outreach programs, including the unavailability of adequate instruments, the use of defective equipment and inadequate infection control. The outreach program also increased the financial burden and workload of supervisors because of inadequate human resources in outreach centers [12,17,18]. Proper planning and pilot testing of programs can be conducted before the program is implemented. Partnerships with the government, local communities and private health centers can be performed to reduce the challenges of budgets and inadequate human resources.

5 CONCLUSION

The utilization of undergraduate dental students in oral outreach programs presents a promising strategy to effectively address the challenges of oral health promotion in the community. With appropriate training, supervision, and support, these students have the potential to make a substantial contribution to enhancing the oral health of a community, while also acquiring valuable experience for their future careers. The development of a curriculum should be performed to compulsorily include outreach programs where dental students should be encouraged to take the lead. These activities can be incorporated from the initial years of dental college, specifically in the third year or fourth year, rather than solely during the internship period, will aid students in becoming familiar with such activities. Dental institutions can also establish mandatory community-based oral health education programs aimed at promoting and preventing oral health issues. Expanding these programs into interdisciplinary forms by incorporating students from various health-related fields can be more effective in terms of learning for students. Proper planning and evaluation of outreach programs should be performed regularly to reduce this gap. Further research assessing the cost-effectiveness of the programs and the long-term impact on dental students is necessary to enhance the effectiveness of these programs.

REFERENCES

[1] Jin L, Lamster I, Greenspan J, Pitts N, Scully C, Warnakulasuriya S. (2016). Global burden of oral diseases: emerging concepts, management and interplay with systemic health. *Oral Disease.* 22(7):609–19.

[2] World Health organization. *Global Oral Health Status Report [Internet].* Geneva. World health Organization. Assessed on: 2024/9/2. Available from https://www.who.int/team/noncommunicable-diseases/global-status-report-on-oral-health-2022

[3] Watt RG. (2005). Strategies and approaches in oral disease prevention and health promotion. Bull World Health Organization. 711–712.

[4] Dagli R, Singh A. (2015). Dental outreach program – how effective it is in reaching out to the community. *Journal of International Oral Health.* 7(5): i–ii.

[5] Subedi K, Shrestha A, Bhagat T, Baral D. (2021). Effectiveness of oral health education intervention among 12–15-year-old school children in Dharan, Nepal: A randomized controlled trial. *BMC Oral Health.* 21(1):525.

[6] Gurav KM, Shetty V, Vinay V, Bhor K, Jain C, Divekar P. (2022). Effectiveness of oral health educational methods among school children aged 5–16 years in improving their oral health status: A meta-analysis. *International Journal of Clinical Pediatric Dentistry.* 15(3):338–49.

[7] Bhat N, Singh A, Asawa K, Tak M, Kahlon H, Gambhir R, *et al.* (2016). Assessment of satisfaction levels of patients during dental outreach programs in rural part of Udaipur, India. *Nigerian Postgraduate Medical Journal.* 23(4):227.

[8] Ferro R, Dainese V, Benacchio L, Besostri A, Olivieri A. (2021). Effectiveness of a portable dental hygiene outreach program in improving the oral health of disabled adults. *Journal of Oral Health and Community Dentistry.* 14(3):88–2.

[9] Habbu SG, Krishnappa P. (2015). Effectiveness of oral health education in children – a systematic review of current evidence (2005–2011). *International Dental Journal.* 65(2):57–64.

[10] Nepal Medical Council. *Accreditation Standard for The BDS Program [Internet].* Kathmandu. Nepal Medical Council. Assessed on: 2024/9/2. Available from: https://nmc.org.np/files/4/ACCREDITATION%20STANDARDS%20FOR%20THE%20BDS.pdf.

[11] Suresan V, Jnaneswar A, Swati S, Jha K, Goutham B, Kumar G. (2019). The impact of outreach programs on academic development, personal development and civic responsibilities of dental students in Bhubaneswar city. *Journal of Education and Health Promotion.* 8(1):188.

[12] Kruger C, Nkambule NR, Bhayat A. (2024). Self-reported experience of Outreach activities among undergraduate Oral Health students at a University in South Africa. *South African Dental Journal.* 79(01):30–5.

[13] Goswami S, Karaharju-Suvanto T, Kaila M, Tseveenjav B. (2024). Community Health Centre-Based Outreach Clinic for undergraduate dental education: Experience in Helsinki over 8 years. *European Journal of Dental Education [Internet].* [cited 2024 Sep 2];22(3). Available from: https://onlinelibrary.wiley.com/doi/10.1111/eje.12295

[14] Behar-Horenstein LS, Feng X, Roberts KW, Gibbs M, Catalanotto FA, Hudson-Vassell CM. (2015). Developing dental students' awareness of health care disparities and desire to serve vulnerable populations through service-learning. *Journal of Dental Education.* 79(10):1189–200.

[15] Major N, McQuistan MR. (2016). An exploration of dental students' assumptions about community-based clinical experiences. *Journal of Dental Education.* 80(3):265–74.

[16] Phlypo I, De Tobel J, Marks L, De Visschere L, Koole S. (2018). Integrating community service learning in undergraduate dental education: A controlled trial in a residential facility for people with intellectual disabilities. *Special Care Dentistry.* 38(4):201–7.

[17] Abuzar MA, Owen J. (2016). A community engaged dental curriculum: a rural indigenous outplacement programme. *Journal of Public Health Research.* 5(1):jphr.2016.668

[18] Verma A, Muddiah P, Krishna Murthy A, Yadav V. (2016). Outreach programs: an adjunct for improving dental education. *The International Journal of Rural and Remote Health Research, Education, Practice and Policy.* [cited 2024 Aug 26]; Available from: https://www.rrh.org.au/journal/article/3848

[19] Sager JJ, Blue CM. (2019). Reflective learning outcomes of community-based experiences: A qualitative study. *Journal of Dental Education.* 2019 May;83(5):530–5.

[20] Smith PD, Mays KA. (2019). Dental students' non-clinical learning during community-based experiences: A survey of u.s. dental schools. *Journal of Dental Education.* 83(11):1289–95.

[21] Coe JM, Best AM, Warren JJ, McQuistan MR, Kolker JL, Isringhausen KT. (2015). Service-learning's impact on dental students' attitude toward community service. *European Journal of Dental Education*;19(3):131–9.

[22] Mays KA, Maguire M. (2018). Care provided by students in community-based dental education: helping meet oral health needs in underserved communities. *Journal of Dental Education*. 82(1):20–8.

[23] McQuistan MR, Mohamad A, Kuthy RA. (2014). Association between dentists' participation in charitable care and community–based dental education. *Journal of Dental Education*. 78(1):110–8.

[24] Nayar P, McFarland K, Lange B, Ojha D, Chandak A. (2014). Supervising dentists' perspectives on the effectiveness of community-based dental education. *Journal of Dental Education*. 78(8):1139–44.

[25] Elsheli J, Patrick A, Stokes C. (2024). Community- based education programs in the context of dental education: A scoping review. *European Journal of Dental Education*. 28:576–590.

[26] Commision on Dental Accrediation. Accreditation Standards for Dental Education Programs. [Internet]. Chicago. Assessed on: 2024/9/2. Available from: https://coda.ada.org/-/media/project/ada-organization/ada/coda/files/predoc_standards.pdf.

[27] Cowpe J, Plasschaert A, Harzer W, Vinkka-Puhakka H, Walmsley AD. (2010). Profile and competences for the graduating European dentist – update 2009. *European Journal of Dental Education*. 14(4):193–202.

 ISBN: 978-1-041-32674-8

Feasibility and Effectiveness of E-Learning during the COVID-19 Pandemic in Interpreting Intraoral Periapical and Panoramic Radiographs: A Hospital-Based Study

Sarju Shrestha
Trishuli Hospital, Nuwakot, Nepal

Jyotsna Rimal and Iccha Kumar Maharjan
Department of Oral Medicine and Radiology, BP Koirala Institute of Health Sciences, Dharan, Nepal

Pragya Regmee
Trishuli Hospital, Nuwakot, Nepal

Ashish Shrestha
Department of Public Health Dentistry, BP Koirala Institute of Health Sciences, Dharan, Nepal

Akunchan Shrestha
Department of Oral Medicine and Radiology, BP Koirala Institute of Health Sciences, Dharan, Nepal

ABSTRACT: **Background:** The coronavirus disease 2019 (COVID-19) pandemic has forced the world into a standstill that includes most of the day-to-day activities and academics, which has led to the search for alternative methods for continuing academic activities. This pandemic opened up the way for this innovative tool in continuing academics. This study aimed to assess the feasibility and effectiveness of e-learning during the COVID-19 pandemic in the interpretation of intraoral periapical and panoramic radiographs.

Materials and Methods: An experimental study was conducted on 41 fourth-year BDS students allocated into conventional learning (20 students) and e-learning groups (21 students). A pretest was performed just prior to the class, after which the students were taught radiographic interpretations of oral conditions/diseases in four consecutive classes, each lasting one hour. A posttest was taken 10 days after the last class, followed by an analysis of the pre- and posttest scores.

Results: When the e-learning group was compared with the conventional teaching group, the pre- and posttest scores were not statistically significant, whereas within each group, the mean improvement between the pre- and posttest scores was significant ($p < 0.001$). Reporting skills improved following academic intervention ($p < 0.001$), and the students agreed on the feasibility of online learning.

Conclusion: The present study demonstrated that e-learning is as effective as conventional teaching and can be used as an alternative to conventional methods when the former method of teaching is not feasible.

Keywords: COVID-19, Effectiveness, E-learning, Feasibility, Radiographic interpretation

1 INTRODUCTION

Year 2020 had been a phase of the coronavirus disease 2019 (COVID-19) pandemic, affecting millions all around the globe in terms of their personal lifestyle, day to day activities. [1] As, people were at risk of developing life-threatening conditions, there were substantial challenges in medical education, such as delivery of the lectures by the instructors safely with ensured integrity and continuity of the medical education process. [2] Although the acute phase of the pandemic has passed, the medical education landscape now faces new challenges. Institutions must adapt to hybrid teaching models, ensuring the safe delivery of lectures while maintaining the integrity and continuity of medical training. The pandemic highlighted the need for resilient educational frameworks capable of addressing future disruptions while supporting the evolving demands of healthcare systems.

During that period, students of B.P. Koirala Institute of Health Sciences (BPKIHS) were confined to their homes, away from campus, which significantly disrupted classroom learning and compromised the quality of education. So as to overcome the challenges in learning, e-learning could be one of the best and most easily approachable or feasible means as an alternative to traditional way of teaching and learning.

Broadly, utilization of the internet for education can be perceived as e-learning [3]. One of the benefits of e-learning is that it allows self-directed or teacher-led learning and can utilize a range of materials in

 DOI: 10.1201/9781042016075-10

the form of text, graphics, animation, audio, and video [4]. E-learning can help address a portion of the difficulties in healthcare education by permitting on demand access, control and learning analytics [5].

Regarding the Bachelor of Dental Surgery (BDS) curriculum of BPKIHS, interpretation of intraoral and panoramic radiographs is an integral part of Oral Medicine and Radiology. Also, interpreting skill of radiographs is one of the essential competency of undergraduate program. With availability of digital images and online surfing, oral and maxillofacial radiology has been particularly explored in the aspect of e-learning and blended learning. Also these images can be used conveniently for testing the students' capabilities to interpretation and radiographic diagnosis of anatomical features or disease conditions [5]. Objective Structured Clinical Examination (OSCE) can be utilized for this purpose as it objectively tests the clinical and practical knowledge and skills acquired during the medical curriculum.

Taking all these in consideration, the aim and objective of this study was to find out the feasibility and effectiveness of virtual learning/ e-learning in the period of crisis along with minimizing the more possible spread of the pandemic in the community level. Also with this study the probability of using e-learning as the alternative to traditional learning can also be sought out for future approach.

2 MATERIALS AND METHODS

An experimental study was conducted from March 2021 to August 2021 among the BDS fourth year students of BPKIHS after obtaining ethical clearance from Institutional Review Committee (IRC), BPKIHS (ref. number: 546/077/078-IRC). The informed written consent was obtained and the students were randomly allocated into two groups, Group 'A' and Group 'B' via fish bowl technique. Students unwilling to participate or not giving consent and not attending either pre-test or post-test were excluded from the study.

The students were taught 4 topics sequentially: a) Systematic way of interpretation of radiograph and anatomic landmarks in OPG b) Interpretation of pulpal, periapical and periodontal conditions/diseases c) Interpretation of cyst and tumors of jaws and d) Interpretation of fibrous-osseous lesions, bony lesions of jaws and fracture.

2.1 *Group 'A': Conventional teaching learning method*

Students allocated in this arm were taught as per the Oral Medicine and Radiology (OMR) portion of BDS curriculum twice weekly for two consecutive weeks via lecture method of teaching learning in lecture hall with all safety precautions.

2.2 *Group 'B': E-learning*

Students allocated in this arm were taught via e-learning method. Online classes were taken via Zoom platform twice a week for two consecutive weeks by the same faculties on the same day. Attendance was taken at end of each class and study resources related to the topic were shared.

Pre-test consisting of 30 MCQs and 2 OSCE (featuring 2 panoramic images) was taken prior to starting the course using Google form with form limiter setting duration of 1 hour and post-test was taken physically 10 days after the end of the course. All questions were compulsory to respond/attempt and there was no negative marking.

The feasibility of the e-learning was assessed in arm 'B' at the end of the final online session with the help of a validated **Watkins and Trainer Questionnaire 2004** [6].

Statistical Package for Social Sciences (SPSS) version 11.5 was used for the analysis of the data.

3 RESULT

Total number of 41 BDS students of VIIth semester were enrolled in this study. 20 of them were allocated in group A (conventional teaching learning) and remaining 21 in group B (e-learning). Out of them, one from group B was excluded who missed the post-test whereas three were excluded from group A (1 missed pre-test and 2 missed post-test).

3.1 *Test response*

Pre-test and post-test: Mean pre-test and post-test score was 21.41 ± 2.98, 32.00 ± 4.73 in group A and 20.45 ± 3.14, 30.93 ± 6.54 in group B. Comparing the mean using Independent 't' test, score in both group was not statistically significant.

Table 1. Comparison of pre and post test score of Group A and B.

	Group A		Group B		
	Mean	SD	Mean	SD	p value*
Pre-test	**21.41**	**2.98**	**20.45**	**3.14**	**0.348**
Post-test	**32.00**	**4.73**	**30.93**	**6.54**	**0.577**

* Independent 't' test, p <0.05: statistically significant

Improvement in the test score: The difference in mean post-test score from the mean pre-test score in each group was statistically significant **(p=0.001)**. However, while comparing the mean improvement in test score in group A and group B, the difference between the groups was not statistically significant. **(p=0.92).**

Reporting skill: Mean post-test score in interpreting the panoramic imaging was 9.28 ± 2.41 while it was 6.65 ± 1.62 in pre-test and mean difference was statistically significant. **(p<0.001)**

3.2 *Feasibility of the e-learning*

The Watkins and Trainer Questionnaire was used for assessing the feasibility. [13] Mean score for each question and domain was calculated considering frequency of response from group B students only in 5-point Likert scale. Although the response was recorded in 5-point Likert scale, it has been brought down to 3-point (Table 2).

Table 2. Assessment of feasibility (Response categorized into 3-Point scale).

DOMAINS	QUESTIONS	Disagree (%)	Not sure (%)	Agree (%)	Mean	SD	Mean ± SD
TECHNOLOGY ACCESS	1. I have access to a computer with an internet connection.	25	10	65	3.65	1.69	3.63 ± 1.52
	2. I have access to a fairly new computer (e.g., enough RAM, speakers, CD-ROM).	15	10	65	3.65	1.50	
	3. I have access to a computer with adequate software (e.g., Microsoft Word, Adobe Acrobat).	25	15	60	3.60	1.60	
ONLINE SKILLS AND RELATIONSHIPS	4. I have the basic skills to operate a computer (e.g. saving files, creating folders).	5	10	85	4.30	1.03	4.11 ± 0.81
	5. I have the basic skills for finding my way around the internet (e.g., using search engines, entering passwords).	10	5	85	4.25	1.12	
	6. I can send an email with a file attached.	5	5	90	4.45	1.00	
	7. I think that I would be comfortable using a computer several times a week to participate in a course.	10	30	60	3.85	1.18	
	8. I think that I would be able to communicate effectively with others using online technologies (e.g., email, chat).	5	20	75	4.05	1.05	
	9. I think that I would be able to express myself clearly through my writing (e.g., mood, emotions, and humor).	15	30	55	3.80	1.15	
	10. I think that I would be able to use online tools (e.g., email, chat) to work on assignments with students who are in different time zones.	5	25	70	4.20	1.01	
	11. I think that I would be able to schedule time to provide timely responses to other students and/or the instructor.	5	20	75	4.10	1.07	
	12. I think that I would be able to ask questions and make comments in clear writing.	10	20	70	4.00	1.17	
MOTIVATION	13. I think that I would be able to remain motivated even though the instructor is not online at all times.	20	40	40	3.15	1.18	3.15 ± 1.14
	14. I think that I would be able to complete my work even when there are online distractions (e.g., friends sending emails or Websites to surf).	35	15	50	3.30	1.26	

(continued)

Table 2. Continued

DOMAINS	QUESTIONS	Disagree (%)	Not sure (%)	Agree (%)	Mean	SD	Mean ± SD
	15. I think that I would be able to complete my work even when there are distractions in my home (e.g., television, children, and such).	40	20	40	3.00	1.45	
ONLINE AUDIO/ VIDEO	16. I think that I would be able to relate the content of short video clips (1-3 minutes typically) to the information I have read online or in books.	10	15	75	3.80	1.01	3.85 ± 0.76
	17. I think that I would be able to take notes while watching a video on the computer.	15	25	60	3.55	1.05	
	18. I think that I would be able to understand course related information when it's presented in video formats.	5	10	85	4.20	0.83	
INTERNET DISCUSSIONS	19. I think that I would be able to carry on a conversation with others using the internet (e.g., internet chat, instant messenger).	15	10	75	3.90	1.29	3.70 ± 0.98
	20. I think that I would be comfortable having several discussions taking place in the same online chat even though I may not be participating in all of them.	25	30	45	3.35	1.18	
	21. I think that I would be able to follow along with an online conversation (e.g., internet chat, instant messenger) while typing.	10	30	60	3.80	1.15	
	22. I sometimes prefer to have more time to prepare responses to a question.	10	15	75	3.75	1.12	
IMPORTANCE TO YOUR SUCCESS	23. Regular contact with the instructor is important to my success in online coursework.	10	25	65	3.70	1.03	3.78 ± 1.07
	24. Quick technical and administrative support is important to my success in online coursework.	15	10	75	3.75	1.21	
	25. Frequent participation throughout the learning process is important to my success in online coursework.	10	10	80	3.90	1.17	
	26. I feel that prior experiences with online technologies (e.g., email, internet chat, online readings) are important to my success with online course.	15	-	85	3.95	1.23	
	27. The ability to immediately apply course materials is important to my success with online courses.	20	10	70	3.60	1.23	

4 DISCUSSION

Educational institutes around the globe had been forced to embrace and adapt online teaching modalities due to the COVID-19 pandemic. Although, e-learning was first introduced in the field of dentistry during 1970s, its use has been up-surged only at the present time of COVID-19. [8] As the radiographic interpretation of various oro-facial condition/disease holds major bulk of BDS curriculum of Oral Medicine and Radiology, VIIth semester students were the best study sample to be included in this study.

This study has shown that e-learning was as effective as the conventional teaching learning. Although, there was non-significant difference in mean pre-test and post-test score between the groups, both pre and post-test score in e-learning group is lower in comparison to conventional teaching learning method. This can be attributed to poor to average internet connection and inconsistent power supply. [7] Moreover, this can also be related to variation in teaching skill of each faculty in two different methodology and individual variation among students in acquiring the knowledge via different media. These assumptions thus opens the path for improvement required in the e-learning method prior to substituting the conventional way.

The studies by Hugenholtz *et al.*, Khatoni *et al.*, Nourian *et al.* has also shown the comparable effectiveness of e-learning to traditional lecture based teaching learning further supporting the outcome of this study [9–11]. Moreover, studies by Moazami *et al.*, Soltainmer *et al.* revealed that virtual learning was more effective in comparison to traditional teaching learning [13,23]. In contrast to this study, students in virtual group scored higher final examination score in these studies.

Unlike this study, studies by Farkhondeh *et al.* 2015, Alpert *et al.* 2016 has shown e-learning to be not as effective as conventional way of teaching learning [14,15].

The reporting skill in this study has been evaluated through interpretation of two OPG images in OSCE section. There was statistically significant improvement in the score signifying that students can gain knowledge and skill irrespective of different teaching methodology considered. Similar findings has also been presented in previous studies [16,23]. Botelho *et al.* supported the previous literature on the benefits of e-learning regarding knowledge and attitude outcome and suggested the need of more focused research of e-learning for in-depth understanding of its benefit [5].

One major strength of this study was that both the theoretical knowledge and reporting skills gained by students were evaluated with regard to radiographic interpretation of bony lesions of the jaw via two educational methods. The weakness was inclusion of only two OPG images. It would have been better had few other IOPAR images along with OPGs been incorporated for the same purpose.

4.1 *Feasibility of the e-learning*

This study has assessed the feasibility of the e-learning based upon the response given by the group B students on a validated questionnaire by Watkins and Trainer [6]. Except for few questions, most of the student's responses on the questions were "agree" inferring that e-learning is feasible.

In a trial by Schneider *et al.* 2016, authors indicated the feasibility of online evidence based practice education on a broad scale but compliance with completion of the online courses and booster lessons was poor. [17] Some other studies doubted on implementation of e-learning in the current scenario [7,18,19].

Correlating with response from the students, they have adequate skills for pursuing online learning indicating the feasibility of the e-learning. However, students felt uncomfortable in using online platform multiple times for participating in the course and communicating effectively among themselves or with teachers. This can be minimized by promoting bi-directional sharing of knowledge during online session or via use of social media whenever feasible. Martin *et al.* 2019 enlisted host of tools and strategies for the online instructor to build meaningful relationships with students and increase satisfaction levels - instructor-created video content, sharing relevant personal experiences, show interest in the lives of students, personalized video feedback, videoconference calls etc [20].

Recent advancements in educational technology have transformed virtual learning, offering innovative ways to enhance students' reporting skills. Interactive platforms like Microsoft Teams and Zoom enable collaborative case-based learning, while simulation tools such as Body Interact and DentSim provide practicality. AI-powered tools like FeedbackFruits and Grammarly deliver personalized feedback, improving documentation accuracy. Collaborative tools such as Padlet and Miro promote peer-assisted learning and critical thinking. Blended learning approach, combining traditional in-person instruction with modern digital tools, has proven highly effective in teaching radiographic interpretation. Hands-on sessions remain essential for direct instructor feedback and skill refinement, while virtual tools like simulators and e-learning platforms offer flexibility and diverse case exposure. This combination fosters critical thinking, peer collaboration, and enhanced diagnostic accuracy.

Overall, the major constraints for implementation of e-learning are infeasible consistency of electricity supply and internet, paying attention, and understanding lessons through the online platform. [21] These can be overcome through managing the uninterrupted source of electricity supply and provision of high speed internet. Also, adding unique and interesting cases in presentation during class might help students in focusing more during the class and motivate for self-directed learning. Moreover, it has been suggested that school/universities should make online courses easily accessible by all students to accommodate learning styles. [22] All these steps would make the e-learning effective and feasible. Also, larger sample size, multi-centric study, longer study duration and modification of the feasibility questionnaire as per the context would add more strength to the study.

5 CONCLUSION

Based upon the findings of this study, it can be concluded that e-learning is as effective as the conventional teaching learning method and is also feasible as conventional teaching learning method in undergraduate program regarding interpretation of IOPAR and panoramic radiographs. And, it can be used as the alternative when conventional method is not feasible. Future research should examine long-term radiographic skill retention, comparing blended learning with traditional methods, and explore the role of AI, VR, and periodic reinforcement in sustaining diagnostic accuracy. However, to be used as substitute to conventional, stronger evidences are required.

REFERENCES

[1] Woolliscroft JO. (2020). Innovation in response to the COVID-19 pandemic crisis. *Acad Med.* 95: 1140–2.

[2] Alsoufi A, Alsuyihili A, Msherghi A, *et al.* (2020). Impact of the COVID-19 pandemic on medical education: Medical students' knowledge, attitudes, and practices regarding electronic learning. *PLoS One*, 15: 1–20.

[3] Ellaway R, Masters K. (2008). AMEE Guide 32: E-Learning in medical education Part 1: Learning, teaching and assessment. *Med Teach* 30: 455–73.

[4] Donnelly P. (2012). *E- learning. What is it? How to succeed at e-learning*. 12th ed: John Wiley & Sons; pp. 5–27.

[5] Botelho MG, Agrawal KR, Bornstein MM. (2019). A systematic review of e-learning outcomes in undergraduate dental radiology curricula—levels of learning and implications for researchers and curriculum planners. *Dentomaxillofacial Radiol* 48: 1–10.

[6] Watkins R, Leigh D, Trainer D. (2004). Assessing readiness for e-learning. *Perform. Improv. Q*. 17: 66–79.

[7] Sarwar H, Akhtar H, Naeem MM, Khan JA, Waraich K, Shabbir S, *et al.* (2020). Self-reported effectiveness of e-Learning Classes during COVID-19 pandemic: A nation-wide survey of pakistani undergraduate dentistry students. *Eur J Dent* 14: S34–S43.

[8] Woelber JP, Hilbert TS, Ratka-Krüger P. (2012). Can easy-to-use software deliver effective e-learning in dental education? A randomised controlled study. *Eur J Dent Educ* 6: 187–92.

[9] Hugenholtz NI, De Croon EM, Smits PB, Van Dijk FJ, Nieuwenhuijsen K. (2008). Effectiveness of e-learning in continuing medical education for occupational physicians. *Occup Med (Lond)*. 58:370–2.

[10] Khatoni A, Nayery ND, Ahmady F, Haghani H. (2011). Comparison the effect of Web-based Education and Traditional Education on Nurses Knowledge about Bird Flu in Continuing Education. *Iran J Med Sci*. 11:140–8

[11] Nourian A, Nourian A, Ebnahmadi A, Akbarzadeh Baghban A, Khoshnevisan MH. (2012). Comparison of E-learning and traditional classroom instruction of dental public health for dental students of shahid beheshti dental school during 2010–2011. *J Dent Sch*. 30:174–83.

[12] Sendra-Portero F, Torales-Chaparro OE, Ruiz-Gómez MJ, Martínez-Morillo M. (2013). A pilot study to evaluate the use of virtual lectures for undergraduate radiology teaching. *Eur J Radiol*. 82:888–93.

[13] Moazami F, Bahrampour E, Azar MR, *et al.* (2014). Comparing two methods of education (virtual versus traditional) on learning of Iranian dental students: A post-test only design study. *BMC Med Educ* 14: 1–5.

[14] Alpert WT, Couch KA, Harmon OR. (2016). A randomized assessment of online learning. *Am Econ Rev* 106: 378–82.

[15] Farkhondeh A, Geist JR. (2015). Evaluation of web-based interactive instruction in intraoral and panoramic radiographic anatomy. *J Mich Dent Assoc*. 97:34–8.

[16] George PP, Papachristou N, Belisario JM, Wang W, Wark PA, Cotic Z, *et al.* (2014). Online eLearning for undergraduates in health professions: a systematic review of the impact on knowledge, skills, attitudes and satisfaction. *J Glob Health*. 4: 010406

[17] Schneider M, Evans R, Haas M, Leach M, Delagran L, Hawk C, *et al.* (2016). The effectiveness and feasibility of an online educational program for improving evidence-based practice literacy: an exploratory randomized study of US chiropractors. *Chiropr Man Ther*. 24:1–11.

[18] Mirzamohammadi MH. (2017). The feasibility of E-Learning Implementation in an Iranian University. *Electron J e-Learning*. 15: 423.

[19] Shama S, Ikbal J. (2020). Education during a pandemic. A feasibility study of online classes in Bangladesh to counteract potential study gaps caused by COVID-19 related lockdowns. *SocArXiv*

[20] Martin J. (2019). Building relationships and increasing engagement in the virtual classroom: Practical tools for the online instructor. *J Educ Online*. 16:n1.

[21] Al-Amin M, Al Zubayer A, Deb B, Hasan M. (2021). Status of tertiary level online class in Bangladesh: students' response on preparedness, participation and classroom activities. *Heliyon*. 7: e05943.

[22] Kaifi BA, Mujtaba BG, Williams AA. (2009). Online college education for computer-savvy students: A study of perceptions and needs. *Journal of College Teaching & Learning (TLC)*. 1: 6

[23] Soltanimehr E, Bahrampour E, Imani MM, *et al.* (2019). Effect of virtual versus traditional education on theoretical knowledge and reporting skills of dental students in radiographic interpretation of bony lesions of the jaw. *BMC Med Educ* 19: 1–7.

 ISBN: 978-1-041-32674-8

Evaluation of Seminars Presented by Undergraduate Dental Students in Oral Medicine and Radiology: An Academic Audit

Abhinaya Luitel
Department of Oral Medicine and Radiology, BP Koirala Institute of Health Sciences, Dharan, Nepal

Harleen Bali
Department of Oral Medicine and Radiology, Kathmandu University School of Medical Sciences, Kavrepalanchowk, Nepal

Kripa Gurung
Saint Mary Dental Health Centre, Kathmandu, Nepal

ABSTRACT: **Purpose:** Educational skills are better accomplished when students direct their own learning. This audit aimed to evaluate and provide feedback to seminar presentations of undergraduate dental students in oral medicine and radiology.

Methods: Academic audits were conducted at the Kathmandu University School of Medical Sciences between August 2021 and June 2022. The seminars of 50 dental students were evaluated, and feedback was provided. The data were entered into an Excel spreadsheet, and descriptive statistics were calculated.

Results: For a given topic, more than 80% of the students were marked good for consulting relevant books and completeness of preparation but had an average understanding of the subject, whereas 50–60% were marked average for consulting other references, clarity of presentation, use of audio™visual aids and ability to answer questions; 76% had good time scheduling.

Conclusions: Overall, the students had average to good presentations. The positive and constructive feedback further helped them improve their seminar preparation and presentation skills.

Keywords: evaluation, medical education, seminar, undergraduate

1 INTRODUCTION

Teaching learning activities in our part is still teacher centered. Learners passively receive information and memorize it. Independent and flexible learning, critical thinking skills and problem solving behavior are the least recognized methods [1].

Small and focused group discussions, short writing exercises, quizzes, field trips, debates, seminar presentation and project-based learning have been widely promoted [2,3]. The aim of active learning methods is to motivate students for high-order thinking tasks such as analysis, synthesis, and evaluation [4,5]. The aim of this academic audit was to evaluate seminars presented by fourth-year dental students in the Department of Oral Medicine and Radiology (OMR).

2 MATERIALS AND METHODS

This academic audit was conducted at the Kathmandu University School of Medical Sciences (KUSMS), Dhulikhel, Nepal, from August 2021 to June 2022. All 50 fourth-year students in Bachelor of Dental Surgery (BDS) were provided with different seminar topics pertaining to OMR and were asked to present them via PowerPoint presentation. A self-designed platform with a five-point Likert scale was used by constant single assessor to evaluate the seminar, and feedback was provided. The data were entered into an Excel spreadsheet, and descriptive statistics were calculated.

3 RESULTS

There were 38 females and 12 males. The mean age of the participants was 24.20 years. For a given topic, 43 (86%) of the students were marked good at consulting relevant books. Thirty (60%) students were marked on average for consultation with other references. With respect to the completeness of preparation, 40 (80%) students were

 DOI: 10.1201/9781042016075-11

considered good. Forty-four (88%) students had average understanding of the subject for the topic provided. For clarity of presentation, 27 (54%) were marked average, and 21 (42%) were marked good. Twenty-eight (56%) students were marked on average for the use of appropriate audio™visual aids. Thirty-eight (76%) students had good time scheduling, whereas 31 (62%) students were marked on average for their ability to answer the questions asked by either the audience or the faculty attending the seminar. The overall results of the evaluation are displayed in Table 1.

Special observations were mentioned in terms of comments in the form of single words or phrases. The positive feedback included "Well presented, well prepared, good seminar, good presentation, informative slides, well organized pictures and videos, interactive seminar." The constructive feedback included "Be loud and more confident, be interactive, face the audience during presentation, know the basics and clinical applications, add/consult more references."

Table 1. Seminar evaluation performance and students' performance on various observations.

S N.	Observation	Poor	Below average, n (%)	Average n (%)	Good n (%)	Very good n (%)	Total N (%)
1	Consultation to relevant books			7 (14%)	43 (86%)		50 (100%)
2	Consultation to other references		7 (14%)	30 (60%)	12 (24%)	1 (2%)	
3	Completeness of preparation			9 (18%)	40 (80%)	1 (2%)	
4	Understanding of the subject			44 (88%)	6 (12%)		
5	Clarity of presentation			27 (54%)	21 (42%)	2 (4%)	
6	Use of appropriate audio-visual aids		6 (12%)	28 (56%)	16 (32%)		
7	Time scheduling			11 (22%)	38 (76%)	1 (2%)	
8	Ability to answer the question		16 (32%)	31 (62%)	3 (6%)		
9	Overall performance			21 (42%)	29 (58%)		
10	Other special observation if any	Variable comment was provided based on individual presentation.					

4 DISCUSSION

Multiple methods of summative and formative assessment have been identified, developed and implemented over time, with a focus on clinical, communication and procedural skills and professionalism. Assessment directs brilliance and leads to the process of precise learning.[1] While preparing seminar, students actively search/research a topic and prepare the presentation. In this process, a student thoroughly gains knowledge about the topic in depth [6]. They also acquire skills such as literature search, relevant book consultation, searching for authentic videos and pictures to maintain presentation, preparing PowerPoint presentation, making the presentation interactive, etc., which helps them learn in an calm and contented way [6,7].

Most of our students were good at consulting relevant books, as the topics provided to them were from common textbooks used for undergraduates in OMR. However, consultation with other references was average. This could be because undergraduate students are not much acquainted with other forms of literature search via search engines. Additionally, they are not proficient in differentiating between the authentic and unauthentic information displayed on the internet [8]. It also shows that we, as faculty, should help them find scientific literature via different search engines.

Most of the students were marked good for completeness of preparation, as they were guided by the faculty before the presentation. Most of the students were marked average for understanding of the subject/their topic of presentation. It was realized that their concepts regarding their topic of presentation and basic and clinical knowledge were not marked. Not being able to defend whatever they presented also reflected the same [8]. Most of them had average to good clarity of presentation. This could be because they had done such presentations previously in other subjects and other fields as well. The use of audio-visual aids was the average for the majority of the students. Most of them were smart enough to include pictures, videos, animations, etc., through reliable sources in their presentation. The time schedule was good among the maximum number of students. They were able to complete their presentation in allotted time, i.e., 45 minutes, and were able to enter into the discussion session. The topics provided to them were short, and they might have practiced before the presentation. The ability to answer the questions during the discussion session was average among the majority of the students. This could be because they thoroughly go through and try to gain in-depth knowledge about their topic of presentation. However, some students lacked the basic and clinical correlation/application of the topic. The overall seminar performance was average to good. Different positive and constructive feedback was also provided, which helped students modify and improvise their further presentation making and presenting skills.[9] However, incorporating students' self-feedback and peer feedback would have added further to the strength of this audit.

Presence of single assessor from within the department and non-blinding of the identity of students might have led to bias during evaluation. These were few limitations of the study which needs to be addressed in future.

5 CONCLUSION

The seminar evaluation of fourth-year BDS students at OMR revealed an overall average-to-good presentation. The positive and constructive feedback provided helped them further improve their seminar preparation and presentation skills.

CONFLICT OF INTEREST:

The authors declare that they have no competing interests.

AKNOWELEDGEMENT

We would like to thank all fourth-year BDS students for their active participation.

REFERENCES

[1] Patel JR, Patel DS, Desai R, Parmar J, Thaker R, Patel ND. (2015). Evaluation of student seminar in medical education: Students' perspective. *Int J Cur Res Rev*. 7(7):6–9. [Full Text]

[2] Sharma D, Gupta R. (2016). Evaluation of usefulness of seminar as a learning tool at medical undergraduate level. *Int J Basic Clin Pharmacol*. 5(5):2143–5. [Full Text | DOI]

[3] Schreiber BE, Fukuta J, Gordon F. (2010). Live lecture versus video podcast in undergraduate medical education: a randomized controlled trial. *BMC Med Educ*. 10:68. [PubMed | Full Text | DOI]

[4] Jain A, Bansal R, Singh K, Kumar A. (2014). Attitude of medical and dental first year students toward teaching methods in a medical college of Northern India. *J Clin Diagn Res*. 8(12):XC05–XC08. [PubMed | Full Text | DOI]

[5] Bonwell C, Eison. (1991). *Active Learning: Creating Excitement in the Classroom AEHE-ERIC Higher Education report No. 1*. Washington DC: Jossey-Bass. [Full Text]

[6] Sabbani P, Sunanda V, Sujatha P. (2020). Effect of students' seminar on learning in 1st year MBBS students. *J. Evid. Based Med. Healthc*. 7(15):787–90. [Full Text]

[7] Panda SP, Bharathi DV, Babu RS, Rao KB. (2016). Perception of 2nd Year MBBS Students Toward Student-Led Seminar as Small Group Teaching Page Method. *Int J Cur Res Rev*. 8(1):6–8. [Full Text]

[8] Spruijt A, Jaarsma ADC, Wolfhagen HAP, Beukelen PV, Scherpbier AJJA. (2012). Students' perceptions of aspects affecting seminar learning. *Med Teach*. 34(2):e129–e35. [PubMed | Full Text | DOI]

[9] Leung SF, Mok E, Wong D. (2008). The impact of assessment methods on the learning of nursing students. *Nurse Educ Today*. 28 (6):711–9. [PubMed | Full Text | DOI]

Navigating Dental Education Trends and Transforming Dental Pedagogy – Abas and Srikant N (Eds)
© 2027 The Author(s), ISBN: 978-1-041-32674-8

Evaluating a Comprehensive Dental Curriculum for the 21st Century: Integrating Technology and Practical Skills: A Qualitative Study

Vaishnavi Jalaj
Manipal College of Dental Sciences Mangalore, Manipal Academy of Higher Education, Manipal, India

Vignesh Kamath
Department of Prosthodontics and Crown and Bridge, Manipal College of Dental Sciences Mangalore, Manipal Academy of Higher Education, Manipal, India

ABSTRACT: This study evaluates the effectiveness and feasibility of incorporating four technological advancements—CAD/CAM, surgical microscopes, intraoral scanners, and 3D printers—into the dental curriculum to improve student learning and clinical proficiency. A qualitative study was conducted with 30 participants, including 20 dental students and 10 educators, from various dental institutions. Structured interviews gathered their perspectives on the advantages, disadvantages, and suitability of these technologies for the undergraduate curriculum. The results revealed strong support for CAD/CAM (100%) and intraoral scanners (96.7%) in the curriculum, with most recommending their inclusion during the 4th year or internships. While awareness of 3D printers was high (86.7%), most participants (96.4%) believed they were unnecessary for the curriculum. Surgical microscopes, though widely recognized, received mixed feedback, with only 36.7% considering them useful for undergraduate training. The study concludes that integrating CAD/CAM and intraoral scanners would significantly enhance dental education, while the inclusion of 3D printers and surgical microscopes requires further consideration. These findings emphasize the need for a balanced curriculum that introduces essential technologies at appropriate stages, ensuring students are well-prepared for 21st-century dental practice.

Keywords: Dental Curriculum, CAD/CAM, Intra-oral scanner, 3D printer

1 INTRODUCTION

The 21st century heralds a transformative era in dental education, driven by technological advancements and the imperative for more integrated, practical, and interprofessional training. Digital dental technology is transforming the landscape of dental education and clinical practice. The integration of advanced tools such as 3D printing, intraoral scanning, and dental operative microscopes offers promising opportunities to enhance both the learning experiences of dental students and patient outcomes.

AI's impact on dental curricula is profound, offering innovative tools for diagnosis, treatment planning, and personalized learning experiences [1]. Pottle (2019) discusses how VR's application in medical education enhances learning and retention, suggesting similar benefits for dental training[2]. Integrating advanced dental technologies enhances education, practice, and patient outcomes [3]. Integrating digital dentistry and AI tools transforms teaching and clinical education [4].

McHarg and Kay (2009) emphasize designing curricula that blend theoretical knowledge with extensive practical training, thereby fostering a deeper understanding and retention of clinical concepts[5]. Additionally, Salian et al. (2022) compare traditional teaching methods with live-field teaching, underscoring the superior performance and retention achieved through practical, real-world experiences[6]. Evaluating modern dental curricula emphasizes integrating technology and practical skills effectively [7]. Studies have shown that dental students respond positively to the inclusion of digital tools, appreciating their accuracy, efficiency, and potential to improve clinical outcomes [8,9].

Similarly, 3D printing in dentistry is expanding the horizons of dental practice by enabling the creation of customized prosthetics and surgical guides with unmatched precision [9]. Intraoral scanners have gained popularity among dental students due to their ability to provide high-quality digital impressions, which are more efficient and patient-friendly compared to traditional methods [10]. Another critical advancement is the use of dental operative microscopes, which enhance visibility and accuracy during restorative procedures, improving both diagnostic capabilities and treatment success [11].

2 AIM

This study aims to systematically evaluate the advantages and disadvantages of four technological advancements in dental skill training that can improve dental learning in India which will ensure graduates are well prepared for 21st century dental practice.

DOI: 10.1201/9781042016075-12

3 OBJECTIVES

- The objective is to determine the effectiveness, feasibility, advantages, and disadvantages of four technological advancements:
  - Utilization of CAD/CAM
  - Utilization of Surgical Microscopes
  - Intraoral scanner
  - 3D Printer

4 MATERIALS AND METHODS

The study (Qualitative study) was carried out in the Department of Prosthodontics and Crown and Bridge, Manipal College of Dental Sciences, Mangalore, on a total of 30 participants out of which 20 participants were students from various dental colleges around Mangalore and 10 were dental educators, including professors and lecturers. Ethical clearance for the study was obtained Institutional Ethics Committee, Manipal College of Dental Sciences, Mangalore. The aim is to gather their insights on proposed modifications to the dental curriculum. During the structured interviews, participants will be presented with information about four distinct curriculum modifications. This information will include detailed descriptions and photographs that highlight the key aspects of each modification, focusing on teaching modalities, advantages, and disadvantages.

Following the presentation, participants will be asked a series of structured questions to explore their perspectives on each modification. The questions will cover their initial thoughts on the modification, perceived advantages and disadvantages, the potential impact on dental education, and whether they believe the modification should be incorporated into the undergraduate curriculum. Additionally, participants will be asked how prepared they feel to integrate these modifications into their teaching or learning processes.

To facilitate data collection, all interviews will be recorded and transcribed. The responses will be carefully categorized and analysed to identify common themes and patterns.

5 RESULTS

				Count	Column N %
Topics	3D printer	Ability to identify the Image	No	4	13.3%
			Yes	26	86.7%
	CAD/CAM	Ability to identify the Image	No	2	6.7%
			Yes	28	93.3%
	Intraoral scanner	Ability to identify the Image	Yes	30	100.0%
	Surgical microscope	Ability to identify the Image	Yes	30	100.0%
Topics	3D printer	Will it be useful in Undergraduate Curriculum?	not Useful	26	96.3%
			Useful	1	3.7%
	CAD/CAM	Will it be useful in Undergraduate Curriculum?	Useful	30	100.0%
	Intraoral scanner	Will it be useful in Undergraduate Curriculum?	not Useful	1	3.3%
			Useful	29	96.7%
	Surgical microscope	Will it be useful in Undergraduate Curriculum?	not Useful	19	63.3%
			Useful	11	36.7%
Topics	3D printer	Should be incorporated in Curriculum	No	29	96.4%
			Optional	1	3.6%
	CAD/CAM	Should be incorporated in Curriculum	Optional	1	3.6%
			Yes	29	96.4%
	Intraoral scanner	Should be incorporated in Curriculum	No	1	3.3%
			Yes	29	96.7%
	Surgical microscope	Should be incorporated in Curriculum	No	20	66.7%
			Yes	10	33.3%
Topics	3D printer	When should the Item be incorporated in the curriculum	Internship	1	100.0%
	CAD/CAM	When should the Item be incorporated in the curriculum	3rd year	2	7.1%
			4th year	4	14.3%
			Internship	22	78.6%
	Intraoral scanner	When should the Item be incorporated in the curriculum	3rd year	3	10.3%
			4th year	23	79.3%
			Internship	3	10.3%

(continued)

Continued

			Count	Column N %
Surgical microscope	When should the Item be incorporated in the curriculum	3rd year	6	54.5%
		4th year	4	36.4%
		Internship	1	9.1%

Thematic analysis will be used to identify and interpret patterns in the qualitative data. Quantitative data (such as the number of participants supporting each modification) will be summarized using descriptive statistics.

In this study, awareness of various dental technologies and their perceived usefulness in the undergraduate curriculum were evaluated.

3D Printer: 86.7% of participants were aware of 3D printers, but 96.3% believed they were not useful for the undergraduate curriculum, with 96.4% opposing its incorporation. Among those who thought it should be included, 100% recommended it for the internship year.

CAD/CAM: A high awareness level was noted, with 93.3% able to identify CAD/CAM technology. All participants (100%) believed it to be useful, and 96.4% supported its inclusion in the curriculum, with 78.6% suggesting it be introduced during the internship.

Intraoral Scanner: Awareness was also high for intraoral scanners, with 100% recognizing them and 96.7% finding them useful. An equal percentage (96.7%) supported their inclusion in the curriculum, with the majority (79.3%) recommending they be introduced in the 4th year.

Surgical Microscope: All participants (100%) recognized the surgical microscope, but only 36.7% found it useful. A third of participants (33.3%) supported its inclusion in the curriculum, with 54.5% suggesting it be introduced in the 3rd year.

6 DISCUSSION

The evolution of dental education is increasingly driven by technological advancements, necessitating the integration of digital tools and innovative methodologies into curricula. This shift prepares students for modern clinical environments. Chatham et al. (2014) advocate incorporating digital technologies into Bachelor of Dental Surgery (BDS) curricula to align education with contemporary standards[8]. Similarly, Turkyilmaz and Wilkins (2021) emphasize 3D printing's potential to revolutionize dentistry with customized, accurate, and cost-effective solutions[9]. Lam et al. (2021) highlight students' preference for intraoral scanners over traditional impression techniques due to their accuracy and ease of use[4], while Bud et al. (2021) underscores the role of surgical microscopes in enhancing visibility and precision during restorative procedures[7].

The integration of tools like surgical microscopes, intraoral scanners, 3D printers, and CAD/CAM systems is reshaping dental practice. Surgical microscopes improve precision and ergonomics, essential in minimally invasive dentistry, despite high costs and the need for specialized training[7]. Intraoral scanners, replacing traditional impression methods, enhance accuracy, patient comfort, and workflow efficiency[4]. 3D printers enable rapid, precise customization of restorations and surgical guides, though costs and perceived non-essentiality hinder widespread undergraduate adoption[9]. CAD/CAM systems streamline prosthetic design, reducing material waste and chair time[8]. Collectively, these technologies ensure graduates are equipped to deliver advanced, patient-centered care, meeting the demands of modern dentistry.

7 CONCLUSION

This study highlights undergraduate students' awareness and perceived usefulness of various dental technologies and their preferences for curriculum integration. CAD/CAM technologies and intraoral scanners were strongly endorsed, with support for their inclusion in the 4th year or during internships, reflecting their practical benefits. In contrast, 3D printers and surgical microscopes received mixed reviews. Despite high recognition, 3D printers were deemed less useful and preferred for internships rather than formal inclusion, while surgical microscopes, though acknowledged, were considered less essential and suggested for the 3rd year. These findings emphasize the need for a balanced curriculum that integrates key technologies without overloading students, aligning with contemporary clinical demands.

ABBREVIATIONS

(1) CAD/CAM -Computer-Aided Design and Computer-Aided Manufacturing
(2) AI- Artificial Intelligence
(3) VR- Virtual Reality

REFERENCES

[1] Thurzo, A.; Strunga, M.; Urban, R.; Surovková, J.; Afrashtehfar, K.I. Impact of Artificial Intelligence on Dental Education: A Review and Guide for Curriculum Update. *Educ. Sci.* 2023, 13, 150. https://doi.org/10.3390/ educsci13020150.

[2] Pottle J. Virtual reality and the transformation of medical education. *Future Healthc J.* 2019 Oct;6(3):181–185. doi: 10.7861/fhj. 2019-0036. PMID: 31660522; PMCID: PMC6798020.

[3] Priyaa NP, Jeevanandan G, Govindaraju L. Practice management in undergraduate dental program: The need among dental students. *J Adv Pharm Technol Res* 2022;13: S594–8.

[4] Kim CS, Samaniego CS, Sousa Melo SL, Brachvogel WA, Baskaran K, Rulli D. Artificial intelligence (A.I.) in dental curricula: Ethics and responsible integration. J Dent Educ. 2023 Nov;87(11):1570-1573. doi: 10.1002/jdd.13337. Epub 2023 Jul 25. PMID: 37489621.

[5] McHarg J, Kay EJ. Designing a dental curriculum for the twenty-first century. Br Dent J. 2009 Nov 28;207(10):493-7. doi: 10.1038/ sj.bdj.2009.1011. PMID: 19942894.

[6] Salian A, Sanal Kumar S, Natarajan S, Lewis AJ, Manaktala N, Naik DG, Boaz K, Kp N, Yellapurkar S. Performance of Dental Students in Understanding and Retention of Oral Pathology Concepts: A Comparative Analysis of Traditional versus Live-Field Teaching Methods. ScientificWorldJournal. 2022 Jul 4; 2022:3257377. doi: 10.1155/2022/3257377. PMID: 35833055; PMCID: PMC9273418.

[7] Abasseri, T., Ha, W. Value of including loupes in prosthodontic and endodontic components of dental degrees: a systematic review. *Br Dent J* (2023).

[8] Chatham, C., Spencer, M.H., Wood, D.J., and Johnson, A. (2014). The introduction of digital dental technology into BDS curricula. *British dental journal*, *217*(11), 639–642.

[9] Turkyilmaz I, Wilkins GN. 3D printing in dentistry - Exploring the new horizons. J Dent Sci. 2021 Jul;16(3):1037-1038. doi: 10.1016/j.jds.2021.04.004. Epub 2021 Apr 20. PMID: 34141126; PMCID: PMC8189864.

[10] Lam, W.Y., Mak, K.C., Maghami, E., and Molinero-Mourelle, P. (2021). Dental students' preference and perception on intraoral scanning and impression making. *BMC medical education*, *21*(1), 501.

[11] Bud M, Jitaru S, Lucaciu O, Korkut B, Dumitrascu-Timis L, Ionescu C, Cimpean S, Delean A. The advantages of the dental operative microscope in restorative dentistry. Med Pharm Rep. 2021 Jan;94(1):22-27. doi: 10.15386/mpr-1662. Epub 2021 Jan 29. PMID: 33629044; PMCID: PMC7880065.

Impact of Anxiety and Depression on Saliva Composition and Oral Health During Summative Assessment: A Comparative Study

Shaila Mulki and Ashika Dechamma
Department of Oral Pathology and Microbiology, KVG Dental College and Hospital, Kurunjibag Sullia

Anitte Shah Mannaparambil
Public Health Officer (Health Protection). Birmingham City Council, United kingdom

Audrey Madonna Decruz
Department of Public Health dentistry, A B Shetty memorial Institutte of Dental Sciences, Deralkatte, mangaluru

Urvashi
Department of Oral Pathology and Microbiology, A B Shetty memorial Institutte of Dental Sciences, Deralkatte, Mangaluru

Jaseela Praveena
Department of Public Health dentistry, KVG Dental College and Hospital, Kurunjibag, Sullia

ABSTRACT: This study aimed to assess the relationship between anxiety and depression levels, as measured by the Hospital Anxiety and Depression Scale (HADS), and the occurrence of oral mucosal changes in students during summative assessments. Changes in salivary pH and flow rate before and after examinations as a response to exam-induced stress were assessed.

Forty consenting healthy dental students, aged 17 to 25, were enrolled in the study. Anxiety and depression levels were assessed using the HADS questionnaire before the students' final summative assessment. Saliva samples were collected from participants at two time points—Pre and postassessment. Salivary pH was measured using a pH meter, and flow rate was determined by timing the collection of 5 ml of saliva. Descriptive statistics, repeated measures ANOVA and Spearman's correlation test were performed using SPSS software. HADS survey revealed that 30 participants had abnormal anxiety levels, 8 were borderline, and 1 had normal levels. For depression, 21 participants had abnormal scores, 14 were borderline, and 4 had normal scores. Repeated measures ANOVA showed no statistically significant difference between the parameters. Correlation was observed between participants with anxiety and depression group and also between preassessment salivary pH and anxiety. These findings necessitate formulation of policies which are directed towards planning and implementation of specialized interventions during the training period of students with integrated coping mechanism.

Keywords: Oral mucosal changes, anxiety, depression, assessment, salivary changes

1 INTRODUCTION

Students experience high stress during assessment for various reasons, such as a lack of preparation, methods of their studies and lifestyle habits. When stress is perceived negatively or becomes excessive, it can lead to anxiety, which ultimately affects academic achievement. Although every physical disease has a psychological effect, how one copes with it varies from person to person. Moreover, women are more likely than men to experience stress, which affects their performance [1]. Professional studies impart great stress among students. More than half of the students pursuing medicine and dentistry reported being stressed [2] The stress level among dental students is considerably higher in third- and final-year undergraduates. [3].

Stress, anxiety, and depression can lead to parafunctional habits in the oral cavity and result in the occurrence and intensity of symptoms in conditions such as RAS (recurrent aphthous stomatitis).[4,5],When stress, anxiety and depression are not perceived well, somatic diseases surface [6]. Acute psychological stress influences both salivary composition and salivary function [7]. The prevalence of aphthous ulcers among professional students is high, and its association with stress as a precipitating factor is well documented [8]. In addition, immunomodulation as a consequence of stress results in a longer time for wounds to heal [9].

The cognitive and psychomotor skills are compromised in students who experience unusual anxiety. Challenge their psychological health imparts general health issues, which may lead to substance abuse and a lack of academic pursuit and passion [10]. Needless to say, assessments pose significant stress to students. It is important to emphasize and evaluate stress, anxiety, depression and physical changes in professional students during assessment so that planning and formulating interventions to manage stress among students can be helpful.

DOI: 10.1201/9781042016075-13

Thus, the present study aimed to evaluate anxiety and depression via the HADS questionnaire during the summative assessment and to analyze its impact on saliva composition before and after the Summative Assessment.

2 MATERIALS AND METHODS

Forty healthy undergraduate dental students aged between 20 and 25 years who appeared for summative assessment at KVG Dental College and Hospital, Sullia were included.

A systematic random sampling method was used to select forty healthy undergraduate dental students aged between 20 and 25 years who presented for a fourth-year summative assessment at KVG Dental College and Hospital, Sullia.

After ethical approval from the Institutional Ethical Committee and informed consent from all the participants of the study were obtained, they participated in the study.

Subjects who complained of dry mouth, those with the habit of tobacco abuse, those with systemic or psychological diseases and those on long-term medication were excluded from the study.

All the participants were administered the Hospital Anxiety and Depression Scale (HADS) to assess anxiety and depression levels on the day of the summative assessment. The HADS has 14 questions divided into two subscales of seven questions each. Each item is rated on a 4-point scale ranging from 0–3, with a maximum score of 21 for anxiety and depression. Scores of 11 or more on either subscale are considered abnormal, whereas scores of 8–10 indicate borderline and scores of 0–7 indicate normal [11].

Furthermore, each participant was subjected to the following procedures one day before and two weeks after the examination.

(1) A complete oral examination was performed to record oral mucosal changes.
(2) Following an oral examination, whole unstimulated saliva was collected via the spitting method. Approximately 5 ml of saliva was collected, and the flow rate was calculated as the volume collected divided by the time required for collection.
(3) A digital pH meter was used to record the pH of the saliva. Salivary pH in unstimulated saliva was measured directly via a pH meter calibrated with buffers with pH values of 4·01 and 7·01.

3 RESULTS

Thirty-nine female participants were included in the study, as one participant was unable to appear for the assessment. Among the 39 participants who responded to the HADS questionnaire survey for anxiety and depression, 30 had abnormal levels of anxiety; the anxiety scores were borderline for 8 participants, and 1 presented with a normal level of anxiety. Moreover, for depression, 21, 14, and 4 participants presented with abnormal,

Table 1. Correlations between salivary parameters and anxiety and depression among the participants were determined via the Spearman correlation test.

				Depression	Pre-Salivary flow rate	Post Salivary flow rate	Pre- salivary pH	Post Salivary pH
Spearman's rho	Anxiety	Correlation Coefficient		.618**	−.128	.048	.364*	−.192
		Sig. (2-tailed)		.000	.436	.771	.023	.243
	Depression	Correlation Coefficient	.618**		−.006	.088	.296	−.308
		Sig. (2-tailed)	.000		.971	.595	.068	.056
	Pre-Salivary flow rate	Correlation Coefficient	−.128	−.006		.639**	−.187	.158
		Sig. (2-tailed)	.436	.971		.000	.254	.338
	Post Salivary flow rate	Correlation Coefficient	.048	.088	.639**		−.143	−.007
		Sig. (2-tailed)	.771	.595	.000		.386	.966
	Pre- salivary pH	Correlation Coefficient	.364*	.296	−.187	−.143		−.087
		Sig. (2-tailed)	.023	.068	.254	.386		.599
	Post Salivary pH	Correlation Coefficient	−.192	−.308	.158	−.007	−.087	
		Sig. (2-tailed)	.243	.056	.338	.966	.599	

**. Correlation is significant at the 0.01 level (2-tailed).
*. Correlation is significant at the 0.05 level (2-tailed).

borderline and normal depression scores, respectively. The data were examined via SPSS, version 21.0. Repeated-measures ANOVA revealed no statistically significant differences between the parameters. Spearman correlation was used (Table 1). Five participants presented with recurrent aphthous stomatitis (RAS) during the preassessment oral examination, which resolved after the assessment.

4 DISCUSSION

Stress is a phenomenon in which every person responds differently. Inter- and intrapersonal, intellectual, and environmental factors usually influence the response to stress [12]. It is during adolescence and early adulthood that anxiety and depressive disorders peak [13].

Anxiety is characterized by persistent intrusive thoughts and concerns that result in perpetual worry and tension. Anxiety has been described as having a disproportionate amount of worry and fear relative to everyday situations, which leads to adverse thoughts and predictions about future events [14].

Depression is a mood disorder that causes a state of sadness or unhappiness, which may continue to such a degree and, for such a length of time, far outweighs the importance of the precipitating factor. This results in a loss of interest in activities which were previously enjoyed [15].

Situation-specific anxiety usually results when students take assessments during professional courses, as the grades they achieve ensure better outcomes in life. The relationship between personality traits and exam-related anxiety in medical students was associated with increased anxiety levels prior to the exam [16]. The assessment of the level of anxiety in chiropractic students and the relationship between test anxiety and academic performance showed that test anxiety, particularly the worry and emotionality components, has an adverse effect on test performance, other parameters, such as performance mediators, may influence performance [17]. Somatization significantly increases across a wide range of symptoms under exam stress. The symptom indices and stress, depression and anxiety scores significantly increased during the exam period when compared with both the before and after baseline values [18].

The findings of the present study are in line with these findings. A significant correlation was observed between anxiety and depression, as expected. Five participants presented with recurrent aphthous stomatitis before the assessment, all of whom healed after the assessment. All the five participants had abnormal anxiety scores, while depression score was abnormal for two participants and borderline for one participant.

Previous studies that evaluated the effects of stress, anxiety and depression in RAS patients concluded that psychological stress is a triggering factor [19]. Focal immune dysfunction involving T-cell-mediated immunity is a key mechanism in the development of the RAS. Stress alters immune function, which could be the probable reason for the occurrence of apthous ulcers during the assessment [20]. Some studies also revealed that wound healing is significantly affected by stress, which might be the reason why these ulcers take time to resolve [21].

Salivary gland function is largely under autonomic control, and the autonomic receptor types that respond to neurotransmitters and other autonomic messenger substances result in protein release that is capable of being differentially regulated among glands [22]. The present study revealed decreased salivary flow before assessment, which increased after assessment; however, this difference was not statistically significant. The salivary flow rate is dependent on the nerve-mediated reflex by the salivary gland, which is influenced by nerve signals from other centers in the central nervous system, which in turn causes hypo salivation during anxiety. Additionally, decreased salivation can be related to increased cortisol levels in saliva after short periods of stress, as evidenced in several studies [23].

Researchers who analyzed dynamic changes in saliva after acute mental stress showed that there was an increase in salivary pH. This is attributed to the bicarbonate in the saliva [24]. Stress induces parafunctional activities, including cheek biting and the chattering of teeth, increases the bicarbonate ion concentration and may be cited as the reason for increased salivary pH during the pre-assessment phase. Postassessment, when stress levels decrease, it results in the resolution of parafunctional activities and decreased bicarbonate ion composition. Thus in the absence of anxiety, salivary pH returns to normal value.

Student performance is a reflection of the cognitive and psychomotor skills acquired throughout a course. Abnormal levels of stress and anxiety during assessment can negatively impact the performance of dental students. Some of the factors reported to cause anxiety were excessive course load, number of attempts, studying all night preassessment and fear of failure [25].

Students with anxiety respond negatively to both academic and treatment-related exercises, resulting in errors in treatment, namely, extraction of the wrong tooth, failure to follow infection control, failure in examination, etc. Students lack confidence and have self-perceived constraints to achieve competency. Increased academic pressure related to professional dental courses and the need to acquire all the skills pertaining to the dental curriculum through quotas have been reported as some of the reasons for this pressure [10,26].

The achievement of cognitive and psychomotor competencies as prescribed by regulatory bodies is mandatory and necessary for achieving outcomes that positively impact the life of health professionals after graduation. Health professionals must realize the responsibilities they need to harbor to serve society with the best of their knowledge and skills. Anxiety levels, which are optimal, are not deterrents to achieve the desired academic success, and they do not impart any deficiencies in physical or mental health [26]. Interventions are needed only when the stress levels reach abnormal levels. Preparatory workshops aimed at decreasing stress levels before dental students take exams have resulted in positive outcomes, as reflected by their improved academic performance [27].

Early intervention and management of stress among students will aid in preventing future adversities such as self-harm and substance abuse.

The present study is the first to analyze the impact of anxiety and depression measured with the HADS during a summative assessment to assess oral mucosal and salivary changes both before and after the assessment. However, the study does not consider socioeconomic factors, and further studies should be planned by including all the parameters that may influence the HADS score.

5 CONCLUSION

The present study evaluated anxiety and depression during a summative assessment in students via the HADS and assessed oral mucosal and salivary changes before and after the summative assessment among final-year dental students. Five participants presented with RAS before the assessment. A correlation was observed between anxiety and depression and between anxiety and preassessment salivary pH. Students who respond to competencies with abnormal levels of anxiety and depression need to be identified and addressed. Policies that are directed toward planning and implementing specialized interventions during the training period of students with integrated coping mechanisms seem to be appropriate initiatives toward the management of stress in students, which in turn will impact the student and, indirectly, the society at large.

REFERENCES

[1] Wadikar SS, Muley PA, Muley PP. (2017). A comparative study of gender difference in reaction time in response to exam stress among first-year medical students. *Natl J Physiol Pharm Pharmacol* 7(2):209–213.

[2] Cohen M, Meir T, Klein E, *et al.* (2011). Cytokine levels as potential biomarkers for predicting the development of posttraumatic stress symptoms in casualties of accidents. *Int J Psychiatry Med.* 42(2):117–131.

[3] Mary AV, Kesavan R, Ranjani D, Alee N, Boopathy S, Lakshme K, *et al.* (2023). Assessment of stress among dental students: A descriptive crosssectional study. *International Journal of Applied Dental Sciences* 9(4):272–276.

[4] Albanidou-Farmaki E, Poulopoulos AK, Epivatianos A, Farmakis K, Karamouzis M, Antoniades D. (2008). Increased anxiety level and high salivary and serum cortisol concentrations in patients with recurrent aphthous stomatitis. *Tohoku J Exp Med* 214:291–6.

[5] Gavic L, Cigic L, Biocina Lukenda D, Gruden V, Gruden Pokupec JS. (2014). The role of anxiety, depression, and psychological stress on the clinical status of recurrent aphthous stomatitis and oral lichen planus. *J Oral Pathol Med* 43:410–7.

[6] Kumar NN, Panchaksharappa MG, Annigeri RG. (2016). Psychosomatic disorders: An overview for oral physician. *J Indian Acad Oral Med Radiol* 28:24–9.

[7] Bosch, Jos A. MSc; Brand, Henk S. PhD; Ligtenberg, Toon J.M. PhD; Bermond, Bob PhD; Hoogstraten, Johan PhD; Amerongen, Arie V. Nieuw PhD. (1996). Psychological stress as a determinant of protein levels and salivary-induced aggregation of streptococcus gordonii in human whole saliva. *Psychosomatic Medicine* 58(4):374–82.

[8] Shiny George, Biju Baby Joseph. (2016). A study onaphthous ulcer and its association with stress among medical students of an Indian medical institution. *International Journal of Contemporary Medical Research* 3(6):1692–1695.

[9] Marucha, Phillip T. DMD, Kiecolt-Glaser, Janice K., Favagehi, Mehrdad DDS. (1998). Mucosal wound healing is impaired by examination stress. *Psychosomatic Medicine* 60 (3): 362–5.

[10] Lakshmi BA, Fammina CJ, Ganesh R. (2016). Clinical anxiety provoking situations among dental students in Chennai. *Indian J Oral Health Res* 2: 77–81.

[11] Snaith RP. (2003). The hospital anxiety and depression scale. *Health Qual Life Outcomes.* 1;1:29.

[12] Raghupathy, Balasubramanian S, Subramaniam G *et al.* (2023). Evaluation of salivary pH and flow rate among exam going students of Karpaga Vinayaga Institute of Dental Sciences. *Eur J Clin Exp Med.* 21(3):534–538. doi: 10.15584/ejcem.2023.3.19.

[13] Altemus M, Sarvaiya N, Neill Epperson C. (2014). Sex differences in anxiety and depression clinical perspectives. *Front Neuroendocrinol.* 35(3):320–30.

[14] Perrotta, G. (2019). Anxiety disorders: definitions, contexts, neural correlates and strategic therapy. 6(1), 15.

[15] World health organization; [Last accessed on 2024 Aug 9]. Depression. Mental health and substanceabuse.Availablefrom: http://www.searo.who.int/en/Section1174/Section1199/Section1567/Section1826.htm. [Google Scholar]

[16] Pahwa B, Goyal S, Srivastava K, Saldanha D, Bhattacharya D. (2008). A study of exam related anxiety amongst medical students. *Ind Psychiatry J.* 17:46–8.

[17] Niu Zhang and Charles N.R. Henderson (2014) Test anxiety and academic performance in chiropractic students. *Journal of Chiropractic Education: Spring* Vol. 28, No. 1, pp. 2–8.

[18] Zunhammer M, Eberle H, Eichhammer P, Busch V (2013) Somatic symptoms evoked by exam stress in university students: The role of alexithymia, neuroticism, anxiety and depression. *PLoS ONE* 8(12): e84911.

[19] Dhopte A, Naidu G, Singh-Makkad R, Nagi R, Bagde H, Jain S. (2018). Psychometric analysis of stress, anxiety and depression in patients with recurrent aphthous Stomatitis-A cross-sectional survey based study. *J Clin Exp Dent.* 10(11):e1109–14.

[20] Gallo Camila de Barros, Mimura Maria Angela Martins, Sugaya Norberto Nobuo. (2009). Psychological stress and recurrent aphthous stomatitis. *Clinics [Internet]*. 64(7): 645–648.

[21] Graykowski EA, Barile MF, Lee WB, Stanley HR. (1966). Recurrent Aphthous Stomatitis: Clinical, Therapeutic, Histopathologic, and Hypersensitivity Aspects. *JAMA*. 196(7):637–644.

[22] Jos A. Boschab, Christopher, RingEco J.C.de GeusEnno C.I., VeermanArie V.Nieuw Amerongen. (2002). Stress and secretory immunity. *International Review of Neurobiology* 52: 213–253.

[23] Gordan B. (2016). Proctor The physiology of salivary secretion. *Periodontology 2000 A Review Article*, 70(1):11–25.

[24] Naumova EA, Sandulescu T, Bochnig C, Al Khatib P, Lee WK, Zimmer S, Arnold WH. (2014). Dynamic changes in saliva after acute mental stress. *Sci Rep*. 4:4884.

[25] Al-Sahman LA, *et al.* (2019). Major factors causing examination anxiety in undergraduate dental students - a questionnaire based cross-sectional study. *Ann Med Health Sci Res*. 691–694.

[26] Gurung, Deepak; Bhardwaj, Vinay Kumar; Fotedar, Shailee. (2023). Assessment of anxiety in dental practice among dental students of himachal pradesh: A cross-sectional study. *Dentistry and Medical Research*. 11(2):75–79.

[27] Deborah A. Dilbone, Xiaoying Feng, Yu Su, Patricia Xirau-Probert, Linda S. Behar-Horenstein, Marcelle M. Nascimento. Influence of preparatory workshops on dental students' academic performance and stress on their first operative dentistry psychomotor exam. *Journal of Dental Education*; 82(6):608–613.

Navigating Dental Education Trends and Transforming Dental Pedagogy – Abas and Srikant N (Eds)
© 2027 The Author(s), ISBN: 978-1-041-32674-8

Future-Proofing Dental Education: Strategies for Innovation and Excellence in Conservative Dentistry and Endodontics

Annapoorna Shenoy, Janina Loren D'Souza, and M Kundabala
Department of Conservative Dentistry and Endodontics, Manipal College of Dental Science Mangalore, Manipal Academy of Higher Education, Manipal, India

ABSTRACT: The introduction of digital technologies has caused a paradigm shift in the practices of dental practitioners, significantly altering the process of making diagnoses, making treatment plans, and carrying out interventions.The way in which dentists treat patients today has been completely transformed by digital dentistry. This Review describes the application of digital technologies to all facets of dentistry, including diagnosis, planning, and restoration. It includes a variety of technologies, such as 3D printing, artificial intelligence, augmented reality, tele dentistry, and CAD/CAM, which is a rapidly developing and revolutionizing field in conservative dentistry and endodontics. Compared with traditional methods, Patients can now enter and exit the clinic with their entire course of treatment completed in much less time because of the speed and ease of use of digital technology. This article explains the different facets of dental care that have benefited from digital technology. The integration of digital tools into everyday dental practice is not only a futuristic concept but also a current reality that is swiftly becoming the standard of care. With digital dentistry, procedures that previously required multiple visits can now be completed within a single appointment, greatly enhancing the patient experience. Compared with traditional techniques, digital tools allow dental practitioners to offer faster, more predictable, and less invasive treatment options, resulting in improved patient satisfaction.

Keywords: Artificial intelligence, Digital dentistry, Tele dentistry, Virtual reality

1 INTRODUCTION

The introduction of digital technologies has caused a paradigm shift in the practices of dental practitioners, significantly altering the process of making diagnoses, making treatment plans, and carrying out interventions [1]. The way in which dentists treat patients today has been completely transformed by digital dentistry. This Review describes the application of digital technologies to all facets of dentistry, including diagnosis, planning and restoration. It includes a variety of technologies, such as 3D printing, artificial intelligence, augmented reality, tele dentistry, and CAD/CAM, which are rapidly developing and revolutionizing fields in conservative dentistry and endodontics [2]. 3D printing reduces the need for endodontic treatments while increasing clinical efficacy by assisting in the negotiation of calcified canals and periapical surgeries [3]. This article explains the different facets of dental care that have benefited from digital technology [4]. The integration of digital tools into everyday dental practice is not only a futuristic concept but also a current reality that is swiftly becoming the standard of care [5]. With digital dentistry, procedures that previously required multiple visits can now be completed within a single appointment, greatly enhancing the patient experience [6]. Compared with traditional techniques, digital tools allow dental practitioners to offer faster, more predictable, and less invasive treatment options, resulting in improved patient satisfaction.

2 METHODS

2.1 *Search strategy*

Keywords were structured using Boolean operators and Medical Subject Headings (MeSH) terms, such as artificial intelligence, digital dentistry, applications in conservative dentistry and endodontics, and virtual reality in dentistry.

2.2 *Time frame*

Electronic databases like Google Scholar, Medline, PubMed, Embase, Web of Science, and Scopus were searched for the literature published in the recent years, from 2018 to 2024.

 DOI: 10.1201/9781042016075-14

2.3 *Inclusion criteria*

- Peer-reviewed journal publications
- New research methods and findings pertinent to endodontics and conservative dentistry

2.4 *Exclusion criteria*

- Articles with insufficient methodology or no full-text access.
- Articles published in non-indexed journals or outside of the chosen time window.

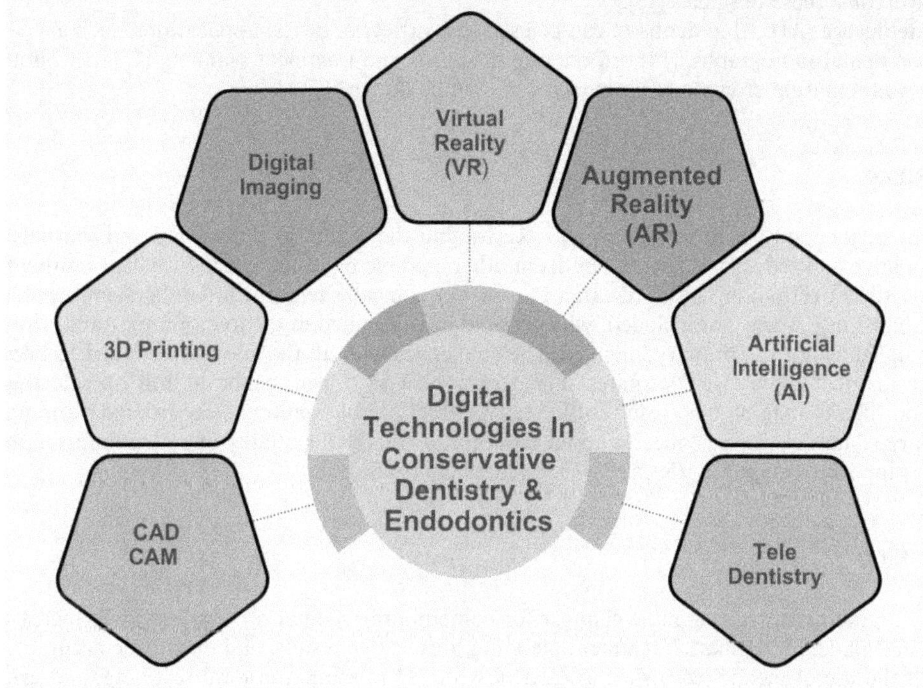

Figure 1. A Venn diagram depicting the digital technologies in conservative dentistry and endodontics.

Applications:

- **Digital Dentistry CAD CAM**
- Dentistry has undergone a transformation owing to computer-aided design and computer-aided manufacturing (CAD/CAM) systems. Traditional impression methods are no longer necessary due to CAD/CAM technology, as intra oral digital scanners are used which also shortens chairside times and improves patient comfort. CAD/CAM guarantees the best possible fit and function by enabling extremely precise and predictable restoration results. The exceptional marginal integrity of such restorations lowers the possibility of bacterial leakage and the problems that may follow. To meet the specific requirements and preferences of each patient, these systems also provide a large variety of material possibilities, including ceramics, composite resins, and metal alloys [7].
- **3D printing**
- The modern educational environment demands innovation, which makes it easier for pupils to learn in an understandable and engaging way. Since they offer educational equality and realistic reproduction of actual teeth, three-dimensional (3D) printing, also known as additive manufacturing, offers an alluring substitute for excised teeth and conventional dental models in the form of 3D-printed teeth [8]. The capacity to produce accurate 3D models of patients' dental anatomy in order to plan and model endodontic procedures, such as root canal therapy or surgery, is one of the keys uses of 3D printing in endodontics [9].
- **Digital Imaging**
- Since digital radiography (DR) produces higher-quality images and allows dentists to perform radiographic exams with reduced radiation exposure, it is becoming increasingly popular as a substitute for conventional radiography (CR). Radiographic diagnosis is critical for root canal therapy. Procedural mistakes, resorptive flaws, and fractures are also found with this approach [10].

- **Virtual reality (VR) & augmented reality (AR)**
- Dental students have historically received training on phantom heads and teeth to hone their clinical abilities prior to treating actual patients. With the help of these simulators, educators may show pupils how to prepare cavities while also working to improve their physical dexterity. Before switching to new treatment methods, students must provide their lecturers with ongoing input regarding their development while using these simulators [11]. These methods are used for cavity design, crown and bridge preparation, canal location, and obturation accuracy [12].
- **Tele dentistry**

Early identification is critical regarding to dental caries, a global public health hazard. Conventional techniques, especially visual inspection, have financial and accessibility issues. To maximize the effectiveness of oral healthcare systems, tele dentistry, an emerging technology, must be given greater attention for evaluation since it has the potential to overcome these obstacles [13].

Artificial intelligence (AI): AI in dentistry can be used in a variety of dental applications, such as the detection of dental caries on dental radiographs, [14] orthodontic diagnosis and treatment planning [15], periodontics [16] and prosthodontics, automating crown margin marking and smile design [17].

3 DISCUSSION

The limitations of the study were the following - Restricting the search to Scopus-indexed journals and specific databases may have omitted significant content from other credible but unindexed journals. Limiting the review to the last decade risks overlooking basic research that is still clinically relevant today. Research published in languages other than English was not included, which would have resulted in the loss of important information from areas where English is not the primary language.The challenges with all the above mentioned technologies which we might face are that high cost , Requires skilled personnel to design, calibrate and operate the equipments Overreliance on digital imaging may result in decreasing ability in interpreting conventional radiographs, AI systems rely on large datasets, raising concerns about the security and confidentiality of patient information and it also requires professionals to adapt for VR ,AR which is time consuming.

4 CONCLUSION

In conclusion, digital dentistry is a game changer for contemporary dental offices, providing increased accuracy, effectiveness, and patient happiness. Treatment planning, restorative results, and diagnostic accuracy have greatly increased with the use of technologies such as CAD/CAM, 3D printing, intraoral scanning, and artificial intelligence. Dental care will undergo even more upheaval in the future with the continuous development of AI-driven diagnostics, robotically aided procedures, and genetically tailored therapies. The integration of digital workflows in clinical and educational settings anticipated to help close the knowledge gap between established practices and cutting-edge technologies. However, challenges remain, including high initial costs, the need for extensive training, and ethical considerations regarding data privacy and AI use. Nonetheless, with ongoing advancements, digital dentistry is poised to play a pivotal role in improving global oral health outcomes.

CONFLICT OF INTEREST

There are no conflicts of interest

FUNDING

No funding

ETHICAL CONSIDERATION

Not- applicable

DATA AVAILABILITY

Data that support the findings of this review are embedded within the manuscript.

REFERENCES

[1] Alshargawi W, Toras F, Almutairi W, Fatiny F, Alhabashi Y, Alyahya F, Felimban A, Alshehri A, Almalki S. The Use of Digital Technologies in Endodontic Diagnosis and Restorative Planning.

[2] Haidar ZS. (2023). Digital dentistry: past, present, and future. *Digital Medicine and Healthcare Technology.* (16).

[3] Alattas MH. (2024). The role of 3D printing in endodontic treatment planning: A comprehensive review. *European Journal of Dentistry.*

[4] Dhawan S, Mandlik J, Gir R, Sinha A, Guru R, Rawal N. (2022). Digitization in conservative dentistry and endodontics: A review. *Journal of Pharmaceutical Negative Results.* 410–4.

[5] Rekow ED. (2020). Digital dentistry: The new state of the art—Is it disruptive or destructive? *Dental Materials.* 36(1):9–24.

[6] Blatz MB, Conejo J. (2019). The current state of chairside digital dentistry and materials. *Dental Clinics.* 63(2):175–97.

[7] Mourouzis P, Tolidis K. (2024). CAD/CAM Systems. In *Digital dentistry: An Overview and Future Prospects.* (pp. 47–66). Cham: Springer International Publishing.

[8] Fayyaz Y, Ali M, Ullah R, Shaikh MS. (2024). Applications of 3D-printed teeth in dental education: A narrative review. *Journal of Taibah University Medical Sciences.*

[9] Oza S, Lai G, Peters OA, Chen J, Karabucak B, Scott R, Galicia JC. (2023). The influence of cone beam computed tomography-derived 3d-printed models on endodontic microsurgical treatment planning and confidence of the operator. *Journal of Endodontics.* 49(5):521–7.

[10] Boreak N, Hakami A, Hakami S, Nahari H, Alhakami M, Al Dira M, Mahdali H, Kariri SF. (2022). A systematic review of traditional radiology: Conservative therapy in endodontics. *Saudi J Oral Dent Res.* 7(12):317–23.

[11] Fahim S, Maqsood A, Das G, Ahmed N, Saquib S, Lal A, Khan AA, Alam MK. (2022). Augmented reality and virtual reality in dentistry: highlights from the current research. *Applied Sciences.* 12(8):3719.

[12] Huang TK, Yang CH, Hsieh YH, Wang JC, Hung CC. (2018). Augmented reality (AR) and virtual reality (VR) applied in dentistry. *The Kaohsiung Journal of Medical Sciences.* 34(4):243–8.

[13] Kargozar S, Jadidfard MP. (2024). Teledentistry accuracy for caries diagnosis: a systematic review of in vivo studies using extraoral photography methods. *BMC Oral Health.* 24(1):828.

[14] Müller A, Mertens SM, Göstemeyer G, Krois J, Schwendicke F. (2021). Barriers and enablers for artificial intelligence in dental diagnostics: A qualitative study. *Journal of Clinical Medicine.* 10(8):1612.

[15] Mohammad-Rahimi H, Nadimi M, Rohban MH, Shamsoddin E, Lee VY, Motamedian SR. (2021). Machine learning and orthodontics, current trends and the future opportunities: A scoping review. *American Journal of Orthodontics and Dentofacial Orthopedics.* 160(2):170–92.

[16] Pitchika V, Büttner M, Schwendicke F. (2024). Artificial intelligence and personalized diagnostics in periodontology: A narrative review. *Periodontology* 2000.

[17] Kong HJ, Kim YL. (2024). Application of artificial intelligence in dental crown prosthesis: A scoping review. *BMC Oral Health.* 24(1):937.

 ISBN: 978-1-041-32674-8

Perceptions of Dental Students About Their Learning Environment in a Dental School in Karnataka, India

Ashwini Rao
Department of Public Health Dentistry, Manipal College of Dental Sciences Mangalore, Manipal Academy of Higher Education, Manipal, India

Arathi Rao
Department of Paediatric & Preventive Dentistry, Manipal College of Dental Sciences Mangalore, Manipal Academy of Higher Education, Manipal, India

Ramya Shenoy
Department of Public Health Dentistry, Manipal College of Dental Sciences Mangalore, Manipal Academy of Higher Education, Manipal, India

Nikita Rungta
University of Michigan, Ann Arbor, USA

ABSTRACT: **Background**: Student learning experiences, academic results, accomplishments, contentment, and success are significantly influenced by the educational environment. What, how, and why students learn is influenced by their educational environment.

Objective: The purpose of this study was to determine how undergraduate dentistry students in a dental school in Karnataka, India felt about their learning environment.

Methodology: A simple demographic questionnaire was utilized in conjunction with the 'Dundee Ready Education Environment Measure' (DREEM) inventory. As a universal diagnostic inventory for assessing the caliber of the learning environment, the DREEM has been proven to be reliable. In the present study, 259 undergraduate dental students in their first, second, third, and fourth years at a dental school in Karnataka, India, were given the DREEM instrument.

Results: An analysis of the students' overall evaluations revealed that approximately 80% of them thought the learning environment was more positive than it was negative, and 12% thought it was excellent. As the course progressed, the rating improved.

Conclusion: In summary, the effectiveness of the learning process is significantly influenced by the educational environment. Consequently, optimizing learning settings would be advantageous for any endeavor seeking to provide students with a more comprehensive educational experience.

Keywords: dental student, DREEM, educational environment, educational perceptions

1 INTRODUCTION

The standard curriculum for dentist training is prescribed by a governmental authority that oversees the dental profession in India. For training to be successful, a learning-friendly workplace is essential. An essential element of a health science program is curriculum renewal and academic upgrading.

Major reforms and innovations have been planned for undergraduate courses in dentistry, such as, the problem-based learning, objective based education (OBE) and other changes in the new national education policy (NEP) and these reforms might influence the learning environments of students.

Since health professions involve highly pressured professional training and education, measuring the environment and climate of higher educational institutions including dental institutions has become important.

The DREEM inventory is one such diagnostic tool used to measure the status of the learning environment and teaching climate in an institution. Using the 'Dundee Ready Education Environment Measure' (DREEM) [1], the medical field has been able to use a significantly greater degree of empirical introspection with respect to the learning environments of its students [2–7].

Although classroom and clinical learning environments are frequently combined in Indian dental health science courses, there is a dearth of empirical data that characterize or assess this current balance or how students view its delivery.

As these students embark on their careers, their proficiency not only speaks volumes about the school they attended but also matters immensely to all of their future patients and the community at large. This study was designed to determine the learning environment and teaching climate in a dental school in Karnataka, India.

 DOI: 10.1201/9781042016075-15

2 METHODOLOGY

This was a cross-sectional study and the subjects were undergraduate dental students studying in the first, second, third and fourth years of their course. In the first- and second-year courses the students are taught preclinical exercises, and in the third- and fourth-year courses they are exposed to clinical experiences.

2.1 *Data collection*

The demographic questionnaire and the DREEM inventory were administered to the students during their college hours, and those who were present and willing to participate were included. They were given 20 minutes to respond to the inventory. Data collection was carried out over a period of two months. The reliability and validity of the questionnaire were measured via Cronbach's alpha by pilot testing on 10 individuals, and a value of 0.8 was obtained which indicated good agreement

Demographic information about age, sex, and course year was collected. The educational atmosphere and environment of the students were evaluated via the DREEM inventory [1]. 'Students' perceptions of learning', 'students' perceptions of course organizers', 'students' academic self-perceptions', 'students' perceptions of the atmosphere', and 'students' social self-perception' are the five subscales that comprise the fifty statements that cover a wide range of topics directly related to the educational climate.

Real positive scores were those that had a mean score of at least 3.5 points. A closer look was given to any item with a mean of two or less, as they suggested potential issue areas. Aspects that had a mean of two to three indicated room for improvement.

2.2 *Ethical considerations*

The Institutional Ethics Committee granted ethical approval. Every subject provided informed consent. The students received a detailed explanation prior to the administration of the questionnaire. The confidentiality of their answers and their anonymity were guaranteed, and students' participation was voluntary.

2.3 *Data management and statistical analysis*

The Statistical Package for the Social Sciences (SPSS, ver. 17.0; SPSS, Inc., Chicago, IL, USA) was used for data analysis. Reports using descriptive statistics have been made by comparing the scale scores and the items. $P < 0.05$ was considered statistically significant.

3 RESULTS

Among the 315 students present on the day of the visits, 259 participated in the study, resulting in a response rate of 82%. Among them, 191 were females, and 68 were males (Table 1).

Table 1. Subscales of the DREEM inventory.

	1 BDS	2 BDS	3 BDS	4 BDS	Total
Students' perception of learning A more positive perception	36 (61)	43(71.7)	57(77)	59(89.4)	195(75.3)
Students' Perception of course organisers Moving in the right direction	45(76.3)	51(85)	65(87.8)	62(94)	223(86)
Students' academic self perception Feeling more on the positive side	34(57.6)	42(70)	54(72.9)	48(72.8)	178(68.7)
Students' perception of atmosphere A more positive attitude	39(66.1)	50(83.4)	55(74.3)	49(74.2)	193 (74.5)
Students' Social Self Perception Not too bad	38(64.4)	41(68.3)	48(64.8)	48(72.7)	175(67.6)
Students' overall rating More Positive than Negative	38 (64.4)	47 (78.3)	60 (81.1)	62 (94)	207(79.9)

3.1 *'Students' perceptions of learning'*

When the questionnaire was analysed, 13.9% of the 259 respondents thought highly of teaching, and 75.3% had a more positive perception of learning. This perception was significantly greater among the clinical students than among the preclinical students ($P<0.05$). When the male and female students were compared, among the

195 students who had a more positive perception of learning, the percentage of female students (77.9%) was greater than that of male students, and this difference was statistically significant (P<0.05) (Table 1).

3.2 *'Students' perceptions of course organizers'*

None of the students perceived the course organizers as abysmal, and 86% of the students perceived them as moving in the right direction. This perception also increased significantly as the students progressed through the course from the first year to the fourth year. (P<0.05). Among the 223 students who felt that the course organizers were 'moving in the right direction', 76.2% were female, and this difference was statistically significant (P<0.05) (Table 1).

3.3 *'Students' academic self-perceptions'*

With respect to their academic self-perceptions, more than 68% were feeling more positive, and 13% were confident about themselves. A higher proportion of final-year students reported feeling more positive than first-year students did when yearwise comparisons were performed, and this difference was statistically significant. (P<0.05) (Table 1). Nonetheless, there were no gender disparities in the students' assessments of their academic self-perceptions..

3.4 *'Students' perception of the atmosphere'*

Approximately 75% of the students reported an atmosphere of 'more positive attitudes'. When the perceptions were analysed yearwise, a significantly greater number of students in the second, third and fourth years of the course perceived a more positive attitude than did first-year students. However, no significant differences were perceived in terms of gender. (P<0.05) (Table 1).

3.5 *'Students' social self perception'*

With respect to their social self-perception, 72.7% perceived it as 'not too bad', and approximately 22.7% perceived it to be 'very good socially'. The yearwise or genderwise differences were not statistically significant (Table 1).

3.6 *'Students' overall rating'*

When the overall rating of the students was analysed, approximately 80% of the students' perceptions of the educational environment were found to be more positive and 12% found it to be excellent. The rating was also found to increase with the advancement of the course.

4 DISCUSSION

In contrast to the current study among dentistry students, Abraham *et* al. [3] in their study of medical students at an Indian medical school, reported that first-year students were more content with the learning environment than were clinical students. Unnikrishnan *et al.* [4] in their study of medical students in coastal Karnataka reported that these students had positive perceptions and more positive scores than negative scores. Sabbagh *et al.* [5] reported that the overall mean score was "more positive than negative" in their study of dental students in Saudi Arabia, which was similar to the findings of the present study. However, they also reported that the mean scores of third-year students were greater than those of fourth-year students which was in contrast to the current study where the scores were found to increase as the course advanced from the first to fourth years.

5 RECOMMENDATION

The periodic administration of a universal diagnostic inventory such as the DREEM, would help identify deficiencies and be instrumental in refining the teaching climate, thus improving the learning environment of dental students.

6 CONCLUSION

Learning environments are becoming increasingly important in higher education. A curriculum's effectiveness appears to be largely determined by the educational environment. There is a need to carry out further research on the educational environment among the dental colleges of the country to provide a more comprehensive student learning experience through more efficient utilization of learning environments.

REFERENCES

[1] Roff S, McAleer S, Harden R, Al-Qahtani M, Ahmed A, Deza H, Groenen G, Primparyon P. (1997). Development and validation of the Dundee Ready Education Environment Measure (DREEM). *Med Teach* 19:295–299.

[2] Mayya S, Roff S. (2004). Students‘ perceptions of educational environment: A comparison of academic achievers and under-achievers at Kasturba Medical College, India. *Educ Health.* 17(3):280–91.

[3] Abraham R, Ramnarayan K, Vinod P and Torke S. (2008). Students' perceptions of learning environment in an Indian medical school. *BMC Medical Education* 8; 20 :1–5

[4] Unnikrishnan B, Rekha T, Mithra PP, Kumar N, Reshmi B. (2012). Perceptions of medical students about their educational environment in community medicine in a medical college of coastal Karnataka. *Indian J Community Med* 37:130–2

[5] Lokuhetty MDS, Warnakulasuriya SP, Perera RIR, De Silva HTR, Wijesinghe HD. (2010). Students' perception of the educational environment in a Medical Faculty with an innovative curriculum in Sri Lanka. *South-East Asian Journal of Medical Education.* 4 (1): 9–16

[6] Sabbagh HJ, Bakhaider HA, Abokhashabah HM, Bader MU. (2020). Students' perceptions of the educational environment at King Abdulaziz University Faculty of Dentistry (KAUFD): A cross sectional study. Sabbagh *et al. BMC Medical Education,* 20:241. https://doi.org/10.1186/s12909-020-02165-7

[7] Almansour M, Abouammoh N, Idris RB, Alsuliman OA, Alhomaidi RA, Alhumud MH, Alghamdi HA . (2024). Exploring medical students‘ experience of the learning environment: a mixed methods study in Saudi medical college. *BMC Med Educ* 24: 723. https://doi.org/10.1186/s12909-024-05716-4

Navigating Dental Education Trends and Transforming Dental Pedagogy – Abas and Srikant N (Eds)
© 2027 The Author(s), ISBN: 978-1-041-32674-8

Enhancing Active Learning Through Team Case-Based Learning: An Indian Dental School Experience

Asavari Desai, Supriya Nambiar, Nidhin Philip Jose, and MV Ashith
Department of Orthodontics & Dentofacial Orthopedics, Manipal College of Dental Sciences Mangalore, Manipal Academy of Higher Education, Manipal, India

1 INTRODUCTION

Active learning has been broadly defined as a type of learning that demands active gathering, processing and application of information rather than passive assimilation of knowledge. [1] This happens when the learning experience is more interactive and there is increased involvement of students with the learning content of the course, encouraging them to enquire rather than passively receive knowledge. In an active learning environment, teachers perform the job of facilitation in learning for students, as it involves self-directed learning from their own experiences and previously acquired knowledge. Numerous teaching strategies have been developed to promote active learning across health professions education, including problem-based learning, case-based learning, flipped learning, team-based learning, and group discussion. Research suggests that students and instructors positively value active learning as it may be more effective than traditional lecture-based teaching in dental education [2,3] Case-based learning (CBL) is an interactive student-centered exploration of real-life situations in which the students initially gain basic knowledge on the topic, and are then encouraged to participate in a problem-solving activity. [4] A case is used as a trigger to initiate the learning and places events in a context or situation that promotes active learning. [5] Cases are generally written as problems that provide the student with the history or background of a patient or as a clinical situation of chair side clinical patient. Additional supporting information such as X-rays and study models are provided.

Dental schools across India offer the Bachelor of Dental surgery (BDS) program which runs for five years as per the curriculum mandated by the Dental Council of India. The first three years are annual programs whereas the final year curriculum is done in two phases Part I and Part II. Students undergo orthodontic training in Final year Part 1. The content delivery in majority of our dental schools is predominantly lecture based with clinical chair side case discussions. Even though the assessment methods probe analytical and reasoning skills a dental student ought to have, they often fall short in assessment of communication and team-based skills. There are a number of educational strategies that are being experimented in CBL which include, self-directed learning (SDL), problem-based learning (PBL), task-based learning (TBL), co-operative learning (CL) and peer assisted learning (PAL). [6–10] But when done individually it fails to give the same result as it does not have peers in the learning process.

The dental curriculum is delivered in a traditional system-based approach. The exponential growth in knowledge has prompted educationists to investigate strategies that would foster better learning styles. To introduce active learning among undergraduate dental students, we decided to modify the existing individual CBL program and incorporate Team based CBL(TB-CBL) sessions in the orthodontic undergraduate curriculum. This was done to assess and compare the academic performance of final year orthodontic students participating in the individual CBL and TB-CBL and to investigate student perceptions on TB-CBL.

2 METHODOLOGY

The study was conducted in the Department of Orthodontics during the final year clinical posting which the students attended on rotation, after obtaining approval from the Institutional ethics committee. (IEC approval number:19062)

The rotation was of approximately one month duration and comprised of 115 students divided into 5 groups of 23 students each.

An orientation program on CBL for faculty was conducted two weeks prior to the commencement of TB-CBL sessions as case taking demonstrations. This program introduced students to the use of case study approaches in Orthodontics and educated them about the need for active learning in the dental curriculum. Issues related to case processes and group dynamics were also dealt with and the need for modifying to TB-CBL was emphasised. The CBL was allotted for the orthodontic case diagnosis exercise and cases for the same were identified before the commencement of each rotation.

In one rotation, the class comprising 20 students was divided into 4 groups of five students each. A patient was allotted to each group with a set of specified orthodontic problem list. The case sheets with history and relevant

 DOI: 10.1201/9781042016075-16

findings were prepared by the students during commencement of CBL. During presentation sessions, the class of five groups had a faculty member from the department of Orthodontics identified as a facilitator for each session. Students were asked to present the learning objectives individually. Role of the facilitator was limited to keep students focused on learning objectives and to ensure group dynamics. Topics discussed during TB-CBL sessions were evaluated by including these contents during sessional examinations, which was conducted at the end of each rotation.

A cross-sectional survey was conducted among the students using a questionnaire to assess the students' perceptions on TB-CBL. The questionnaire comprising of questions shown in Table 1 contained finalized after a focus group discussion. These included items regarding CBL and TB-CBL and how it linked to their learning, analytical and communication skills. It also probed into the validity of CBL in better understanding of orthodontic subject matter, examination performance and promotion of cooperative learning. The responses were in the YES/NO pattern. The purpose of the questionnaire was explained in detail to the participating students and confidentiality of the results was assured.

To assess the academic performance of students in the topics covered during individual CBL and TB-CBL, we compared the average scores obtained by the students for the TB-CBL portions with their average scores obtained in the individual CBL exercise. To find the effect of TB-CBL on the academic performance, we compared student scores of the batch that had used TB-CBL (Group B) with their immediate senior batch (Group A) that had undergone training through individual CBL alone. The same faculty participated in the content delivery to both the batches and the assessment pattern was also standardized. Performance of these groups in the orthodontic diagnosis & treatment plan exercise was compared, by analysing the mean scores obtained in each year.

3 STATISTICAL ANALYSIS:

The scores obtained by students in the topic covered during the TB- CBL sessions and individual CBL sessions were compared using Paired t test. The average scores obtained by the students before and after the introduction of TB-CBL sessions were compared by independent samples t test. Statistical analyses of the results were performed using SPSS 20 software for windows.

4 RESULTS

Among the 114 students who participated in the survey, 61 (54%) opined that their group members showed responsibility and respect towards the tutorial process and learning skills. 48(42.5%) felt that their group members were able to process the information from the tutorial at the clinical setting and 52(46%) felt that their teammates participated well in the critical analysis of the case history, clinical examination and diagnosis. 43(38.4%) felt their teammates were able to achieve the desired learning requirements after the chair side case-based learning. 55(48.7%) rated the interaction and collaboration among group members as very good. 39(34.8%) opined that group based CBL has helped change their attitude and 38(33.9%) felt that group based CBL improved their learning process. 27(24.1%) rated their analytical skills in CBL as good and 29(25.9%) rated themselves as good in communication skills post CBL. (Table 1)

Table 1. Response of participants towards TB-CBL.

	Strongly agree	Moderately agree	Agree	Disagree	Strongly disagree
1. Did you feel all your group members showed responsibility and respect towards the tutorial process?	54.00%	22.10%	21.20%	1.80%	0.90%
2. Were your group members able to process the information from the tutorial at the clinical setting?	42.50%	24.80%	24.80%	6.20%	1.80%
3. Do you think your teammates were able to achieve the desired learning requirements after the chair side case-based learning?	38.40%	29.50%	23.20%	6.20%	2.70%
4. How well did your teammates participate in the critical analysis of the case history, clinical examination and diagnosis?	46.00%	38.90%	11.50%	0.90%	2.70%
5. How do you rate interaction and collaboration among your group members?	48.70%	35.40%	11.50%	2.70%	1.80%
6. Do you think the group based CBL has helped you change your attitude?	34.80%	31.20%	26.80%	4.50%	2.70%
7. Do you think the group based CBL has helped you change your learning process?	33.90%	29.50%	26.80%	7.10%	2.70%
8. How did you rate your analytical skills in CBL	24.10%	52.70%	18.80%	2.70%	1.80%
9. How do you rate yourself in communication skills post CBL?	25.90%	52.70%	16.10%	1.80%	3.60%

While comparing the average marks obtained in the topics covered during CBL sessions and TB-CBL sessions, the mean scores obtained by students in the topics that were covered during TB-CBL sessions was found to be significantly higher than the scores obtained in CBL sessions (P value = <0.0001).

5 DISCUSSION

CBL has been widely used in medical education and a recent meta-analysis has shown that it is an effective strategy to enhance their clinical reasoning skills.[11] However, literature pertaining to its application in dental education and specifically in Orthodontics is scant. This study explored the impact of CBL on the learning experiences of final year undergraduate students in orthodontics. Among the broad educational domains, a critical approach, research-oriented attitude and communication skills are some of the most important for dental students. While it is widely agreed upon that problem solving skills are essential in the practice of medicine and dentistry, there is a widespread skepticism to transform educational strategies in this direction. This is particularly true in the Indian context. Most of the activities which foster student centered learning have been tried, purely on an experimental basis. Previous studies [12,13] have shown that students prefer structured learning activities and assessment schemes and by introducing TB-CBL, we were challenging an existing curricular framework.

Students' approach towards learning is influenced by several factors such as the curriculum, teaching characteristics, departmental characteristics, and assessment methods. Literature states that the chances of better learning are there if it is centred around a realistic problem. Cases used during CBL necessarily shift the focus of student learning beyond the facts and stimulate the students to utilize scientific knowledge to frame questions and to answer them. In the process, they also learn to locate and manage information, develop reasonable answers to the questions and provide support for their conclusions. [13] In addition, TB-CBL improves peer interaction thereby improving on the communicative and collaborative skills. Collaborative learning takes place when the participants are mutually dependent, they share responsibilities and strive together to achieve a common goal. In a TB-CBL, learners are encouraged to interact with each other as these interactions positively influence learning. It is heartening to note that attributes of cooperative learning incorporated in the questionnaire were highly appreciated by the participants. Our study corroborates the findings of previous studies suggesting that TB-CBL is an effective technique for enhancing student learning through active group learning. [14] The instructor's role in TB-CBL is that of a facilitator who actively participates in the session to offer constructive feedback. Orientation programs should be conducted for faculty, stressing the need for implementing teaching approaches that would stimulate higher order thinking among the learners. Faculty apprehensions are common when one deviates from the routine. However, in our study, faculty had a positive approach towards the curricular change.

6 CONCLUSION

TB-CBL is learner-centred teaching method, where the students collaboratively address problems using an analytical approach. Our study showed that TB-CBL used instead of an individual case-based learning method in a traditional curriculum, can promote active learning among dental students. The information gathered will help us in planning strategies that direct learners to more self-directed learning which will be more of an inquiry driven, collaborative, student centered approach.

REFERENCES

[1] Arnaldo Perez *et al.* (2023). Active learning in undergraduate classroom dental education- a scoping review. *PLoS ONE* 1–21

[2] Reimschisel T, Herring AL, Huang J, Minor TJ. (2017). A systematic review of the published literature on team-based learning in health professions education. *Med Teach.* 39(12):1227–1237

[3] Hew KF, Lo CK. (2018). Flipped classroom improves student learning in health professions education: a meta-analysis. *BMC Med Educ.* 18(1):38

[4] Chowaniec JA, Doubleday AF, LeHew CW, *et al.* (2018). Timing of case-based discussions and educational outcomes for dental students. *J Dent Educ.* 82(5): 510–514.

[5] Gade S, Chari S. (2013). Case-based learning in endocrine physiology: An approach toward self-directed learning and the development of soft skills in medical students. *Adv Physiol Educ.* 37(4):356–60.

[6] Ciraj A.M, Vinod P, Ramnarayan K; (2010). "Enhancing active learning in microbiology through case based learning: Experiences from an Indian medical school; *Indian Journal of Pathology and Microbiology* - 53(4).

[7] Neda Mehrdada, Shoaleh Bigdelib *et al.* (2012). A comparative study on self, peer and teacher evaluation to evaluate clinical skills of nursing students"; *Procedia - Social and Behavioral Sciences* 47:1847–1852

[8] Tracey Papinczak, Louise Young, Michele Groves & Michele Haynes. (2007). An analysis of peer, self, and tutor assessment in problem-based learning tutorials, *Medical Teacher*, 29:5, e122–e132

[9] VP Patil *et al.* (2017). "Case based earning in biochemistry-an innovative criterion based module for effective learning among MBBS Phase 1 students in India. *Indian Journal of Medical Biochem* 21(1) 62–68.

[10] Donkin R, Yule H and Fyfe T. (2023). "Online case-based learning in medical education: a scoping review. *BMC Medical Education* 23,564

[11] Cen XY, Hua Y, Niu S, *et al.* (2021). Application of case-based learning in medical student education: a meta-analysis. *Eur Rev Med Pharmacol Sci.* **25**(8): 3173–3181.

[12] Du GF, Li CZ, Shang SH, Xu XY, Chen HZ, Zhou G. (2023). Practising case-based learning in oral medicine for dental students in China. *Eur J Dent Educ.* 17:225–8.

[13] Gali S, Shetty V, Murthy NS, Marimuthu P. (2015). Bridging the gap in 1st year dental material curriculum: A 3-year randomized cross over trial. *J Indian Prosthodont Soc.* 15:244–9.

[14] Ulfa Y, Igarashi Y, Takahata K, Shishido E, Horiuchi S. (2021). A comparison of team-based learning and lecture-based learning on clinical reasoning and classroom engagement: A cluster randomized controlled trial. *BMC Med Educ.* 21(1): 444

 ISBN: 978-1-041-32674-8

An Analysis of the Motivations Influencing the Choice of Dental Higher Education Degree Programs Among Dental Students: A Pilot Study

Ankita Singh
Senior Lecturer, Department of Conservative Dentistry and Endodontics, Manipal College of Dental Sciences Mangalore, Manipal Academy of Higher Education, Manipal, India

Karthik Shetty
Department of Conservative Dentistry and Endodontics, Manipal College of Dental Sciences Mangalore, Manipal Academy of Higher Education, Manipal, India

N Srikant
Department of Oral Pathology, Manipal College of Dental Sciences Mangalore, Manipal Academy of Higher Education, Manipal, India

Nandita Shenoy
Associate Professor, Department of Oral Medicine and Radiology, Manipal College of Dental Sciences Mangalore, Manipal Academy of Higher Education, Manipal, India

ABSTRACT: This pilot study investigates the factors influencing the decision-making processes of postgraduate dental students in India when their MDS programs and institutions are selected. The purpose of the study was to analyze the key motivations, including intrinsic factors such as personal interest in the field; extrinsic factors like job prospects, financial considerations, and the influence of mentors, parents, and institutional reputation. A cross-sectional online survey was conducted among 107 postgraduate dental students, and data on the significance of these factors were gathered. The results revealed that personal interest in the field and job prospects were the most prominent motivators, with financial considerations also playing a major role. External influences, including parental guidance and mentor recommendations, were significant for a large portion of the students. The reputation of the institution was another critical factor. Additionally, the majority of the students reported challenges during the decision-making process, although their satisfaction with their chosen programs remained high. These findings highlight the need for educational institutions to address both practical considerations and academic aspirations when attracting prospective students. The study's conclusions suggest that improved support services and clearer communication regarding financial aid, career prospects, and institutional reputation could better guide students in their decisions.

Keywords: Postgraduate dental education, decision-making, motivation, India, career guidance

1 INTRODUCTION

In the evolving field of dental education, understanding the factors that influence students' choices of degree courses is crucial. Aspiring dental professionals face a range of decisions, from selecting specialties to evaluating institutional factors. The decision-making process is multifaceted; and shaped by individual motivations and external information sources. This understanding is vital for educational institutions aiming to attract students and for policymakers seeking to enhance educational guidance systems.

Students' choices can be significantly influenced by their personal interests, career goals, and the perceived value of the degree in the job market. Previous studies have highlighted how intrinsic motivations, such as a genuine interest in the subject, often compete with extrinsic factors such as job prospects and earning potential. [1,2] Similarly, parental guidance and societal expectations can also be identified as key influences, particularly in developing countries such as India. [3,4]

As university selection is often a carefully considered decision, institutional factors, such as academic reputation, location, and facilities, may also be crucial in shaping student preferences. [5] Fuller and Delorey's study in Maritime Canada further highlighted the importance of program-specific factors such as faculty expertise and research opportunities in attracting students. [5]

A study of the Spanish public university system, emphasized the quality of education and career outcomes offered, as significant factors in degree choice selection. [6] In India however, the interplay between personal aspirations and institutional offerings is particularly pronounced, as shown in a comprehensive analysis of student preferences in higher education. [4]

 DOI: 10.1201/9781042016075-17

In summary, the decision to pursue a university degree may be shaped by a complex interaction of motivational factors, information sources, and institutional characteristics. Understanding these influences is essential for tailoring educational programs to better meet student needs and for developing more effective guidance and support systems.

To date, there have been few attempts to identify the individual reasons that drive university degree choices and more so, there are limited data for dental student motivators. This study aims to provide valuable insights into the same topic.

1.1 *AIM*

To analyze the motivations influencing the choice of higher education degree programs among dental students.

1.2 *Objectives*

1) To analyze the decision-making process of a dental student while determining the postgraduate course to pursue.
2) To analyze the decision-making process of a dental student while determining which dental college to opt for while pursuing postgraduate training.

2 MATERIALS AND METHODS

2.1 *Study design*

Cross sectional study

Inclusion criteria

- Dental postgraduate students from India
- Students in the age group of 20-35 years

Exclusion criteria

- Under graduate/postgraduate students of Bachelors in Science, Commerce, Arts.

2.2 *Sample size*

For the pilot study approximately 100 students were given the online questionnaire. The final sample size will be subsequently calculated on the basis of the pilot study.

2.3 *Method of evaluation*

This study was conducted among dental postgraduate students pursuing MDS in India. A well-structured online questionnaire was prepared and distributed among the postgraduate students. The questionnaire was validated by four expert dentists. The questionnaire comprised a covering letter with study-related details (participant information sheet) and consent from the participants followed by demographic details; and multiple-choice questions to understand the participants' motivations influencing their choice of dental higher education degree programs and the colleges to pursue the same. The collected data was compiled in an MS excel spreadsheet.

2.4 *Statistical analysis*

This cross-sectional study utilized a questionnaire consisting of approximately 20 questions designed to assess the motivations influencing the selection of college and dental courses among students. To analyze the data, tests of proportions were applied, with frequencies and percentages calculated to identify the most common or preferred reasons for college and course selection.

The chi-square test was used to assess associations between categorical variables, whereas the independent t-test was used to compare mean differences in continuous variables between genders. Statistical significance will be set at an appropriate level (e.g., $p < 0.05$), and all analyses will be performed via SPSS software, version 11.5.

2.5 *Data collection method*

The questionnaire was shared with postgraduate students pursuing different dental specialties.

2.6 *Budget*

No budget is needed. Online circulation of the questionnaire.

3 RESULTS

A total of 107 respondents participated in this study, with 50.5% being under 30 years old and 49.5% being over 30. In terms of sex, 63.6% were female, and 36.4% were male.

When considering factors that influenced the choice of an MDS course, 33.6% of the participants indicated that parental influence was very important, whereas 28.0% found it important. Regarding interest in the field, 50.5% rated it as very important, and 32.7% rated it as important. Job prospects were seen as very important by 49.5% and important by 29.9%. The influence of mentors or guides was rated as very important by 43.9%, and the reputation of the college was deemed very important by 47.7%.

Financial considerations were also crucial for 49.5% of the respondents, with an additional 29.0% finding them important. The location of the college was very important for 32.7% of the respondents, with 26.2% finding it important. Prior experience in the field played a significant role, with 47.7% indicating that it influenced their decision to some extent, and 30.8% finding it to be a significant factor.

When deciding on the course, 36.4% of the respondents made their choice within 1-3 months, and 34.6% took less than a month. Most respondents (43.0%) considered multiple dental specialty courses before deciding. Rankings such as the National Institutional Ranking Framework (NIRF) influenced 45.8% of the respondents, whereas 39.3% did not consider rankings.

Challenges during the decision-making process were reported by 60.7%, with 18.7% describing them as significant. Looking back, 49.5% would definitely make the same choice again, and 40.2% would probably do so. Satisfaction with their MDS course was high, with 48.6% very satisfied and 38.3% satisfied.

Factors such as infrastructure, location, cost, faculty expertise, and course reputation were important for the majority of respondents, while academic performance and college ranking were also significant considerations. In contrast, research opportunities and alumni placement were less frequently cited as decisive factors.

4 DISCUSSION

The findings of this study underscore the multifaceted nature of these decisions, where intrinsic motivation (interest in the field) and extrinsic factors (job prospects, financial considerations, parental and mentor influences) intersect. The predominance of intrinsic motivation, such as interest in the field, suggests that students are deeply committed to their professional aspirations. However, external influences, such as parental involvement and mentor guidance, are not insignificant, revealing the strong familial and academic networks that shape these decisions. The role of institutional reputation highlights how external validation, such as college standing, reinforces these choices, pointing to the need for students to balance personal ambition with perceived prestige.

4.1 *Implications of the findings*

These findings have significant implications for both dental education institutions and policymakers. Institutions must recognize that students are looking for more than just academic quality—they want assurance that their future professional and financial prospects will be secure. The significance of financial concerns, in particular, suggests that education cost and return on investment are major factors that students weigh when choosing a program. This calls for transparent communication about financial aid options, career services, and job placement support. Additionally, the fact that many students rely on the guidance of mentors and family members suggests broader implications for career counseling services that can be more proactive in guiding students, especially in regard to navigating multiple factors such as costs, prospects, and institutional standing.

4.2 *Significance of the study*

This study is significant because it addresses a gap in the literature concerning the motivations behind postgraduate dental education choices in India. Understanding why students select certain programs can help shape educational offerings, marketing strategies, and institutional policies to better meet student needs. By identifying the most important factors influencing decision-making, institutions can tailor their programs, facilities, and outreach efforts. The results also provide actionable insights for educators and policymakers who aim to attract a diverse and committed student populations.

4.3 *Limitations of the study*

Despite its insights, the study has several limitations. The sample size is relatively small and regionally specific, which may limit the generalizability of the findings to the broader population of dental students in India. Additionally, this study focused on dental postgraduate students, which means that the motivations and challenges for undergraduate students remain unexplored. Future research could address these limitations by expanding the sample size and including students from a broader range of educational levels and regions, providing a more comprehensive understanding of student decision-making in dental education.

5 CONCLUSION

This pilot study highlights the complex interplay of intrinsic and extrinsic factors influencing the choice of post-graduate dental programs among students in India. The findings reveal that personal interest, job prospects, and financial considerations significantly shape decision-making processes. By recognizing the importance of parental and mentor influences, educational institutions can enhance their support services to better guide prospective students. Ultimately, this study underscores the need for tailored strategies that address both academic aspirations and practical considerations, contributing valuable insights to the field of dental education and informing future research directions.

REFERENCES

[1] Skatova A, Ferguson E. (2014). Why do different people choose different university degrees? Motivation and the choice of degree. *Frontiers in Psychology*, 13;5:1244.

[2] Sadjail SI, Sansawi D, Matolo MA. (2022). Factors influencing students in choosing their college course. psychology and education. *A multidisciplinary Journal*. 2022;3(8):697–700.

[3] Areces Martínez D, Rodríguez Muñiz LJ, Suarez Alvarez J, Roca Pascual YD, Fernández Cueli MS. (2016). Information sources used by high school students in the college degree choice. *Psicothema*.

[4] Reddy M. (2011). Determinants of student choice of business schools in India: A factor analytic investigation. *International Journal of Management*. 28(3):751.

[5] Fuller MA, Delorey R. (2016). Making the choice: University and program selection factors for undergraduate management education in Maritime Canada. *The International Journal of Management Education*. 14(2):176–86.

[6] Peró M, Soriano PP, Capilla R, i Olmos JG, Hervás A. (2015). Questionnaire for the assessment of factors related to university degree choice in Spanish public system: A psychometric study. *Computers in Human Behavior*. 47:128–38.

 ISBN: 978-1-041-32674-8

Oral and General Health Care Integration Through Interprofessional Education: An Overview

Lakshmi Puzhankara
Department of Periodontology, Manipal College of Dental Sciences Manipal, Manipal Academy of Higher Education, Manipal, India

Asavari Desai
Department of Orthodontics, Manipal College of Dental Sciences Mangalore, Manipal Academy of Higher Education, Manipal, India

Madhurya N Kedlaya and Namratha Nayak
Department of Periodontology, Manipal College of Dental Sciences, Manipal, Manipal Academy of Higher Education, Manipal, India

ABSTRACT: Integrated oral and general health care delivery is essential for achieving the development of holistic health care systems. Interprofessional education (IPE), which involves students from different healthcare professions working together to improve patient care, can help achieve integrated health care delivery through the dissemination of knowledge about oral health care among other disciplines and the development of collaborative skills. The objective of this paper is to perform a scoping review on modalities for integrated health care delivery systems that involve an altered curriculum with interprofessional education. A search was performed on the databases PUBMED, SCOPUS, EMBASE, Web of Science and Google Scholar via the following search terms: oral healthcare OR dental health OR oral health OR oral care AND primary healthcare OR general health AND integrated disease prevention OR integration OR collaborative practice AND interprofessional education. The initial search yielded 13,252 results. A total of 1253 duplicates were removed. Title and abstract screening resulted in the elimination of 11,910 papers. Of the 89 papers that underwent full-text screening, 32 were included in the review. Although there is a drive to promote IPE, the practical application of IPE has not been achieved. It would be beneficial for the overall health of the populace if interprofessional education with practical perspectives is brought into effect, as it would serve as an essential tool for integrated health care delivery. An altered curriculum focused on themes instead of disciplinary boundaries may help in developing an appropriate IPE curriculum and promote interprofessional care delivery.

Keywords: Collaboration, Interprofessional education, Integrated healthcare

1 INTRODUCTION

Oral health maintenance is a critical element for general health improvement, and there is a significant impact of oral diseases on the healthcare economy of developed and developing nations. Yearly, oral health care utilizes US $110 billion in the USA [1]. In India, in 2017-18, catastrophic healthcare expenditure (CHE), was at 63.6%. [2] The out-of-pocket expenditure for dental care has been estimated to be 14% in Organization for Economic Cooperation and Development (OECD) countries. [3]

Integrated preventive programs for oral health promotion are economical and reduce payments for hospital visits pertaining to systemic health conditions. [4] The Health Resources and Services Administration (HRSA) has described initiatives with six levels of integration for uniting oral health with primary medical care, utilizing communication, the proximity of care delivery areas and practice changes as tenets for change. [5] In India, it would be favorable to consider the integration of oral and general health care through knowledge of integrated health care imparted at the time of basic training in health care through interprofessional education (IPE). [6]

The various methods of achieving IPE should be assessed to understand the modalities of integrating healthcare. This paper aims to review approaches for integrated health care delivery systems that involve interprofessional education with or without curriculum modification.

2 METHODS

An initial search of MEDLINE and SCOPUS was undertaken to identify articles on the topic. Text words contained in titles and abstracts of relevant articles were used to develop a full search strategy for *Web of Science,*

 DOI: 10.1201/9781042016075-18

EMBASE. The search terms used were 'Oral healthcare OR Dental health OR oral health OR oral care AND primary healthcare OR general health AND Integrated disease prevention OR integration OR Collaborative practice AND Interprofessional education'. The reference lists of the included sources of evidence were screened for additional studies.

3 RESULTS

The initial search yielded 13,252 results. A total of 1253 duplicates were removed. Title and abstract screening resulted in the elimination of 11,910 papers. Of the 89 papers that underwent full-text screening, 32 were included in the review.

Among the papers related to oral health integration that were selected, ten had pre- and posttest designs. Three papers were observational/descriptive, and one was a case study (Table 1).

Table 1. Details of target professional groups and IPE interventions employed.

Author	Target professional groups	IPE Intervention
Hartnett, E *et al* [7]	Nurses, students of medicine and dentistry	Collaboration in: Reviewing patient Oral assessment, fluoride varnish application, education and guidance
Hallas, D *et al.* [8]	Pediatric dental students, residents, and Pediatric Nursing students	Interprofessional education, Clinical practice, and Professional socialization
Dsouza R *et al.* [9]	Accelerated Bachelor of Nursing (ASBN) students	Clinical simulation and didactic sessions on oral health screening, counseling, referral to dentist
Cooper D, *et al.* [10]	Students in nursing, medicine, dentistry.	Education on children's oral health and inequities in low-income groups in relation to oral health and needs
Haber J, *et al.* [11]	Nurse practitioner/midwifery, dental, and medical students'	Interprofessional clinical simulation session. Case study experience to help develop interprofessional core competencies in oral-systemic health factors.
Farokhi MR, *et al.* [12]	Patients who were refugees, medical students, nursing students, and community/parish members	Educational intervention on oral health literacy.
Ditmyer MM, *et al.* [13]	Dental students and dental care providers	Changes in curriculum: Conversion of previously siloed to two-year combined courses Course delivery by groups of faculty members that constitutes an interprofessional team. Decrease in total curriculum credit/contact hours to accommodate additional courses.
Nadershahi NA, *et al.* [14]	Dental students and health care providers	Development of Pacific Dental Helix Curriculum. Five major content areas known as "strands": Integrated Medical, Preclinical, Clinical Sciences, Clinical Practice, and Personalized Instructional Program.
Braun, P. A *et al* [15]	Primary health care providers	Oral health education was delivered on caries risk assessment, oral examination and health instruction, application of fluoride varnish
Mowat, S.*et al.* [16]	Health care professionals	Lectures and round-table discussions
Kanan C, *et al.* [17]	Primary Health care professionals	Collaborative learning session
Haber J *et al.* [18]	Nurse practitioner/midwifery, dental, medical, and pharmacy (PharmD) students.	Interprofessional oral health and simulated clinical experience with case study
Haresaku, S *et al*, [19]	Dental and nursing students	Nursing and oral healthcare training programmes with one-to-one training of students and discussion.
Mohammed CA *et al.* [20]	Students of Dentistry	Readiness for Interprofessional Learning Scale was utilized to determine subscales of learning and roles and responsibilities toward interprofessional education of dental students.

4 DISCUSSION

Education is one of the basic means of enhancing healthcare workforce awareness of the importance of oral health care and achieving sustainable oral health. [21] One of the shortcomings of the traditional model of healthcare education is the siloed approach to delivering content. To ameliorate the problems associated with this, IPE may be used. [22,23] IPE is based on the basic principles of respect for interprofessional practice (IP), allotment of responsibilities and their effective execution by a multidisciplinary team through effective communication and collective effort of the group. [16,18,19,24] The goals of IPE include changing the course structure to learn about other professions, from and with other professionals, to achieve better patient outcomes. [13–15,25,26]

The heads of various dental schools believe that future curricula should be arranged around themes with an amalgamation of clinical sciences with basic sciences. [27] Although interest in the use of IPE in the curriculum of dental schools has increased [20], very few schools are satisfied with the expertise of their students in IPE and IP by graduates. [25]

Studies on IPE in the medical field were explored to identify additional methods for the incorporation of IPE in oral healthcare. (Table 2)

Table 2. Methods utilized for incorporation of IPE in oral healthcare.

Author	IPE Intervention
Barcelo A [28]	Education program-Plan™do™study™act
Brown JB. [29]	Team-work to form an action plan with interactive discussions, role playing and didactic learning.
Campbell JC [30]	
Helitzer DL. [31]	Patient-focused communication Simulated patients-clinician interaction with feedback on it, Workshops
Nielsen PE [32]	Creation and structuring interprofessional teams at intervention site
Strasser DC [33]	Interactive workshop, development of action plans, utilization of performance feedback to create strategies for improvement of the interprofessional care process.
Taylor CR. [34]	Redistribution of tasks, standardized methods of communication along with appropriate decision-support systems.

In India, a traditional teaching model, which does not involve IPE, is largely followed. The most common problem associated with adopting IPE is changing curricula and class schedules. Moreover, many institutions have medical and dental units in separate campuses, which precludes colocation for IPE. [24] The use of an outcome-based education curriculum in dental schools in India is useful for promoting a broader outlook toward patient care. However, practical application of IPE is still in its infancy in the Indian scenario.

5 CONCLUSION

There is a need to promote IPE and practice among healthcare practitioners. The development of an integrated curriculum with mandatory IPE on oral health and case study clinical simulation experience with appropriate task redistribution, standardized communication methods and decision-support tool development may be utilized to facilitate the robust growth of IPE and practice in the Indian context.

REFERENCES

[1] Facts, Figures and Stats. *FDI World Dental Federation.* Accessed October 22, 2020. https://www.fdiworlddental.org/oral-health/ask-the-dentist/facts-figures-and-stats

[2] Verma VR, Kumar P, Dash U. (2021). Assessing the household economic burden of non-communicable diseases in India: evidence from repeated cross-sectional surveys. *BMC Public Health.* 21(1):881. doi:10.1186/s12889-021-10828-3

[3] Health at a Glance 2023. OECD; 2023. doi:10.1787/7a7afb35-en

[4] Stearns SC, Rozier RG, Kranz AM, Pahel BT, Quiñonez RB. (2012). Cost-effectiveness of preventive oral health care in medical offices for young medicaid enrollees. *Arch Pediatr Adolesc Med.* 166(10):945–951. doi:10.1001/archpediatrics.2012.797

[5] White paper: Integrating oral health with primary health care. *Association of state and territorial dental directors* (ASTDD). December 2016. Accessed October 22, 2020. https://www.astdd.org/www/docs/integrating-oral-health-with-primary-health-care.pdf

[6] Puzhankara L, Janakiram C. (2021). Medical-dental integration-achieving equity in periodontal and general healthcare in the Indian Scenario. *J Int Soc Prev Community Dent.* 11(4):359–366. doi:10.4103/jispcd.JISPCD_75_21

[7] Hartnett E, Haber J, Catapano P, *et al.* (2019). The impact of an interprofessional pediatric oral health clerkship on advancing interprofessional education outcomes. *J Dent Educ.* 83(8):878–886. doi:10.21815/JDE.019.088

[8] Hallas D, Fernandez JB, Herman NG, Moursi A. (2015). Identification of pediatric oral health core competencies through interprofessional education and practice. *Nurs Res Pract.* 2015:1–7. doi:10.1155/2015/360523

[9] Dsouza R, Quinonez R, Hubbell S, Brame J. (2019). Promoting oral health in nursing education through interprofessional collaborative practice: A quasi-experimental survey study design. *Nurse Educ Today.* 82:93–98. doi:10.1016/j.nedt.2019.07.010

[10] Cooper D, Kim J, Duderstadt K, Stewart R, Lin B, Alkon A. (2017). Interprofessional oral health education improves knowledge, confidence, and practice for pediatric healthcare providers. *Front Public Health.* 2017;5. doi:10.3389/fpubh.2017.00209

[11] Haber J, Hartnett E, Allen K, *et al.* (2017). The impact of oral-systemic health on advancing interprofessional education outcomes. *J Dent Educ.* 81(2):140–148. doi:10.1002/j.0022-0337.2017.81.2.tb06259.x

[12] Farokhi MR, Muck A, Lozano-Pineda J, Boone SL, Worabo H. (2018). Using interprofessional education to promote oral health literacy in a faculty-student collaborative practice. *J Dent Educ.* 82(10):1091–1097. doi:10.21815/JDE.018.110

[13] Ditmyer MM, Mobley CC, Davenport WD. (2014). Evaluation of an integrative model for professional development and research in a dental curriculum. *J Dent Educ.* 78(3):368–379.

[14] Nadershahi NA, Bender DJ, Beck L, Alexander S. (2013). A case study on development of an integrated, multidisciplinary dental curriculum. *J Dent Educ.* 77(6):679–687.

[15] Braun P, Widmer Racich K, Ling S, *et al.* (2015). Impact of an interprofessional oral health education program on health care professional and practice behaviors: a RE-AIM analysis. *Pediatric Health Med Ther.* Published online July 2015:101. https:doi.org/10.2147/PHMT.S79826

[16] Mowat S, Hein C, Walsh T, MacDonald L, Grymonpre R, Sisler J. (2017). Changing health professionals' attitudes and practice behaviors through interprofessional continuing education in oral-systemic health. *J Dent Educ.* 81(12):1421–1429. doi:10.21815/JDE.017.102

[17] Kanan C, Ohrenberger K, Bayham M, Raskin SE, Tranby EP, Boynes S. (2020). MORE Care: an evaluation of an interprofessional oral health quality improvement initiative. *J Public Health Dent.* 80(S2). doi:10.1111/jphd.12407

[18] Haber J, Hartnett E, Cipollina J, *et al.* (2021). Attaining interprofessional competencies by connecting oral health to overall health. *J Dent Educ.* 85(4):504–512. doi:10.1002/jdd.12490

[19] Haresaku S, Naito T, Aoki H, *et al.* (2024). Development of interprofessional education programmes in nursing care and oral healthcare for dental and nursing students. *BMC Med Educ.* 24(1):381. doi:10.1186/s12909-024-05227-2

[20] Mohammed CA, Narsipur S, Vasthare R, Singla N, Yan Ran AL, Suryanarayana JP. (2021). Attitude towards shared learning activities and Interprofessional education among dental students in South India. *European Journal of Dental Education.* 25(1):159–167. doi:10.1111/eje.12586

[21] Fisher J, Berman R, Buse K, *et al.* (2023). Achieving oral health for all through public health approaches, interprofessional, and transdisciplinary education. *NAM Perspectives.* 2023;2(13). doi:10.31478/202302b

[22] Mays KA. (2021). Designing oral health curriculum that facilitates greater integration of oral health into overall health. *Frontiers in Dental Medicine.* 2. https://doi.org/10.3389/fdmed.2021.680520

[23] Reeves S, Perrier L, Goldman J, Freeth D, Zwarenstein M. (2013). Interprofessional education: effects on professional practice and healthcare outcomes. *Cochrane Database of Systematic Reviews.* 2018(8). doi:10.1002/14651858.CD002213.pub3

[24] Vasthare R, Mansingh P, Gupta K. (2018). Inter-Professional education and collaboration in dentistry-Current issues and concerns, in India: A narrative review. *Indian J Public Health Res Dev.* 9(10):261. doi:10.5958/0976-5506.2018.01352.9

[25] Jiang T, Tavares MA, Ticku SH, *et al.* (2020). Interprofessional education in dental schools: Results of a national survey. *J Interprof Educ Pract.* 18:100256. doi:10.1016/j.xjep.2019.04.001

[26] Do H, Calache H, Darby I, Lau P. (2021). The effectiveness of interprofessional education for the management of diabetes and oral health: A systematic review. *J Interprof Care.* 35(3):454–463. doi:10.1080/13561820.2020.1758046

[27] Haden NK, Hendricson WD, Kassebaum DK, *et al.* (2010). Curriculum change in dental education, 2003–09. *J Dent Educ.* 74 (5):539–557. doi:10.1002/j.0022-0337.2010.74.5.tb04901.x

[28] Barceló A, Cafiero E, de Boer M, *et al.* (2010). Using collaborative learning to improve diabetes care and outcomes: The VIDA project. *Prim Care Diabetes.* 4(3):145–153. doi:10.1016/j.pcd.2010.04.005

[29] Brown JB, Boles M, Mullooly JP, Levinson W. (1999). Effect of Clinician Communication Skills Training on Patient Satisfaction. *Ann Intern Med.* 131(11):822. doi:10.7326/0003-4819-131-11-199912070-00004

[30] Campbell JC, Coben JH, McLoughlin E, *et al.* (2001). an evaluation of a system-change training model to improve emergency department response to battered women. *Academic Emergency Medicine.* 8(2):131–138. doi:10.1111/j.1553-2712.2001.tb01277.x

[31] Helitzer DL, LaNoue M, Wilson B, de Hernandez BU, Warner T, Roter D. (2011). A randomized controlled trial of communication training with primary care providers to improve patient-centeredness and health risk communication. *Patient Educ Couns.* 82(1):21–29. doi:10.1016/j.pec.2010.01.021

[32] Nielsen PE, Goldman MB, Mann S, *et al.* (2007). Effects of Teamwork Training on Adverse Outcomes and Process of Care in Labor and Delivery. *Obstetrics & Gynecology.* 109(1):48–55. doi:10.1097/01.AOG.0000250900.53126.c2

[33] Strasser DC, Falconer JA, Stevens AB, *et al.* (2008). Team Training and Stroke Rehabilitation Outcomes: A Cluster Randomized Trial. *Arch Phys Med Rehabil.* 89(1):10–15. doi:10.1016/j.apmr.2007.08.127

[34] Taylor CR, Hepworth JT, Buerhaus PI, Dittus R, Speroff T. (2007). Effect of crew resource management on diabetes care and patient outcomes in an inner-city primary care clinic. *Qual Saf Health Care.* 16(4):244–247. doi:10.1136/qshc.2006.019042

 ISBN: 978-1-041-32674-8

Comparison of Jigsaw-Based Learning and Didactic Lecture-Based Learning on Dental Students' Knowledge Acquisition and Retention: A Randomized Controlled Trial

Pooja J Shetty and A Nusrath Raeesa Fathima
Department of Public Health Dentistry, A.J. Institute of Dental Sciences, Kuntikana, Mangalore

ABSTRACT: The purpose of this study was to evaluate and compare the effectiveness of Jigsaw-based learning and didactic lecture-based learning on dental students' knowledge acquisition and retention. This interventional study was carried out among 3rd-year undergraduates at a dental college in Mangalore. The sample size was calculated to be 30 per group. The students were randomly divided into 2 groups: Group1-Jigsaw method, and Group2–Didactic lecture. 1 week after sensitization of the topic, a pre-intervention test was conducted for all the students on "Pit and Fissure Sealants". Group-1 students received a PowerPoint-lecture class. The Group-2 Students were subdivided into groups of 5 members each and were given 5 different subtopics to learn. All those who received the same topic formed an expert-group and discussed key points. During the 2nd-week, expert group students taught their respective sub-topics to their home-group members. A post-intervention test was conducted for all the students. 2 weeks after the post-intervention test, a retention test was conducted for all the students. Both the pre-intervention test, post-intervention test, and retention test scores were analyzed via the SPSS–v.23, using independent and paired t-tests. Among the 60 study participants, 81.4% were females. The analysis revealed that there was a significant difference between the pre-intervention test and post-intervention test scores of the Jigsaw-group (p=0.02). A significant difference was also observed between the pre-intervention test and post-intervention test scores of didactic-group (p=0.03). The knowledge acquisition and retention of the Jigsaw-group were significantly better than those of didactic-group (p<0.05). From the study, it can be concluded that the Jigsaw method of learning is associated with higher levels of academic performance among students, than traditional lecture classes. It also creates opportunities for active participation, and innovative exchanges of learning and teaching ideas.

Keywords: Jigsaw method, Didactic lecture, Dental Students, Active participation, Knowledge acquisition

1 INTRODUCTION

Most educational institutes follow the didactic method of teaching and do not involve students in learning activities, leading to a decrease in students' perceived knowledge. To overcome this problem, Aronson and his students introduced the Jigsaw method, in which a classroom is well structured, with a cooperative learning situation, to develop interpersonal skills, motivation in learning, and increased achievements by the students. [1] The jigsaw method of learning has great potential for enabling students to learn a large amount of information in a short period. In this method, the students act as blocks of the jigsaw puzzle, learn cooperatively, and act as both teachers and learners. [2]

Medical education is a complex process. Dental students must apply basic scientific concepts in clinical practice. Dental education should also improve individual responsibility and positive social skills. Although didactic lectures are widely practiced, they do not improve students' ability to make their own decisions. [3] In this continuously updating curriculum, there is much interest among the faculties and students in innovative methods of learning. One of the core components is to make it student-centric with an emphasis on group learning rather than individual learning. [4]

Many studies have used the Jigsaw method of learning in collaborative teaching. In a 2024 study by Moin et al, knowledge acquisition among medical students in Islamabad, Pakistan was higher in the jigsaw group than in the control group. [5] Krishnan et al (2021) compared the jigsaw method with didactic lecture method in medical students in Kerala, India. [2] They reported substantial improvements in knowledge acquisition and retention in the jigsaw group. A study by Eachempati (2017) on dental students in Malaysia, revealed significant differences in knowledge acquisition and retention between jigsaw groups and lecture-based groups. [6] Sagsoz et al (2015) compared the jigsaw method and didactic lecture-based method among dental students in Turkey, and reported a statistically significant improvement in knowledge acquisition in the jigsaw group. [3]

While there have been previous studies involving short-group learning, fewer studies have been conducted on Indian students, and even fewer studies have been conducted on the Jigsaw method of learning among dental

 DOI: 10.1201/9781042016075-19

students. Hence, the purpose and objective of this study is to fill this void by evaluating and comparing the effectiveness of Jigsaw-based learning and didactic lecture-based learning on dental student's knowledge acquisition and retention.

2 MATERIALS AND METHODS

2.1 *Study design, setting, and participants*

A single-blinded randomized controlled trial was conducted. The study participants were selected from among the third-year undergraduate students of a dental college in Mangalore. After ethical clearance was obtained, students who provided informed consent were included in the study. The study participants were randomized into 2 groups via computer generated randomization.

Group 1: The Jigsaw group was the experimental group who received the Jigsaw method of learning.

Group 2: The Didactic group was the control group who received only the didactic lectures.

Sample size:

The sample size was calculated using data from a study by Sagsoz et al [3]. Considering a 20% attrition, it was determined to be 30 per group and 60 in total.

2.2 *Methodology*

The students and faculty facilitators were sensitized regarding the study. During the first week, a traditional lecture class was taken on "Pit and Fissure Sealants" for all the students. During the second week, a pre-intervention test was conducted to assess the existing knowledge on the chosen topic, with 25 Multiple Choice Questions (MCQ) on Google Forms, with each correct answer awarded 1 point. After the pre-intervention test, the didactic group students were sent to a different classroom, where a repeat lecture was taken on the same topic. During the same session, the Group Jigsaw students were divided into 6 subgroups: A, B, C, D, E, and F. Each subgroup (homegroup) consisted of 5 students, and each student in the homegroup was given a different sub-topic. The distribution of subgroups and subtopics is given in the illustration below:

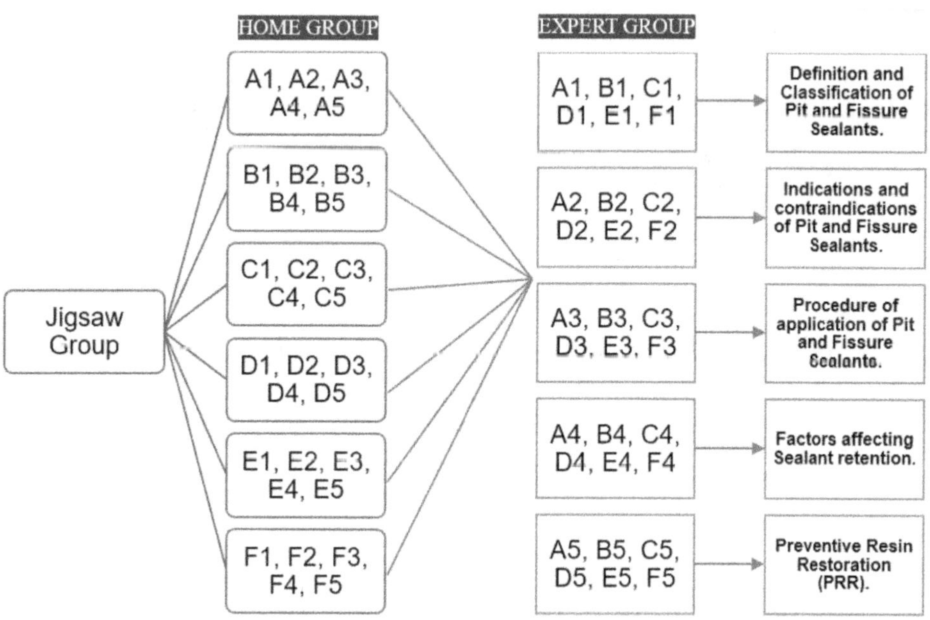

Each person who received the same subtopic formed a new group called the Expert Group. The expert group members were asked to write assignment on their respective topics by referring the textbook "Essentials of Public Health Dentistry: by Soben Peter; 7th edition". Their assignments were assessed by the faculty and necessary corrections were made. Based on the assignment, the home group students discussed key points and planned how to learn, simplify, and teach their topics to others in their home group. During the third week, the Jigsaw group was asked to sit in a separate class from the Didactic group. The expert group members of Jigsaw returned to their home subgroup and taught the members their respective topics. Once every member finished teaching, they discussed and cleared their doubts among themselves, and unclear doubts were still discussed with the faculty. For the didactic group, doubt-clearing session was conducted in the third week. Once the doubt-clearing sessions of both the groups were done, a post-intervention test with 25 MCQ questions was given to all the students, on Google Forms. Two weeks after the post-intervention test, a retention test with 25 MCQ questions on Google Forms was conducted on the same topic to assess how well the two groups had retained the knowledge.

2.3 *Statistical analysis*

The data obtained were entered into the Statistical Package for Social Sciences (SPSS) -v.23. The frequency distribution of males and females was determined. The mean score with a standard deviation of the pre-intervention test, post-intervention test and retention-test scores was calculated. Paired t-test was used to compare the scores before and after intervention. Independent t-test was performed to test the significance of difference in knowledge acquisition and retention between the two groups. A p-value <0.05 was considered significant.

3 RESULTS

Among the study participants, 81.4% were females. Table 1 lists the results of the paired t-test. The analysis, revealed that there was a significant difference between the pre-intervention test and post-intervention test scores of the Jigsaw-group (p=0.02). A significant difference was also observed between the didactic group's pre-intervention test and post-intervention test scores (p=0.01). A significant improvement was seen from the pre-intervention test to the retention test scores in both the groups ($p<0.05$) *[not mentioned in table]*. This analysis proves that both the methods are effective in knowledge acquisition and retention.

Table 2 discusses the results of independent t-test. On analysis, the pre-intervention test scores show no significant difference between the two groups ($p>0.05$), indicating that the existing knowledge of both the groups is almost similar. But, the knowledge acquisition of the Jigsaw-group was significantly better than that of the didactic-group (p=0.000). On analysis of knowledge retention test conducted after 2 weeks of post-intervention test, a significant improvement was found in the jigsaw group (p=0.02) than the didactic group. This analysis proves that though both the methods are respectively effective in knowledge acquisition and retention, the jigsaw method proves to be significantly better than the didactic method.

Table 1. Comparison of pre-intervention and post-intervention test scores within the jigsaw and didactic learning groups using paired t-test.

Learning Method	Tests	Mean score	Standard Deviation	Paired t-test p-value
Jigsaw	Pre-intervention test	14.12	2.604	**0.02**
	Post-intervention test	19.54	2.983	
Didactic	Pre-intervention test	13.85	2.931	**0.01**
	Post-intervention test	15.59	3.411	

Table 2. Comparison of pre-intervention, post-intervention, and retention test scores between the Jigsaw and didactic learning groups using independent t-test.

Learning Method	Tests	Mean score	Standard Deviation	Independent t-test p-value
Jigsaw	Pre-intervention test	14.12	2.604	0.711
Didactic		13.85	2.931	
Jigsaw	Post-intervention test	19.54	2.983	**0.000**
Didactic		15.59	3.411	
Jigsaw	Retention test	17.16	3.244	**0.02**
Didactic		14.90	4.147	

4 DISCUSSION

This study's findings demonstrate that Jigsaw is a very effective method of learning, in which the students assume individual responsibility, cooperate, learn, and teach each other. The mean pre-intervention test scores of the two groups showed no statistical difference ($p>0.05$). But the study revealed a significant difference in knowledge attainment and retention between the two groups. A significant difference was also observed between the pre-intervention test and post-intervention test scores in both groups indicating that both the Jigsaw and didactic lecture methods are effective on the chosen topic. These findings are supported by several previous studies. A study by

Krishnan et al revealed a significant difference in posttest and retention test scores between the two groups. [2] Dat conducted similar studies on two different populations and reported that the mean posttest and retention test scores in both studies were significantly greater in the jigsaw group. [7,8] In a study by Eachempati, there was a significant difference between the jigsaw and didactic groups in the posttest and retention test scores. [6] Sagsoz et al reported a significant difference in the retention scores between the jigsaw and lecture groups, but no significant difference was found in the immediate posttest scores between the two groups. [3] Many studies have compared only the posttest scores, between the jigsaw and lecture methods, and have found statistical significance. [4,5,9–11]

5 CONCLUSION

In the context of dental education, the curriculum has been continuously undergoing reform. There is a need to move from traditional lecture-based lessons to more student-focused methods, which require students to be actively involved in the discussions with their peers, thereby promoting student achievements and interest in learning. The study findings concluded that the Jigsaw method of learning is associated with higher levels of academic performance among students than traditional lecture classes are. It has also created opportunities for active participation and innovative exchange of learning and teaching ideas.

ACKNOWLEDGMENTS

We thank the Head of our department for her recommendation and critical appraisal of the study. We also thank the 3rd-year students for actively participating in the session.

REFERENCES

[1] Kolhekar SP, Alone AS, Bendle SS, Bhasme AS, Bhoge RS, Bhoyar K. (2020). *A Study to Assess the Effectiveness of the Jigsaw Reading Technique in Improving the Reading Skills among High School Children.* JCDR [Internet]. Available from: https://jcdr.net/article_fulltext.asp?issn=0973-709x&year=2020&volume=14&issue=12&page=LC01&issn=0973-709x&id=14303

[2] Krishnan DG, Keloth AV, Ubedulla S, Mohandas P. (2021). *Effectiveness of Jigsaw Active Learning Method in Promoting Knowledge Gain and Retention among Medical Students: A Quasi-experimental Study.* JCDR [Internet]. [cited 2024 Aug 13]; Available from: https://jcdr.net/article_fulltext.asp?issn=0973-709x&year=2021&volume=15&issue=12&page=JC05&issn=0973-709x&id=15779

[3] Sagsoz O, Karatas O, Turel V, Yildiz M, Kaya E. (2017). Effectiveness of Jigsaw learning compared to lecture-based learning in dental education. *Eur J Dent Educ.* 21(1):28–32.

[4] Uppal V, Uppal N. (2020). Flipped jigsaw activity as a small group peer-assisted teaching learning tool in Biochemistry department among indian medical graduate: An experimental study. *Biochem Mol Biol Educ.* 48(4):337–43.

[5] Moin H, Majeed S, Zahra T, Zafar S, Nadeem A, Majeed S. (2024). Assessing the impact of jigsaw technique for cooperative learning in undergraduate medical education: Merits, challenges, and forward prospects. *BMC Medical Education.* 24(1):853.

[6] Eachempati P, KS KK, Ismail. (2017). Cooperative learning through jigsaw classroom. *MedEdPublish.* Available from: https://mededpublish.org/articles/6-88

[7] Tran VD. (2014). The effects of cooperative learning on the academic achievement and knowledge retention. *International Journal of Higher Education.* 3(2):131–40.

[8] Dat TV. (2016). The effects of jigsaw learning on students' knowledge retention in vietnamese higher education. *International Journal of Higher Education.* 5(2):236–53.

[9] Arslan A. (2016). Effect of jigsaw i technique on teaching turkish grammar. *Educational Research and Reviews.* 11(8):635–41.

[10] Kılıç D. (2008). The effect of the jigsaw technique on learning the concepts of the principles and methods of teaching. *World Applied Sciences Journal.* 4:109–14.

[11] Maden S. (2010). The effect of Jigsaw IV on the achievement of course of language teaching methods and techniques. *Educational Research and Reviews.* 5.

Navigating Dental Education Trends and Transforming Dental Pedagogy – Abas and Srikant N (Eds)
© 2027 The Author(s), ISBN: 978-1-041-32674-8

A Novel Innovative Approach by Incorporating ICD-11 Coding in Routine Biopsy Reports and its Comparative Analysis: A Retrospective Study

Eva Rachel Koshy
Department of Oral & Maxillofacial Pathology, Pushpagiri College of Dental Sciences, Thiruvalla, Kerala, India

Reuben Abraham Jacob, Shruti Nayak, and Riaz Abdulla
Department of Oral Pathology & Microbiology, Yenepoya Dental College, Yenepoya (Deemed to be University), Mangalore, Karnataka, India

ABSTRACT: The International Classification of Diseases (ICD), developed by the WHO, provides a common language for the classification of diseases, injuries and causes of death and for the standardized reporting and monitoring of health conditions. This study aimed to assign the International Classification of Diseases, 11th Revision (ICD-11) and Application of the International Classification of Diseases for Dentistry and Stomatology (ICD-DA) codes to oral lesional diagnosis obtained from the archived cases and to study ICD coding's clinical and histopathological correlation and disparity. The ICD-11 and ICD-DA codes were assigned to 250 histopathological diagnoses obtained from archived cases. The results revealed significant differences between the two coding systems, with some uncoded lesions and inconsistencies in coding patterns across different ICD versions. Although the ICD-11 standardizes oral disease classification, it lacks coverage for many histological terms, highlighting the need for a dedicated WHO database for histological diagnoses. Moreover, the ICD-11 can be included in the dental curriculum to develop essential clinical skills and communicate about oral health conditions. It can provide dental students with an understanding of museum archives and career options in medical coding and dental transcription.

Keywords: International Classification of Diseases, Pathology, Biopsy, Dentistry

1 INTRODUCTION

The International Classification of Diseases (ICD) was developed by the WHO. It serves as a global framework for recording, analyzing, and comparing mortality and morbidity data systematically. It offers a common language for standardising the reporting and monitoring of health conditions as well as for classifying illnesses, injuries, and causes of death. [1] The ICD-11 is a digitally updated classification system that has a lot more cases than diseases.

The ICD-11 contains 120,000 clinical terms (and can code millions of terms), thousands of new categories, updated classification schemes, disorders, injuries, external causes, signs and symptoms, substances, medications, anatomy, devices, histopathology, severity, and many more. The ICD converts medical diagnoses from spoken words into an alphanumeric code, making it simple to store, retrieve, and analyse data. Various histological diagnoses of oral lesions are translated by the ICD.[2,3]

The International Classification of Diseases to Dentistry and Stomatology (ICD-DA) provides a practical and convenient basis for the classification and coding of data by all those working in the field of oral and dental disorders, derived from the ICD-10 as a companion volume.[4]

The ICD-11 provides a standardized language and framework for dental students to learn and communicate about oral health conditions. By becoming familiar with the WHO's ICD-11, students can accurately diagnose and classify diseases, ensuring consistency in treatment planning and record-keeping. This standardized system facilitates effective communication and collaboration among dental professionals.

In addition to its role in teaching and learning, the ICD-11 can also be integrated into dental education to enhance students' understanding of museum archives and career options in the field of dentistry. The ICD-11 can also be a valuable tool for dental students considering their careers in medical coding and dental-transcription. By understanding the ICD-11, dental transcriptionists can accurately translate spoken medical information into written documents, ensuring that patient records are complete and accurate.[3]

The purpose of this study was to determine whether any oral lesions are left uncoded in the new ICD-11 classification system and compare it with ICD-DA, thereby aiding in the refinement and evaluation of the ICD-11 classification system.

DOI: 10.1201/9781042016075-20

2 MATERIAL AND METHODS

A total of 250 biopsy reports from a period of one year (January 2023-December 2023) were taken from the archives of the Department of Oral Pathology & Microbiology, Yenepoya Dental College, Mangalore. Reports with a definitive description of the diagnosis were chosen for the study. Incomplete reports and uncertain or ambiguous diagnoses were excluded. The diagnosed lesions were classified into 13 categories for analysis and were assigned codes obtained from the ICD-11 electronic database (https://icd.who.int/en) and the ICD-DA database. A comparative analysis of the ICD-11 codes with the ICD-DA codes was performed.

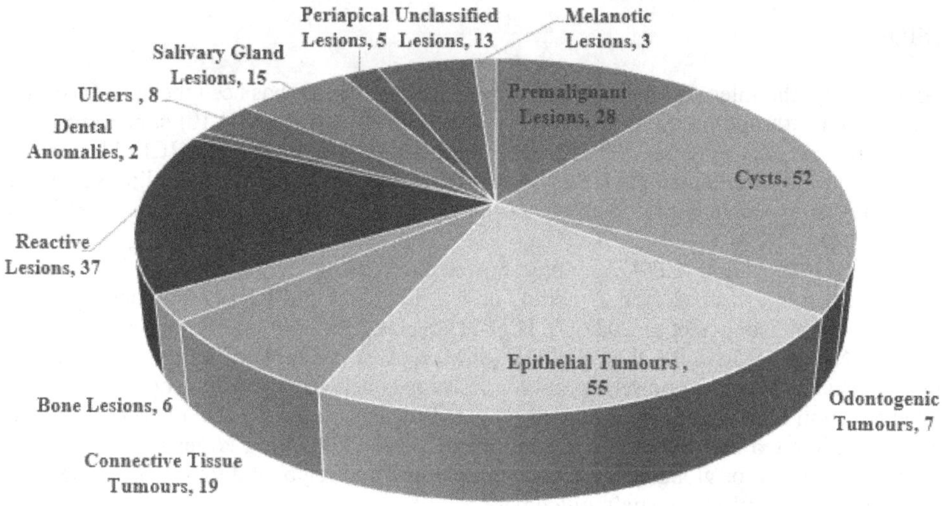

Figure 1. Categories of lesions.

3 RESULTS

Compared with ICD-DA, the integration of ICD-11 coding into routine biopsy reports demonstrated a notable improvement in coding accuracy and comprehensiveness. The biopsy reports were categorized into 13 categories (Figure 1). The results revealed that ICD-11 coding captured more lesions, with a total of 162 coded cases, whereas ICD-DA coded only 130 cases. Notably, ICD-11 coding performed better in categorizing connective tissue tumours (19 vs 16), bone lesions (5 vs 2), and reactive lesions (27 vs 11). This finding suggests that the updated classification scheme for the ICD-11 more accurately captures the intricate details of these lesion types. Premalignant lesions (14 vs. 14), cysts (40 vs. 40), odontogenic tumours (7 vs. 7), and salivary gland lesions (15 vs. 15) were equally coded (Table 1). This finding might suggest that the ICD-DA classification scheme still applies to some types of lesions. However, significant differences in assigned codes were noted in the ICD-11 classification compared with the ICD-DA.

Table 1. Comparison between ICD-11 & ICD-DA.

Type of lesion	ICD-DA		ICD-11	
	Coded	Non-coded	Coded	Non-coded
Premalignant Lesions	14	14	14	14
Cysts	40	12	40	12
Odontogenic Tumours	7	0	7	0
Epithelial Tumours	18	37	19	36
Connective Tissue Tumours	16	3	19	0
Bone Lesions	2	4	5	1
Reactive Lesions	11	26	27	10
Dental Anomalies	1	1	1	1
Ulcers	6	2	6	2
Salivary Gland Lesions	15	0	15	0
Periapical Lesions	0	5	5	0
Unclassified Lesions	0	13	1	12
Melanotic Lesions	0	3	3	0
Total	**130**	**120**	**162**	**88**

The greater number of noncoded cases in the ICD-DA (88) than in the ICD-11 (20) highlights the limitations of the older classification system. The more comprehensive and updated coding structure of the ICD-11 allows for more accurate and detailed reporting of lesion types.

The presence of unclassified lesions in both systems suggests that there is still room for improvement in lesion classification and coding. ICD-11's compatibility with electronic health records also plays a role in supporting data sharing and interoperability, allowing healthcare providers to access and use data more effectively across different care settings. This can lead to better data tracking, research, and patient care.[4]

Further studies can explore the long-term benefits and potential refinements of ICD-11 coding in biopsy reporting.

4 DISCUSSION

For more than a century, the International Classification of Diseases (ICD) has been the main basis for comparable statistics on causes of death and nonfatal diseases. [1] The Tenth Revision (ICD-10) came into effect in January 1993; it consists of three separate volumes. The WHO published the latest version, the ICD-11, which was officially adopted in May 2019 by all WHO member states for recording and reporting causes of illness and death. [2,3] The ICD-DA is one of several manuals that were developed by the Oral Health Unit of the WHO, Geneva, in its epidemiology subprogram [5] [6].

In the present study, ICD-11 and ICD-DA coding showed marked differences, and some histological lesions were left uncoded. A similar trend was observed in a study in which ICD-11 and ICD-O, an oncology derivation of the ICD-10, were compared (Yicong X et al, 2022)[7]. ICD-11 involves the addition of more parameters that were not included in earlier versions (Harrison J E et al, 2021).[8] Moreover, the implementation of extension codes in the ICD-11 coding system has become a powerful tool for assisting coders in generating code clusters and guiding the postcoordinated selection of relevant extension codes related to a stem code clinical concept.[9] The present study was conducted with a limited number of cases; a more extensive study with a larger sample size would be more effective. The ICD-11 aims to be globally applicable, but cultural and regional differences in disease manifestation and diagnostic practices can affect the study outcomes.

5 CONCLUSION

This study highlights the advantages of integrating ICD-11 coding into routine biopsy reports, with notable improvements in coding accuracy, detail, and comprehensiveness compared to ICD-DA. The results demonstrate ICD-11's ability to capture a broader range of oral lesions, particularly for connective tissue tumours, bone lesions, and reactive lesions. The significant reduction in non-coded cases with ICD-11 underscores its enhanced capacity for detailed classification. However, the presence of unclassified lesions in both systems suggests ongoing opportunities for refinement.

The compatibility of ICD-11 with electronic health records also offers considerable benefits in data sharing, improving access across various healthcare settings. These findings emphasize that ICD-11 could support more robust data tracking, patient care, and research outcomes. Further studies may explore the long-term impact and potential refinements of ICD-11 coding in oral pathology to ensure comprehensive and precise documentation across diverse lesion types.

ABBREVIATIONS

WHO: World Health Organization; ICD: International Classification of Diseases; ICD10: International Classification of Diseases, 10th revision; ICD-11: International Classification of Diseases, 11th revision; ICD-DA: Application of the International Classification of Diseases to Dentistry and Stomatology; ICD-O: International Classification of Diseases for Oncology

ACKNOWLEDGMENT

Nil

REFERENCES

[1] World Health Organization. (2022). *Classification of Diseases [Internet]*. Geneva, Switzerland: World Health Organization; [cited 2024 July 26].Available from: International Classification of Diseases (ICD) (who.int)

[2] World Health Organization. (no date) *ICD-11 Reference Guide [Internet].* Geneva, Switzerland: World Health Organization; [cited 2024 July 26]. Available from: ICD-11 Reference Guide (who.int)

[3] World Health Organization. (2023). *ICD-11 Implementation or Transition Guide [Internet].* Geneva, Switzerland: World Health Organization; [cited 2024 July 26]. Available from: ICD-11 Implementation and Transition Guide_Draft_v105.edited.pages (who. int)

[4] CareCloud. (2023).*Navigating the Transition to ICD-11: Benefits and Challenges [Internet].* 2023 [cited 2024 Nov 14]. Available from: https://www.carecloud.com/continuum/navigating-the-transition-to-icd-11-benefits-and-challenges/

[5] Bezroukov V. (1979). The application of the international classification of diseases to dentistry and stomatology. *Community Dentistry and Oral Epidemiology*. 7(1):21–4.

[6] World Health Organization. (2018). *International Classification of Diseases (ICD-11) [Internet].* Geneva, Switzerland: World Health Organization. [cited 2024 Aug 27]. Available from: Application of the international classification of diseases to dentistry and stomatology (who.int)

[7] Yicong X, Jingya Z, Yi W. (2022). The novel and powerful ICD-11 classification system for neoplasm coding: a comparative study with the ICD-O. *BMC Medical Informatics and Decision Making (Web)*. 22(1):1–8.

[8] Harrison JE, Weber S, Jakob R, Chute CG. (2021). ICD-11: An international classification of diseases for the twenty-first century. *BMC Medical Informatics and Decision Making*. 21:206.

[9] Stefanie W. (2021). ICD-11 extension codes support detailed clinical abstraction and comprehensive classification. *BMC Medical Informatics and Decision Making (Web)*. 21(6):1–9.

 ISBN: 978-1-041-32674-8

Emerging Trends and Challenges in Dental Curriculum: Navigating New Horizons

Neetha Shenoy, Sandya Kini, and Shashirashmi Acharya
Department of Conservative Dentistry and Endodontics, Manipal College of Dental Sciences, Manipal

ABSTRACT: **Objective:** To evaluate the integration of advanced technologies and innovative pedagogical strategies in dental education, focusing on their impact on student engagement, skill development, and educational outcomes.

Rationale: The field of dentistry is undergoing significant transformation due to technological advancements and the need for adaptive teaching methods. These developments address challenges in traditional dental education, including limited hands-on practice, variability in learning styles, and the demand for precision in diagnostics and treatment.

Approach: This review explores the incorporation of cutting-edge technologies such as AI-powered adaptive learning platforms, which personalize educational content using quizzes and interactive modules tailored to individual progress. Additionally, AI applications for diagnostic training provide instant feedback on x-ray analysis, enhancing diagnostic accuracy. The use of AI-driven virtual reality (VR) and augmented reality (AR) is also assessed, particularly their role in creating immersive 3D models of dental anatomy and simulated clinical environments for practicing procedures and interacting with virtual patients.

Conclusion: The integration of advanced technologies and modern pedagogical approaches is transforming dental education, offering promising solutions to current challenges. These innovations enhance student engagement, practical skills, and learning outcomes, underscoring their effectiveness in improving the quality of dental training.

Keywords: Adaptive Learning Platforms, Artificial Intelligence (AI), Virtual Reality (VR), Augmented Reality (AR), Dental Curriculum

1 INTRODUCTION

The field of dentistry is rapidly evolving with advancements in technology and pedagogical approaches. Emerging trends in dental education are increasingly centered around the integration of advanced technologies to enhance learning and skill development [1]. Adaptive learning platforms are at the forefront, utilizing AI algorithms to customize educational content based on individual progress and learning styles, thereby providing personalized quizzes and interactive modules. Concurrently, AI applications are revolutionizing diagnostic training by analyzing images like x-rays and offering instant feedback to improve students' diagnostic accuracy. Additionally, AI-driven virtual reality (VR) and augmented reality (AR) technologies are transforming traditional methods by offering immersive 3D models of dental anatomy and simulated clinical environments, enabling students to practice procedures and interact with virtual patients in a dynamic and engaging way [2,3]. These innovations collectively contribute to a more effective and personalized educational experience, preparing students for the complexities of modern dental practice. This review aims to explore the integration of innovative technologies and educational methods in dental education into dental curricula, with a focus on their impact on student engagement, practical skills, and educational outcomes. The significance of this topic lies in understanding how these innovations can address current challenges in dental education and improve the overall quality of training.

2 METHODS

To conduct this review, a comprehensive search of the literature was performed using several academic databases, including PubMed, Scopus, and Google Scholar. The search terms included key words such as VR, AR, 3D printing, active learning, and simulation in dental education. Studies were selected based on their relevance to the topic, methodological rigor, and publication date, with a focus on articles published within the last decade (2013–2023) to ensure the inclusion of the most recent and relevant findings. Inclusion criteria involved peer-reviewed articles, reviews, and case studies that discussed the application and impact of these innovations in dental education. Exclusion criteria encompassed studies outside the specified scope or lacking empirical data.

 DOI: 10.1201/9781042016075-21

3 RESULTS

The review revealed several key findings regarding the integration of innovative technologies and methods in dental education:

(1) **Technological Integration:** VR and AR technologies have been shown to enhance students' spatial understanding and procedural skills by providing immersive, interactive learning experiences. 3D printing has facilitated hands-on practice with realistic dental models and prosthetics [2].
(2) **Active Learning**: Problem-Based Learning (PBL) and Team-Based Learning (TBL) are increasingly used to foster critical thinking and collaborative skills. The flipped classroom model encourages deeper understanding by reversing traditional teaching methods, allowing more time for practical application during class [4].
(3) **Simulation-Based Training:** Advanced simulators and Objective Structured Clinical Examinations (OSCEs) have become essential for providing realistic practice opportunities and assessing clinical competencies [3].
(4) **Interprofessional Education (IPE):**

Simulation-based scenarios involving collaboration with other healthcare professionals are promoting a holistic, patient-centered approach to care [5].

Table 1. Summary of findings.

Innovation/Method	Benefits	Challenges
Virtual Reality (VR) and Augmented Reality (AR)	Enhanced spatial understanding, improved procedural skills	High cost, need for technical support
3D Printing	Realistic models for hands-on practice	Requires significant investment in equipment and training
PBL/TBL	Encourages critical thinking, fosters teamwork	Demands extensive curriculum redesign and faculty training
Flipped Classroom	Promotes deeper learning and practical application	Needs effective pre-class content delivery and student buy-in
Simulation-Based Training	Realistic practice, effective assessment of clinical skills	Requires high-fidelity equipment and robust infrastructure
IPE	Enhances collaboration and patient-centered care	Complexity in coordinating interdisciplinary activities

4 DISCUSSION

The integration of virtual and augmented reality, 3D printing, and active learning methodologies into dental education represents a significant shift towards more engaging and effective learning environments. These cutting-edge technologies are ushering in a new era of dental training and patient care, gaining recognition for their ability to enhance both learning experiences and clinical outcomes [6]. Pulijala *et al.* [7] compared the traditional training methods using PowerPoint presentations versus immersive virtual reality (iVR) via Oculus Rift and Leap Motion devices for surgical training. The study highlights the potential of VR technologies to enhance surgical training by offering a realistic and immersive environment that improves learning, boosts self-confidence, and better prepares trainees for real surgical procedures. Casap *et al.* [8] highlighted the need of balanced approach combining traditional and innovative methods such as VR to maximize training effectiveness and efficiency.

In dental education, the flipped classroom model can be integrated by having students review online materials, such as recorded lectures or interactive modules, before attending in-person sessions. This preparatory work allows students to familiarize themselves with foundational concepts, enabling face-to-face time to focus on active learning through discussions, case-based problem solving, and hands-on activities like simulations or clinical exercises. By priming students with relevant background knowledge, the flipped approach enhances their understanding and application of complex dental procedures, improving their clinical reasoning, manual dexterity, and confidence in practical settings. [9]

Inter professional Education (IPE) plays a pivotal role in preparing future dentists to collaborate effectively within multidisciplinary healthcare teams, ensuring holistic patient care. Dentistry is inherently connected to overall health, with oral health influencing and being influenced by systemic conditions such as diabetes, cardiovascular disease, and more. [10] IPE enables dental students to understand the roles of other healthcare professionals, such as physicians, pharmacists, nurses, and dietitians, fostering communication and teamwork skills essential for coordinated care. By learning alongside peers from other disciplines, dental students develop a comprehensive perspective on patient care, improve their ability to address complex cases, and contribute to better health outcomes, aligning oral health with broader public health priorities. [11]

4.1 *Challenges*

Adapting innovative technologies like Virtual Reality (VR), Augmented Reality (AR), 3D printing, and Inter professional Education (IPE) in dental education presents several challenges, including the high cost of acquiring and maintaining advanced equipment and software, which can strain institutional budgets. Additionally, the integration of these technologies requires significant faculty development to ensure instructors are proficient in their use and capable of leveraging them effectively for teaching. Robust infrastructure, including reliable internet access, specialized facilities, and technical support, is essential but often lacking in many educational settings. Furthermore, the incorporation of IPE demands careful coordination across disciplines, curriculum alignment, and overcoming logistical barriers such as scheduling conflicts. These obstacles highlight the need for strategic planning, resource allocation, and institutional commitment to maximize the potential of these innovations in enhancing dental education. [12].

Table 2. Appropriate BDS year to introduce each of the specified techniques.

Technique	BDS Year	Justification
Virtual Reality (VR) and Augmented Reality (AR)	2nd Year	VR/AR provides immersive learning for anatomy and basic dental procedures, enabling safe practice and skill development without involving patients.
3D Printing	2nd Year & Internship	Introduce basics in the 2nd year for creating models and understanding the process. Advanced applications like surgical guides can be practiced during the internship.
Problem-Based Learning (PBL) / Team-Based Learning (TBL)	1st Year onwards	Early introduction develops critical thinking, collaboration, and problem-solving skills that are essential throughout the curriculum.
Flipped Classroom	1st Year onwards	This method encourages self-directed learning and active participation, ideal for foundational courses and progressively more complex topics.
Simulation-Based Training	1st Year onwards	Early exposure to simulation builds manual dexterity and confidence, gradually progressing to more advanced simulations in higher years.
Interprofessional Education (IPE)	4th Year & Internship	Introduced later when students are more proficient, enabling collaborative learning with other healthcare disciplines to enhance teamwork and holistic care.

4.2 *Clinical implications*

The integration of technologies like VR, AR, 3D printing, and IPE in dental education has significant clinical implications, as these tools enhance students' practical skills, clinical decision-making, and ability to work collaboratively in multidisciplinary teams. By simulating real-world scenarios and enabling hands-on practice in a controlled environment, these innovations better prepare students for the complexities of clinical practice, improving patient safety and care outcomes [13]. However, addressing the associated challenges is crucial to fully realize these benefits and ensure equitable access to advanced training across educational institutions.

4.3 *Future research directions*

Future research should focus on longitudinal studies to evaluate the long-term impact of these innovations on dental practice outcomes. Investigating cost-effective solutions for implementing new technologies and developing best practices for faculty training and curriculum integration will be crucial. Additionally, exploring the effectiveness of combining multiple innovative approaches in a cohesive educational framework could provide valuable insights [9–13].

5 CONCLUSION

This review underscores the transformative potential of VR/AR, 3D printing, and active learning methodologies in dental education. By enhancing student engagement and practical skills, these innovations promise to improve the quality of dental training. Addressing the identified challenges and gaps is essential for maximizing the benefits of these advancements. Future research should continue to explore and refine these approaches to ensure they effectively contribute to the development of proficient and well-prepared dental professionals.

ACKNOWLEDGMENTS

The authors would like to thank the team ICDECC 6.0 for encouragement and support.

REFERENCES

[1] Spielman AI. (2024). Dental education and practice: past, present, and future trends. *Front Oral Health.* 5:1368121.

[2] Kwon HB, Park YS, Han JS. (2018). Augmented reality in dentistry: a current perspective. *Acta Odontologica Scandinavica.* 76 (7):497–503.

[3] Li Y, Ye H, Ye F, Liu Y, Lv L, Zhang P, *et al.* (2021). The current situation and future prospects of simulators in dental education. *J Med Internet Res.* 2021;23(4):e23635.

[4] Lin GS, Tan WW, Tan HJ, Khoo CW, Afrashtehfar KI. (2023). Innovative pedagogical strategies in health professions education: active learning in dental materials science. *International Journal of Environmental Research and Public Health.* 20(3):2041.

[5] Hallas D, Fernandez JB, Herman NG, Moursi A. (2015). Identification of pediatric oral health core competencies through interprofessional education and practice. *Nursing Research and Practice.* 2015(1):360523.

[6] Zheng M, Bender D, Nadershahi N. (2017). Faculty professional development in emergent pedagogies for instructional innovation in dental education. *European Journal of Dental Education.* 21(2):67–78.

[7] Pulijala Y, Ma M, Pears M, Peebles D, Ayoub A. (2018). Effectiveness of immersive virtual reality in surgical training—a randomized control trial. *Journal of Oral and Maxillofacial Surgery.* 76(5):1065–72.

[8] Casap N, Nadel S, Tarazi E, Weiss EI. (2011). Evaluation of a navigation system for dental implantation as a tool to train novice dental practitioners. *Journal of Oral and Maxillofacial Surgery.* 69(10):2548–56.

[9] Vanka A, Vanka S, Wali O. (2020). Flipped classroom in dental education: A scoping review. *European Journal of Dental Education.* 24(2):213–26.

[10] Olsson TO, Dalmoro M, da Costa MV, Peduzzi M, Toassi RF. (2022). Interprofessional education in the dentistry curriculum: analysis of a teaching-service-community integration experience. *European Journal of Dental Education.* 26(1):174–81.

[11] Coleman AJ, Finn GM, Nattress BR. (2018). Interprofessional education in dentistry. *British Dental Journal.* 225(3):257–62.

[12] Walker MP, Duley SI, Beach MM, Deem L, Pileggi R, Samet N, Segura A, Williams JN. (2008). Dental education economics: challenges and innovative strategies. *Journal of Dental Education.* 72(12):1440–9.

[13] Ghassan A, Shukr I, Sadiq N, Ahsan R. (2021). Current trends in dental education. *Pakistan Armed Forces Medical Journal.* 71 (3):1107–3.

 ISBN: 978-1-041-32674-8

Engage or Enrage? The Double-edged Sword of Games in Learning

Jessica Sonal Monteiro, Charisma Thimmaiah, and Arathi Rao
Department of Pediatric and Preventive Dentistry, Manipal College of Dental Sciences Mangalore, Manipal Academy of Higher Education, Manipal, India

ABSTRACT: **Purpose**: Playing is more than just fun, it ignites curiosity, powers skill-building and entwines motivation into learning. In today's digital world, games have become a key educational tool, leaderboards, badges and points are elements that are utilized to boost motivation and participation. Nevertheless, there are certain drawbacks to this, such as high levels of stress, self-confidence, and quality of education, which calls for a more thorough investigation of how it affects learning results. This review explores how games in learning affects learning objectives

Methods: A search strategy was applied across databases such as PubMed, Scopus and Google scholar. Keywords like "game-based learning", "gamification", "gamification AND education", and "gamification AND learning outcomes was utilized. Manual screening to discover appropriate studies, reviews and conference papers followed this.

Results: The findings show a paradox in gamification's influence on education, with research noting both favorable and adverse outcomes. Although gamification can improve inspiration, learning efficacy and participation, it also has possible downsides such as increased anxiety, surface level knowledge and cognitive strain, implying that its benefits are highly context-sensitive.

Conclusion: Researchers and academics must carefully weigh intrinsic and extrinsic intent, versatility of gamification mechanisms, and the psychological repercussions for students. Only through such thoughtful and subtle integration can gamification be transformed into a potent vehicle for realistic educational change instead of a fleeting trend that distracts more than it educates.

Keywords: dental education, innovative teaching, gamification, game based learning

1 INTRODUCTION

Every day, we find ourselves grappling with a myriad of tasks, racing against time, and competing not only with ourselves but also with the relentless march of technology. From dawn to dusk our screens dominate, and much of our work and daily routines have become gamified. Game-based learning adopts games as educational tools whereas gamification involves integrating game design elements into non-game contexts [1], subtly altering behavior of the user. Over the past few years, gamifying education has emerged as a trendsetter among researchers and academics.

Games are celebrated for their ability to captivate, engage and entertain, tapping into the intrinsic human drives of competence, immersion and mastery [2]. From the addictive appeal of Candy Crush to the strategic allure of Clash of Clans, digital games have become a ubiquitous part of our everyday life, transcending age and demographic boundaries. While the use of games in education is not new, gamification remains a relatively young concept [3], typically characterized by fragmented knowledge and limited quantifiable evidence. The true potential lies in understanding the concept intricately to achieve optimal outcomes.

Badges, rewards and scores are some design elements that align student behavior with intended learning objectives. This increased integration has sparked both enthusiasm and skepticism. While some studies showcase that gamification excites and engages students, others reveal a darker side: heightened anxiety, cognitive load and demotivation [2,4]. This review critically examines existing literature, dissecting the double-edged nature of gamification to understand when it serves as a win or a loss.

2 METHODS

A comprehensive search strategy was undertaken across databases PubMed, Scopus and Google scholar. Keywords like "game-based learning", "gamification", "gamification AND education", and "gamification AND learning outcomes was utilized. A manual screening to discover appropriate studies, reviews and conference papers followed this. To ensure the applicability, inclusion criteria was meticulously chosen to include papers published in English

 DOI: 10.1201/9781042016075-22

that particularly investigated the usage of gamification in educational contexts. Given the intricate connection between gamification and information technologies, suitable research from this domain were added. The search was narrowed with an emphasis on the type of results recorded. Conversely, studies exploring gamification outside the realm of education, such as those in marketing and business management, were excluded, as they did not align with educational objectives. Additionally, studies published in languages other than English were omitted to maintain ease in data interpretation.

3 RESULTS

In education, gamification is used more intuitively to promote learning and are often structured to facilitate the practice of skills [2]. Gamification incorporates key elements into systems to achieve psychological or behavioral outcomes via affordances [3]. Affordances in this context refer to the various components within games that foster gameful experiences. The experiences often include a sense of freedom, familiarity, enjoyment and engagement. Consequently, the behavioral outcomes may include increased physical activity or enhanced learning in educational setups. In addition, gamification can also result in negative outcomes. The highly competitive environment can increase the cognitive strain on students; this can further lead to superficial learning of the subject. The Figure (1) illustrates the positive and negative outcomes of gamification as a pedagogical approach in learning. (Figure 1)

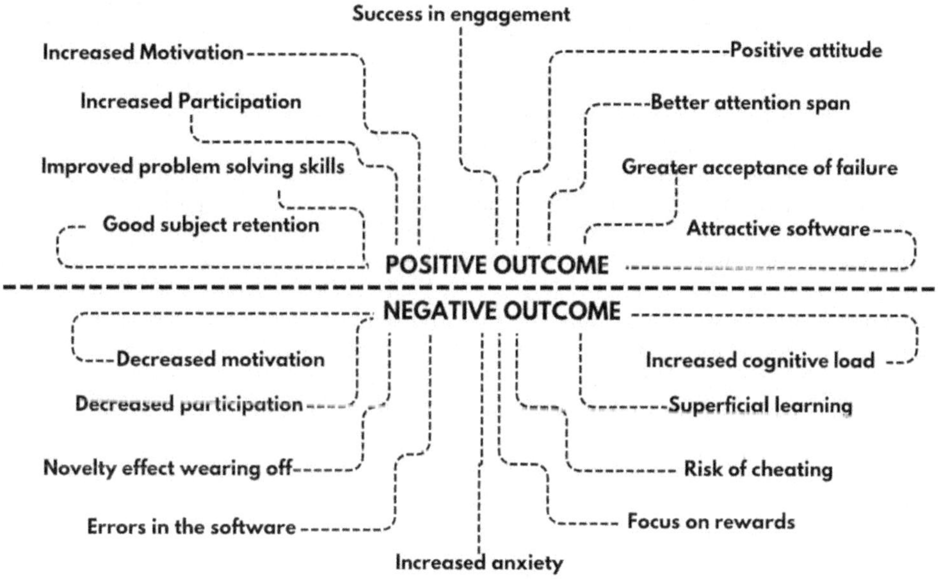

Figure 1. A schematic diagram outlining the dual nature of games in learning.

The dichotomy of gamification's impact: its ability to both engage and enrage, stems from its core design principles and the different ways in which students interact with these elements. The increase in motivation and participation, positive attitude towards learning, better attention span and recall of the subject are some of the positive outcomes. In contrast, cognitive strain, increased anxiety, lack of deeper learning and software errors are negative aspects that can hamper gamified learning.

4 POSITIVE OUTCOMES

Based on studies, gamification can be used to provide positive reinforcement and to ensure that students achieve the intended learning outcome. Games enable individuals to enhance their problem-solving skills by spending lots of time playing it. Studies have also demonstrated that gamification promotes motivation, participation and increases learning level [3,5]. In a study conducted on university students, an online application was developed which showed an increase in participation [6]. Students showed a positive attitude towards gamification and suggested that as a frequent teaching method. A systematic review indicated that the use of combined game elements generally had a positive impact on learning outcomes[7]. The involvement of students in a competitive class environment and the opportunity to win rewards boosted their attention span and positively affected their learning [7,8]. A review of 41 studies revealed that 12 demonstrated conclusive evidence of positive outcomes, including improved learning, increased motivation, greater participation, enhanced engagement, better time management, and superior learning simulations [9].

In another study, a mobile web application was developed, with an intervention and control group set up over two consecutive years. The first year saw significant learning success, with the intervention group using the game app, outperforming the control group. The game app notably improved student learning compared to traditional methods [10]. Another good example is AntibioGame®, a serious game intended as a novel educational tool that mimics real-world medical events in an enjoyable and informative manner. It is claimed to have a major impact on the comprehension of antibiotic use. It has also been linked to increased student interaction and better information recall [11].

5 NEGATIVE OUTCOMES

Studies have found a negative association between ages and simplicity of use of gamified applications, implying that mature learners might have trouble with these tools [8]. Three of the 41 research reviewed had negative findings, including no impact on test scores, less autonomy, and more grave degrees of contentment.The competitive characteristic of gamification can create psychological concerns such as raised stress and anxiety because of the obligation to achieve superior scores. This increased fret, which is connected to efficiency, might divert intellectual energy, reducing a student's concentration. The cognitive strain, when coupled with intense demands, may cause lowered concentration and increased mental effort [9].

AntibioGame® also identified significant drawbacks. Design features like scoreboards and points can cause students to be more anxious and shift their focus from learning to winning. This method of teaching may promote superficial learning where students memorize the answers instead of understanding the material thoroughly. The demand to stay ahead might aggravate students with varying learning paces and impair their grasp of real-life scenarios [11]. Hanus *et al.* (2015) investigated the effects of gamification on student involvement and academic success over a 16-week period, discovering that students in gamified programs had poorer drive, fulfilment, and accomplishment than those enrolled in standard courses [12].

A comprehensive analysis of the negative consequences of gamification identified numerous recurring difficulties, notably a lack of impact, poor performance, comprehension, and ambition. Ethical obstacles, such as cheating caused by technology defects or fiercely competitive conditions, were regularly mentioned. The competitive atmosphere of gamification can additionally deter students who despise competing or find themselves lagging, causing them to drop out instead of striving for progress. Non-gamers described perceptions of estrangement, apprehension and aggravation. Another possible limitation is the "novelty effect," which occurs when initial excitement for gamified learning fades gradually, reducing its beneficial impact. Teaching professionals and programmers confront substantial hurdles, such as system maintenance, software reliability issues, and expenditure—all of which contribute to the burden and difficulty of incorporating gamification into education [13].

A study assessing gamified training management systems to traditional strategies discovered that, while gamification elevated participation, those trained in traditional settings performed better, which the researchers credited to their acquaintance and ease with conventional strategies [14].

A literature review of 20 papers found that while adaptive gamification can enhance learning experiences, its effects might not be universally sustained. The novelty effect, inconsistencies in measuring motivation, and varying benefits for different learners were highlighted. Many studies relied on feedback tools that may not accurately capture the depth of student engagement. Moreover, educators' over-reliance on gamification for its ability to boost participation might overshadow other critical pedagogical strategies, potentially leading to a superficial understanding of course material [15].

6 DISCUSSION

The allure of gamification lies in its promise to make learning fun and rewarding but the unintended consequences can be equally powerful. A framework commonly used to understand motivation is the self-determination theory, according to which human motivation is intrinsically or extrinsically motivated. Gamification often aims to leverage intrinsic motivators such as autonomy, mastery and relatedness. When learners perceive game-based rewards as obligatory, their intrinsic motivation diminishes. Instead of engaging with the content for its own sake, students may begin to focus solely on external rewards, which can detract from deep learning. This can be detrimental in educational environments when proficiency and comprehension are the primary objectives. If students become overly focused on their gaming skills rather than learning goals, they may acquire an operational outlook, about education as a means of collecting rewards rather than acquiring wisdom [2]. Furthermore, individual variables between learners, such as type of motivation and gaming experiences complicate the assessment of gamifications efficacy. According to studies not all learners connect with gamified content in the same manner; some might find it stimulating while others may encounter a cognitive overload or heightened anxiety especially in a competitive set up [4]. Research frequently discusses the disparity of gamification's role in academic performance.

Domínguez (2013) found no significant effect on student achievement among university students, highlighting that not all gamified interventions lead to improved performances [6]. An evaluation of 41 study results indicated that 26 had unreliable results, which were frequently prompted by systematic faults such as short study durations, limited number of samples, and the absence of controls [9]. Hanus *et al.*, (2015) discovered that gamified programs led to lesser motivation, performance and enjoyment than traditional teaching. This implies that the initial appeal of gamification may wear off and external factors may impede learning [12]. A rigorous mapping of negative consequences highlighted difficulties such as inadequate achievement, moral concerns such as cheating and individuals distaste of competition, all of which could cause dissociation. Researchers also face challenges with generalization and correlation because some studies employ qualitative approaches whereas others depend on quantitative indicators [13].

Additionally, a review of the literature on adaptive gamification found that less extensive trials have greater favorable implications than larger research, which frequently yields ambiguous outcomes [15]. This implies that, while gamification's initial appeal can increase involvement, the novelty impact may wane over time, and long-term advantages cannot be ensured. The inconsistent results in studies can be associated to the varying assessment techniques, like the use of surveys against statistical participation rates [15]. Future research should focus on longitudinal studies to understand the long-term effects of gamification, particularly as the novelty effect wears off. Employing, mixed methods approaches that combine qualitative insights with quantitative data can offer a more comprehensive understanding of learner motivation. Standardized surveys built on well-known frameworks—like the Hexad player types—might be able to classify students based on their psychological traits and reveal the ways in which distinct gamification components affect different learner types [15].

7 CONCLUSIONS

The investigation of gamification in educational settings reveals a multifaceted environment where games have the potential to both engage and enrage students, serving as a double-edged sword. Although gamification has great potential as a teaching aid, the state of the research suggests that its implementation should be treated cautiously. There are many benefits to using it, such as greater motivation, engagement, and tailored learning experiences, but there are also serious concerns, such as increased anxiety, cognitive overload, and learning outcomes that are shallow. A few key criteria that impact the effectiveness of gamification are the length of the research, the heterogeneity of each learner, and the type of gamified features used. To prove the educational advantages of gamification, the field needs longer, more controlled trials, well-defined control groups, and more conceptually driven research. There is no one-size-fits-all approach when it comes to gamification efficacy; it significantly hinges on the learner, the environment, and the careful incorporation of incentive components. The harmony between intrinsic and extrinsic motives, the versatility of gamification systems, and the psychological effects on students are all important factors educators and researchers need to consider. Only through such thoughtful and subtle integration can gamification be transformed into a potent vehicle for realistic educational change instead of a fleeting trend that distracts more than it educates.

ACKNOWLEDGEMENTS

Nil.

REFERENCES

[1] Caponetto I, Earp J, Ott M. (2014). Gamification and education: A literature review. In *European Conference on Games Based Learning* (Vol. 1, p. 50). Academic Conferences International Limited.

[2] Koivisto J, Hamari J. (2019). The rise of motivational information systems: A review of gamification research. *International Journal of Information Management*. 45:191–210.

[3] Hamari J, Koivisto J, Sarsa H. (2014). Does gamification work?–a literature review of empirical studies on gamification. In *2014 47th Hawaii International Conference on System Sciences* (pp. 3025–3034). IEEE.

[4] Turan Z, Avinc Z, Kara K, Göktas Y. (2016). Gamification and Education: Achievements, cognitive loads, and views of students. *Int. J. Emerg. Technol. Learn.*. 11(7):64–9.

[5] Cheong C, Cheong F, Filippou J. Quick quiz: A gamified approach for enhancing learning.

[6] Domínguez A, Saenz-de-Navarrete J, De-Marcos L, Fernández-Sanz L, Pagés C, Martínez-Herráiz JJ. (2013). Gamifying learning experiences: Practical implications and outcomes. *Computers & Education*. 63:380–92.

[7] van Gaalen AE, Brouwer J, Schönrock-Adema J, Bouwkamp-Timmer T, Jaarsma AD, Georgiadis JR. (2021). Gamification of health professions education: A systematic review. *Advances in Health Sciences Education*. 26(2):683–711.

[8] Koivisto J, Hamari J. (2014). Demographic differences in perceived benefits from gamification. *Computers in Human Behavior*. 35:179–88.

[9] Dichev C, Dicheva D. (2017). Gamifying education: what is known, what is believed and what remains uncertain: a critical review. *International Journal of Educational Technology in Higher Education.* 14:1–36.

[10] Lemos M, Wolfart S, Rittich AB. (2023). Assessment and evaluation of a serious game for teaching factual knowledge in dental education. *BMC Medical Education.* 23(1):521.

[11] Tsopra R, Courtine M, Sedki K, Eap D, Cabal M, Cohen S, Bouchaud O, Mechaï F, Lamy JB. AntibioGame®: A serious game for teaching medical students about antibiotic use. *International Journal of Medical Informatics.* 136:104074.

[12] Hanus MD, Fox J. (2015). Assessing the effects of gamification in the classroom: A longitudinal study on intrinsic motivation, social comparison, satisfaction, effort, and academic performance. *Computers & Education.* 80:152–61.

[13] Almeida C, Kalinowski M, Uchôa A, Feijó B. (2023). Negative effects of gamification in education software: Systematic mapping and practitioner perceptions. *Information and Software Technology.* 156:107142.

[14] De-Marcos L, Domínguez A, Saenz-de-Navarrete J, Pagés C. (2014). An empirical study comparing gamification and social networking on e-learning. *Computers & Education.* 75:82–91.

[15] Hallifax S, Serna A, Marty JC, Lavoué É. (2019). Adaptive gamification in education: A literature review of current trends and developments. In *Transforming Learning with Meaningful Technologies: 14th European Conference on Technology Enhanced Learning*, EC-TEL 2019, Delft, The Netherlands, September 16–19, 2019, Proceedings 14 (pp. 294–307). Springer International Publishing.

Leveraging Mind Maps in Dental Education: A Pathway to Better Learning

M Chaithra and P Anupama Nayak
Department of Pediatric and Preventive Dentistry, Manipal College of Dental Sciences Mangalore, Manipal Academy of Higher Education, Manipal, India

1 INTRODUCTION ADDED IN A CONCISE MANNER

The use of numerous supplementary resources, such as charts and models, has replaced teacher-centered and blackboard instruction in the education system. Most of the time, kids memorize the data rather than comprehending the concept. The primary objective of today's educational system is to develop the student's ability to access information rather than only imparting it. Despite the abundance of instructional strategies available, students still struggle greatly with organizing and remembering the material they have learned. [1]

Step A, B, C, and so on is the typical sequence in which we teach at dental school, and this is how students prefer to study. The issues and connections in the health sciences are not linear, despite the fact that this is the "easier" method of instruction. Teachers may be able to better understand how students conceive the connections between technological processes and biologic outcomes—a topic that can be challenging for students to grasp—by using mind maps. [2]

British psychologist Buzan T first coined the term "mind mapping" at the close of the 1960s. Since its beginnings, it has been applied in a variety of ways across learning streams to develop and produce positive outcomes. Mind mapping is a very valuable learning tool that students should get familiar with and utilize often. This strategy helps people "organize facts and thoughts." [3] Concept mapping is a visual approach that asks students to reflect on how well they grasp a subject and how the many components of that understanding fit together. [4]

2 METHOD HAS BEEN ELABORATED

Widespread electronic search was performed across several databases, including PubMed and Google Scholar to identify pertinent articles published. The search utilized a range of key words such as "dentistry, dental education and mind map" respectively. Boolean operators such as 'AND' and 'OR' were employed to refine the search within each database.

Studies were selected based on their relevance to dental education and were limited to those involving dental students or educators. Dental and medical education system were the inclusion criteria. Non-dental and general population were excluded.

More evidences added A study conducted by Grazziotin *et al.* thirteen second-year students were instructed to create a mind map on root canal cleaning and shaping. Eighteen weeks later, they were asked to create another mind map about root canal obturation. Faculty used a qualitative method—a multi-layered theme analysis process—to visually examine the mind maps. To find out if students could articulate relevant and fact-based thoughts on the subjects (accuracy of relationships and depth of material offered), codes and themes were developed. For every task, two of the mind maps with the highest and two with the lowest grades were directly compared. The identical student's progress from the first to the second mind map was also assessed using originality and trend/style. They concluded that the students with various learning styles can benefit from the use of mind maps in dentistry education, and the teacher can use them to determine the degree of conceptualization a student has formed on a given topic. [2]

REFERENCES

[1] Lamba G. MIND mapping–a learning strategy to acquire knowledge. *Dental Education Technology*. 7.

[2] Grazziotin-Soares R, Curtis DA, Ardenghi DM. (2021). Use of mind maps in dental education: An activity performed in a preclinical endodontic course. *Journal of Dental Education*. 85(5):623–33.

DOI: 10.1201/9781042016075-23

[3] Muchhal M, Patthi B, Singla A, Gupta R, Malhi R, Chaudhary D. (2018). Effectiveness of mind mapping as a learning tool among dental students. *Journal of Indian Association of Public Health Dentistry*. 16(2):122–6.

[4] Kinchin, I.M. and Cabot, L.B., (2009). An introduction to concept mapping in dental education: the case of partial denture design. *European Journal of Dental Education*, *13*(1), pp.20–27.

[5] Farrand P, Hussain F, Hennessy E. (2002). The efficacy of the mind map study technique. *Medical Education*. 36(5):426–31.

[6] Yan Y, Yuehong W, Kun L, Hongbo Z, Hongyu Z, Yingming Y, Zhili Z. (2023). Implementation of mind mapping with problem-based learning in prosthodontics course for Chinese dental students. *BMC Medical Education*. 23(1): 530.

[7] Abdel-Hamid GA. (2017). Mind maps as a new teaching strategy for medical students. *MOJ Anat & Physiol*. 3(3): 00090.

[8] Khodabandeh F. (2021). The comparison of mind mapping-based flipped learning approach on introvert and extrovert EFL learners' speaking skill. *Iranian Journal of English for Academic Purposes*. 10(1):35–53.

Navigating Dental Education Trends and Transforming Dental Pedagogy – Abas and Srikant N (Eds)
© 2027 The Author(s), ISBN: 978-1-041-32674-8

Revolutionizing Dental Education: The Impact of Artificial Intelligence

Komal Singh and YM Karuna

Department of Paediatric and Preventive Dentistry, Manipal College of Dental Sciences Mangalore, Manipal Academy of Higher Education, Manipal, India

ABSTRACT: In earlier times, education was mainly based on teacher-student interaction and learning was confined to books but in the changing modern era with advancement of technology students have access to newer and more diverse interactive methods of learning. One of the newest additions to it is Artificial Intelligence.

Artificial intelligence is a branch of computer science that uses computational models to perform tasks that previously required human intelligence which includes machine learning, neural network /deep learning, cognitive system, perception robotics, and natural language processing.

After the era of COVID-19, When the need to come up with newer teaching methods were required, alternative ways have come up to simulate patient interaction, Artificial Intelligence has come into the limelight and since then has accelerated its transformation and incorporation in Dental Education.

This review explores the opportunities and challenges in dental education incorporating Artificial Intelligence as a mode of learning in dental curriculum.

The article reviews the impact of Artificial Intelligence 1. on theoretical learning aspect in dentistry and 2. on clinical aspect of learning in dentistry through Virtual Reality, Augmented Reality and Mixed Reality.

Keywords: artificial intelligence, dental education, teaching, dentistry, distance education, virtual reality, augmented reality

1 INTRODUCTION

As we advance further into the era of cutting-edge technology, our dependence on digital tools for learning and teaching has significantly increased. Data-driven tools have become integral to our daily routines. [1] In healthcare, including dentistry, digital transformation encompasses every aspect of patient care—from initial assessments and diagnostics to treatment planning, execution, and ongoing support. [2] As dental practice and education rapidly evolve with new diseases, diagnostic methods, and treatment plans, traditional teaching methods struggle to keep up with the ever-expanding curriculum. [3]

Dental education, aimed at training future dentists to prevent, diagnose, and treat oral diseases, typically combines non-clinical instruction with hands-on clinical experience. However, the COVID-19 pandemic disrupted both components, leading to a shift towards online teaching, remote learning, and virtual interactions between students and instructors. [4] This transition, while necessary, has highlighted the need for innovative solutions to bridge the gap between theoretical knowledge and practical skills. This has led to a reliance on digital tools to manage and access the wealth of information needed for effective learning and patient care.

Recently, artificial intelligence (AI)-driven tools have been increasingly integrated into dental training. [5] Existing literature indicates a surge in research involving digital technologies in implantology, restorative dentistry, and oral anatomy, highlighting their role in improving clinical performance and advancing early interventions. [6] The rapid integration of AI and immersive technologies like virtual reality (VR), augmented reality (AR), and mixed reality (MR) offers promising new avenues to enhance dental education effectively. [4–7]

This literature review aims to evaluate and explore the current uses of the various aspects of artificial intelligence domains as they pertain to dental digital literacy to help students concerning preclinical and clinical aspects of learning.

2 METHODOLOGY

Widespread electronic search was performed across several databases, including PubMed, Google Scholar, and Web of Science, to identify pertinent articles published from January 2014 to August 2024. The search utilized a range of keywords, including 'artificial intelligence', 'dental education', 'teaching', 'dentistry', 'distance education', 'virtual reality' and 'augmented reality'. Boolean operators such as 'AND' and 'OR' were employed to refine the search within each database.

Studies were selected based on their relevance to dental education and were limited to those involving dental students or educators. Articles focusing exclusively on the general population or non-dental student samples were excluded. Additionally, certain studies that fell outside the primary research scope were excluded.

From the initial search of 174 articles, 12 met our inclusion criteria after screening titles and abstracts. These studies were relevant to AI and immersive tools in dental education. However, upon full-text review, 7 of these articles were excluded. Ultimately, we included 5 articles that explored the integration of AI and immersive learning tools in clinical or nonclinical dental education (Table 1).

Table 1. List of included studies with teaching medium used and mode of learning assessed.

		Mode of learning assessed	
Author/year	AI teaching medium	Theoretical	Clinical
Dave 2023	VR	Yes	Yes
Huang 2018	VR AR		Yes
Danesh 2023	ChatGPT	Yes	
Xhang 2021	VR	Yes	Yes
Mahrous 2021	AR		Yes

3 RESULTS

Innovative AI applications in dental education in theoretical teaching, and clinical decision-making are now being researched in dentistry. Due to the ongoing development of artificial intelligence and its implications for dentistry, dental schools should assess the benefits and drawbacks of AI and investigate current and future ethical issues in the field.

3.1 *Impact on clinical aspects*

3.1.1 *Positive outcomes*

Dave and Patel (2023) highlight that virtual simulations are helpful for dental students as they enable practice of complex procedures like fillings and root canals without putting real patients at risk. This hands-on approach is flexible, allowing students to practice at their own pace and repeat techniques until mastery is achieved. The incorporation of Virtual Reality for training of dental students in preclinical training and complex dental procedures proves beneficial. [8] Similar to this, Huang *et al.* (2018) highlight the ways in which VR and AR systems improve skills and hand-eye coordination in addition to integrating learning and teaching frameworks. [7] According to their research, VR and AR technologies can be proven helpful in postural correction and skill enhancement as well as can save faculty in charge providing training up to five times to conventional preclinical teaching methods, which makes these systems great to be included for independent learning.

3.1.2 *Negative outcomes*

In contrast, Dave (2023) emphasizes that involving Artificial Intelligence in dental education has its own setbacks. There are worries that human empathy may be lost in diagnosis and treatment, and that students may become unduly reliant on AI, which could harm their capacity for critical thought and problem-solving. [8] Furthermore, problems with the impartiality and accuracy of AI algorithms may result in inaccurate diagnosis or treatment recommendations, indicating that AI should be utilized in addition to conventional methods of teaching rather than as a substitute.

3.2 *Impact on theoretical aspects*

3.2.1 *Positive outcomes*

According to Danesh (2023), ChatGPT and allied AI technologies can produce precise dental content, giving dental students useful resources for producing material about dental topics. [9] Zhang (2021) mentions in study that dental students face difficulty switching from theoretical to clinical training. According to the study, clinical practice can be assisted by using VR and AR technology to integrate theoretical knowledge with practical training. [10]

3.2.2 *Negative outcomes*

According to Dave and Patel (2023), there can be an unwanted outcome of Artificial Intelligence as it can be used in academic deceitfulness. The integrity of the educational system may be jeopardized if students make use of AI in unethical ways, for as by utilizing cheating software or automated essay generators. For educational institutes to maintain their standing and academic integrity, these issues must be focused on. [8] Mahrous (2021) also highlights some of the difficulties that come with using AR in dental anatomy instruction as it exists today. The necessity of head-mounted displays (HMDs) to provide an immersive augmented reality (AR) experience poses a challenge to the broad acceptance and serviceability of AR technologies, potentially hampering their successful incorporation into educational settings. [11]

4 DISCUSSION

Artificial intelligence (AI) in dental education is technological integration and involvement that is a great advancement in dental teaching and learning. This discussion looks at how AI technology affects several aspects of dental education, considering both the advantages as well as drawbacks of using it. It also considers how artificial intelligence (AI), and virtual and augmented reality (VR and AR) fit into dental education.

Studies show that integrating AI with VR and AR has a significant positive impact on dental education. Immediate feedback and possibilities for repeated practice are made possible by these advancements, which gives better results at skillfulness and clinical procedural outcomes. The immersive qualities of VR and AR help students become more skillful technically and better equipped for therapeutic settings in the real world.

Dave and Patel (2023) emphasize how Artificial Intelligence can revolutionize dental education. They showcase cutting-edge uses, like test questions created by AI for unbiased evaluation and virtual patients driven by AI for practical experience. [8] But training AI systems need high-quality data, which presents a big barrier. The intricacy, privacy issues, and strict laws governing healthcare data make this a substantial barrier to the mainstream use of AI in dental education.

Future research structured clinical examinations (OSCEs) for dental education may include AR or VR simulations with real-time feedback and objective evaluation elements, according to additional research by Huang (2018) and Zhang (2021). Further advancements in AR and VR can give large scale benefits in clinical training of all dental department programs. With these tools, postgraduate students and young professionals should be able to practice on their own and advance their academic and clinical expertise. Artificial intelligence (AI) in virtual simulations has the potential to improve healthcare results by improving hand-eye coordination and facilitating repeated practice in preclinical settings. Conversely, because AI might be abused for unethical work as an example to create fake assignments, educational institutions must safeguard academic integrity. [7,10]

Danesh (2023) highlights the prominence of using AI tools like ChatGPT with caution. Dental students should consider such tools as complementary resources rather than primary sources of information. [9] Future research should continue to evaluate the efficacy and accuracy of AI models in dental education to fully understand their role and improve their functionality.

Mahrous (2021) points out difficulties with the practical implementation of AR in dental education. All dental students may not be able to take full use of these technologies due to the high expense of VR headsets and other AR gear. [11] The vast adoption of AR for theoretical learning and clinical practice is limited for cost issue being, indicating the need for more cost-effective alternatives or different approaches to integrate AR into dentistry education.

In brief, while AI, VR, and AR have great potential for improving dental education, their application faces obstacles such as accessibility, data quality and academic integrity. Further research and development are essential for advancements in these technologies and overcoming their limitations to improve educational outcomes in the profession of dentistry.

5 CONCLUSION

As Artificial Intelligence along with Virtual Reality and Augmented Reality holds great power to contribute to dental education, facilitate access to theoretical learning materials, and grant for repeated practice of clinical procedure learning, artificial intelligence is a great complement to teaching methods. Dental education has commitment to be proactive and forward-thinking when it comes to utilising AI safely and ethically for the benefit of students, patients, and future providers.

While an over-reliance on artificial intelligence may result in a decline in creative thinking, problem-solving, and assignment cheating, students still need to possess the requisite knowledge and abilities to understand and utilise this technology. Because of this, artificial intelligence needs to be utilised in addition to traditional teaching techniques, not as an alternative to them.

REFERENCES

[1] Schwendicke F, Chaurasia A, Wiegand T, Uribe SE, Fontana M, Akota I, Tryfonos O, Krois J. (2023). ADR e-oral health network and the ITU/WHO focus group AI for health. Artificial intelligence for oral and dental healthcare: Core education curriculum. *J Dent*. 128:104363. doi: 10.1016/j.jdent.2022.104363. Epub 2022 Nov 21. PMID: 36410581.

[2] Islam NM, Laughter L, Sadid-Zadeh R, Smith C, Dolan TA, Crain G, Squarize CH. (2022). Adopting artificial intelligence in dental education: A model for academic leadership and innovation. *J Dent Educ*. 86(11):1545–1551. doi: 10.1002/jdd.13010. Epub 2022 Jul 3. PMID: 35781809

[3] Saghiri MA, Vakhnovetsky J, Nadershahi N. (2022). Scoping review of artificial intelligence and immersive digital tools in dental education. *J Dent Educ*. 86(6):736–750. doi: 10.1002/jdd.12856. Epub 2021 Dec 28. PMID: 34962645.

[4] Haroon Z, Azad AA, Sharif M, Aslam A, Arshad K, Rafiq S. (2020). COVID-19 Era: Challenges and solutions in dental education. *J Coll Physicians Surg Pak*. 30(10):129–131. doi: 10.29271/jcpsp.2020.supp2.129. PMID: 33115587

[5] Li B, Cheng L, Wang H. (2022). Challenges and opportunities for dental education from COVID-19. *Dent J (Basel)*. 10(10):188. doi: 10.3390/dj10100188. PMID: 36285998; PMCID: PMC9600572.

[6] Edwards PC. (2015). The future of dental education: toward disruptive innovation or incremental improvements? *Oral Surg Oral Med Oral Pathol Oral Radiol*. 119(3):257–9. doi: 10.1016/j.oooo.2014.12.006. Epub 2015 Jan 6. PMID: 25660827

[7] Huang TK, Yang CH, Hsieh YH, Wang JC, Hung CC. (2018). Augmented reality (AR) and virtual reality (VR) applied in dentistry. *Kaohsiung J Med Sci*. 34(4):243–248. doi: 10.1016/j.kjms.2018.01.009. PMID: 29655414.

[8] Dave M, Patel N. (2023). Artificial intelligence in healthcare and education. *Br Dent J*. 234(10):761–764. doi: 10.1038/s41415-023-5845-2. Epub 2023 May 26. PMID: 37237212; PMCID: PMC10219811

[9] Danesh A, Pazouki H, Danesh F, Danesh A, Vardar-Sengul S. (2024). Artificial intelligence in dental education: ChatGPT's performance on the periodontic in-service examination. *J Periodontol*. 95(7):682–687. doi:10.1002/JPER.23-0514. Epub 2024 Jan 10. PMID: 38197146

[10] Zhang J, Xing J, Zheng M, Sheng J, Zhang K, Zhang B. (2021). Effectiveness of virtual simulation and jaw model for undergraduate periodontal teaching. *BMC Med Educ*. 21(1):616. doi: 10.1186/s12909-021-03064-1. PMID: 34906125; PMCID: PMC8672555

[11] Mahrous A, Elgreatly A, Qian F, Schneider GB. (2021). A comparison of pre-clinical instructional technologies: Natural teeth, 3D models, 3D printing, and augmented reality. *J Dent Educ*. 85(11):1795–1801. doi: 10.1002/jdd.12736. Epub 2021 Jul 2. PMID: 34216032.

Assessment of Dental Students' Perceptions of Teaching Methodologies Across the Dental Curriculum: A Mixed Method

Nikhil Ajabrao Bomble
Department of Public Health Dentistry, YCMM & RDF Dental College and Hospital, Ahilyanagar, Maharashtra, INDIA

ABSTRACT: **Background:** Effective dental education relies on student feedback to refine teaching methodologies. Advances in digital technology have transformed these methods, necessitating an understanding of students' perceptions to enhance learning. This study aimed to evaluate dental students' views on various teaching methods and their knowledge of these methods.

Objective: 1) To assess dental students' perceptions of teaching methodologies across the dental curriculum. 2) To assess the knowledge of dental students regarding teaching methodologies across the dental curriculum.

A mixed-methods study was conducted at a private dental institute from May to July 2024. Then, ethical protocols were followed. Among the 480 students, 400 responded to a questionnaire. The focus group discussions involved 12 participants per group, with 8 consenting to qualitative analysis. Data collection included audio recordings and handwritten notes, with demographic details noted. Thematic analysis was used to analyze the data.

Results: Only 15% of the students demonstrated knowledge of teaching methodologies. The analysis revealed 21 initial codes, which were condensed into 6 subthemes through axial and selective coding. Students preferred flipped teaching, focus group discussions, and activity-based learning for theoretical classes. For clinical preclinical training, favored methods include simulation-based learning, case-based discussions, OSCE/OPSE, and demonstrations.

Conclusion: Student-centric teaching methods, particularly those incorporating interactive and practical elements, are deemed most effective in enhancing learning outcomes in dental education.

Keywords: Knowledge, Teaching, Dental, Education

1 INTRODUCTION

Learning styles are defined as "the way in which people choose to approach a learning situation or are inclined to do so". [1] In ancient India during the Vedic Age, education was seen as a means of enlightenment, guiding individuals to live successful and honorable lives. Education was considered a tool for personal growth and improvement. However, in contemporary India, education is viewed as a process that facilitates learning and the acquisition of knowledge, skills, values, beliefs, and habits. [2]

Modern educational methods now encompass group discussions, debates, teaching, training, and research. The dental education system in India is structured to train professionals who can provide high-quality oral healthcare. In dental education across India, teaching methodologies are evolving to include a mix of traditional and innovative approaches. [3] The various teaching methodologies employed in dental schools include lecture-based instruction, practical demonstrations, focused group discussion, problem-based learning (PBL), simulation-based learning, case-based learning, a flipped classroom, direct clinical training, flash cards, and process-oriented guided inquiry learning (POGIL) [4].

These innovative approaches boost team and collaborative learning, enhance students' self-confidence, and foster their critical thinking, creativity, problem-solving, and communication skills [1]. Today, education is considered a crucial element for achieving excellence. As a result, teaching and learning have shifted from teacher-centric to student-centric approaches [5]. Given the rapid changes in information and technology, education must evolve alongside these advancements and continue to grow through innovative learning methods [6].

In dentistry, modern learning techniques that are quickly spreading across the world are not well known. Effective dental education relies on student feedback to refine ongoing teaching methodologies. Advances in digital technology have transformed these methods, necessitating an understanding of students' perceptions to enhance learning. In today's rapidly evolving world, students' perceptions and thought processes have shifted, necessitating more varied and interactive teaching methods to meet their diverse educational needs [7]. Hence, this study was conducted to evaluate dental students' views on various teaching methods and their knowledge of these methods .

1.1 *Objective*

1) To assess dental students' perceptions of teaching methodologies across the dental curriculum.
2) To assess the knowledge of dental students regarding teaching methodologies across the dental curriculum.

DOI: 10.1201/9781042016075-25

2 METHODOLOGY

A mixed-methods study (qualitative study followed by a cross-sectional study) was conducted at a private dental institute from May to July 2024. Institutional ethics committee approval was taken-YCDC/IES-IRC/7-A/2024-25. Following ethical protocols, the students were informed in the reading hall about the study. Those willing to participate provided written informed consent and completed a standardized, prevalidated structured questionnaire. The principal investigator collected the questionnaires the same day. Among the 480 students, 400 responded, resulting in an 83.33% response rate. The data were entered into Microsoft Excel 2010 and analyzed via SPSS version 29.

To gain in-depth perceptions of teaching methodologies, focus group discussions (FGDs) were conducted. Three groups were formed: Group 1 (1st- and 2nd-year students) for preclinical teaching methodologies, Group 2 (3rd- and 4th-year students) for theoretical teaching methodologies, and Group 3 (interns) for clinical teaching methodologies. Each group included 12 participants. FGDs were led by the principal investigator, with discussions recorded and transcribed verbatim. Handwritten notes were taken by an assistant. The data were coded into 21 initial codes, which were condensed into 6 subthemes through axial and selective coding.

Predefined questionnaire for focus group discussion
1 Which teaching method would you prefer?
2 What are the positive traits of teaching methods?
3 What are the negative traits of teaching methods?
4 How does your level of understanding compare when using traditional teaching methods versus modern teaching methods?
5 What are the suggestions from you about teaching methodology?

Results: All the study participants were aware of the teaching methodology. The mean age of the study participants was 23.46±52 years. A maximum of 89% (n=356) of the females were enrolled in this study. A maximum of 42.3% (n=169) of the study participants were from the 1^{st-} and 2nd year classes, whereas only 25.3% (n=101) were from internships. A total of 31.3% (N=125) of the students felt that the didactic teaching method was best for understanding the subject. Similarly, 31% (n=124) of the students felt that the flipped method was better at learning the subject. A total of 51.8% of the students agreed that demonstrations are useful for learning in preclinical classes. However, only 20% (n=83) feel that the OSCE/OSPE method is beneficial for learning in the preclinical setting. Most 38% (n=152) of the students reported that discussion-based learning was effective in learning in the clinical class whereas 31% (n=123) of the students still believed that simulation-based demonstrations were effective. Very few (11.5%, n=46) agreed that the OSCE/OPSE could be used to better understand the clinical class. Compared with traditional versus modern teaching methods, 76.3% (n=305) agreed that modern teaching methods could better understand the subject and clarify concepts (Table 1). For an in-depth understanding of the perceptions of the students, 3 focus group discussions (the theory group, preclinical group and clinical group) were held verbatim. Twenty-one codes were generated (Table 2). We obtained the following 6 themes: 1) engagement and interaction; 2) modern and traditional methods; 3) visual aids and digital tools; 4) preparation and reinforcement; 5) preference and practical methods; and 6) adaptability and flexibility (Table 3).

3 DISCUSSION

This study evaluated the perceptions of dental students regarding various teaching methodologies, highlighting their preferences and the effectiveness of different approaches in enhancing learning outcomes. The analysis revealed that students favored interactive and practical teaching methods, particularly those incorporating digital tools and simulations.

Our findings indicate that 76.3% of the students preferred modern teaching methods over traditional methods, a sentiment echoed in other studies. For example, Rhythm Bains *et al.* (2023) [6] reported that students favor a combination of audio-visual and blackboard teaching for better engagement in classroom settings. Similarly, (8) noted that flipped classrooms significantly enhance student learning by promoting interactive learning and increasing knowledge retention nearly threefold.

A notable demographic trend observed in this study was the high percentage of female participants (89%). This trend aligns with the increasing number of female dentists globally, as reported by [2], who reported a similar female predominance in their study. This shift may influence the study results, as gender differences in learning preferences have been documented in the dental education literature.

In preclinical and clinical settings, students showed a strong preference for simulation-based learning and demonstrations, with 51.8% and 38% favoring these methods, respectively. These findings are consistent with those of the study by [4], which demonstrated the effectiveness of simulations and digital tools in practical skill acquisition. Additionally, the use of case-based discussions was highlighted as an effective strategy for clinical education, promoting critical thinking and real-world application of knowledge.

Table 1. Distribution of study participants and perception of teaching methodologies.

Sr. No.	Parameters	Variables	No. of study participants	Percentage
1	Gender	Male	44	11%
		Female	356	89%
2	Year of studying	1st and 2nd year	169	42.3%
		3rd and 4th year	130	32.5%
		Internship	101	25.3%
3	Awareness regarding teaching methodology	Yes	400	100%
4	Theory class perception	Flipped	124	31%
		Focus Group	45	11%
		Activity based learning	106	26.5%
		Didactic Teaching	125	31.3%
5	Preclinical class perception	Simulation based learning	110	27.5%
		Demonstration	207	51.8%
		OSCE/OSPE	83	20.8%
6	Clinical class perception	Simulation based learning	123	30.8%
		Case based discussion	152	38%
		OSCE/OSPE	46	11.5%
		Demonstration	79	19.8%
7	Traditional class vs Moder class	Traditional	95	23.8%
		Modern	305	76.3%

Table 2. Codes and Interpretation from focus group discussions.

Code No	Codes	Interpretation
Theory classes		
1	Interactive sessions help maintain attention during theory classes.	Students prefer active engagement during lectures, which enhances focus and participation.
2	Adding humor (jokes) during sessions makes learning more enjoyable.	Humor in teaching can lighten the mood, making learning less stressful and more memorable.
3	Animations are effective for understanding complex concepts.	Visual aids like animations simplify complex topics, making them easier to grasp.
4	Some students appreciate eye contact in traditional teaching.	Direct eye contact fosters a personal connection, enhancing communication and attentiveness.
5	Students dislike online learning due to lack of engagement and eye contact.	Online learning lacks interactive elements and personal connection, leading to decreased motivation.
6	Flipped classrooms are preferred but not feasible for all topics.	While flipped classrooms encourage active learning, they may not be suitable for all subjects or contexts.
7	Digital tools can cause screen fatigue and irritation.	Excessive screen time can lead to discomfort, affecting students' ability to concentrate.
8	"Chalk and talk" method is favored for its simplicity and engagement.	Traditional methods like "chalk and talk" are appreciated for being straightforward and interactive.
9	Reinforcement through questions about past and current lectures improves retention.	Frequent review questions help reinforce learning and facilitate long-term memory retention.
Preclinical and Clinical Class		
10	Simulation-based learning (3D models) preferred for practical understanding.	Simulations, especially 3D models, provide hands-on experience, which is crucial for clinical education.
11	Demonstrations are effective for learning practical skills.	Demonstrations offer direct observation and practice opportunities, enhancing practical skills.
12	Case-based discussions are highly effective for clinical learning.	Case-based discussions foster critical thinking and application of knowledge in real-world scenarios.
13	OSCE/OSPE methods are valued for their structured approach.	OSCE/OSPE provides a standardized way to assess clinical competence and practical skills.
14	Group discussions benefit collaborative and self-directed learning.	Group discussions encourage peer learning, teamwork, and communication skills development.
15	Hands-on experiences are preferred over theoretical learning for clinical skills.	Direct, hands-on activities are essential for mastering clinical competencies and skills.

(*continued*)

Table 2. Continued

Code No	Codes	Interpretation
Suggestions for Improvement		
16	Pre reading assignments before lectures help prepare students better.	Pre reading enables students to familiarize themselves with the material, leading to more productive lectures.
17	A combination of multiple methods is recommended for effective teaching.	A diverse mix of teaching methods can cater to different learning styles and needs, enhancing overall effectiveness.
18	Mixed feelings about modern methods: engaging but can cause fatigue; traditional methods provide direct contact.	Modern methods offer dynamic content but may also lead to burnout, while traditional methods support personal interaction.
Additional insights		
19	Engagement	Methods that engage students actively are preferred.
20	Interactivity	Interactive methods are seen more effective for learning.
21	Adaptability	Teaching methods should be adaptable to cater to different learning preferences.

Table 3. Themes and sub-themes of student perceptions about theory, preclinical, and clinical classes.

Theme	Sub-Theme	Theory Class	Preclinical or Clinical Class
Engagement and Interaction	Positive Interactions	Interactive sessions and humor improve engagement in theory classes.	Group discussions enhance collaborative learning and engagement.
	Mixed Feelings about Modern Methods	Digital tools engage but can cause screen fatigue and lack of eye contact.	Collaborative methods like simulations, case-based discussions, and demonstrations promote practical understanding and active learning.
Modern vs. Traditional Methods	Preference for Modern Tools	Animations and digital tools help understanding but may cause screen fatigue.	Simulation-based learning (3D models) is preferred for practical skills; hands-on activities and visual tools are effective.
	Drawbacks of Traditional Methods	Traditional methods may seem monotonous but allow for direct eye contact.	Traditional methods like demonstrations are well-received for skill-building; OSCE/OSPE provides structured assessments.
Visual Aids and Digital Tools	Use of Visual Aids	Animations and digital photos simplify complex concepts.	Digital tools (e.g., 3D models) and simulations enhance practical understanding.
Preparation and Reinforcement	Memory Retention Strategies	Review questions on past and current lectures reinforce learning.	Regular practice, hands-on activities, and structured assessments reinforce preclinical and clinical knowledge.
Preference for Practical Methods	Combination of Teaching Methods	A blend of flipped classrooms, interactive sessions, and digital tools is recommended.	Combination of simulations, demonstrations, case-based discussions, and hands-on practice is effective.
Adaptability and Flexibility	Adaptive Teaching Approaches	Methods should be adaptable to different learning preferences and topics.	Flexibility in combining different teaching methods is needed to address diverse clinical situations effectively.

However, the study also highlighted some challenges with modern teaching methods. While digital tools and online learning offer numerous benefits, they also present issues such as screen fatigue and a lack of personal interaction, which can negatively impact student motivation and engagement. This duality underscores the need for a balanced approach, that integrates both modern and traditional methods to cater to diverse learning preferences.

Another significant observation was the importance of interactive and engaging teaching methods. The students reported that interactive sessions and humor in teaching enhanced their focus and made learning more enjoyable. This aligns with findings from the Journal [3], which emphasized the role of active engagement in improving learning outcomes.

4 STRENGTHS AND LIMITATIONS

One of the strengths of this study is its high response rate (83.33%) and the inclusion of a large sample size (n=400), which enhances the generalizability of the findings. Compared with purely quantitative studies, the mixed-methods design, which incorporates both quantitative and qualitative data, allowed for a more comprehensive exploration of student perceptions. The qualitative component, particularly the focus group discussions, provided deeper insights into student preferences and the reasons behind them.

However, the study has several limitations. The sample was drawn from a single private dental institute, which may limit its generalizability to other settings. Additionally, the study's cross-sectional design does not allow for the assessment of changes in perceptions over time. Potential bias due to the high proportion of female respondents should also be considered, as gender differences in learning preferences might influence the overall findings.

5 CONCLUSION

Every student has a unique mindset and level of understanding, which must be taken into consideration while imparting various teaching methods in the dental curriculum. Student-centric teaching methods, particularly those incorporating interactive and practical elements, are deemed most effective in enhancing learning outcomes in dental education.

REFERENCES

[1] Olabisi Hajarat O, Balogun M, Pugsley H. (2024). Exploring dental students' perceptions of their clinical learning environment: A qualitative study to evaluate the curriculum. *International Journal of Research in Education and Science.* 10(2):279–98.

[2] Kunduru Sushma Reddy KVNRP, T. Madhavi Padma3, V. Shiva Kalyan, P. Srikanth. (2019). Knowledge and attitude on teaching methods among dental students. *International Journal of Research in Engineering, Science and Management.* 2,(10):242–245.

[3] Singh R, Gupta N, Singh G. (2016). Learning style and teaching methodology preferences of dental students. *Journal of the Anatomical Society of India.* 65(2):152–5.

[4] Varughese A, M R, S D, Ramanarayanan V, Varghese AA, G VK. (2024). effectiveness of different teaching methods in enhancing dental undergraduate students' knowledge and restorative cement manipulation skills. *Cureus.* 16(8):e67999.

[5] Tulbah HI, Alhamdan EM, Alqahtani AS, Alduhayan GA, Albedaiwi LS. (2024). Dental students' preferences regarding teaching methods in Riyadh. *Saudi Journal of Oral Sciences.* 6(2).

[6] Bains R, Parikh V, Pandey P. (2023). Undergraduate students' perception of the Indian dental curriculum: A focus-group based, multicentric questionnaire survey. *Journal of Oral Biology and Craniofacial Research.* 13(2):230–5.

[7] Gopinath V, Nallaswamy D. (2017). A systematic review on the most effective method teaching dentistry to dental students compared to video based learning. *American Journal of Educational Research.* 2017;5(1):63–8.

[8] Singh V, Sahai A. (2023). Implementation of Competency Based Medical Education in Anatomy with Poor Teacher™Student Ratio: The Utopia 2023.

Awareness and Attitudes of Dental Practitioners in Implementing Tobacco Cessation Programme Among Patients and the Need for Curriculum Changes

Ria Sinha
Intern, Manipal College of Dental Sciences Mangalore, Manipal Academy of Higher Education, Manipal, Karnataka, India

K David
Department of Periodontology, Manipal College of Dental Sciences Mangalore, Manipal Academy of Higher Education, Manipal, Karnataka, India

Tanya Bharadwaj
Intern, Manipal College of Dental Sciences Mangalore, Manipal Academy of Higher Education, Manipal, Karnataka, India

Sangeeta Umesh Nayak and Mranali K Shetty
Department of Periodontology, Manipal College of Dental Sciences Mangalore, Manipal Academy of Higher Education, Manipal, Karnataka, India

ABSTRACT: **Objectives:** The objectives of this study were to review a questionnaire to assess the awareness and attitudes of private dental practitioners in implementing a tobacco cessation program in patients visiting their clinic in and around Mangalore.

Methods: A cross-sectional study was conducted. A series of questionnaires were given to private dental practitioners in and around Mangalore, with a sample size of 54.

Results: The results of the questionnaire were divided into academic and nonacademic private dental practitioners, of which 50 were academic practitioners and 4 were nonacademic practitioners. Most of the practitioners agreed that, owing to the reward pathway and adrenaline rush, quitting tobacco for their patients was difficult, despite them advising the users to quit tobacco.Lack of awareness of tobacco cessation methods and a lack of resources, many practitioners were not able to implement the program.

Conclusions: Tobacco addiction is emerging as a major threat. Dental teams in primary care are aware of the importance of offering tobacco cessation advice and, with further training, could guide many of their patients who smoke towar a successful quitting journey. Tobacco tobacco issues in developing countries are usually taught nonsystematically as well as when the topic arose. The counseling and treatment of nicotine addiction are important components of the tobacco education module. Dental educators should consider improving dental curricula to train future dentists in the prevention and cessation of tobacco. The World Health Organization and Global Health Professional Student Survey (GHPSS) has suggested including an integrated tobacco module in dental school curricula.

Keywords: tobacco cessation, dental practitioners, questionnaire study

1 INTRODUCTION

Tobacco is the primary factor responsible for numerous conditions that affect millions of people worldwide. Despite several initiatives implemented to mitigate the intake of tobacco, its usage continues to increase. [1] The prevalence of aggressive marketing strategies for tobacco products, the lack of strict regulations for the sale of tobacco products, and the addictive properties of tobacco products may have all played a role in the increasing use of tobacco products. [2] The prevalence of tobacco-related diseases is widespread among people residing in developing and poor nations. These countries suffer from a clear scarcity of resources, particularly in regard to providing healthcare. India is one of the foremost countries with the highest prevalence of tobacco-related disorders globally. According to Asma *et al.*, [3] 41% of adults aged 15 years or older regularly use some type of tobacco. The findings of the Global Adult Tobacco Survey (GATS 2) revealed that the overall prevalence of tobacco use in India decreased from 34.6% in 2009–10 to 28.6% in 2016–17, according to the Tata Institute of Social Sciences and the Ministry of Health and Family Welfare of the Government of India. [4] Nevertheless, the prevalence of tobacco use in India continues to be quite high. The trends of tobacco-related conditions in India suggest that they

DOI: 10.1201/9781042016075-26

disproportionately affect the disadvantaged population. One of the most significant public health challenges currently confronting India is the prevalence of tobacco-related conditions. [5] Tobacco cessation is the act of refraining from smoking cigarettes and other tobacco products for a minimum of 6 months but ideally for 1 year. [6] This abstinence is verified by measuring the levels of expired carbon monoxide or other objective tests. Tobacco cessation interventions can be categorized into three main types: behavioral, pharmaceutical, and alternative. Several studies have revealed that the majority of doctors infrequently provide guidance and support to tobacco users in their efforts to quit tobacco. [7] This is mostly attributed to their insufficient training, lack of expertise, and low confidence in conducting smoking cessation treatments. Additionally, there are other barriers that hinder doctors from effectively carrying out such interventions. Nicotine replacement treatment (NRT) can be obtained via prescription in various nations. Physicians play crucial roles in providing educational material, counseling, and nicotine replacement therapy (NRT) to patients. It is necessary for them to have a thorough understanding of the proper use, contraindications, and adverse effects of NRT. [8] The objective of this survey was to evaluate the knowledge and attitudes of private dentistry practitioners in and around Mangalore city, Karnataka, with respect to providing guidance on smoking cessation.

2 MATERIALS AND METHODS

A survey was conducted among private dental practitioners in and around Mangalore city via a questionnaire-based approach. The researchers directly approached the respondents and requested their participation in answering the questionnaire while being observed by the researcher. Participants who met the criteria were invited to participate in the survey after providing informed consent.

A validated survey was used to assess the comprehension, attitudes, and execution of smoke cessation methods among private dental professionals. The questionnairecomprises ten validated questions, which were assessed by two professionals. The survey was distributed to independent dental practitioners. The responses supplied by the participants were subjected to statistical analysis.

Given a population proportion of 95%, a confidence interval of 95%, an error margin of 0.05, and an anticipated population size of 200, the sample size needed was determined to be 54.

Approval was received from the Institutional Ethical Committee. Prior to conducting the survey, the respondents provided informed consent.

3 STATISTICAL ANALYSIS

The questionnaires that were received were categorized and evaluated. The results were quantified as numerical values and percentages of participants for each question. The data were analyzed via the SPSS Version 17 program. A chi-square test was conducted for inferential analysis, with a predetermined level of statistical significance established at $P < 0.05$.

4 RESULTS

The questionnaire study aimed to measure the level of awareness among private dental practitioners of tobacco cessation programs and assess their attitudes toward establishing such programs for patients who visit their clinics. A total of 54 dental practitioners in private practice took part in the survey. The study revealed that 98.1% of private dental practitioners who had an academic background believed that it is within the scope of dental practice to recommend that patients stop using tobacco. Approximately 48% of private dental practitioners in academic settings occasionally documented the tobacco consumption history of patients, as opposed to nonacademic private dental practitioners. Approximately 59.3% of dental practitioners occasionally believe that they are capable of offering tobacco cessation assistance. A total of 83.3% of private dental practitioners in academics consistently recommend that patients cease tobacco use, whereas 75% of private dental practitioners outside of academic settings provide the same advice.

Nonaffiliated private dentistry practitioners utilize behavioral counseling as their strategy for tobacco cessation. The same strategy is used by 68% of private practitioners in the academic field. The survey indicated that 37% of nonacademic private dental practitioners suggest the use of nicotine gums at a dosage of 2–4 mg for a period of 8–16 weeks. Almost 72% of private dental practitioners outside of academic contexts perceive motivating patients as not being time-consuming, whereas only 28% of private dental practitioners in academic settings share this belief. Almost half (48.1%) of the participants considered the adrenaline rush as the main obstacle in their patients efforts to quit tobacco. Gratification and the reward pathway trail closely behind, accounting for 40.7% and 11.1%, respectively. Our survey revealed that 75.9% of nonacademic private practitioners do not consider the fear of losing patients be the primary hindrance to achieving successful tobacco cessation. Conversely, 24.1% of academic private dental practitioners believe that fear is the main obstacle to successfully achieving tobacco cessation. On the basis of statistics, 40.7% of private dental practitioners who are not employed in academic settings recommend nicotine replacement therapy (NRT) to tobacco users as a method to quit the habit, whereas 25.9% of nonacademic private practitioners do not prescribe NRT.

5 DISCUSSION

The current study was a survey-based investigation that attempted to gauge the awareness and attitudes of private dental practitioners regarding tobacco cessation programs. This study highlights the crucial function of dentists in assisting their patients in smoking cessation. However, our study emphasizes the propensity among numerous dentists to disregard the documentation of their patients' tobacco use history. Tobacco counseling is a crucial part of the early stage of the treatment plan, requiring that all patients who use any type of tobacco receive assistance and support to quit the habit. However, a study conducted in 2010 by Lisa Szatkowsk *et al.* reported that the smoking status of 74.2% of adults was not documented. [9]

Among private dental practitioners in academic settings, 83.3% regularly provided counseling to promote smoking cessation, whereas 75% of their counterparts in nonacademic settings offered similar guidance. In a study conducted by K. R. Thankappan [10], two intervention groups were compared. The minimal intervention group received counseling from doctors to aid in smoking cessation, whereas the enhanced intervention group received additional brief counseling for smoking cessation from a qualified nonmedical health professional. After a three-month follow-up, the study reported cessation rates of 16% in the minimal intervention group and 21% in the increased intervention group.

Our study results show that 75.9% of nonacademic private practitioners do not consider the fear of losing patients to be a significant obstacle in attaining successful tobacco cessation. On the other hand, 24.1% of private dental practitioners who are into academics say that fear is the main barrier to achieving success in tobacco cessation. In a 2021 study conducted by Jazia A. Alblowi, [11] a shortage of time was discovered to be a major obstacle preventing individuals from participating in tobacco counseling and cessation (TCC). This factor accounted for 48.4% of the reported difficulties.

The results of this survey reveal that 68% of private dental practitioners, both those not associated with academic institutions and those in the academic sector, utilize behavioral counseling as their primary approach for helping patients quit tobacco use. On the other hand, a study carried out by Gholamreza Heydari *et al* [12] proposed three main approaches to stop smoking: NRT, Champix (varenicline), and smoking cessation education.

The study findings indicate that 37% of nonacademic private dental practitioners recommended that their patients use nicotine gum at a dosage of 2–4 mg for a period of 8–16 weeks. In contrast, a previous study suggested the use of 4 mg of nicotine gum. [13] Our survey revealed that 40.7% of private dental practitioners who are not associated with academic institutions suggest NRT as a recommended approach for individuals who want to quit the tobacco habit. In the same vein, half of nonacademic private practitioners also support the utilization of NRTs for the purpose of quitting tobacco. Prabhu *et al.*14 reported that 37.8% of participants reported prescribing chewing gum in the form of NRT, whereas 37.4% reported prescribing sublingual pills. The remaining percentage of participants reported prescribing other kinds of NRT.

According to our analysis, 48.1% of participants attributed the adrenaline surge as the main barrier to quitting tobacco. On the other hand, a 2022 study by the American Cancer Society indicated that emotional reliance acts as a substantial obstacle for people seeking to stop tobacco. [15]

6 CONCLUSION

Our research indicates that the attitudes and behaviors of private dental practitioners toward tobacco cessation programmes reveal both praiseworthy efforts and areas that require improvement. The importance of dentists in assisting patients in quitting tobacco has been confirmed; however, there are still difficulties in implementing comprehensive cessation programs in both academic and nonacademic environments. To increase the effectiveness of tobacco cessation interventions in dental settings, it is important to promote the integration of evidence-based practices, provide continuing education programs, and encourage open discussions among practitioners. Dental educators should consider improving dental curricula to train future dentists in the prevention and cessation of smoking. The World Health Organization and Global Health Professional Student Survey (GHPSS) has suggested including an integrated tobacco module in dental school curricula.

Table 1. Response from question number 1 to 7.

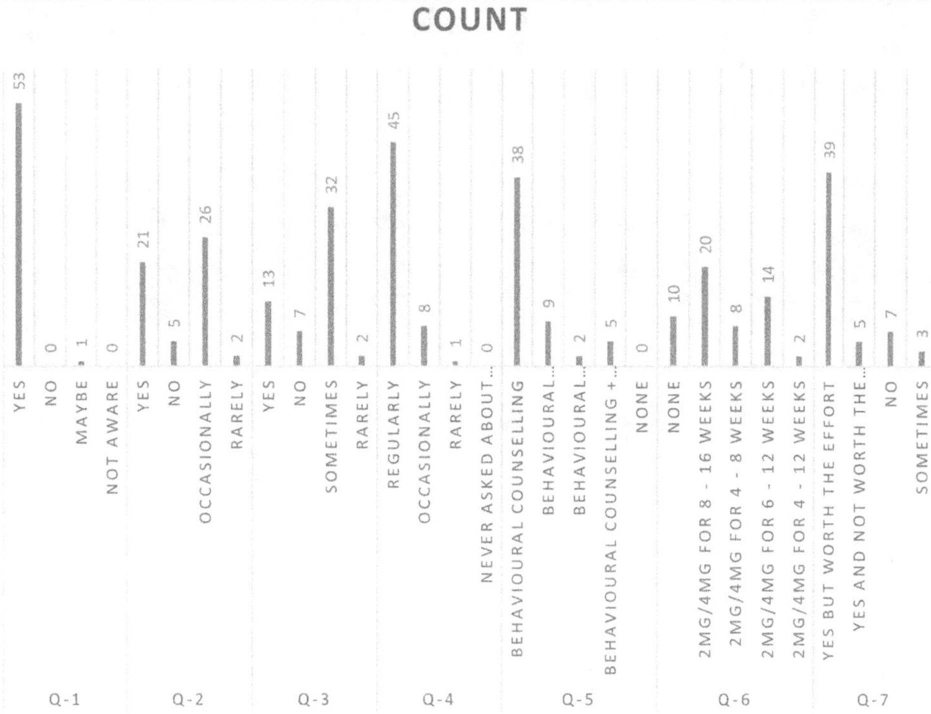

Table 2. Response for question number 8.

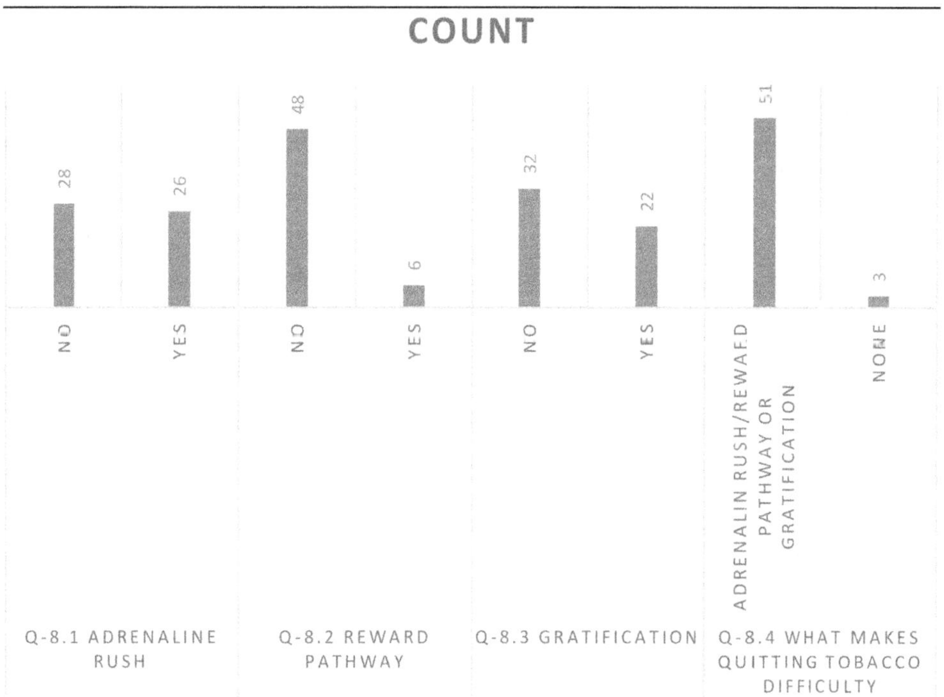

Table 3. Response for question number 9.

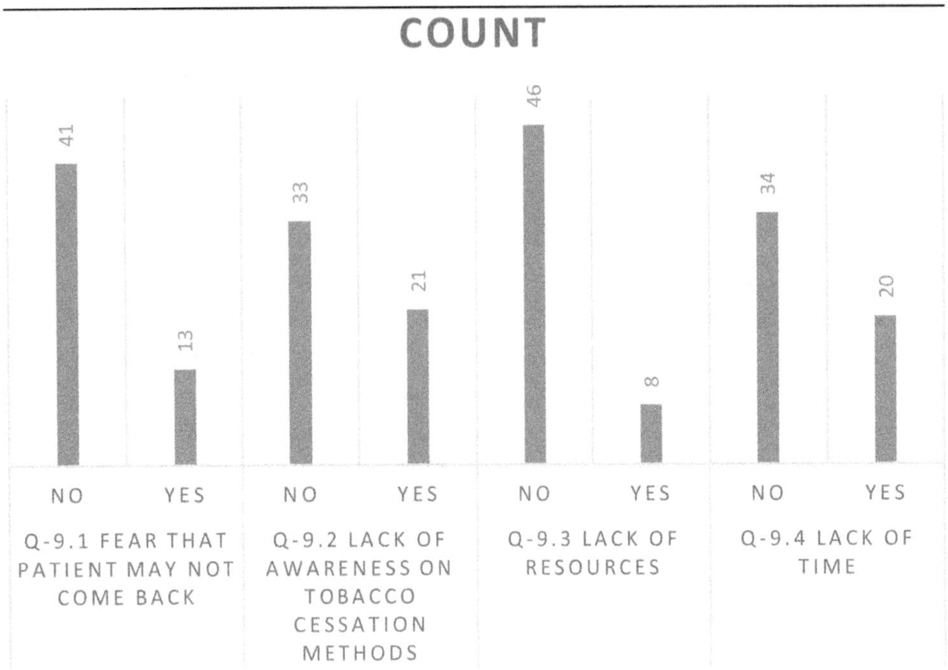

Table 4. Response for question number 10.

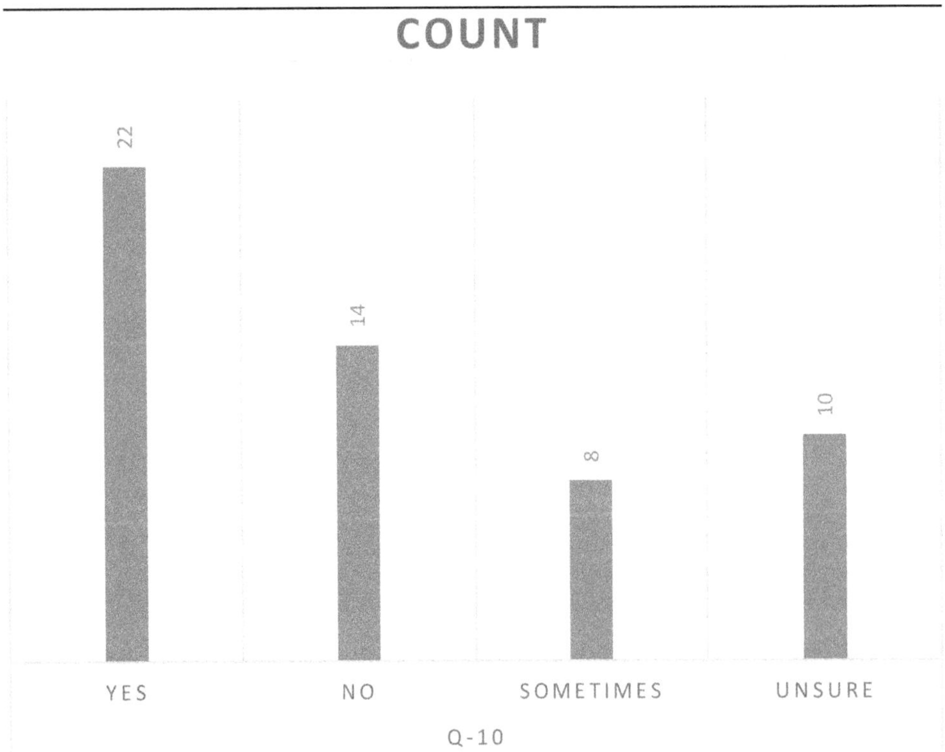

Table 5. Academic and Non-academic partitioners percentage.

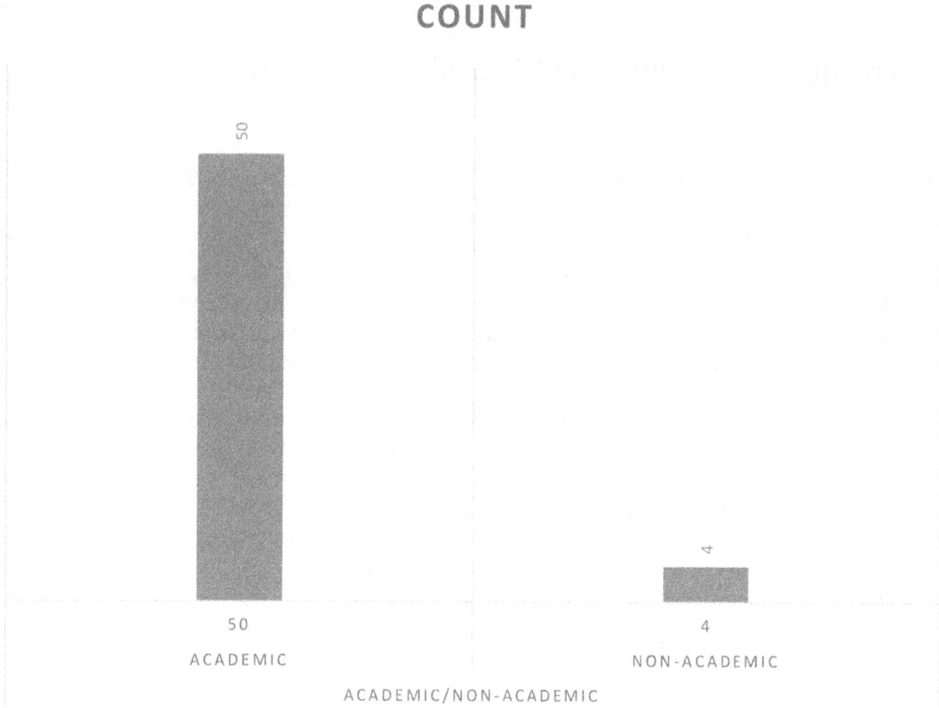

REFERENCES

[1] World Health Organization (WHO) (2017). *WHO Report on the Global TOBACCO Epidemic, 2017*, World Health Organization. Available at: http://apps.who.int/iris/bitstre/10665/255874/1/9789241512824-eng.pdf?ua=1&ua=1

[2] Göktalay T, Coşkun AŞ, Havlucu Y, Horasan GD. (2020). Use of tobacco products in turkish children and young people: Is there an alarm for hookah use? *Turk Thorac J.* 21(4):234–241.

[3] Asma S, Mackay J, Song SY, et al. (2015). *The GATS Atlas. CDC Foundation* 30–31

[4] Tata Institute of Social Sciences and Ministry of Health and Family Welfare, Government of India (2017). *Global Adult Tobacco Survey GATS 2 India 2016-2017 Report.* Available at: https://mohfw.gov.in/sites/default/files/GlobaltobacoJune2018.pdf

[5] Mishra GA, Pimple SA, Shastri SS. (2012). An overview of the tobacco problem in India. *Indian J Med Paediatr Oncol.* 33(3): 139–45.

[6] Desalu OO, Adekoya AO, Elegbede AO, Dosunmu A, Kolawole TF, Nwogu KC. (2009). Knowledge of and practices related to smoking cessation among physicians in Nigeria. *J Bras Pneumol.* 35:1198–203.

[7] United States Public Health Service Office of the Surgeon General; National Center for Chronic Disease Prevention and Health Promotion (US) Office on Smoking and Health. Smoking Cessation: A Report of the Surgeon General [Internet]. Washington (DC): US Department of Health and Human Services; 2020. Chapter 6, Interventions for Smoking Cessation and Treatments for Nicotine Dependence. Available from: https://www.ncbi.nlm.nih.gov/books/NBK555596/

[8] Thawani V, Pande S, Turankar A. (2003). Pharmacotherapy for treating tobacco dependence. *Indian J Pharmacol.* 35:402–3.

[9] Szatkowski L, Lewis S, McNeill A, Coleman T. (2010) Is smoking status routinely recorded when patients register with a new GP? *Fam Pract.* 27(6):673–5.

[10] Thankappan KR. (2014). Tobacco cessation in India: a priority health intervention. *Indian J Med Res.* 139(4):484–6.

[11] Alblowi JA. (2021) Perception of tobacco counseling and cessation among dental practitioners. *J Smok Cessat*:6692525.

[12] Heydari G, Masjedi M, Ahmady AE, Leischow SJ, Lando HA, Shadmehr MB, Fadaizadeh L. (2014) A comparative study on tobacco cessation methods: a quantitative systematic review. *Int J Prev Med.* 5(6):673–8.

[13] Olson CK, Sherwood N, Berkane M, Gilligan K, McKinney WJ Jr. (2023) Perceptions, intentions, and actual use of a consumer nicotine gum. *Harm Reduct J.* 20(1):132.

[14] Prabhu A, Jain JK, Sakeenabhi B, Kumar PGN, Imranulla M, Ragher M. (2017). Smoking Cessation Advice: Knowledge, Attitude, and Practice among Clinical Dental Students'. *J Pharm Bioallied Sci.* 9(Suppl 1):S117–S120.

[15] Hartmann-Boyce J, Lindson N, Butler AR, McRobbie H, Bullen C, Begh R, Theodoulou A, Notley C, Rigotti NA, Turner T, Fanshawe TR, Hajek P. (2022). Electronic cigarettes for smoking cessation. *Cochrane Database Syst Rev.* 11(11):CD010216.

 ISBN: 978-1-041-32674-8

Modern Techniques of Teaching and Learning: A Review

Madna Shilpa
Department of Public Health Dentistry, A. J Institute of Dental College, Mangalore. Karnataka

ABSTRACT: Education is an ever-evolving and active process in which the students and teachers have to work mutually to make this knowledge-sharing process enjoyable and easier for comprehension and that requires periodic refinement. Nowadays, in every country education and training are of particular importance due to their role in various scientific, cultural, social, political, and economic fields. Thus, the objective of this review is to describe and assess the alternative teaching-learning methods to promote active student involvement and expedite a smooth flow of information. Various modern learning methodologies were identified, including Case-Based learning, Evidence-Based medicine, Problem-Based learning, Simulation-Based learning, Peer-Assisted learning, Observational learning, Team-Based learning, and Flipped classrooms. These various teaching and learning methods are well-validated, and discussed to attend to individual learning differences allowing students to broaden their thinking and professional knowledge Early introduction of integrative approaches develops students‘ competency and leadership, preparing them for a seamless transition into clinical practice. Given technological advancements and the broader implications of medical information Students require innovative skills through interprofessional learning. The method of discussion in small groups is more influential. Regarding students' level of learning and satisfaction, encouragement is given to participate in discussions and dialogues. Thus, it becomes essential to utilize an approach to teaching and learning that best meets the specific needs of the students.

Keywords: Medical education, Techniques and methods, Case-Based learning, Evidence-Based medicine, Problem-Based Learning, and Flipped classrooms.

1 INTRODUCTION

Education and training are essential due to their role in various scientific, cultural, social, political, and economic fields. medical education plays a crucial role in developing compassionate healthcare professionals. [1]

Learning is teaching the students using educational principles and learning theory. It is a dynamic, two-way communication process between teachers and students. In India, however, medical education faces challenges related to poor quality and limited contributions to research. The medical curriculum is often inadequate in preparing students for future challenges, primarily due to a lack of innovative teaching methods. [2]

The importance of problem-based learning (PBL) was highlighted at a symposium by the World Federation of Medical Education. The symposium aimed to inform educators from undergraduate, postgraduate, and continuing medical education programs about this novel approach. Following this, the World Health Organization (WHO) recognized PBL as a highly valued educational method. [3]

1.1 *Objective*

This review aims to explore and evaluate alternative teaching-learning methods designed to increase student engagement and facilitate the smooth transfer of knowledge.

1.2 *Methods*

A comprehensive literature review was conducted using databases like PubMed, ResearchGate, and Google Scholar, utilizing keywords related to alternative learning, modern teaching techniques, and medical education. Various articles on each teaching technique and its implementation were examined. Inclusion criteria consisted of peer-reviewed, open-access studies published between 2009 and 2023, and written in English. Non-English literature was excluded from the review. [4]

1.3 *Results*

The literature search identified eight modern teaching techniques that are well-established and widely used to achieve specific educational goals. These methods were reviewed to assess their effectiveness, challenges in implementation, and suggestions for overcoming those challenges. [5]

 DOI: 10.1201/9781042016075-27

2 MODERN TEACHING AND LEARNING TECHNIQUES

2.1 *Case-based learning*

This is a student-centered approach in which learners analyze and discuss detailed scenarios, applying their knowledge to each case. Students typically engage in group discussions or individual assessments of realistic or hypothetical cases, which helps them develop critical thinking, problem-solving, and decision-making skills. This approach is particularly valuable in medical education, as it allows students to integrate theory with practice, fostering an understanding of real-world applications. However, the effectiveness of case-based learning depends on the relevance and quality of the cases, as well as the facilitation skills of the instructors. [6]

2.1.1 *Limitations*

This learning technique can be time-consuming, as it requires students to identify problems, decompose them into components, and develop effective solutions.

2.1.2 *Recommendation*

This method proves to be more effective when implemented in small group sessions, with active participation from engaged learners and cases that are closely aligned with clinical scenarios. [7]

2.2 *Evidence-based learning*

Evidence-based Medicine (EBM) provides students with the necessary skills to learn, comprehend, and assess medical research. It involves five essential steps: a) transforming unclear information into a clear, answerable question, b) identifying the most relevant evidence, c) critically evaluating the evidence for its reliability, d) integrating the findings into clinical practice, and e) assessing the outcomes.

2.3 *Limitations*

- Despite its crucial role in modern education, integrating Evidence-Based Medicine (EBM) into the medical curriculum requires careful guidance to meet its goals. It should be tailored to individual training and experience.
- Challenges include gaps in knowledge and experience in research, as well as the need for students to be proficient with computers and trained in effective research techniques using online databases.

2.4 *Recommendation*

- Evidence-based medicine (EBM) should be thoroughly integrated into both undergraduate and postgraduate education to overcome challenges and equip students with the skills needed to effectively use this learning strategy. [8]

3 PROBLEM-BASED LEARNING

It is a student-focused method where learners work in groups to address open-ended problems, fostering motivation and deepening their learning. In addition to covering the course content, PBL promotes the development of critical thinking, problem-solving, and communication skills. Typically, Problem-based learning is delivered through small group tutorials, where the teacher acts as a facilitator. These sessions usually involve discussing specific problems, with time allocated for self-directed research and information gathering. This method encourages students to build a strong foundation in self-directed learning.

3.1 *Limitations*

- Evaluating students' performance during Problem-Based Learning (PBL) sessions can be challenging, requiring clear and effective evaluation methods.

3.2 *Recommendations*

- Students need to come prepared for each class with prior knowledge of the subject to address any misconceptions and fill knowledge gaps.
- Students should also be encouraged to participate in peer assessments to promote peer learning. [9]

4 SIMULATION-BASED LEARNING

Simulation-based learning is a teaching method that not only conveys course concepts but also provides students with the opportunity to apply new skills, knowledge, and ideas in a realistic practice setting. It involves creating artificial representations of real-world processes to achieve educational goals through hands-on learning. Simulation tools serve as substitutes for real patients, allowing trainees to make and learn from mistakes without causing harm to actual patients. This approach enables students to develop crucial skills through trial and error in a safe, controlled environment before applying them in real-world situations. [10]

4.1 *Limitations*

- Simulation-Based Learning (SBL) requires coordination, patience, collaboration, and effective guidance.
- Preparing and organizing sessions can be time-consuming and demands sufficient equipment to ensure all students have equal opportunities.

4.2 *Recommendations*

- Simulation-based learning should be introduced early in basic sciences to provide hands-on, pseudo-clinical experience.
- Smaller groups with limited instructional guidance can boost student enthusiasm, allowing them to manage tasks independently and increase participation and peer discussions.

5 PEER-ASSISTED LEARNING

Peer-assisted learning (PAL) is a collaborative approach where individuals develop skills and knowledge through mutual support among equals. It is an informal, team-based learning method in which motivated students assist each other, with both tutors and tutees having similar educational backgrounds. This approach involves selecting students with appropriate teaching qualities to facilitate learning and practice medicine. [11]

5.1 *Limitations*

- Challenges such as perceived stigma regarding Factors such as peer knowledge, lack of motivation, and limited willingness to collaborate can pose significant limitations. [12]

5.2 *Recommendations*

- Peer tutors should develop strong communication skills and confidence to ensure their success.

6 OBSERVATIONAL LEARNING

Which involves learning through demonstration, is especially important in the medical field, where "patient safety first" is the top priority. Mastering motor skills is a crucial component of medical expertise and requires effective teaching and practice. Many medical procedures, such as Oro-tracheal intubation and surgical suturing, are considered open skills because they demand physicians to adapt to unpredictable and dynamic environments. [13]

6.1 *Limitations*

- Observational learning presents several challenges, especially when incorporating it into the curriculum. Instructors may find it difficult to assess students' interest in observing certain techniques or skills.

6.2 *Recommendations*

Therefore, it is essential to complement observational learning with other teaching methods to minimize bias and address any gaps that may arise from relying on a single approach. [14]

7 TEAM-BASED LEARNING

In modern medical education, Team-Based Learning (TBL) is a widely adopted and popular teaching method. Many healthcare faculties worldwide have incorporated Team-Based Learning (TBL) in various combinations across different settings and subject areas. It is an innovative, student-centered approach that complements the flipped classroom model in healthcare education. [15]

7.1 *Limitations*

- Despite its many benefits, implementing Team-Based Learning (TBL) presents several challenges. Managing group dynamics can be complex, as students may vary in their levels of commitment, engagement, and communication styles.
- Some students may dominate discussions, while others might be more passive, making it difficult to ensure equal participation from all team members.

7.2 *Recommendations*

- Provide comprehensive training for both instructors and students to ensure effective implementation of TBL. This includes familiarizing participants with TBL components such as pre-class preparation and individual and team readiness assessments.

8 FLIPPED CLASSROOM

The flipped classroom model has attracted significant interest in medical education. In this approach, students review pre-class materials independently, while class time is used for active learning, discussions, and problem-solving activities. It also addresses strategies for effective implementation and potential challenges. Research shows that the flipped classroom enhances student perceptions, learning outcomes, critical thinking skills, and motivation when compared to traditional lecture-based methods. [16]

8.1 *Limitations*

- The main challenges associated with the flipped classroom model include self-regulated learning difficulties, a heavy workload, and a lack of immediate support.

8.2 *Recommendations*

- A key challenge in implementing a student-centric learning model is the necessity for extra training and resources to properly equip teachers with the skills needed for effective student-centered instruction.

9 DISCUSSION

Traditionally, lectures have been central to pre-clinical medical education, serving as the primary method for instructors to deliver information. However, this didactic approach has faced significant challenges, prompting the need for modern learning techniques. Traditional lectures often lack interactivity and fail to engage students in active learning, leading to reluctance to participate beyond the classroom. Contemporary educational methods emphasize student-centered learning, where learners take an active role in their education. These modern approaches are designed to actively involve students, improving their understanding, and clinical reasoning. [17]

Integrating these techniques addresses diverse learning styles and enhances student performance across various aspects of medical sciences. Techniques like Peer-Assisted Learning (PAL) and observational learning offer practical, real-world skills and immediate feedback, while simulations allow for safe, reflective practice.

Learning is inherently an active, personal process that benefits from a motivational environment. Promoting self-directed learning and creating a motivational atmosphere—through social relationships, goal fulfillment, and professional growth—enhances student engagement and participation. [18]

10 CONCLUSION

Learning is a continuous process, and it is important to recognize that students have diverse learning styles. Modern teaching methods in medical education, such as Case-Based Learning (CBL), Evidence-Based Medicine (EBM), Problem-Based Learning (PBL), Simulation-Based Learning (SBL), Peer-Assisted Learning (PAL), observational learning, the flipped classroom model, and team-based learning, provide student-centered alternatives. These innovative approaches promote critical thinking, encourage meaningful knowledge acquisition, and help develop essential skills, competencies, and leadership qualities in the medical profession. As a result, medical education must remain flexible, incorporating multidisciplinary teaching models effectively and appropriately from the pre-clinical years onward.

REFERENCES

[1] Ataei M, Hamedani SS, Zameni F. (2020). Effective methods in medical education: from giving lecture to simulation. *Journal of Advanced Pharmacy Education and Research.* 10(1):36–42.

[2] Hidayati D, Komariah A, Mirfani AM. (2020). The effect of information technology on the quality of teaching learning process in junior high school in bandung. *ICEPP* 65–67.

[3] Walton, H.J., and Matthews, M.B. (1989). Essentials of problem-based learning. *Medical Education, 23*(6), 542–558.

[4] Williams B. (2005). Case-based learning–a review of the literature: is there scope for this educational paradigm in prehospital education? *22*(8), 577–581

[5] Archana BR, Sangeetha S. (2023). E-learning in medical education: 12(2):108–12.

[6] Singhal A. (2017). Case-based learning in microbiology: observations from a North West Indian Medical College. 7(1): 47–51.

[7] Thistlethwaite, J.E., Davies, D., Ekeocha, S., Kidd, J.M., *et al.* (2012) The effectiveness of case-based learning in health professional education. *A BEME Systematic Review*: 34(6), e421–e444.

[8] Gagliardi JP, Stinnett SS, Schardt C. (2012). Innovation in evidence-based medicine education and assessment: An interactive class for third-and fourth-year medical students. 100(4):306.

[9] Ubbink DT, Guyatt GH, Vermeulen H. (2013). Framework of policy recommendations for implementation of evidence-based practice. 3(1): 1–12.

[10] Ledingham IM. (1998). Twelve tips for setting up a clinical skills training facility. *Medical Teacher.* 20(6):503–507.

[11] Awasthi S, Yadav KK. (2015). Assessment of the acceptance and effectiveness of peer-assisted learning in pediatrics. *International Journal of Applied and Basic Medical Research.* 5(1): S3–6.

[12] Scicluna HA, O'Sullivan AJ, Boyle P, Jones PD, McNeil HP. (2015). Peer learning in the UNSW Medicine program. *BMC Medical Education.* 15:1–9.

[13] Cordovani L, Cordovani D. (2016). A literature review on observational learning for medical motor skills and anesthesia teaching. 21:1113–21.

[14] Van Gog T, Paas F, Marcus N, Ayres P, Sweller J. (2009). The mirror neuron system and observational learning: Implications for the effectiveness of dynamic visualizations 21:21–30.

[15] Burgess A, Bleasel J, Haq I, Roberts C, Garsia R, Robertson T, Mellis C. (2017). Team-based learning (TBL) in the medical curriculum: better than PBL? 17:1.

[16] Gilboy MB, Heinrichs S, Pazzaglia G. (2015). Enhancing student engagement using the flipped classroom. 47(1):109–14.

[17] Hernández-Torrano D, Ali S, Chan CK. (2017). First-year medical students' learning style preferences and their correlation with performance in different subjects within the medical course. 17:1–7.

[18] McCombs BL. (1991). Motivation and lifelong learning. *Educational Psychologist.* 26(2):117–27.

Navigating Dental Education Trends and Transforming Dental Pedagogy – Abas and Srikant N (Eds)
© 2027 The Author(s), ISBN: 978-1-041-32674-8

BUDDY System: An Innovative Learning Strategy

Anand Badavannavar, Roopa Jatti, and Adithi Rao
Department of Orthodontics and Dentofacial Orthopaedics, KLE V K Institute of Dental Sciences, KAHER University, India

Aarti Sethia
Private Practitioner and Consultant Orthodontist, Mumbai, India

Atrey Pai Khot
Department of Public Health Dentistry, Goa Dental College, Goa

Zameera Naik
Department of Oral Medicine and Radiology, KLE V K Institute of Dental Sciences, KAHER University, India.

Sumedh Koderi
Department of Orthodontics and Dentofacial Orthopaedics, KLE V K Institute of Dental Sciences, KAHER University, India

Jasleen Thakkar
Department of Periodontics, KLE VK Institute of Dental Sciences, KAHER University, India

1 INTRODUCTION

Orthodontics is a speciality of dentistry that requires an advanced understanding of craniofacial growth and occlusal development. It requires critical understanding and skill to learn, which is difficult for a postgraduate student to attain due to increased stress and fear of failure. Therefore, there is a need for a good framework to build teamwork and close the knowledge gaps.

2 MATERIALS AND METHODS

A total of 30 students participated during the piloting of this study. Twelve post-graduate students participated in semi-structured interviews. Amongst these 90.16% were alumni and 9.8% were current post-graduates in the Department of Orthodontics. The first phase consisted of Semi-structured qualitative interviews with 12 consecutive postgraduate students. The qualitative interviews were designed following guidelines for qualitative research by Mays and Pope.10 Interviews were carried out by the first author in a non-clinical setting informally with no time pressure through Google Forms. The information thus gathered via these interviews was used to construct the questionnaire. The second phase consisted of piloting the questionnaire on 30 participants. The typical time taken to complete the consent and questionnaire was approximately 5–10 minutes. The questionnaire was then subjected to reliability testing.

The generated data then underwent content analysis where key themes and concepts were identified in the transcripts and categorized by the author. The data were analyzed by the second author to check the subjective biases in analyses. A five-point Likert scale was used for the evaluation of these questions. During the content validity by the experts, three irrelevant and open-ended questions were eliminated to avoid any ambiguity.

3 RESULTS

There was good agreement in understanding the subject concepts and exchange of study material in terms of research work and books however the same wasn't appreciated in terms of literature search. All 30 post-graduate students as well as alumni reverted back for the test-retest through Google Forms. Responses from the first test were compared with the responses given through retest and were correlated using the Kappa test. The responses recorded on these two occasions were statistically significant using the Kappa test and were statistically significant ($p<0.001$) suggesting that scores are reliable over time. Test-retest reliability of all the questions was analyzed using weighted Kappa because of their ordinal nature. A weighted Kappa (Kw) was used to measure the level of agreement between time 1 and time 2 which accounts for near misses in agreement. Weights were

DOI: 10.1201/9781042016075-28

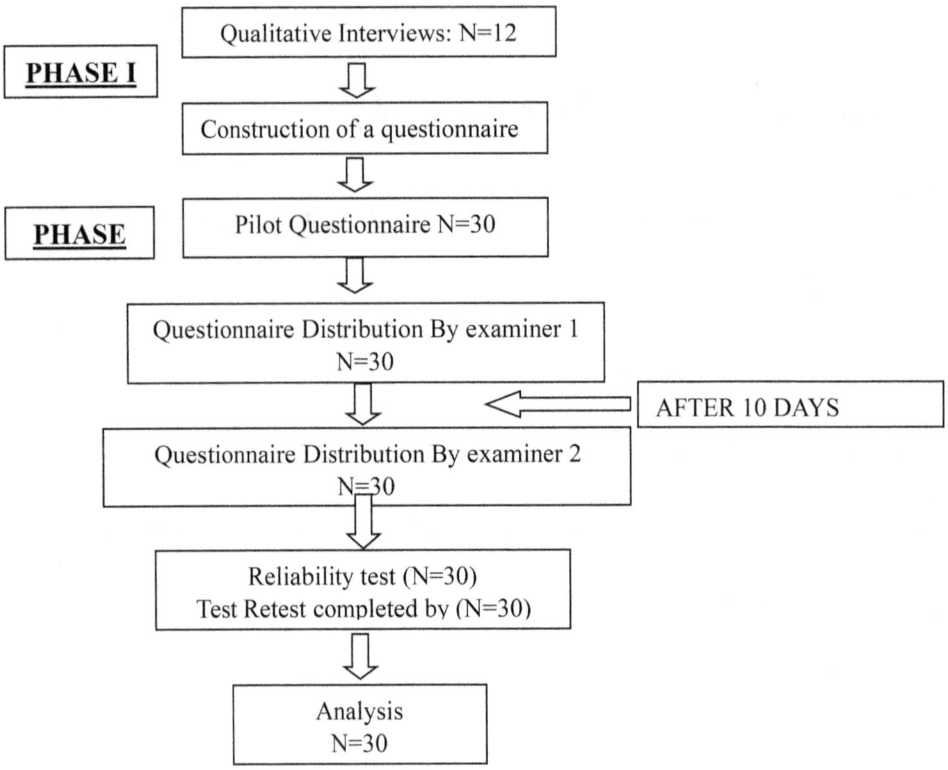

assigned according to the method described by Altman. [12] There was little to moderate consensus on whether the buddy system improved clinical practice and knowledge, but early clinical exposure helped grasp case scenarios

4 DISCUSSION

The Buddy system is an educational method whereby there is the acquisition of knowledge and skills through active helping and supporting among status equals or matched companions. In the current study, there was good agreement in understanding the subject concepts and exchange of study material in terms of research work and books however the same wasn't appreciated in terms of literature search. These findings were in congruence with observations by Hunt *et al.* [15] and Freret *et al.* [16] Wherein peer-assisted learning methods led to reciprocal learning, allowing tutors to gain a deeper understanding of topics previously learnt, providing a good recap of information, helping identify their learning styles, as well as streamline the knowledge they had acquired throughout the course. There was little to moderate consensus on whether the buddy system improved clinical practice and knowledge, but early clinical exposure helped grasp case scenarios. Varghese *et al.* [7] in their study on peer-assisted learning in a dental environment reported that such methods help build confidence among students and help them with management and conversation skills both of which are equally important in routine clinical practice.

5 CONCLUSION

The benefit of the Buddy system is not only to the post-graduate students but also an investment in the intellectual capital and capacity of teachers and leaders of various fields. The long-term effects on the outcomes of resident postgraduates has to be explored.

ACKNOWLEDGEMENTS

Principal/Dean, KLE VK Institute of Dental Sciences, Belagavi and Staff and postgraduate students, Department of Orthodontics and Dentofacial Orthopedics, Department of Prosthodontics and Department of Oral Medicine and Radiology.

No external funding received.

REFERENCES

[1] Ravindra Nanda, Madhur Upadhyay, (2013), Skeletal and dental considerations in orthodontic treatment mechanics: a contemporary view, *European Journal of Orthodontics*, Volume 35, Issue 5, Pages 634–643

[2] Jheon AH, Oberoi S, Solem RC, Kapila S. (2017), Moving towards precision orthodontics: An evolving paradigm shift in the planning and delivery of customized orthodontic therapy. *Orthodontics & Craniofacial Research*. 20:106–13.

[3] Isherwood G, Taylor K, Burnside G, Fitzgerald R, Flannigan N. (2020), Teaching orthodontic emergencies using the "flipped classroom" method of teaching—A mixed methods RCT. *European Journal of Dental Education*. 24(1):53–62.

[4] Schönwetter DJ, Lavigne S, Mazurat R, Nazarko O. (2006), Students' perceptions of effective classroom and clinical teaching in dental and dental hygiene education. *Journal of Dental Education*. 70(6):624–35.

[5] Tangade PS, Mathur A, Gupta R, Chaudhary S. (2011), Assessment of stress level among dental school students: an Indian outlook. *Dental Research Journal*. 2011;8(2):95.

[6] Acharya S. (2003), Factors affecting stress among Indian dental students. *Journal of Dental Education*. 67(10):1140–8.

[7] Varghese AM, Zijlstra-Shaw S. (2021), Teaching to learn: Using peer-assisted learning to complement the undergraduate dental curriculum. *European Journal of Dental Education*. 25(4):762–7.

[8] Roche R, Manzi J, Kruithoff BC. (2021), The benefits of being a "Buddy": Exploring the medical student experience as mentor to minority high-school students. *Health Equity*. 5(1):1–7.

[9] Hall S, Harrison CH, Stephens J, Andrade MG, Seaby EG, Parton W, McElligott S, Myers MA, Elmansouri A, Ahn M, Parrott R. (2018), The benefits of being a near-peer teacher. *The Clinical Teacher*. 15(5):403–7.

[10] Casey EC. (1972), The buddy system reexamined. *Journal of the National Medical Association*. 64(5):452.

[11] Mays N, Pope C. (1995), Qualitative research: rigour and qualitative research. *Bmj*. 311(6997):109–12.

[12] Sayers MS, Newton JT. (2006), Patients' expectations of orthodontic treatment: part 1–development of a questionnaire. *Journal of Orthodontics*. 33(4):258–69.

[13] Altman DG. (1990), Practical statistics for medical research. *Chapman and Hall/CRC*.

[14] Topping K, Ehly S. (1998), Introduction to Peer-Assisted Learning, in. In: Topping K, Ehly S, editors. *Hrsg. Peer-assisted learning. Mahwah*, NJ, US: Lawrence Erlbaum Associates Publishers; p. 1–23.

[15] Capstick S. (2004), Benefits and Shortcomings of Peer Assisted Learning (PAL) in higher education: an appraisal by students. In, *Peer Assisted Learning Conference* .

[16] Hunt T, Jones TA, Carney PA. (2019), Peer-assisted learning in dental students' patient case evaluations: an assessment of reciprocal learning. *J Dent Educ*. 84:343–349.

[17] Freret T, Rana J, Schwartzstein RM, Gooding HC. (2017), Twelve tips for implementation of "student-as-teacher" programs. *Med Teach*. 39(12):1221–1226.

[18] Herrmann-Werner, A., Gramer, R., Erschens, R., Nikendei, C., Wosnik, A., Griewatz, J., Zipfel, S. and Junne, F., (2017). Peer-assisted learning (PAL) in undergraduate medical education: An overview. *Zeitschrift für Evidenz, Fortbildung und Qualität im Gesundheitswesen*, 121, pp.74–81.

[19] Darling-Hammond L, Flook L, Cook-Harvey C, Barron B, Osher D. (2020), Implications for educational practice of the science of learning and development. *Applied Developmental Science*. 24(2):97–140.

[20] Ten Cate O,Durning S. (2007), Peer teaching in medical education: twelve reasons to move from theory to practice. *Medical Teacher* 29:591–9.

[21] Kaufman A, Klepper D, Obenshain SS, Voorhees JD, Galey W, Duban S, *et al.* (1982), Undergraduate medical education for primary care: a case study in New Mexico. *South Med J* 75(9): 1110–17.

Navigating Dental Education Trends and Transforming Dental Pedagogy – Abas and Srikant N (Eds)
© 2027 The Author(s), ISBN: 978-1-041-32674-8

Gaming the Curriculum: Advancing Dental Education Through Gamification

Ann Sales
Department of Prosthodontics and Crown and Bridge, Manipal College of Dental Sciences Mangalore, Manipal Academy of Higher Education, Manipal, India

Amoli Singh
Department of Orthodontics and Dentofacial Orthopaedics, Manipal College of Dental Sciences Mangalore, Manipal Academy of Higher Education, Manipal, India

ABSTRACT: As dental education adapts to the evolving demands of healthcare, innovative teaching strategies such as gamification are essential for preparing future professionals. This paper explores the integration of gamification into the dental curriculum, emphasizing its potential to enhance student engagement, knowledge retention, and clinical skill development. Gamification incorporates game design elements such as points, badges, and leaderboards into educational content, transforming traditional learning into interactive, engaging experiences. This approach motivates students, to enjoy learning while fostering essential skills such as collaboration and healthy competition.

This paper reviews case studies from dental programs that have successfully implemented gamified learning modules, demonstrating improvements in both theoretical knowledge and practical skills. Gamification supports competency-based education, allowing students to progress at their own pace and achieve a deeper understanding of key concepts. Additionally, the integration of gamification offers opportunities for continuous assessment and personalized feedback, enabling educators to tailor teaching methods to individual student needs. However, the paper also addresses challenges such as barriers to implementation, the need for faculty training, and the potential risk of overemphasizing competition.

By synthesizing these insights, the paper provides practical recommendations for effectively integrating gamification into dental curricula, ensuring that it complements traditional methods and aligns with educational goals. Finally, the review suggests areas for future research, particularly the need for longitudinal studies to assess the long-term impact of gamification on student performance and professional competency.

Keywords: gamification, artificial intelligence, educational innovation, dental curriculum advancements

1 INTRODUCTION

Gamification in education has become a topic of growing interest across various fields, and dental education is no exception. As dental curricula evolve to meet the ever-changing demands of modern healthcare, traditional lecture-based methods are struggling to fully engage today's tech-savvy learners [1]. Gamification, which involves the use of game design elements in nongame settings, offers a promising alternative [2]. The incorporation of interactive features such as points, leaderboards, and simulations, creates a more engaging and immersive learning environment. This innovative approach redefines how dental education is delivered, encouraging active participation and increasing motivation [3]

The advantages of gamification go beyond simply making learning more engaging. It has been shown to improve critical thinking, enhance knowledge retention, and provide a bridge between theoretical concepts and practical application [4]. Technologies such as virtual reality (VR), artificial intelligence (AI), and serious games have further expanded its reach and effectiveness [5,6]. This review delves into the applications, benefits, challenges, and future possibilities of gamification in dental education, drawing on insights from evidence based studies to present a well-rounded perspective.

2 APPLICATIONS OF GAMIFICATION IN DENTAL EDUCATION

2.1 *Enhancing theoretical learning*

Gamification has the unique ability to turn dry theoretical concepts into dynamic and enjoyable learning experiences. For example, Aboalshamat *et al.* [7] found that gamified board games significantly improved the understanding of antimicrobial resistance (AMR) among both dental students and the public. Their study revealed that

 DOI: 10.1201/9781042016075-29

these games were more effective than traditional lectures for long-term knowledge retention. Similarly, Amir *et al.* [8]developed a serious game called "HistoRM," which was designed to teach oral histology. Compared with those taught via conventional methods, students using this tool not only scored higher on assessments but also reported greater satisfaction.

Escape games have also shown promise in dental education. Aubeux *et al.* [9]introduced an endodontic-themed escape game where students solved clinical puzzles under time constraints. This creative approach helped participants apply theoretical knowledge to practical scenarios while building teamwork and problem-solving skills.

2.2 *Bridging the gap between theory and practice*

Simulation-based learning, a key element of gamification, plays a crucial role in connecting theory to real-world applications. For instance, Azhari *et al.* [10]used VR to create a simulated environment for tooth preparation. Students who practiced in this setting demonstrated significant improvement in their practical skills and showed a positive attitude toward the integration of technology in their education. Similarly, Krause *et al.* [11] designed the METIS platform, which is a dual-player simulation that combines competition and collaboration to deepen students' understanding of operative dentistry.

In the area of dental practice management, Peanchitlertkajorn *et al.* [12] developed a virtual clinic that allowed students to experience real-world challenges in a safe and controlled environment. This tool increased their confidence and preparedness for future clinical practice.

2.3 *Promoting Skill Development in specialized fields*

Gamification has also been found in specialized areas of dentistry. Mahrous *et al.* [13] explored the use of AI-driven gamified platforms for teaching removable partial denture design. These platforms provide automated feedback, enhancing students' critical thinking and decision-making skills. Similarly, Lakshmikantha [14] highlighted the effectiveness of game-based learning in orthodontics, particularly in improving student engagement and retention of information.

In oral pathology, Pisal *et al.* [15] demonstrated how gamified approaches could simplify complex topics such as odontogenic cysts, making them easier for students to grasp and retain.

3 BENEFITS OF GAMIFICATION IN DENTISTRY

3.1 *Boosting engagement and motivation*

One of the most notable benefits of gamification is its ability to actively engage students and keep them motivated. [16] For example, Nguyen *et al.* [17] reported that gamified quizzes such as Kahoot capture students' attention more effectively than traditional teaching methods do, particularly in the early stages of their training. Similarly, Friedrich *et al.* [18] observed that Jeopardy-style games not only made learning fun but also encouraged greater participation.

3.2 *Enhancing knowledge retention*

Gamified methods have proven to be highly effective for long-term retention of knowledge. Aboalshamat *et al.* [7] found that gamified board games helped students retain AMR-related information more effectively than traditional approaches did. Moreover, Moreira *et al.* [19] reviewed gamified oral hygiene apps and reported that interactive games significantly improved children's understanding of proper oral care habits.

3.3 *Supporting practical skill development*

Interactive simulations and serious games provide a safe environment for students to practice complex dental procedures. Tools such as Azhari *et al.*'s [10]VR tooth preparation module and Mahrous *et al.*'s [13] AI-powered denture design platform enable students to refine their practical skills without the stress of real-world consequences.

4 CHALLENGES IN IMPLEMENTING GAMIFICATION

4.1 *High resource requirements*

One of the greatest hurdles to adopting gamification is the investment it requires in technology, infrastructure, and faculty training. Lakshmikantha [14] noted out that the high costs of tools such as VR and AI can be a significant barrier for many institutions. Mehrotra [20] argued for the development of more affordable and accessible solutions to help overcome these limitations.

4.2 *Striking a balance between competition and collaboration*

While a sense of competition can motivate students, placing too much emphasis on performance metrics may lead to stress and diminished intrinsic interest in learning. Amir *et al.* [8] emphasized the need for a balanced approach that combines both competitive and collaborative elements to create a healthy learning environment.

4.3 *Addressing ethical and technical concerns*

The use of advanced technologies in gamification brings its own set of challenges, including issues related to data privacy, accessibility, and technical proficiency. Chauhan *et al.* [21] stressed the importance of addressing these concerns to ensure that gamified tools are equitable and sustainable.

5 FUTURE DIRECTIONS AND INNOVATIONS

5.1 *Personalizing learning through AI*

AI has the potential to transform gamification by tailoring learning experiences to individual students' needs. For instance, Mahrous *et al.* [13] demonstrated how AI-powered platforms could adapt to learners' progress, allowing them to advance at their own pace.

5.2 *Expanding health promotion initiatives*

Gamification is not limited to academic settings. Moreira *et al.* [19] reviewed oral hygiene apps that use gamification to promote better brushing habits among children and adolescents. These tools highlight the potential of gamification to encourage positive behaviors beyond the classroom.

5.3 *Leveraging emerging technologies*

The future of gamification lies in advanced technologies such as virtual and augmented reality. Examples such as Azhari *et al.*'s [10] VR modules and Peanchitlertkajorn *et al.*'s [12]virtual dental clinic demonstrate how these tools can enhance both theoretical understanding and practical skills.

6 EMPIRICAL EVIDENCE AND KNOWLEDGE GAPS

Despite its promising potential, there are still gaps in our understanding of gamification's long-term impact. Zaror *et al.* [22] noted the absence of standardized evaluation methods and the need for longitudinal studies to measure its sustained effectiveness. Song *et al.* [23] highlights the importance of scalability and robustness to ensure that gamified tools can be applied across diverse educational contexts.

7 CONCLUSION

Gamification is transforming dental education by making learning more engaging, interactive, and effective. By integrating innovative tools and techniques, educators can enhance knowledge retention, foster skill development, and better prepare students for the demands of modern dental practice. However, challenges such as resource constraints, ethical considerations, and the need for further research must be addressed to fully realize its potential.

REFERENCES

[1] van Gaalen AEJ, Brouwer J, Schönrock-Adema J, Bouwkamp-Timmer T, Jaarsma ADC, Georgiadis JR. (2021). Gamification of health professions education: a systematic review. *Advances in Health Sciences Education. Springer Science and Business Media B. V.*; Vol. 26, p. 683–711.

[2] Tubelo RA, Branco VLC, Dahmer A, Samuel SMW, Collares FM. (2015). The influence of a learning object with virtual simulation for dentistry: A randomized controlled trial. *Int J Med Inform.* 85(1):68–75.

[3] Germa A, Gosset M, Gaucher C, Valencien C, Schlumberger M, Colombier ML, *et al.* (2021). OSCEGame: A serious game for OSCE training. *European Journal of Dental Education.* 25(4):657–63.

[4] Khorasanchi M, Hoseinzadeh M, Khadem Rezaeian M, Kazemian A, Moradi A, Sarabadani J. (2024). The development of a serious game for laser applications in dentistry and the evaluation of dental students' satisfaction. *BMC Med Educ.* 24(1).

[5] Mladenovic R, Mladenovic K. (2024). From boring to engaging: Using gamification to transform dental education and practice. In: *Augmented Reality Games II.* Springer International Publishing; p. 223–41.

[6] Pereira AC, Walmsley AD. (2019). Games in dental education: playing to learn or learning to play? *Br Dent J.* 227(6):459–60.
[7] Aboalshamat K, Khayat A, Halwani R, Bitan A, Alansari R. (2020). The effects of gamification on antimicrobial resistance knowledge and its relationship to dentistry in Saudi Arabia: A randomized controlled trial. *BMC Public Health.* 20(1).
[8] Amir LR, Dewatmoko SN, Leonardy IC, Yanuar R, Suniarti DF, Idrus E, *et al.* (2024). Perceived Enablers of and Barriers to Serious Game as Oral Histology Learning Strategy for Undergraduate Dental Students. *Dent J (Basel)*;12(9):280.
[9] Aubeux D, Blanchflower N, Bray E, Clouet R, Remaud M, Badran Z, *et al.* (2020). Educational gaming for dental students: Design and assessment of a pilot endodontic-themed escape game. *European Journal of Dental Education.* 24(3):449–57.
[10] Azhari AA, Ashy Y, Abulhamail L, Sharshar H, Ahmed WM. (2024). Integrating virtual–reality into restorative dentistry training: A study on the acceptability and effectiveness of tooth preparation simulations. *J Dent Educ.*
[11] Krause F, Horn B, Braun A, Fedrowitz S, Bell L, Lemos M. (2024). Who learns more: the impact of dual-player and single-player modes in a serious game on dental students' factual knowledge. *BMC Med Educ.* 24(1).
[12] Peanchitlertkajorn S, Reynolds PA, Chaisawas M, Krungthong Y, Boonkaew B, Sipiyaruk K. (2024). The impact of an online gamified virtual tour on cognitive enhancement in dental practice management. *Sci Rep.* 14(1):26975.
[13] Mahrous A, Botsko DL, Elgreatly A, Tsujimoto A, Qian F, Schneider GB. (2023). The use of artificial intelligence and game-based learning in removable partial denture design: A comparative study. *J Dent Educ.* 87(8):1188–99.
[14] Lakshmikantha HT. (2024). Leveling up orthodontic education: Game-based learning as the new frontier in orthodontic curriculum. *Research and Development in Medical Education [Internet].* 13:13. Available from: https://rdme.tbzmed.ac.ir/Article/rdme-33205
[15] Pisal E, Bommanavar S, Agarwal R, Baad R, Vibhute N, Belgaumi U. Game Based Learning Approach (Gbl) To Improve Student's Learning Performance in Dental Academics [Internet]. Vol. 2022, *Journal of Positive School Psychology.* Available from: http://journalppw.com
[16] El Tantawi M, Sadaf S, AlHumaid J. (2018). Using gamification to develop academic writing skills in dental undergraduate students. *European Journal of Dental Education.* 22(1):15–22.
[17] Nguyen LM, Le C, Lee VD. (2023). Game-based learning in dental education. *J Dent Educ.* 87(5):686–93.
[18] Friedrich S, Moeltner A, Ruttermann S, Szep S. (2019). Game-based learning "Jeopardy" in dental education: A pilot study. *Journal of Dental Problems and Solutions.* 6(2):044–8.
[19] Moreira R, Silveira A, Sequeira T, Durão N, Lourenço J, Cascais I, *et al.* (2024). Gamification and Oral Health in Children and Adolescents: Scoping Review. *Interact J Med Res.* 13:e35132.
[20] Mehrotra P. (2020). Edutainment in dental curriculum-A systematic review. Vol. 10, *Journal of Oral Biology and Craniofacial Research. Elsevier B.V.*; p. 417–21.
[21] Chauhan A, Angadi PV. (2024). Metaverse in Dentistry: Assessment of knowledge regarding its application among dental students and dental professionals. *Annals of Dental Specialty.* 12(2):6–14.
[22] Zaror C, Mariño R, Atala-Acevedo C. (2021). Current state of serious games in dentistry: A scoping review. Vol. 10, *Games for Health Journal. Mary Ann Liebert Inc.*; p. 95–108.
[23] Song YL, Foo LH, Ong MAM. (2023). Exploring gamified learning for inculcating patient safety concepts in dentistry: A mixed-methods study. *European Journal of Dental Education.* 27(3):662–78.

Navigating Dental Education Trends and Transforming Dental Pedagogy – Abas and Srikant N (Eds)
© 2027 The Author(s), ISBN: 978-1-041-32674-8

Augmented and Virtual Reality: A Boon or Bane for Dental Education?

Sandipan Mukherjee
Department of Prosthodontics and Crown & Bridge, Manipal College of Dental Sciences Mangalore, Manipal, India

Digital technology and its advancements have significantly propelled progress within dentistry. In addition to considering the impending problems in digitalization, which embraces robotics and artificial intelligence, the thorough examination seeks to uncover the fascinating potential applications of virtual, augmented and mixed realities in dentistry. These technologies are indispensable in educational technology, enhancing students' learning experiences and facilitating their training in clinical settings. Additionally, Augmented Reality and Virtual Reality serve as indispensable tools in clinical practice. Augmented Reality facilitates the seamless integration of digital data with real-life clinical information, offering a comprehensive and immersive experience for healthcare professionals. However, with a comprehensive digital wax-up, virtual reality offers an engrossing preliminary rendering of the ultimate outcome of the therapy, allowing for a deeper understanding and study of the treatment outcome. The advancements in these technologies offer the potential to help patients overcome dental phobia, improve patient education, and facilitate better communication between dentists, patients, and technicians. Artificial Intelligence shows promise in advancing dental diagnoses and providing more accurate prognoses for dental conditions. Meanwhile, Robotics has the potential to enhance various aspects of daily clinical practice within the field of dentistry. [1, 2]

1 EXPLORING THE UTILITY OF DENTAL MORPHOLOGY IN EDUCATIONAL SETTINGS

Static 2D pictures are frequently employed in anatomy studies. However, comprehending spatial relationships could be challenging because anatomical structures are three-dimensional. Three-dimensional virtual models provide a more interesting learning environment for dental students. Additionally, dental morphology and tooth features may be better understood with the use of AR and VR, which has the advantages of including increased student immersion. [3–7]

2 PRE-CLINICAL EDUCATION

Dental education places a great focus on teaching clinical skills through the use of lifelike patient simulators. Students' fine motor skills and coordination of the hand and eye Students' fine motor skills and coordination of the hand and eye can be greatly enhanced by these simulators. Considering the COVID-19 pandemic, educators are turning to cutting-edge methods like AR, VR, and MR to educate pupils and give them timely feedback. The performance of both inexperienced and seasoned dental practitioners has shown notable gains because of these technologies, which include digital models, handpieces, and real-time feedback. There are a lot of advantages to optimizing lab training time and enhancing hand dexterity before patient interactions. [8–12]

3 CLINICAL PRACTICE

A variety of surgical procedures, such as neurosurgery, laparoscopic surgery, cosmetic surgery, and dental treatments including orthognathic and dental implant surgery, are the primary focus of AR integration in the medical area. Augmented reality devices reduce surgical risks by seamlessly integrating medical data and images into real-world scenarios. This allows real-time intraoperative information to be provided. Interestingly, AR has shown great value in the domains of dental implant placement and orthognathic surgery, while VR has been used for instruction in orthognathic surgery. In the medical industry, AR is mostly being used for a variety of surgical procedures, such as neurosurgery, laparoscopic surgery, cosmetic surgery, and dental treatments including orthodontic and dental implant surgery. AR devices reduce surgical risks by seamlessly integrating medical data and images into real-world scenarios. This allows real-time intraoperative information to be provided. Notably, VR has been utilized for orthognathic surgery education, whilst the use of AR has shown substantial value across the fields of dental implant placement and orthognathic surgery. [13–23]

DOI: 10.1201/9781042016075-30

4 CAN DENTAL PHOBIA BE OVERCOME?

Approximately 50-60% of people are afraid or anxious about dental operations. When dealing with such issues, Virtual Reality Exposure Therapy (VRET) and In Vivo Exposure Therapy (IVET) are helpful. To increase the success of a technique, VRET is a safer one that strengthens the sense of presence in a virtual environment. When dealing with such issues, Virtual Reality Exposure Therapy (VRET) and In Vivo Exposure Therapy (IVET) are helpful. To increase the success of a technique, VRET is a safer one that strengthens the sense of presence in a virtual environment. Several strategies have been recognized as beneficial in reducing pain and suffering during dental operations, including cognitive-behavioral therapy, nitrous gas, intravenous sedatives, and distraction with visual media. Furthermore, Virtual Reality (VR) has shown usefulness in relieving dental pain by diverting patients' attention. Incorporating 3D audio in VR, particularly in binaural format, enhances the sensation of immersion and realism inside the virtual environment, creating a mood of tranquillity and relaxation. [24–38]

5 VR AND AR FOR PATIENT EDUCATION

Through instructional and motivating techniques, people may successfully learn about their oral health situation, including oral ailments that damage oral tissues. This strengthens their resolve to provide oral treatment at home. Notably, oral health education increases patients' attitudes and habits around mouth cleanliness. It gives useful tools and procedures for controlling dental plaque, perhaps improving periodontal health and lowering the risk of dental cavities. [39, 40].

VR and AR offer instructional tools that can be beneficial to patients of all ages. The goal of using VR and AR in oral home care is to give patients—of all ages—a digital platform for adopting improved dental hygiene habits. Consequently, this promotes more engaging teaching experiences and makes it easier to prevent oral infections. Furthermore, the teaching and learning process may be greatly improved by incorporating instructional interfaces or game components into VR and AR technologies. Although there isn't much research on VR's application in patient education, it's clear that the technology is a useful and interesting teaching tool. Patients who have participated in pertinent research have stated that they view it as helpful in knowing their current state of health. [41, 42]. Regarding kid oral health care, the application of a game has the benefit of giving the patient visual feedback when they are not appropriately doing the brushing method. As a result, this gives the patient the ability to adjust as needed. It is imperative to do more study to fully investigate the possibilities of virtual reality in the future to improve oral health care and education.

6 AS DENTIST-PATIENT COMMUNICATION TOOLS

Healthcare practitioners create thorough treatment plans using a range of instruments, such as physical exams, radiography, and photos. Still, some patients could find it difficult to understand the suggested course of action. New technology in digital dentistry have made it possible to facilitate post-visit analysis, improve communication, and provide images more quickly. Anticipating the results of therapy in advance fosters better communication and a higher level of trust with patients. [43, 44]

7 AI AND ROBOTICS

AI and robotics offer two examples of how these technological advances are transforming conventional dental processes. The use of AI improves computers' abilities speed, accuracy, precision, and resource efficiency by enabling them to execute tasks that people can and to solve issues using data. Machine learning, a crucial component of AI, employs algorithms to forecast outcomes based on datasets. Artificial neural networks also act in a manner like to that of the human brain. These are interconnected neural networks that draw inspiration from organic nervous systems. [45, 46].

In the fields of diagnosis and outcome prediction, AI is being used extensively in medicine. By utilizing data from evaluations made by medical experts, AI plays a major role in medical decision-making by aiding in diagnosis and prognosis. In the construction of caries prediction models guided by clinical observations and demographic/lifestyle parameters, for example, machine learning algorithms—which are drawn from the experience of dental professionals—have shown remarkable usefulness. Data mining has several essential applications, including comparing and identifying causal relationships within existing information. AI is essential to dentistry because it can extract important information from large medical records, including predicting how long dental restorations will last depending on the materials used. Additionally, AI is being used in dentistry to analyse several imaging modalities, including CT and MRI images. The development of software meant to expedite data management and diagnosis in dentistry, notably in the areas of clinical decision support and aesthetically pleasing mock-ups, is also greatly aided by AI-driven systems. [47–50]

AI has become a vital tool in dentistry, helping to advance diagnosis, treatment planning, and prognosis prediction. Its importance has increased significantly in tandem with the growth in data processing and the availability of large patient datasets, making it easier to analyse radiological exams to improve oral pathology and disease diagnosis and treatment. The diagnosis of dental cavities, the computation of working lengths in endodontics, and the detection of instances of oral squamous cell carcinoma have all shown considerable promise when it comes to AI.

In addition, the incorporation of robots is a noteworthy frontier in dentistry. In the early 2000s, human-controlled robots demonstrated the ability to perform a variety of dental tasks, such as endodontic treatments, crown and bridge preparations, and dental caries removal. These robotic devices have shown to be accurate and effective, matching—and often even exceeding—the abilities of human dentists in terms of tooth preparation. Additionally, robotics advancements have led to the development of a mobile wire-bending machine that can create orthodontic retainers using intraoral scan data in just four minutes. Robotics is also the foundation of computer-assisted surgery, in which the attending dentist uses a navigation system to track the placement of surgical tools in real-time while seeing digital photographs with instructions projected onto them. Nowadays, optical tracking systems based on light-emitting diodes are the most widely used technology in this industry. Soon, the possibility of virtual robotic surgery might indeed enable remote surgical procedures, signifying a significant breakthrough in dental treatment. [51–65]

8 CONCLUSION

Numerous disciplines have looked at the application of AR and VR in dentistry. Literature assessing its real-world implementation is few, nevertheless. To support clinical practice in the fields of endodontics, prosthodontics, orthodontics, and oral and maxillofacial surgery, this paper tries to emphasize the advantages of virtual and augmented reality. Practitioners can use virtual reality technology to teach patients what to expect from therapy before they do any treatments. Furthermore, dental students may benefit from enhanced pre-clinical training and instruction using AR and VR technologies. These technologies also appear to be promising in treating dental anxiety, especially in younger patients. To integrate AR/VR technology into dentistry, future research must concentrate on creating rigorous data-backed technological standards and creating devices that have been scientifically tested.

Comparison of different dental simulators.

	PerioSim®	Dentsim™	IDEA	Simodont®	Voxel Man	CDS
Teeth Used	Animated	Plastic teeth	Animated	Animated	Animated	Animated
Right and Left Operation	Available	Available	Available	Available	Available	Available
Reported Real Life Experience	Tactile sensation is realistic for teeth but not for gingiva	Realistic experience using plastic teeth on a real manikin	Tactile sensation still needs to be tuned to simulate a genuine sensation	3D images are realistic. However, the texture of healthy decayed and restored tooth structure still needs improvement	/	/
Ergonomic Postures	No	Yes	No	Yes	No	Yes
Direct Transfer of Data to Program Instructor/ Tutor	Not available	Yes Run time control. Application enables the instructor to control run time grades.	Yes The software contains a replay mode. Upon completion of a specified task, it can be watched in full by the student or the instructor.	Yes Allows the instructor to watch six simulators live at once and record all preparations for evaluation in order to give feedback later.	Yes	Yes Operating procedures are recorded and can be reviewed to facilitate in training, grading and verifying.
Instant Feed Back	No	Yes	Yes	Yes	Yes	Yes
Exam Simulation	Yes	Yes	No	Yes	Yes	Yes

REFERENCES

[1] Monterubbianesi, R.; Tosco, V.; Vitiello, F.; Orilisi, G.; Fraccastoro, F.; Putignano, A.; Orsini, G. Augmented, virtual and mixed reality in dentistry: A narrative review on the existing platforms and future challenges. *Appl. Sci.* 2022, 12, 877.

[2] Fahim, S.; Maqsood, A.; Das, G.; Ahmed, N.; Saquib, S.; Lal, A.; Khan, A.A.G.; Alam, M.K. Augmented reality and virtual reality in dentistry: Highlights from the current research. *Appl. Sci.* 2022, 12, 3719.

[3] Iwanaga, J.; Kamura, Y.; Nishimura, Y.; Terada, S.; Kishimoto, N.; Tanaka, T.; Tubbs, R.S. A new option for education during surgical procedures and related clinical anatomy in a virtual reality workspace. *Clin. Anat.* 2021, 34, 496–503. [Google Scholar] [CrossRef] [PubMed]

[4] Küçük, S.; Kapakin, S.; Göktaş, Y. Learning anatomy via mobile augmented reality: Effects on achievement and cognitive load. *Anat. Sci. Educ.* 2016, 9, 411–421. [Google Scholar] [CrossRef] [PubMed]

[5] Uruthiralingam, U.; Rea, P.M. Augmented and virtual reality in anatomical education—A systematic review. *Adv. Exp. Med. Biol.* 2020, 1235, 89–101. [Google Scholar] [CrossRef] [PubMed]

[6] Reymus, M.; Liebermann, A.; Diegritz, C. Virtual reality: An effective tool for teaching root canal anatomy to undergraduate dental students—a preliminary study. *Int. Endod. J.* 2020, 53, 1581–1587. [Google Scholar] [CrossRef]

[7] Chiodera, G.; Orsini, G.; Tosco, V.; Monterubbianesi, R.; Manauta, J.; Devoto, W.; Putignano, A. essential lines: a simplified filling and modeling technique for direct posterior composite restorations. *Int. J. Esthet. Dent.* 2021, 16, 168–184. [Google Scholar]

[8] Roy, E.; Bakr, M.M.; George, R. the need for virtual reality simulators in dental education: A review. *Saudi Dent. J.* 2017, 29, 41–47. [Google Scholar] [CrossRef] [Green Version]

[9] Moussa, R.; Alghazaly, A.; Althagafi, N.; Eshky, R.; Borzangy, S. Effectiveness of virtual reality and interactive simulators on dental education outcomes: Systematic review. *Eur. J. Dent.* 2021. [Google Scholar] [CrossRef]

[10] Suvinen, T.I.; Messer, L.B.; Franco, E. Clinical simulation in teaching preclinical dentistry. *Eur. J. Dent. Educ.* 1998, 2, 25–32. [Google Scholar] [CrossRef]

[11] Ball, C.; Huang, K.-T.; Francis, J. Virtual reality adoption during the COVID-19 pandemic: A uses and gratifications perspective. *Telemat. Inform.* 2021, 65, 101728. [Google Scholar] [CrossRef]

[12] Tabatabai, S. COVID-19 impact and virtual medical education. *J. Adv. Med. Educ. Prof.* 2020, 8, 140–143. [Google Scholar] [CrossRef]

[13] Eve, E.J.; Koo, S.; Alshihri, A.A.; Cormier, J.; Kozhenikov, M.; Donoff, R.B.; Karimbux, N.Y. Performance of dental students versus prosthodontics residents on a 3D immersive haptic simulator. *J. Dent. Educ.* 2014, 78, 630–637. [Google Scholar] [CrossRef]

[14] de Boer, I.R.; Wesselink, P.R.; Vervoorn, J.M. Student performance and appreciation using 3D vs. 2d vision in a virtual learning environment. *Eur. J. Dent. Educ.* 2016, 20, 142–147. [Google Scholar] [CrossRef]

[15] Kwon, H.-B.; Park, Y.-S.; Han, J.-S. Augmented reality in dentistry: A current perspective. *Acta Odontol. Scand.* 2018, 76, 497–503. [Google Scholar] [CrossRef] [PubMed]

[16] Vávra, P.; Roman, J.; Zonča, P.; Ihnát, P.; N⊠mec, M.; Kumar, J.; Habib, N.; El-Gendi, A. recent development of augmented reality in surgery: A review. *J. Healthc. Eng.* 2017, 2017. [Google Scholar] [CrossRef]

[17] Yamaguchi, S.; Ohtani, T.; Ono, S.; Yamanishi, Y.; Sohmura, T.; Yatani, H. Intuitive surgical navigation system for dental implantology by using retinal imaging display. *Implant. Dent. Rapidly Evol. Pract.* 2011. [Google Scholar] [CrossRef] [Green Version]

[18] Durham, M.; Engel, B.; Ferrill, T.; Halford, J.; Singh, T.P.; Gladwell, M. Digitally augmented learning in implant dentistry. *Oral Maxillofac. Surg. Clin. N. Am.* 2019, 31, 387–398. [Google Scholar] [CrossRef]

[19] Jo, Y.-J.; Choi, J.-S.; Kim, J.; Kim, H.-J.; Moon, S.-Y. Virtual Reality (VR) Simulation and Augmented Reality (AR) navigation in orthognathic surgery: A case report. *Appl. Sci.* 2021, 11, 5673. [Google Scholar] [CrossRef]

[20] Ayoub, A.; Pulijala, Y. The application of virtual reality and augmented reality in oral & maxillofacial surgery. *BMC Oral Health* 2019, 19, 238. [Google Scholar] [CrossRef] [Green Version]

[21] Choi, J.-W.; Lee, J.Y. Virtual surgical planning and three-dimensional simulation in orthognathic surgery. In *The Surgery-First Orthognathic Approach: With Discussion of Occlusal Plane-Altering Orthognathic Surgery*; Choi, J.-W., Lee, J.Y., Eds.; Springer: Singapore, 2021; pp. 159–183. ISBN 9789811575419. [Google Scholar]

[22] Fushima, K.; Kobayashi, M. Mixed-reality simulation for orthognathic surgery. *Maxillofac. Plast. Reconstr. Surg.* 2016, 38, 13. [Google Scholar] [CrossRef] [Green Version]

[23] Kim, Y.; Kim, H.; Kim, Y. Virtual reality and augmented reality in plastic surgery: A review. *Arch. Plast. Surg.* 2017, 44, 179. [Google Scholar] [CrossRef] [PubMed] [Green Version]

[24] Arikatla, V.S.; Tyagi, M.; Enquobahrie, A.; Nguyen, T.; Blakey, G.H.; White, R.; Paniagua, B. High fidelity virtual reality orthognathic surgery simulator. *Proc. SPIE Int. Soc. Opt. Eng.* 2018, 10576, 1057612. [Google Scholar] [CrossRef]

[25] Khanagar, S.B.; Al-Ehaideb, A.; Vishwanathaiah, S.; Maganur, P.C.; Patil, S.; Naik, S.; Baeshen, H.A.; Sarode, S.S. Scope and performance of artificial intelligence technology in orthodontic diagnosis, treatment planning, and clinical decision-making—A systematic review. *J. Dent. Sci.* 2021, 16, 482–492. [Google Scholar] [CrossRef] [PubMed]

[26] Weinstein, P.; Milgrom, P.; Getz, T. Treating fearful dental patients: A practical behavioral approach. *J. Dent. Pract. Adm.* 1987, 4, 140–147. [Google Scholar]

[27] Berggren, U. Reduction of fear and anxiety in adult fearful patients. *Int. Dent. J.* 1987, 37, 127–136. [Google Scholar] [PubMed]

[28] Hoffman, H.G.; Sharar, S.R.; Coda, B.; Everett, J.J.; Ciol, M.; Richards, T.; Patterson, D.R. Manipulating presence influences the magnitude of virtual reality analgesia. *Pain* 2004, 111, 162–168. [Google Scholar] [CrossRef] [PubMed]

[29] Hoffman, H.G.; Garcia-Palacios, A.; Patterson, D.R.; Jensen, M.; Furness, T.; Ammons, W.F. The effectiveness of virtual reality for dental pain control: A case study. *Cyberpsychol. Behav.* 2001, 4, 527–535. [Google Scholar] [CrossRef]

[30] Gujjar, K.R.; Sharma, R.; Jongh, A.D. Virtual reality exposure therapy for treatment of dental phobia. *Dent. Update* 2017, 44, 423–435. [Google Scholar] [CrossRef] [PubMed] [Green Version]

[31] Gujjar, K.R.; van Wijk, A.; Sharma, R.; de Jongh, A. Virtual reality exposure therapy for the treatment of dental phobia: A controlled feasibility study. *Behav. Cogn. Psychother.* 2018, 46, 367–373. [Google Scholar] [CrossRef]

[32] Heidari, E.; Newton, J.T.; Banerjee, A. Minimum intervention oral healthcare for people with dental phobia: a patient management pathway. *Br. Dent. J.* 2020, 229, 417–424. [Google Scholar] [CrossRef]

[33] Felemban, O.M.; Alshamrani, R.M.; Aljeddawi, D.H.; Bagher, S.M. Effect of virtual reality distraction on pain and anxiety during infiltration anesthesia in pediatric patients: A randomized clinical trial. *BMC Oral Health* 2021, 21, 321. [Google Scholar] [CrossRef]

[34] Getka, E.J.; Glass, C.R. Behavioral and cognitive-behavioral approaches to the reduction of dental anxiety. *Behav. Ther.* 1992, 23, 433–448. [Google Scholar] [CrossRef]

[35] Gauthier, J.; Savard, F.; Hallé, J.-P.; Dufour, L. Flooding and coping skills training in the management of dental fear. scand. *J. Behav. Ther.* 1985, 14, 3–15. [Google Scholar] [CrossRef]

[36] Raghav, K.; Van Wijk, A.J.; Abdullah, F.; Islam, M.N.; Bernatchez, M.; De Jongh, A. Efficacy of virtual reality exposure therapy for treatment of dental phobia: A randomized control trial. *BMC Oral Health* 2016, 16, 25. [Google Scholar] [CrossRef] [PubMed] [Green Version]

[37] Krijn, M.; Emmelkamp, P.M.G.; Olafsson, R.P.; Biemond, R. Virtual reality exposure therapy of anxiety disorders: A Review. *Clin. Psychol. Rev.* 2004, 24, 259–281. [Google Scholar] [CrossRef]

[38] Baus, O.; Bouchard, S. Moving from virtual reality exposure-based therapy to augmented reality exposure-based therapy: A review. *Front. Hum. Neurosci.* 2014, 8, 112. [Google Scholar] [CrossRef] [Green Version]

[39] Custódio, N.B.; Costa, F.D.S.; Cademartori, M.G.; da Costa, V.P.P.; Goettems, M.L. Effectiveness of virtual reality glasses as a distraction for children during dental care. *Pediatr. Dent.* 2020, 42, 93–102. [Google Scholar]

[40] Vassend, O.; Willumsen, T.; Hoffart, A. Effects of dental fear treatment on general distress. The role of personality variables and treatment method. *Behav. Modif.* 2000, 24, 580–599. [Google Scholar] [CrossRef] [PubMed]

[41] Hendrix, C.; Barfield, W. The sense of presence within auditory virtual environments. *Presence Teleoperators Virtual Environ.* 1996, 5, 290–301. [Google Scholar] [CrossRef]

[42] Rajguru, C.; Obrist, M.; Memoli, G. Spatial soundscapes and virtual worlds: Challenges and opportunities. *Front. Psychol.* 2020, 11, 569056. [Google Scholar] [CrossRef]

[43] Stein, C.; Santos, N.M.L.; Hilgert, J.B.; Hugo, F.N. Effectiveness of oral health education on oral hygiene and dental caries in schoolchildren: Systematic review and meta-analysis. *Community Dent. Oral Epidemiol.* 2018, 46, 30–37. [Google Scholar] [CrossRef] [PubMed]

[44] Ghaffari, M.; Rakhshanderou, S.; Ramezankhani, A.; Noroozi, M.; Armoon, B. Oral health education and promotion programmes: Meta-analysis of 17-year intervention. *Int. J. Dent. Hyg.* 2018, 16, 59–67. [Google Scholar] [CrossRef]

[45] Jimenez, Y.A.; Cumming, S.; Wang, W.; Stuart, K.; Thwaites, D.I.; Lewis, S.J. Patient Education using virtual reality increases knowledge and positive experience for breast cancer patients undergoing radiation Therapy. *Support. Care Cancer* 2018, 26, 2879–2888. [Google Scholar] [CrossRef]

[46] Bekelis, K.; Calnan, D.; Simmons, N.; MacKenzie, T.A.; Kakoulides, G. Effect of an immersive preoperative virtual reality experience on patient reported outcomes: A randomized controlled trial. *Ann. Surg.* 2017, 265, 1068–1073. [Google Scholar] [CrossRef]

[47] Moussa, C.; Hardan, L.; Kassis, C.; Bourgi, R.; Devoto, W.; Jorquera, G.; Panda, S.; Abou Fadel, R.; Cuevas-Suárez, C.E.; Lukomska-Szymanska, M. Accuracy of dental photography: Professional vs. smartphone's Camera. *BioMed Res. Int.* 2021, 2021, e3910291. [Google Scholar] [CrossRef]

[48] Grischke, J.; Johannsmeier, L.; Eich, L.; Griga, L.; Haddadin, S. Dentronics: Towards robotics and artificial intelligence in dentistry. *Dent. Mater.* 2020, 36, 765–778. [Google Scholar] [CrossRef] [PubMed]

[49] Lombardi, R.E. The principles of visual perception and their clinical application to denture esthetics. *J. Prosthet. Dent.* 1973, 29, 358–382. [Google Scholar] [CrossRef]

[50] Nguyen, T.T.; Larrivée, N.; Lee, A.; Bilaniuk, O.; Durand, R. Use of artificial intelligence in dentistry: current clinical trends and research advances. *J. Can. Dent. Assoc.* 2021, 87, l7. [Google Scholar] [PubMed]

[51] Abouzeid, H.L.; Chaturvedi, S.; Abdelaziz, K.M.; Alzahrani, F.A.; AlQarni, A.A.S.; Alqahtani, N.M. Role of robotics and artificial intelligence in oral health and preventive dentistry—knowledge, perception and attitude of dentists. *Oral Health Prev. Dent.* 2021, 19, 353–363. [Google Scholar] [CrossRef] [PubMed]

[52] Park, W.J.; Park, J.-B. History and application of artificial neural networks in dentistry. *Eur. J. Dent.* 2018, 12, 594–601. [Google Scholar] [CrossRef] [PubMed]

[53] Tandon, D.; Rajawat, J.; Banerjee, M. Present and future of artificial intelligence in dentistry. *J. Oral Biol. Craniofacial Res.* 2020, 10, 391–396. [Google Scholar] [CrossRef]

[54] Schwendicke, F.; Krois, J. Data dentistry: How data are changing clinical care and research. *J. Dent. Res.* 2021, 220345211020265. [Google Scholar] [CrossRef]

[55] Lee, J.-H.; Kim, D.-H.; Jeong, S.-N.; Choi, S.-H. Detection and diagnosis of dental caries using a deep learning-based convolutional neural network algorithm. *J. Dent.* 2018, 77, 106–111. [Google Scholar] [CrossRef] [PubMed]

[56] Gürel, G.; Paolucci, B.; Iliev, G.; Filtchev, D.; Schayder, A. The fifth dimension in esthetic dentistry. *Int. J. Esthet. Dent.* 2021, 16, 10–32. [Google Scholar] [PubMed]

[57] Schwendicke, F.; Elhennawy, K.; Paris, S.; Friebertshäuser, P.; Krois, J. Deep learning for caries lesion detection in near-infrared light transillumination images: A pilot study. *J. Dent.* 2020, 92, 103260. [Google Scholar] [CrossRef]

[58] Casalegno, F.; Newton, T.; Daher, R.; Abdelaziz, M.; Lodi-Rizzini, A.; Schürmann, F.; Krejci, I.; Markram, H. Caries detection with near-infrared transillumination using deep learning. *J. Dent. Res.* 2019, 98, 1227–1233. [Google Scholar] [CrossRef] [Green Version]

[59] Ahmed, N.; Abbasi, M.S.; Zuberi, F.; Qamar, W.; Halim, M.S.B.; Maqsood, A.; Alam, M.K. Artificial intelligence techniques: Analysis, application, and outcome in dentistry—A systematic review. *BioMed Res. Int.* 2021, 2021, 9751564. [Google Scholar] [CrossRef]

[60] Johari, M.; Esmaeili, F.; Andalib, A.; Garjani, S.; Saberkari, H. Detection of vertical root fractures in intact and endodontically treated premolar teeth by designing a probabilistic neural network: an ex vivo study. *Dentomaxillofacial Radiol.* 2016, 46, 20160107. [Google Scholar] [CrossRef] [Green Version]

[61] Ekert, T.; Krois, J.; Meinhold, L.; Elhennawy, K.; Emara, R.; Golla, T.; Schwendicke, F. Deep learning for the radiographic detection of apical lesions. *J. Endod.* 2019, 45, 917–922.e5. [Google Scholar] [CrossRef] [PubMed]

[62] Fukuda, M.; Inamoto, K.; Shibata, N.; Ariji, Y.; Yanashita, Y.; Kutsuna, S.; Nakata, K.; Katsumata, A.; Fujita, H.; Ariji, E. Evaluation of an artificial intelligence system for detecting vertical root fracture on panoramic radiography. *Oral Radiol.* 2020, 36, 337–343. [Google Scholar] [CrossRef]

[63] Hung, M.; Voss, M.W.; Rosales, M.N.; Li, W.; Su, W.; Xu, J.; Bounsanga, J.; Ruiz-Negrón, B.; Lauren, E.; Licari, F.W. Application of Machine Learning for Diagnostic Prediction of Root Caries. *Gerodontology* 2019, 36, 395–404. [Google Scholar] [CrossRef]

[64] Udod, O.A.; Voronina, H.S.; Ivchenkova, O.Y. Application of neural network technologies in the dental caries forecast. *Wiadomosci Lek. Wars. Pol.* 2020, 73, 1499–1504. [Google Scholar] [CrossRef]

[65] Aubreville, M.; Knipfer, C.; Oetter, N.; Jaremenko, C.; Rodner, E.; Denzler, J.; Bohr, C.; Neumann, H.; Stelzle, F.; Maier, A. Automatic classification of cancerous tissue in laserendomicroscopy images of the oral cavity using deep learning. *Sci. Rep.* 2017, 7, 11979. [Google Scholar] [CrossRef] [Green Version]

 ISBN: 978-1-041-32674-8

Photographic Feedback and Self-Evaluation with Modified Dental Operator Posture Assessment Instrument (M-DOPAI) to Assess Improvement in Ergonomic Scores in Dental Students: Randomized Controlled Trial

Subha Anirudhan, Eraiyanbu, and V Keerthana
Department of Conservative Dentistry and Endodontics, Sri Ramakrishna Dental College and Hospital, Coimbatore, TN Dr. MGR Medical University

Pavithra Ramanath
GKNM Hospital, Coimbatore

ABSTRACT: **Aim**: To assess the influence of photographic feedback and self-assessment at regular intervals in improving ergonomics and the operator position among dental students using M-DOPAI

Methodology: This was a single centre, randomized controlled trial study where the operator positions and ergonomics among 100 dental students were analyzed. The participants were randomly divided into 2 groups with 50 participants in each group. At the outset, all the study participants were educated about correct operator position while performing dental procedures. For a period of four weeks, one group was shown weekly photos of their posture and instructed to use M-DOPAI to self-evaluate their ergonomics; the other group did not receive any feedback. Final evaluation of ergonomic scores for both groups was done by two raters at the end of four weeks using M-DOPAI.

Result: Ergonomics scores improved for students in both the groups after receiving ergonomic training. At four weeks, in each aspect of the M-DOPAI, the group that received photographic feedback obtained better scores as compared to the non-feedback group. Statistical analysis found these differences to be statistically significant ($p<0.05$).

Conclusion: Photographic feedback and self-assessment are successful in motivating good ergonomic posture among dental students while performing dental procedures. A system like this can increase a person's motivation to enhance the ergonomic aspects during dental procedures and maintain good posture throughout their lifetime and delaying the onset of occupational musculoskeletal issues that could cause early retirement

Keywords: assessment, dental education, dental students, educational technology, ergonomics, self-assessment, photography

1 INTRODUCTION

Musculoskeletal disorders are an unwelcome reality for many dentists, whether they are new to the profession or have years of experience. Despite advances in dental equipment and ergonomic design, poor posture and operator positioning during treatments continue to cause aches, pains, and significant musculoskeletal disorders. Lower back pain, neck strain, and carpal tunnel syndrome are all conditions that can have a substantial influence on a dentist's quality of life and career longevity. [1,2]

Interestingly, while over 60% of dentists are aware of basic ergonomic practices, roughly 74% continue to suffer from musculoskeletal problems. [3] This disconnect often arises because the primary focus in dentistry is on clinical outcomes—how well a procedure is performed—rather than how it is done in terms of posture. Dentists, particularly those who are still learning, frequently disregard their own comfort and positioning until pain or discomfort forces them to alter, when it is usually too late. [4,5]

While most dental professionals receive ergonomics training during their entry-level education, it does not always translate into clinical practice as there is a lack of feedback and self-motivation. If students lack understanding and do not take ownership of ergonomic difficulties, improvements may not be sustained even when faculty members step in and offer ergonomic feedback. A powerful method to improve students' awareness of ergonomics is with self-assessment.

Visual feedback through photographs and objective self-assessment can motivate students to improve their posture and prevent musculoskeletal problems, thus reinforcing ergonomic behaviour. According to the theory of reasoned action, individuals are more likely to engage in a particular behaviour when they perceive it as being beneficial or positive. [6–8]

 DOI: 10.1201/9781042016075-31

Our study aimed to explore whether photographic feedback, combined with self-assessment using the Modified Dental Operator Posture Assessment Instrument (M-DOPAI), could help dental students improve their posture and ergonomics over a time of 4 weeks and also if the students continued to maintain correct ergonomics after stopping feedback, one year from commencement of the study.

1.1 *Objectives*

(1) To assess the effect of photographic feedback on compliance towards ergonomic principles among dental students.
(2) To assess effect of objective self-assessment through M-DOPAI in improvement of ergonomic scores

2 MATERIAL AND METHODOLOGY

This study was conducted as a single-centre, randomized controlled trial involving 100 dental students from our institution. The students were randomly divided into two groups of 50 participants each. We used Modified- Dental Operator Posture Assessment Instrument (M- DOPAI) for student self- assessments and later evaluations. [5] Each component of the scale was rated based on their posture as: acceptable (one point), compromised (two points), or harmful (three points). An ideal posture would receive the lowest score of 12 and the most harmful posture would receive the maximum score of 32. The study design was structured to evaluate the operator positions and ergonomics of the participants using photographic feedback and self-assessment with M-DOPAI over a period of four weeks. The study commenced after obtaining Ethical Clearance from Sri Ramakrishna Hospital Ethical Committee (EC/2023/1005/CR-39), and informed consent of the participants.

Dental students above 18 years of age, regularly attending college and interested in participating in the study were included in the study. Students with pre-existing musculoskeletal problems and who were frequently absent in the institution were excluded.

At the beginning of the study, all participants received instruction from a dental ergonomics expert regarding proper operator positions during various dental procedures. This was done to ensure that all students had a foundational understanding of appropriate posture and positioning techniques. After the initial training, participants were randomized into two groups using randomization sequence generated in randomizer.org for block randomization:

Group I (Intervention Group): Participants in this group were photographed discreetly while performing dental procedures in the first week. These photographs were shown to the students weekly, and they were instructed to self-evaluate their posture using the M-DOPAI scale. This process was repeated for four weeks, with new photos taken and reviewed each week.

Group II (Control Group): Participants in this group were also photographed while performing procedures, but the photographs were not shown to them for self-assessment. They did not receive any feedback during the study period.

At the end of four weeks, all participants' ergonomic scores were evaluated by two independent evaluators using the M-DOPAI scale. The faculty evaluators were blinded to the random assignment during data collection. The results of both groups were then compared to determine the impact of photographic feedback and self-assessment on ergonomic improvement. The participants of both the groups were again photographed and scored after a period of one year to assess continued compliance to ergonomic principles during dental procedures.

3 RESULTS

The descriptive statistics of the participants are presented in Table 1. Of the 100 participants who were enrolled initially, 97 completed the study; 48 in Group I and 49 in Group II. Progression of individual scores were assessed in each group and repeated measures ANOVA was used as test of significance. Baseline scores calculated for both groups did not have statistically significant differences. After ergonomic training, at 4 weeks and one year the M-DOPAI ergonomic scores showed statistical improvement irrespective of the group, in comparison to baseline data, showing that ergonomic training actually improved posture while operating. Intergroup comparison revealed that, at 4 weeks, students who received photographic feedback and self-evaluation questionnaire had statistically significantly better scores than the non-feedback group implying more self-awareness and adherence to ergonomic principles while performing procedures. After one year, there was again a regression in the scores of both the groups, though the scores remained superior in the feedback and self-assessment group. (Figure 1)

Table 1. Descriptive statistics comparing M-DOPAI scores at baseline, 4 weeks and one year between groups.

Assessment	Baseline	4 weeks	1 year	p-value
Group I (n=48)	27.9±1.98	16.8±2.11	23.2±3.45	$<0.001^*$
Group II (n=49)	28.1±1.99	24.1±2.52	26.2±1.9	

*Repeated measures ANOVA

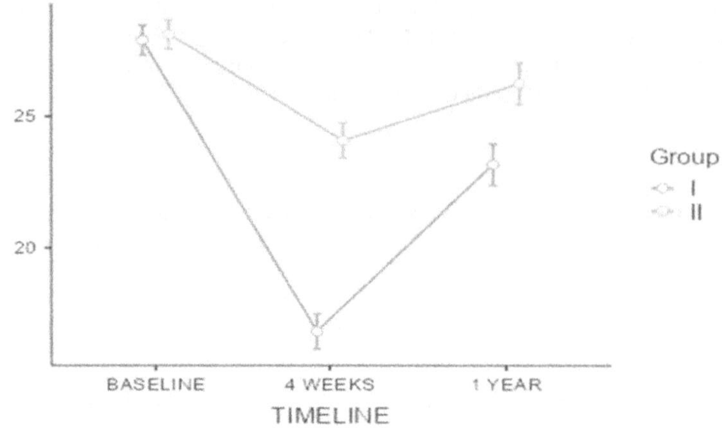

Figure 1. Assessment of ergonomic scores using M-DOPAI at baseline, 4 weeks and one year between groups.

4 DISCUSSION

Previous research has indicated that any improvement in ergonomic ratings can be advantageous since dental operators are more susceptible to work-related musculoskeletal disorders (WMSDs). [9] This study adds credence to the idea that although a dental operator may comprehend the theoretical basis of neutral positioning, it may not always be possible to implement and sustain neutral postures, hence the theoretical standards may not translate into clinical application.

Michalak-Turcotte observed that simply being aware of undesirable habits helped to prevent the eventual advancement into acquired behaviors and advocated the formulation of an ergonomic action plan to provide feasible solutions. [10]

The results of our study imply that self-evaluation along with photographic feedback can successfully enhance the dental students' posture and ergonomics. Students in the feedback group were able to correct their ergonomic faults more successfully than those who did not receive feedback because they were able to routinely assess their own postures and think on what needed improvement. The capacity of visual input to heighten self-awareness is what gives it its potency. Students are more likely to identify poor posture and make corrections when they can see it in themselves. [11] According to the idea of reasoned action, which holds that people are more inclined to engage in behaviors they regard as viable and advantageous, self-awareness is a major factor in behavior change. [8]

The findings of our study coincide with recent studies that assessed the impact of self-evaluation using photography among dentists and dental hygienists and evinced an improvement in ergonomic scores among operators receiving feedback. [4,12,13] A recent study showed that working on certain quadrants especially the fourth one may be at a higher ergonomic risk to working posture among endodontists. [14] In future studies attention to quadrant specific ergonomic compliance can be investigated to understand difficulties in ergonomic compliance with specific quadrants.

Furthermore, our study underlines the value of continual feedback in maintaining ergonomic standards. While initial training offers the requisite knowledge, continuous reinforcement through feedback and self-assessment is required to translate that knowledge into consistent practice. According to Gadbury-Amyot et al, the use of self-assessment in the clinical learning setting enabled the independent and competent dental clinician to exercise self-direction and self-regulation. This not only encourages students to acquire correct habits early on, but it also develops a culture of self-care and career longevity. [15]

Numerous countries have made a second-year course that teaches the fundamentals of dental ergonomics mandatory. Incorporating proper clinical working posture into the student evaluation process could serve as enough incentive to apply ergonomic practices, which should be applied throughout the training years rather than simply during the dental ergonomics module. Thus, separate modules on dental ergonomics, both theoretical and practical, should be introduced into the undergraduate dental training curriculum. [16]

5 CONCLUSION

Photographic feedback and self-assessment are successful in motivating good ergonomic posture among dental students while performing dental procedures. However, the feedback should not stop with the initial feedback. There is a necessity to give periodic photographic feedback and encourage self-assessment to ensure continued adherence to ergonomic principles. A system like this can increase a person's motivation to maintain good posture throughout their lifetime and delaying the onset of occupational musculoskeletal issues that could cause early retirement.

FUNDING

nil

REFERENCES

[1] Adulyawat W, Chokechanachaisakul U, Janwantanakul P. (2022). Poor neck posture and longer working duration during root canal treatment correlated with increased neck discomfort in dentists with <5-years' experience in endodontics. *J Occup Health.* 64(1).

[2] Batham C, Yasobant S. (2016). A risk assessment study on work-related musculoskeletal disorders among dentists in Bhopal, India. *Indian Journal of Dental Research.* 27(3):236–41.

[3] Rafeemanesh E, Jafari Z, Kashani FO, Rahimpour F. (2013). A study on job postures and musculoskeletal illnesses in dentists. *Int J Occup Med Environ Health [Internet].* 2013 [cited 2024 Sep 11];26(4):615–20. Available from: https://pubmed.ncbi.nlm.nih.gov/24142742/

[4] Partido BB, Henderson R. (2021). Reducing the risks for musculoskeletal disorders utilizing self-assessment and photography among Dentists and Dental Hygienists. *J Dent Hyg.* 95(2):36–41.

[5] Partido BB. (2017). Ergonomics calibration training utilizing photography for dental hygiene faculty members. *J Dent Educ* [Internet]. [cited 2024 Sep 11];81(10):1187–93. Available from: https://pubmed.ncbi.nlm.nih.gov/28966183/

[6] Moodley R, Naidoo S, Wyk J van. (2018). The prevalence of occupational health-related problems in dentistry: A review of the literature. *J Occup Health.* 60(2):111–25.

[7] Jackson SC, Murff EJT. (2011). Effectively teaching self-assessment: preparing the dental hygiene student to provide quality care. *J Dent Educ.* 75(2):169–79.

[8] Montaño D, Kasprzyk D. (2008). Theory of reasoned action, theory of planned behavior, and the integrated behavioral model. *The SAGE Encyclopedia of Industrial and Organizational Psychology*, 2nd edition.

[9] Mulimani P, Hoe VC, Hayes MJ, Idiculla JJ, Abas AB, Karanth L. (2018). Ergonomic interventions for preventing musculoskeletal disorders in dental care practitioners. *Cochrane Database Syst Rev.* 10(10):CD011261.

[10] Michalak-Turcotte C. (2000). Controlling dental hygiene work-related musculoskeletal disorders: the ergonomic process. *J Dent Hyg.* 74(1):41–8.

[11] Colthart I, Bagnall G, Evans A, Allbutt H, Haig A, Illing J, *et al.* (2008). The effectiveness of self-assessment on the identification of learner needs, learner activity, and impact on clinical practice: *BEME Guide no. 10. Med Teach [Internet].* [cited 2024 Sep 11];30 (2):124–45. Available from: https://pubmed.ncbi.nlm.nih.gov/18464136/

[12] Partido BB. (2017). Dental hygiene students' self-assessment of ergonomics utilizing photography. *J Dent Educ [Internet].* [cited 2024 Sep 11];81(10):1194–202. Available from: https://pubmed.ncbi.nlm.nih.gov/28966184/

[13] Partido BB, Wright BM. (2018). Self-assessment of ergonomics amongst dental students utilising photography: RCT. *Eur J Dent Educ [Internet].* 22(4):223–33. Available from: http://www.ncbi.nlm.nih.gov/pubmed/29498176

[14] Feige S, Holzgreve F, Fraeulin L, Maurer-Grubinger C, Betz W, Erbe C, *et al.* (2024). Ergonomic analysis of dental work in different oral quadrants: A motion capture preliminary study among endodontists. *Bioengineering (Basel) [Internet].* [cited 2024 Sep 11];11(4). Available from: http://www.ncbi.nlm.nih.gov/pubmed/38671821

[15] Mays KA, Branch-Mays GL. (2016). A systematic review of the use of self-assessment in preclinical and clinical dental education. *J Dent Educ.* 80(8):902–13.

[16] Talpos-Niculescu IC, Farkas AZ, Lungeanu D, Argeşanu V, Anghel MD, Nagib R. (2022). Perception and knowledge of dental ergonomics among romanian dental students. *Int J Environ Res Public Health.* 19(24).

 ISBN: 978-1-041-32674-8

Insightful Evaluation of Public Health Dentistry Syllabus with Regards Education 4.0 Principles and Sustainable Development Goal 4

Pradnya Pramod Hegde and Parag Rishipathak
Symbiosis Centre for Health Skills (SCHS), Symbiosis International (Deemed University), Pune, India

ABSTRACT: **Purpose**: To assess whether the syllabus at the Higher Education Institution (HEI) for Public Health Dentistry is compliant with Education 4.0 principles and has incorporated the Sustainable Development Goal (SDG) target 4.7 in the form of global citizenship education (GCED) and lifelong learning and to compare the syllabi between colleges with different university affiliation.

Methods: A descriptive content analysis study was performed. Among the 318 recognized dental colleges in India, 10% (n=31) were selected. Using the lottery method, the dental colleges were selected based on the geographical direction of India, and affiliation with the university. Scientific committee and ethics committee approval was obtained. The syllabus of the selected colleges was retrieved from their college website, and the content analysis was performed via a checklist. For any doubt, clarification was sought from the faculty of the respective college. Duplicate analysis was performed on 20% of the data.

Results: A 100% sample aligns with the DCI-recommended curriculum. Meagre number of colleges have embraced the principles of Education 4.0 (range 2–8), with limited integration of GCED (n=1) and lifelong learning (n=3). Notably, teamwork and collaboration for student assignment are followed by the majority of the colleges (n=20). Deemed university colleges are faring ahead of other types of university affiliations.

Conclusion: HEIs must adapt to the evolving educational landscape by incorporating cutting-edge technologies and forward-looking concepts such as Education 4.0 and SDG 4.7. As technology bridges physical distance, fostering global connections and providing students with exposure and training are imperative for shaping education in the future.

Keywords: SDG, Lifelong learning, Education 4.0, GCED

1 INTRODUCTION

Technology has permeated every aspect of life, including education. The current dental education curriculum, however, has remained largely unchanged for five decades, failing to keep pace with the latest advancements and developments in the field. [1] In contrast, recent educational frameworks such as the National Education Policy (NEP) 2020, [2] Education 4.0, and Sustainable Development Goal [3] (SDG) 4.7 are more forward-looking, aiming to make learning dynamic, personalized, and student centric.

Today's students, belonging to Generation Z, are digital natives for whom technology is an extension of their minds and hands. They seek greater involvement in their own knowledge development, preferring teamwork and interactive learning. [4] Unlike the traditional education approach, Education 4.0 is a response to the digitalization and globalization driven by Industry 4.0. [5] It promotes principles such as learning anywhere anytime, personalized learning pathways, project-based and hands-on learning, and unconventional assessment methods that incorporate student feedback.

Similarly, the Sustainable Development Goals (SDGs), a set of 17 globally relevant objectives designed by the United Nations in 2015, specifically address "Quality Education" under SDG 4 with lifelong learning. [3,6] The targets of this goal, particularly SDG 4.7, emphasize the importance of global citizenship education (GCED), which fosters values such as humanity, peace, sustainability, and respect for diversity. [7]

There is a clear need to align the curriculum with the latest advancements and educational frameworks to ensure that it is dynamic, personalized, and student-centric while also incorporating Education 4.0, global citizenship and lifelong learning principles.

Against this literature background, it is clear that there is a change needed in the present curriculum. Thus, the aim of the study is to understand the existing learning environment in-order to recommend transforming educational measures by incorporating futuristic constructs. The objectives are : 1. To assess whether the syllabus at the Higher Education Institution (HEI) for Public Health Dentistry is compliant with Education 4.0 (E 4.0) principles and has incorporated the Sustainable Development Goal (SDG) target 4.7 in the form of global citizenship education (GCED) and lifelong learning and 2. To compare the syllabi between colleges with different university affiliation.

 DOI: 10.1201/9781042016075-32

2 MATERIALS AND METHODS

A descriptive content analysis study was performed. The curricula uploaded on the website by the Public Health Dentistry Department of the selected dental colleges were assessed. A checklist was prepared for content analysis. Any doubt while assessing was resolved by speaking to the faculty of the college. Scientific and ethics committee approval was obtained prior to starting the study. There are a total of 318 recognized dental colleges in India. [7] The sample size for the study was fixed at 10% of the total number of dental colleges, i.e., n=31. The selection of dental colleges was based on the geographical direction of India and university affiliation. The distribution of the colleges is as follows: North=69, South=135, West=69 and East=24. Proportionate sampling was used to fix the number of dental colleges. Simple random sampling was employed to select the states according to the geographical direction. Since the highest number of dental colleges are in South India, the number of selected sites in south are more compared to the others. The final number of dental colleges selected according to geographic distribution is North Zone=6, South Zone=13, East Zone=3, West Zone=7 and Central Zone=2. The data were collected, analyzed and expressed as numbers and percentages. Duplicate analysis was performed on 20% of the data to check for any intra-examiner variation.

3 RESULTS

Content analysis was performed for 31 dental colleges. Among the 31 colleges, two were autonomous institutions, three were affiliated with central universities, 17 were affiliated with state universities, and 9 were affiliated with Deemed-to-be universities respectively. One of the two autonomous colleges, all three central affiliate colleges and eight of the 17 state affiliate colleges did not have a curriculum uploaded on their website. All nine colleges affiliated with the deemed to be universities uploaded the curriculum to their websites. One hundred percent of the sample aligns with the DCI-recommended curriculum. Few colleges have embraced the principles of Education 4.0, with limited integration of GCED (n=1) and lifelong learning (n=3). The principles of E4.0 include learning anywhere anytime (n=2), critical thinking (n=8), newer methods of examination (n=6), problem-solving activities (n=16), involving students in designing curricula (n=2) and student-centric curricula (n=2). Notably, teamwork and collaboration for student assignments are followed by the majority of the colleges (n=20). Deemed university colleges are faring ahead of other university type affiliations.

4 DISCUSSION

Presently, all (100%) the dental colleges in India follow the curriculum proposed by the DCI. [7] This is the minimum standard to be followed by the dental colleges. However, comparative analysis of the curriculum across different dental colleges indicates that very few colleges have adopted futuristic constructs.

Gen Z is the cohort who were born between 1996 and 2010. These present-day learners are always almost connected to technology. Their way of learning is different, and they want the teacher as the guide (facilitator) by the side. The motive is now to "adopt and adapt to the technology" for effectively teaching the Gen Z learner cohort. [8] This highlights the principles of Education 4.0 for teaching and learning. Stamenkovic D *et al.* [9], in their paper regarding the impact of the fourth industrial revolution (IR) in the field of dentistry, reported that the use of sophisticated IR technologies has led to instant and accurate diagnoses of oral diseases. In dentistry, new courses have been introduced to provide virtual education. IR has benefited dentistry in many ways, thus assisting in achieving a sustainable future in dentistry. Education 4.0 is a promising concept for learning in higher education. Edutech is a merger of digital systems and traditional education. In the 21st century, education should be online based but should also support classroom teaching and add more research components. [10]

The main themes of GCED are humanity, peace, fair justice, sustainability, respect for diversity and globalization. The University Grant Commission (UGC) has proposed that GCED can be incorporated into the normal teaching learning process through training trainers, by transforming the curriculum and through innovative pedagogy. [11] Global citizenship in dentistry (GCD) was initiated by universities in Egypt, Hong Kong, Malaysia, the UK, and the United States, which developed a portfolio of restorative procedures in simulation laboratories and uploaded them to an online platform. The students in this program welcomed the GCD program and benefitted from global academic exchange, the development of critical thinking, the enhancement of professional communication skills, and opportunities for cultural exchange. [12]

Schutte IW *et al.* [13] conducted a study among 25 undergraduate Honors students in the Netherlands, where they studied GCED in their course for 112 hours. This was a theory-based course, and the results indicated that the students experienced constructive and encouraging impacts. A systematic review investigating effective teaching and learning for sustainable development and global citizenship revealed positive changes in one's knowledge, attitudes/beliefs and behaviors. [14]

Lifelong learning (adult education, adult learning, lifelong education, Adult Life long Education, ALE) is accepted globally and is a formula for preparing individuals for "Uncertainty" in the future. [15,16] In the field of higher education, lifelong learning in the form of continuing professional development (CPD) is noted. [9] It is recommended by SDG 4 and has also been incorporated into the NEP 2020. [2] It can be formal, informal or nonformal. In the presence of digitalization, it can be taken up as microcredentials for skills enhancement. Universities should offer courses to their students, alumni and teachers. Professional associations also play an important role in CPD. [17]

Overall, the study results indicate that the curriculum followed does not include the futuristic constructs. The colleges should plan to include beyond more than the minimum recommended by the DCI. The colleges with affiliation to the deemed- to- be university, NAAC accredited and with higher NIRF rankings have an enriched curriculum and are better aligned with E 4.0. compared to the other university affiliated colleges. GCED and life-long learning components are far from being achieved among all the colleges irrespective of the university affiliation.

The strength of the study is that it is the first of its kind to provide baseline data about the inclusion of futuristic constructs in the curriculum. However, the drawback of this study is that the content analysis method was followed to assess the curriculum on the website. Many times, if the website is not updated, then the results may be understated.

5 CONCLUSION

The study results indicate that the Public Health Dentistry curriculum is not yet aligned to the futuristic constructs. HEIs must adapt to the evolving educational landscape by incorporating cutting-edge technologies and forward-looking concepts such as Education 4.0 and SDG 4.7. As technology bridges physical distance, fostering global connections and providing students with exposure and training are imperative for shaping education in the future.

REFERENCES

[1] Sharma S, Vijayaraghavan V, Tandon P, Kumar DRV, Sharma H, Rao Y. (2012). Dental education: current scenario and future trends. *The Journal of Contemporary Dental Practice* 13:107–10.

[2] National Education Policy 2020. *Ministry of Human Resource Development. Government of India.* [Online] Available from https://www.education.gov.in/sites/upload_files/mhrd/files/NEP_Final_English_0.pdf (accessed on 1-9-2024)

[3] Sustainable development goals. Sustainable development, united nations. [Online] Available from: https://sdgs.un.org/goals/goal4 (accessed on 1-9-2024)

[4] Nandhakumar R. (2019). A study on the Learning Pattern of Generation- Z (Gen-Z) and their perception on Curriculum, Course Deliverance and Infrastructure. *International Journal of Management and Social Sciences.* 9: 625–34.

[5] Bonfield CA, Salter M, Longmuir A, Benson M, Adachi C. (2020). Transformation or evolution? : Education 4.0, teaching and learning in the digital age. *Higher Education Pedagogies* 5: 223–46.

[6] Kakodkar PV, Manivasakan S. (2022). National Education Policy 2020 compliant multidisciplinary education and research universities for dental education in India - A road map. *J Med Evid* 3:60–3

[7] BDS Course Regulation 2007. [Online] Available from: https://dciindia.gov.in/Rule_Regulation/Revised_BDS_Course_Regulation_2007.pdf (accessed on 1-9-2024)

[8] Kakodkar P. (2018). Gen Z Students: Newer Teaching Methods and its Application in Dentistry. *J Dent Res Rev* 5:103–4.

[9] Stamenkovic D, Obradovic-Duricic K, Stamenkovic D, Grbovic A, Dordevic I. (2021). The Fourth Industrial Revolution's impact on dentistry. *Srp Arh Celok Lek* https://doi.org/10.2298/SARH210130037S

[10] Ossiannilsson E, Altinay F, Altinay Z. (2016). MOOCs as change agents to boost innovation in higher education learning arenas. *Education Sciences.* 6:25–30.

[11] University Grants Commission. Educational framework for global citizenship in higher education. (2021). New Delhi. Deeya Media Arts. Available at https://www.ugc.ac.in/e-book/GCED%20Book_WEB.pdf

[12] Yiu FSY, Yu OY, Wong AWY, Chu CH. (2021). Perspective of students in the Global Citizenship in Dentistry as an international peer learning experience. *J Dent Educ.* 85(11):1721–1728.

[13] Schutte IW, Kamans E, Wolfensberger MVC, Veugelers. (2017). Preparing students for Global citizenship: The effects of a Dutch undergraduate Honors course. *Education Research International.* https://doi.org/10.1155/2017/3459631

[14] Chiba M, Sustarsic M, Perriton S, Edwards DB. (2021). Investigating effective teaching and learning for sustainable development and global citizenship: Implications from a systematic review of the literature. *International Journal of Educational Development,* 81. https://doi.org/10.1016/j.ijedudev.2020.102337.

[15] Elfert, M. (2019). Lifelong learning in Sustainable Development Goal 4: What does it mean for UNESCO's rights-based approach to adult learning and education? *Int Rev Educ* 65: 537–56. doi.org/10.1007/s11159-019-09788-z

[16] Webb S, Holford J, Hodge S, Milana M, Waller R. (2019). Conceptualizing lifelong learning for sustainable development and education 2030, *International Journal of Lifelong Education.* 38: 237–40, doi: 10.1080/02601370.2019.1635353

[17] Heuvel Jos, Plasschaert Alphons. (2005). Lifelong learning in dentistry; from quality assurance to quality development. *Community Dental Health.* 22;130–2.

Navigating Dental Education Trends and Transforming Dental Pedagogy – Abas and Srikant N (Eds)

Case-Based Discussions as Workplace-Based Formative Assessments for Postgraduate Training in Prosthodontics Specialty

Sivaranjani Gali
Department of Prosthodontics and Crown & Bridge, Faculty of Dental Sciences, M.S.Ramaiah University of Applied Sciences, Bangalore, India

ABSTRACT: **Objectives:** Clinical competency is an expected outcome of dental postgraduate trainees in the discipline of Prosthodontics. Workplace-based assessments (WPBA) are a form of competency-based formative assessment. The objective of the study is to evaluate the feasibility of conducting Case-based discussions as WPBA for post-graduate training in the Prosthodontics Specialty.

Methods: Monthly progress review meetings were conducted for postgraduates wherein students were instructed to present their faculty-supervised clinical cases. A decision was made to conduct around twelve case-based discussions (Case-based discussion) annually and one Case-based discussion monthly (3-4 weeks). Each Case-based discussion lasted 25–30 minutes with the last 5–10 minutes for feedback. The assessor underwent basic teacher training workshops on providing effective feedback to students. Feedback was given to each of the students with a focus on the clinical and analytical skills of professional training in WPBA such as improving their procedural competencies, diagnostic reasoning, and treatment plan, with the quality of case documentation.

Results: Most of the students expressed that case-based discussions helped them improve case documentation, self-reflection of their clinical competencies, organizational and managerial skills, and clinical case reasoning.

Conclusions: Case-based discussions can be recommended as workplace-based formative assessments in the prosthodontics specialty as part of the postgraduate training curriculum.

Keywords: Workplace-based assessments, case-based discussions, postgraduate training, Prosthodontics

1 INTRODUCTION

Clinical competency is an expected outcome for dental postgraduate trainees in the discipline of prosthodontics. Competency is defined as when a student can begin performing the required chair-side clinical procedures independently without supervision. Competency combines knowledge, experience, critical thinking, problem-solving skills, professionalism, and ethical values, with technical and procedural skills. [1–5] Workplace-based assessments (WPBA) are a form of competency-based formative assessment. WPBA is designed to encourage a self-reflective process for postgraduate trainees by providing feed-forward feedback on knowledge, understanding, skills, and professional attitudes. [6]

During the clinical training of dental postgraduates in the discipline of Prosthodontics, chair-side procedures are supervised by the faculty, wherein the students are given immediate feedback on their clinical work by the faculty. However, following clinical supervision, neither the implementation of faculty feedback by the student nor the assessment of student clinical performance is followed up, often cited due to multiple patient appointments, lack of time, and the busy schedule of patient load in the clinics. There is a compulsive need for formative assessments that not only enhance clinical skills, and provide meaningful feedback but also deliver a scope for self-reflection.

WPBA typically can be of observation of clinical counters using direct procedural skills (DOPs) or Mini-Clinical Examination (Mini-CEX), Case-based Discussions (Case-based discussions), and multi-source feedback. Case-based discussions (Case-based discussions), typically involve the discussion of a clinical case in a semi-structured way. The Academy of Medical Royal Colleges recommends that the Case-based discussions should be conducted as a face-to-face discussion of a case, to probe the reasoning behind any decisions made while offering constructive feedback to the trainee. [7] Case-based discussions have proven to demonstrate the ability for case documentation, reasoning, and diagnostic competency and as WPBA, help to evaluate the trainee's understanding and rationale for the treatment provided. [6,8,9] Further, when combined with feedback, student-reflective learning has been shown to increase student performance. [10–12] Case-based discussions are a form of formative clinical assessment with a semi-structured and detailed discussion between students and clinical teachers on the treatment provided to patients. As the current postgraduate curriculum in

DOI: 10.1201/9781042016075-33

the Prosthodontics Specialty does not include Case-based discussions for formative assessment in clinical training, the objective of the study is to evaluate the feasibility of conducting Case-based discussions for post-graduates as a WPBA.

2 METHODS

The study was carried out in the Department of Prosthodontics and Crown & Bridge, Faculty of Dental Sciences, Ramaiah University of Applied Sciences, Bangalore, India between June 2023 and May 2024. This intervention was intended to assess the clinical work of post-graduates in training for complete dentures, removable partial dentures, and fixed partial dentures. The postgraduate clinical cases are supervised by the faculty in the department comprising of Assistant Professors, Associate Professors, and Professors. The postgraduates show their clinical procedures to the faculty and take their feedback and further work on the patient. Monthly progress review meetings were conducted by the Head of the Department as a Case-based discussion for postgraduates wherein they were instructed to present their faculty-supervised clinical cases.

Format of Case-based discussions: WPBA typically can be of observation of clinical counters using direct procedural skills [DOPs] or Mini-Clinical Examination [Mini-CEX], Case-based Discussions [Case-based discussions], and multi-source feedback. Case-based discussions were chosen due to their feasibility and ease of implementation in our clinical setting.

A decision was taken to conduct around twelve Case-based Discussions [Case-based discussion] annually, and one Case-based discussion every month [3-4 weeks]. Each Case-based discussion lasted for about 25–30 minutes with the last 5–10 minutes for feedback. The assessor was the Head of the Department who underwent basic teacher training workshops on providing effective feedback to students. Feedback was given to each student with a focus on the clinical and analytical skills of professional training in WPBA such as improving their procedural competencies, diagnostic reasoning, and treatment plan, with the quality of case documentation.

The feedback emphasized the areas for improvement to provide constructive feedback with reflective learning on what went well and what could have been done better. This was also fulfilled as documentation for reflective learning. The best clinical cases among the students were selected as the *Case of the Month.* Scores of excellent (03), good (02), and average (01) were given based on rubrics. The rubrics were devised based on the quality of photographic documentation, case distinctiveness, and uniqueness of the treatment approach.

Student feedback on Case-based discussions: The intervention was evaluated using the Kirkpatrick hierarchy model. The first level of the Kirkpatrick model typically evaluates how the students feel about the training. The first level of evaluation was done using Google Forms with a questionnaire.

Post-graduate curriculum consists of a three-year course of pre-clinical with basic clinical, intermediate clinical, and advanced clinical courses. At the end of the course (annual), clinical exams are conducted. These clinical exams include assessment of border molding with the secondary impression for first-year students or tooth preparation for mid-year students. The scores were assessed based on rubrics of average, good, and excellent. The scores of the intervention of Case-based discussion were compared with those of clinical exam scores (mid-year and first-year students).

Statistical analysis: A paired t-test was done to compare the clinical exam scores with Case-based discussion.

3 RESULTS

The study was planned for 10 mid-year and first-year postgraduates [n=5 each]. The intervention was evaluated using the Kirkpatrick hierarchy model. The first level evaluates how the students feel about the training, and the second level on to what extent the students improve their knowledge, skills, and attitude. The third level is on how extent participants change their behavior in the workplace during training and the fourth level is on organizational benefits from the training.

The first level of evaluation was done using Google Forms with a questionnaire. The feedback is presented in Figure 1. About 40% of students strongly agreed and 60% of students agreed case of the month helped record case documentation and in the self-reflection of clinical competencies. About 60% of the students strongly agreed it helps improve managerial and organizational skills, agreed that it helps in clinical case reasoning, and recommended it be part of the postgraduate curriculum. Students gave suggestions to improve their approach to cases, to discuss them beforehand, and to receive demonstrations of procedures before starting the case. Post-operative evaluations were suggested as they would be more meaningful when clinical protocols are followed. Students also recommended using digital cameras and photography courses to standardize photographs for case documentation. However, clinical exam scores before and after Case-based discussions did not show any statistically significant differences ($p>0.05$).

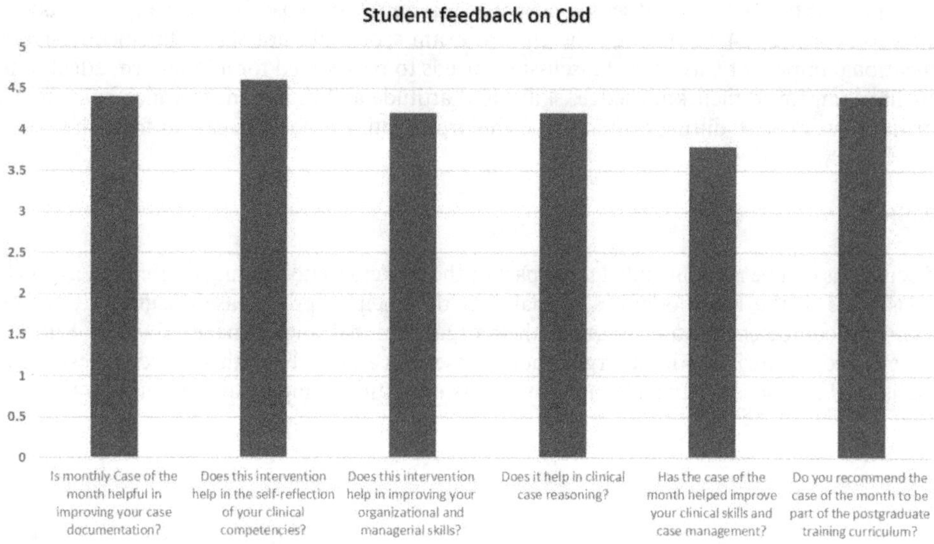

Figure 1. Feedback given by postgraduates on Case-based discussion.

4 DISCUSSION

The introduction of Case-based discussions as a workplace-based formative assessment is a new initiative in the Department of Prosthodontics. Assessments typically are required to gather information from diverse sources to develop an understanding of what the student knows and can do with his or her knowledge as a result of their educational experience.

Case-based discussions enhance learning through exploratory talk, student questions, and scaffolding. Feed forward is typically used in formative assessments, while feedback is for summative assessments. Feed-forward focuses on future improvements, helping students understand what they need to learn, assess their current progress, and plan how to reach their goals. This approach encourages students to take an active role in their learning and become self-directed learners. [13]

Case-based discussion is another form of formative clinical assessment. The discussion focuses on what has been done, rather than hypothetical scenarios. Case-based discussions assess clinical reasoning skills and what the trainee has done, while case presentations evaluate what the trainee says they would do. Both methods evaluate different competencies and are complementary, not interchangeable. [14,15]

Feedback is crucial in case-based discussions (Case-based discussions) and is best delivered using the sandwich approach: positive reinforcement, areas for improvement, and specific, actionable suggestions. [16–18] By the end of a session, students should have addressed Sadler's three steps: understanding the goals, comparing their current progress, and taking steps to bridge any gaps. Initially, trainers lead the conversation, but as trainees advance, they take more control, with trainers adopting a coaching role. This progression helps learners become self-directed. Case-based discussions focus on discussing the management of real patient cases, evaluating the trainee's understanding and treatment rationale, and covering as many competencies as possible. [19–21]

Workplace-based assessments (WPBA) score high in validity because it evaluates students in real-life settings with authentic tasks. Studies consistently show that WPBA correlates well with other clinical competence measures, reinforcing its validity. Although WPBA tools may seem subjective, their reliability is strong due to multiple encounters in various settings with different assessors. While standardization across departments is challenging, this isn't a major issue since WPBA is primarily used for formative purposes. These tools are feasible but require additional effort and faculty training for effective implementation. [14] Case-based discussions are known to have excellent face and construct validity as they focus on the performance of postgraduates in clinical settings and work environments. However, Case-based discussions have limited content and predictive validity as they focus on one type of assessment and do not entirely represent real-life clinical scenarios. Case-based discussions also tend to have low reliability due to a lack of standardization and subjectivity of the assessor. Their reliability can be improved using rating scales and standardized feedback forms with measured inter-examiner reliability using kappa agreement. [22]

A feedback questionnaire on Case-based discussions was taken from students on their effectiveness on their perception of the trainees in Newcastle Hospital. The WBPA was considered more realistic than the current format of the Australian Medical Council clinical examination. The candidates felt that the WBPA did not disrupt their clinical duties. Most candidates mentioned that they received constructive feedback and that the program was effective in stimulating learning and served as an appropriate assessment tool. [23]

One of the limitations of Case-based discussions is that it requires an expansion of the pool of assessors and it is time-consuming to conduct. [24,25] Though the clinical exam scores did not show statistically significant differences, the educational impact of Case-based discussions needs to be assessed for a long-term effect in terms of how much students have improved their knowledge, skills, and attitude and the extent to which students have changed their behavior in the workplace during training, and the organizational benefits gained from the training.

5 CONCLUSIONS

Case-based discussions can be recommended to be part of the postgraduate training curriculum as workplace-based formative assessments in the Prosthodontics specialty as they help improve case documentation, facilitate self-reflection of clinical competencies, and improve their organizational and managerial skills. Future studies can expand the Case-based discussions with a larger pool of assessors and evaluate their effectiveness in improving the knowledge, skills, and attitudes of students, and further its educational impact and benefits to the organization.

REFERENCES

[1] Albino JE, Young SK, Neumann LM, Kramer GA, Andrieu SC, Henson L, *et al.* (2008). Assessing dental students' competence: best practice recommendations in the performance assessment literature and investigation of current practices in predoctoral dental education. *J Dent Educ.* 72:1405–35.

[2] Hendricson WD, Kleffner JH. (1998). Curricular and instructional implications of competency-based dental education. *J Dent Educ* 62:183–96.

[3] Gerald G, Peter E, Thomas E, Zelda G, Wendy K, William N, *et al.* (1980). On competence: A critical analysis of competence-based reforms in higher education. *Am J of Educ.* 88: 245–50.

[4] Grussing PG. (1987). Curricular design: competency perspective. *Am J Pharm Educ* 51:414–9.

[5] Alkhodary, MA, Farah, RI, Ghobashy, AI. (2020). Competency-based education in undergraduate clinical prosthodontics: A paradigm shift in training. *Competency-based Education.* 5:e01220. https://doi.org/10.1002/cbe2.1220.

[6] Haber RJ, Lingard LA. (2001). Learning oral presentation skills: a rhetorical analysis with pedagogical and professional implications. *J Gen Intern Med.* 16:308–314.

[7] Fish C, Coles C. (2005). *Medical Education: Developing a Curriculum for Practice.* Maidenhead: Open University Press.

[8] Bordage G. (1999). Why did I miss the diagnosis? Some cognitive explanations and educational implications. *Acad Med.* 74(10) (suppl):S138–S143.

[9] Oetting TA, Lee AG, Beaver HA, *et al.* (2006). Teaching and assessing surgical competency in ophthalmology training programs. *Ophthalmic Surg Lasers Imaging* 37:384.

[10] Boehler ML, Rodgers DA, Schwind CJ, *et al.* (2006). An investigation of medical student reactions to feedback: a randomized controlled trial. *Med Educ* 40:746–9.

[11] Boud D. (1999). Avoiding the traps: Seeking good practice in the use of self-assessment and reflections in professional courses. *Social Work Educ* 18:121–32.

[12] Kaufman DM. (2003). *Applying educational theory in practice. BMJ* 326:213–6.

[13] Jyothirmayi R. (2012). Case-based discussion: assessment tool or teaching aid? *Clin Oncol (R Coll Radiol).* 24:649–53. doi: 10.1016/j.clon.2012.07.008.

[14] Singh T, Sood R. (2013). Workplace-based assessment: measuring and shaping clinical learning. *Natl Med J India.* 26:42–6. PMID: 24066996.

[15] Accreditation Council for Graduate Medical Education (ACGME) and American Board of Medical Specialties (ABMS). Toolbox of assessment methods. 2000 Version 1.1.

[16] Primhak R, Gibson N. (2019). Workplace-based assessment: how to use case-based discussion as a formative assessment. *Breathe* 15: 163–166.

[17] Mehta F, Brown J, Shaw NJ. (2013). Do trainees value feedback in case-based discussion assessments? *Med Teach* 35: e1166–e1172.

[18] Mohanaruban A, Flanders L, Rees H. (2018). Case-based discussion: perceptions of feedback. *Clin Teach* 15: 126–131.

[19] Gavriel Jennifer. (2013). Assessment for learning: a wider (classroom-researched) perspective is important for formative assessment and self-directed learning in general practice, *Education for Primary Care.* 24: 93–96.

[20] *Toward competency-based curriculum: Application of workplace-based assessment tools in the National Saudi Arabian Anesthesia Training Program.* Academy of Medical Royal Colleges. Improving Assessment. London: Academy of Medical Royal Colleges; 2008.

[21] Uma E. (2020). Workplace-based assessment: A valuable tool in undergraduate dental education. *Int J App Basic Med Res* 10:223–5.

[22] J M L Williamson and A J Osborne. (2012). Critical analysis of case-based discussions. *BJMP* 5:a514

[23] Nair BR, Hensley MJ, Parvathy MS, Lloyd DM, Murphy B, Ingham K, Wein JM, Symonds IM. (2012). A systematic approach to workplace-based assessment for international medical graduates. *Med J Aust.* 196:399–402. doi: 10.5694/mja11.10709.

[24] Field, JC, Walmsley, AD, Paganelli, C, *et al.* (2017). The graduating european dentist: contemporaneous methods of teaching, learning and assessment in dental undergraduate education. *Eur J Dent Educ.* 21(Suppl. 1): 28–35.

[25] Kirton J, Palmer N, Grieveson B, Balmer M. (2013). A national evaluation of workplace-based assessment tools (WPBAs) in foundation dental training: a UK study. *Br Dent J.* 214:305–309.

 ISBN: 978-1-041-32674-8

Opinion of Oral Health Professionals Regarding Comprehensive Care Clinic/ Practice: A Multi-Nation Questionnaire-Based Study

Aayush Anand Poddar
Manipal College of Dental Sciences Mangalore, Manipal Academy of Higher, Education, Manipal, Karnataka, Manipal, India

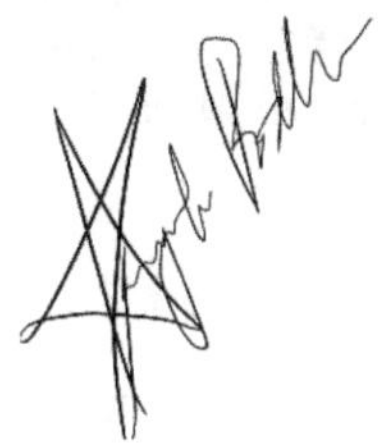

Rakshita Chalotra and Ramya Shenoy
Department of Public Health Dentistry, Manipal College of Dental Sciences Mangalore, Manipal Academy of Higher, Education, Manipal, Karnataka, Manipal, India

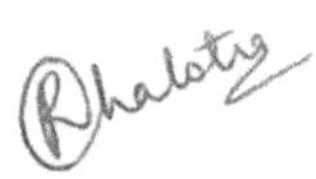

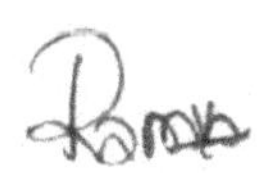

Tarinee Puri
Manipal College of Dental Sciences Mangalore, Manipal Academy of Higher Education, Manipal, Karnataka, Manipal, India

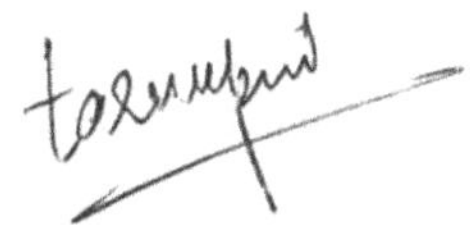

Manuel Thomas
Department of Conservative Dentistry, Manipal College of Dental Sciences Mangalore, Manipal Academy of Higher Education, Manipal, Karnataka, Manipal,India

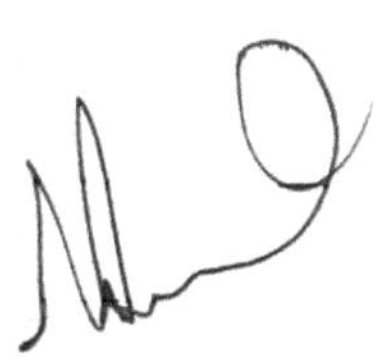

Violet D'Souza
Department of Dental Clinical Sciences, Faculty of Dentistry, Dalhousie University

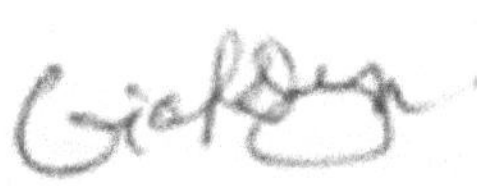

DOI: 10.1201/9781042016075-34

ABSTRACT: **Purpose:** The present study was carried out among dental graduates to know their opinion regarding comprehensive care clinic in dental college hospital. Also to know if the oral health professionals felt a need of presence of a comprehensive care clinic during their course of training. **Methods:** A cross-sectional analytical study was conducted using a questionnaire and circulated among oral health professionals using google forms. The link generated was shared with oral health professionals from India, Malaysia, Brazil, Thailand and United States. The final population consisted of dental interns, graduates and oral health professionals. **Results:** A total of 225 active oral health care professionals completed the questionnaire regarding comprehensive clinic. Among the participants, 93(41.3%) had got exposed to the comprehensive dental clinic in their dental college hospital while 132(58.7%) did not. **Conclusion:** Majority of the oral health professionals lacked the exposure to comprehensive care and felt a need of presence of a comprehensive care clinic during their course of training.

Keywords: Comprehensive Health Care, Dentists, Oral Health, Practice

1 INTRODUCTION

As per the need of the growing population, the demand for general dental practitioners are increasing day by day. A substantial proportion of the dental graduates all over the world work as general practitioners by providing primary dental care services [1,2]. To do so better and effectively, they must have undertaken their dental training in a setting that provides holistic and comprehensive dental care approach. It will lead to development of better personal and professional skills improving the confidence of dental graduates to practise independently. A comprehensive care is an approach in which all the treatment procedures are carried out by the same professional. It is convenient for older adults with special care needs. There is less delay in the treatment due to reduced waiting time. [3]

The dental curriculum of institutions need to be more patient and student centric. This would depend on various institutional factors that could be structural or functional, namely, infrastructure, faculty, the departments, administration, finances, equipments and materials. [4,5] In the present scenario, the students get to know about different dental specialities. This helps the dental student to gain proper knowledge and have proper training and work experience. The disadvantage is that they come out unprepared for the general dental practice [1,6]. Hence, reshaping the clinical aspect of the educational program will help improve both patient care and student learning. [7]

But in developing countries like India and Pakistan only few dental colleges have comprehensive dental care clinic [8,9]. There is no mandatory provision of a comprehensive care unit posting in the BDS curriculum under DCI guidelines in India [8]. On the other hand about 80% of dental schools in USA have approved the comprehensive care clinic in the dental curriculum. This has showed improvement in education goals and patient care [10–12].

So present study was carried out among dental graduates to know their opinion regarding comprehensive care clinic in dental college hospital. We also wanted to know if the oral health professionals felt a need of presence of a comprehensive care clinic during their course of training.

2 METHODS

2.1 *Study design, study population and data collection*

The present study was cross-sectional type of analytical study. This was conducted using a questionnaire and circulated among oral health professionals using google forms (https://docs.google.com/forms/d/e/1FAIpQLSenptTuxTGCv79cCrBei9Z-wlmzf1ogteSvpeByeqq9tlfbXw/viewform?usp=sf_link).This link was shared with oral health professionals from India, Malaysia, Brazil, Thailand and United States. The final population consisted of dental interns, graduates and oral health professionals who logged in and filled the questionnaire.

At 90% confidence interval, 5% of margin of error with population proportion 50%, at least 225 google forms had to be filled as per the sample size calculation. Data collection was started after obtaining approval from the Institutional Ethics Committee of XXX (Protocol No.20012 dated 16 March 2020) and the study was completed within a period of six months. Consent from each participant was documented, confidentiality of the participants was maintained. The link was sent for three times in one-month interval using WhatsApp, Facebook messenger and email id to complete the questionnaire.

2.2 *Validity and reliability of data instrument*

The content and construct validity of the questionnaire were checked by five subject experts in dentistry field. Reliability of the questionnaire was achieved by pre-testing the questionnaire on ten dental graduates. The kappa statistic obtained was 0.96.

2.3 *Data management and statistical analysis*

The data was coded and analysed using jamovi 1.6.3 (Free software available at www.jamovi.org).

3 RESULT

A total of 225 active oral health care professionals completed the questionnaire, out of which 204 (90.7%) were from India, 20 (8.9%) were from Malaysia and 1(0.4%) was from USA. Among the participants 74(33%) were interns, 73(32.6%) were dental graduates, 34(15.2%) were post-graduates, 20(8.9%) were practitioners, and 23 (10.3%) were academicians. Also 93(41.3%) had got exposed and 132(58.7%) had never got exposed to comprehensive dental care clinic. Out of the exposed participants 53(51.5%) had 30 days or less duration of posting ,7 (6.8%) had 45 days or less duration of posting and 36(41.7%) had 60 day or more duration of posting in the clinic. Those participants who did not have a comprehensive dental care clinic in their hospital were asked if the presence of comprehensive care department is needed for which 182(86.3%) agreed ,4(1.9%) disagreed and 25(11.8%) gave a neutral response.

When the participants were asked about their opinion on comprehensive approach to treatment, majority of them i.e. 189(84%) agreed to having better developmental skills , 170(75.6%) said it to be time saving , 173(76.9%) agreed it would deliver quality treatment, 194(86.2%) agreed for a development of skills to run a private practice and 191(84.9%) said it would help to develop a better treatment plan for the patient. Majority [191(84.9%)] said older adults and patients with special needs got more benefited and189(84%) participants told that patient experience will be more comfortable. (Table 1)

Table 1. Responses to questions regarding comprehensive approach.

	QUESTIONS: Comprehensive approach to dental care required for	RESPONSE Agree	Neutral	Disagree
1.	Development of better skills	189 (84%)	33 (14.7%)	3 (1.3%)
2.	Time saving	170 (75.6%)	51 (22.7%)	4 (1.7%)
3.	Deliver quality of treatment	173 (76.9%)	45 (20%)	7 (3.1%)
4.	Development of skills to run a private practice	194 (86.2%)	29 (12.9%)	2 (0.9%)
5.	Better treatment plan for the patient	191 (84.9%)	31 (13.8%)	3 (1.3%)
6.	Older adults and patients with special needs	191 (84.9%)	27 (12%)	7 (3.1%)
7.	Patient's experience more comfortable	189 (84%)	34 (15.1%)	2 (0.9%)

4 DISCUSSION

Traditional dental educational model does not help the students to be self-sufficient as they often lack confidence to manage a clinic independently. Comprehensive clinical model focus on treatment planning and treatment delivery to boost the confidence of students. [2] According to Sang E. Park *et al.* [7], the shift from a student centric to a patient centric comprehensive clinic model increased student interest in a clinical setting, it drove them to attend clinics with increased enthusiasm, thereby, increasing their attendance. Complete oral health is thought to be best achieved through comprehensive dental care. [13,14]

As per the study by Mascarenhas AK [11], comprehensive care model was better than traditional care model. In our study (86.3 %) of participants agreed with this. As per Johnson G [12], students had better understanding of clinical care management and 84% of participants in our study also agreed with the same. As per Johnson G [12], the time management was better among students posted in the clinics and in our study 75.6% of the participants agreed the same.

In our study 84.9% of participants agreed that older patients have more complex needs and benefit more by this model. When asked if they had any other comments , one of the participants wrote, "Comprehensive dental care clinic is really important for an overall development for dental practitioners." Another wrote, "Comprehensive care is absolutely necessary in today's time. It gives the opportunity to treat the patient as a whole and not just his only symptom of pain. It is essential for learning process as a student because a single student is made responsible for the entire dental treatment of the patient."

The shift to a comprehensive care model depends on various institutional factors such as structural or functional, namely, infrastructure (physical and internal), faculty, the departments, administration, finances, equipments and materials. [4,5] Licari FW *et al.* [13], faced certain challenges and limitations while implementing this model. According to them, the transition from a checker to a mentor was rather hard for the faculty, since this model had more person to person as well as interdisciplinary teaching. The model, also, required complete documentation of the histories, records as well as the procedures performed on the patients. They suggested an electronic patient record. According to Johnson [12], managing the faculty was more of a struggle than managing the students. The students got accustomed to it better than the teachers. It was hard to attain a multidisciplinary approach due to the lack of interdisciplinary experience among staff.

The present study has certain limitations. Bias inherent in questionnaire studies such as response bias, social desirability bias might be found in this study.

5 CONCLUSION

Most of the oral health professionals lacked the exposure to comprehensive care. The dental graduates felt a need of presence of a comprehensive care clinic during their course of training.

ACKNOWLEDGMENTS

This is not a funded study

REFERENCES

[1] Ghani F, Salim I. (2010). Comprehensive dental care teaching clinics. A concept of inculcating general dental practice skills in BDS students. *JPDA*. 19(2); 75–77.

[2] DePaola DP, Slavkin HC. (2004). Reforming dental health professions education: a white paper. *J Dent Educ*. 68(11):1139–50.

[3] Karuveettil V, Janakiram C, Krishnan V, Mathew A, Venkitachalam R, Varma B. (2021). Perceptions of a comprehensive dental care teaching clinic among stakeholders in a dental teaching hospital in South India: A baseline assessment. *Med J Armed Forces India*.:S195–S201. Epub 2021 Feb 2.

[4] Chambers DW. (1994). Competencies: a new view of becoming a dentist. *J Dent Educ*. 58(5):342–5.

[5] Chuenjitwongsa S, Oliver RG, Bullock AD. (2018). Competence, competency-based education, and undergraduate dental education: a discussion paper. *Eur J Dent Educ*. 22(1):1–8.

[6] Ireland RS, Dawber S. (1999). Introducing undergraduate dental students to the wider rôle of the primary care team. *Eur J Dent Educ*. 3(4):145–7.

[7] Park SE, Susarla HK, Nalliah R, Timothé P, Howell TH, Karimbux NY. (2012). Does a case completion curriculum influence dental students' clinical productivity? *J Dent Educ*. 76(5):602–8.

[8] Tandon S. (2004). Challenges to the oral health workforce in India. *J Dent Educ*. 68 7 Suppl:28–33.

[9] Ghani F. (2005). Mid-level diplomas in dentistry: which one is relevant. *J Pak Dent Assoc*. 14:54–55.

[10] Kilgore TB, Casada JP. (1994). Clinic educational management systems in United States and Canadian dental schools. *J Dent Educ*. 58(10):775–7.

[11] Mascarenhas AK. (2001). Patient satisfaction with the comprehensive care model of dental care delivery. *J Dent Educ*. 65 (11):1266–71.

[12] Johnson G. (1999). A comprehensive care clinic in Swedish dental undergraduate education: 3-year report. *Eur J Dent Educ*. 3 (4):148–52.

[13] Licari FW, Knight GW. (2003). Developing a group practice comprehensive care education curriculum. *J Dent Educ*. 67(12):1312–5.

[14] K Puneet, C Batra, B Chandni. (2022). Review of the comprehensive public health dentistry approach towards total oral health. *IJFANS*. 11(9): 2784–89.

Navigating Dental Education Trends and Transforming Dental Pedagogy – Abas and Srikant N (Eds)

Future Directions for Artificial Intelligence Enhanced Dental Simulation Training: Emerging Trends and Technologies

Prakyath Malli
Department of Prosthodontics, Yenepoya Dental College, Deralkatte, Mangalore

ABSTRACT: Artificial intelligence (AI) is rapidly transforming dental education through the integration of intelligent simulation, adaptive learning systems, virtual reality (VR), haptic feedback technologies, and natural language processing–based tutoring platforms. This review examines emerging trends and technological advancements shaping AI-enhanced dental simulation training across multiple disciplines, including operative dentistry, endodontics, periodontics, prosthodontics, oral surgery, orthodontics, pediatric dentistry, and oral radiology. AI-driven systems provide real-time performance analytics, automated assessment, and personalized feedback based on quantitative metrics such as angulation, depth control, force application, and surface morphology. These capabilities support competency-based progression, reduce assessor subjectivity, and promote deliberate psychomotor skill acquisition. In addition, intelligent tutoring systems and NLP-powered virtual patients enhance diagnostic reasoning and cognitive skill development beyond technical training. Despite demonstrated benefits—including improved procedural accuracy, reduced learning curves, and enhanced standardization—significant challenges remain related to cost, infrastructure, validation of simulation-to-clinic transfer, faculty training, ethical governance, and data privacy. Future directions emphasize augmented reality integration, AI-driven digital twins, predictive analytics, and scalable cloud-based platforms. Strategic and evidence-based implementation of AI-enhanced simulation may redefine dental education by fostering personalized, data-driven, and patient-centered competency development.

Keywords: Artificial Intelligence, Dental Education, Simulation Training, Virtual Reality, Educational Technology

1 INTRODUCTION

Artificial intelligence (AI) is progressively transforming healthcare education through intelligent tutoring systems, predictive analytics, automated assessments, and immersive virtual environments that enhance clinical reasoning and technical skills. In medical education, AI supports adaptive e-learning, virtual patient simulations, diagnostic training modules, and competency-based assessments with real-time analytics, enabling standardized evaluation and personalized feedback that promote self-directed, mastery-based learning [1,2]. Dental education has followed a parallel evolution—from digitized radiography and CAD/CAM systems to virtual case repositories, haptic simulators, and virtual reality platforms—with recent advances highlighting AI-driven analytics and machine learning algorithms capable of objectively assessing tooth preparations, radiographic interpretation, and diagnostic decision-making [3]. Given the procedural, tactile, and visually intensive nature of dentistry, which requires precise psychomotor skills measurable through parameters such as angulation, depth, convergence, marginal integrity, and force application, AI-integrated simulation offers a uniquely powerful framework for real-time objective analysis [4]. Combined with immersive technologies, these systems enable standardized skill assessment, personalized progression, and competency validation, positioning dental education as one of the most promising areas for scalable AI integration in healthcare training.

2 ARTIFICIAL INTELLIGENCE ENHANCED SIMULATION ACROSS DENTAL DISCIPLINES

Artificial intelligence–enhanced simulation in dental education is not a uniform technological intervention but a discipline-sensitive framework tailored to the procedural, cognitive, and tactile demands of individual specialties. Each branch of dentistry presents distinct technical challenges, and AI-driven simulation platforms are increasingly being calibrated to address these unique competencies with precision and specificity.

2.1 *Operative and restorative dentistry*

Operative and restorative dentistry represent the most extensively studied domains for AI-based simulation, particularly through platforms such as Simodont Dental Trainer. In these disciplines, the focus centers on cavity preparation geometry, marginal integrity, depth control, wall convergence, and smoothness of finish lines [5]. AI-enabled simulators

DOI: 10.1201/9781042016075-35

generate real-time deviation maps that compare student preparations with ideal digital templates, quantifying discrepancies in millimeters and angular deviations. The incorporation of haptic feedback allows learners to internalize correct tactile sensations associated with enamel versus dentin cutting resistance, reinforcing spatial awareness and bur angulation control. By tracking longitudinal performance data, AI systems identify recurring preparation errors and support iterative refinement, contributing to measurable improvements in procedural accuracy [6].

2.2 *Endodontics*

Endodontics is a high-stakes specialty where precision directly influences long-term tooth survival. AI-enhanced VR and haptic simulators are increasingly applied in access cavity preparation, working length estimation, and canal instrumentation training. These systems replicate the tactile sensation of negotiating curved canals and varying dentinal resistance, enabling students to practice delicate hand movements in a risk-free environment [7]. Machine learning algorithms monitor canal path deviation, excessive dentin removal, and force application patterns that may predispose to perforation, ledging, or transportation—errors that are difficult and costly to manage clinically. By providing real-time corrective feedback, AI platforms reduce procedural mishaps during early skill acquisition and enhance preparedness before patient-based endodontic procedures [8].

2.3 *Periodontics*

In periodontics, AI simulation emphasizes force modulation, instrument angulation, and subgingival adaptation during scaling and root planing. Pressure-sensitive haptic systems train students to maintain optimal lateral force without causing root surface trauma [9]. Real-time alerts notify learners of excessive pressure or improper curette positioning, reinforcing controlled instrumentation techniques. Beyond psychomotor skills, AI-assisted diagnostic tools are increasingly integrated into training modules, particularly for radiographic interpretation and staging and grading of periodontitis. By analyzing clinical parameters and radiographic bone levels, AI systems enhance diagnostic consistency and strengthen students' ability to correlate clinical findings with disease progression [10].

2.4 *Prosthodontics*

Prosthodontic training benefits substantially from AI-driven geometric analysis. Crown preparation simulation platforms evaluate taper angles, axial wall height, occlusal reduction depth, and finish line configuration with precision that often surpasses traditional visual faculty assessment [11]. Quantitative feedback enables students to refine convergence angles and achieve uniform occlusal clearance prior to clinical application. Emerging developments in digital prosthodontics further integrate AI into complete denture fabrication workflows, guiding impression evaluation, border molding simulation, and occlusal scheme design [12]. As CAD/CAM technologies become central to restorative practice, AI simulation bridges the gap between conventional preparation techniques and digital prosthetic workflows [13].

2.5 *Oral Surgery and Exodontia*

In oral surgery and exodontive procedures, AI-enhanced simulators provide safe environments for practicing extraction techniques, flap design, suturing, and basic implant placement. VR platforms replicate bone density variations and periodontal ligament resistance, allowing students to rehearse force vectors required for luxation and elevation without risk of jaw fracture or soft tissue injury [14]. Augmented reality overlays are increasingly incorporated to assist in surgical planning simulations, offering anatomical guidance and depth visualization during implant positioning exercises. AI algorithms analyze applied forces and angulation patterns, helping learners refine technique while minimizing traumatic extraction tendencies [15].

2.6 *Orthodontics*

Orthodontic applications of AI simulation focus on bracket placement accuracy, wire bending practice, and digital treatment planning. AI-powered systems evaluate bracket positioning in three dimensions, measuring deviations from ideal torque and angulation parameters. Simulation modules also allow virtual wire bending exercises with feedback on force application and alignment precision [16]. Additionally, AI-driven cephalometric analysis tools are embedded into orthodontic training environments, enabling students to practice growth assessment, skeletal pattern analysis, and malocclusion classification using automated landmark identification and predictive modeling. This integration strengthens diagnostic acumen alongside mechanical skill development [17].

2.7 *Pediatric dentistry*

Pediatric dentistry presents unique dual challenges: technical proficiency and behavior management. AI simulation in this discipline includes training modules for primary tooth morphology recognition, pulp therapy procedures, and stainless steel crown placement. VR environments replicate the anatomical differences between primary and permanent dentition, enhancing procedural adaptation. Notably, emerging virtual patient simulations incorporate behavioral variability—such as anxiety, limited cooperation, or sudden movement—introducing a communication and behavioral management component to technical training. This layered approach reflects the holistic skill set required in pediatric practice [18].

2.8 *Oral radiology and diagnosis*

Among all dental disciplines, oral radiology and diagnostic training represent one of the most advanced applications of AI in education. Deep learning models trained for detection of dental caries, periapical pathology, periodontal bone loss, and anatomical landmark identification are increasingly incorporated into instructional platforms [19]. Students can compare their interpretations with AI-generated heat maps and probability scores, refining pattern recognition and diagnostic confidence. By providing objective benchmarking and immediate correction, AI-assisted radiographic training enhances interpretative accuracy and supports evidence-based decision-making. As validated models continue to evolve, AI integration in radiology education exemplifies the broader potential of intelligent systems to standardize and elevate diagnostic training across dental curricula [20].

3 CHALLENGES AND LIMITATIONS

Despite its transformative potential, AI-enhanced dental simulation faces several significant challenges that limit widespread adoption and seamless integration into curricula. High initial costs of procurement, maintenance, and software upgrades—particularly for advanced VR and haptic systems such as the Simodont Dental Trainer—pose substantial financial barriers, especially for institutions in resource-constrained settings. Infrastructure requirements, including dedicated simulation laboratories, technical support teams, and high-performance computing systems, further compound implementation difficulties [21]. Additionally, the absence of standardized performance metrics and interoperability across different platforms results in variability in assessment criteria, limiting cross-institutional benchmarking and curriculum harmonization. Concerns also persist regarding the validity of skill transfer from simulated environments to real clinical settings, as long-term, large-scale evidence demonstrating consistent simulation-to-clinic translation remains limited [22].

Faculty-related factors represent another critical barrier. Resistance to adopting AI-driven systems may stem from unfamiliarity with emerging technologies, apprehension about reduced pedagogical control, or skepticism regarding automated assessment replacing expert judgment. Effective integration therefore requires structured faculty development programs and calibration workshops to ensure that AI tools function as adjuncts rather than substitutes for clinical mentorship [23]. Ethical considerations further complicate implementation, particularly in relation to algorithmic transparency, potential bias in AI-based grading systems, and over-reliance on automated decision-making. The collection and storage of granular student performance data raise additional concerns regarding data privacy, consent, and cybersecurity compliance. Together, these technical, pedagogical, and ethical limitations underscore the need for robust validation studies, regulatory frameworks, and evidence-based implementation strategies to ensure responsible and equitable deployment of AI in dental education [24].

4 FUTURE DIRECTIONS

The future of AI-enhanced dental simulation is likely to be shaped by deeper integration of augmented reality (AR), predictive analytics, and intelligent digital ecosystems. AR overlays embedded within simulation units have the potential to project real-time anatomical guidance, ideal preparation outlines, and dynamic error alerts directly onto operative fields, bridging the gap between virtual training and live clinical procedures. Beyond isolated task simulation, the emergence of AI-driven "digital twins" — virtual replicas of individual patients constructed from radiographic, intraoral scanning, and clinical datasets — may enable highly personalized case simulations. These models could allow students to rehearse procedures on anatomically accurate digital counterparts before performing them clinically, enhancing preparedness and procedural confidence. Simultaneously, gamification strategies incorporating performance dashboards, milestone achievements, adaptive difficulty levels, and peer benchmarking may increase learner motivation and engagement, aligning educational design with contemporary cognitive and behavioral science principles [5].

At a systemic level, AI simulation platforms are expected to align more closely with competency-based accreditation frameworks, enabling automated documentation of skill acquisition mapped to defined learning outcomes. Predictive analytics derived from longitudinal performance data may facilitate early identification of struggling students, allowing timely remediation and personalized academic support. Importantly, cloud-based AI systems could expand access to high-quality simulation training in remote or resource-limited settings, reducing disparities in educational infrastructure. The growing role of large language models in dental education further broadens this horizon, supporting case-based reasoning, clinical documentation training, literature synthesis, and interactive tutoring. As these technologies mature, the integration of AR, intelligent patient modeling, adaptive analytics, and conversational AI may transform dental education into a fully interconnected, data-driven learning environment that supports technical precision, diagnostic reasoning, and equitable access on a global scale.

5 CONCLUSION

Artificial intelligence–enhanced dental simulation represents a paradigm shift in preclinical and early clinical education, moving beyond static mechanical rehearsal toward intelligent, data-driven, and competency-based training ecosystems. From adaptive learning systems and real-time performance analytics to VR-haptic environments and NLP-powered intelligent tutoring, AI technologies are redefining how psychomotor skills, diagnostic reasoning, and clinical decision-making are cultivated. By reducing assessor subjectivity, standardizing evaluation metrics, and enabling personalized progression pathways, AI-enhanced platforms address long-standing limitations of traditional phantom head–based instruction. Across disciplines—including operative dentistry, endodontics, periodontics, prosthodontics, oral surgery, orthodontics, pediatric dentistry, and oral radiology—AI integration demonstrates the potential to enhance procedural precision, accelerate learning curves, and strengthen simulation-to-clinic transfer, ultimately contributing to improved patient safety.

However, responsible implementation requires careful attention to validation, cost-effectiveness, faculty calibration, ethical governance, and data privacy safeguards. Large-scale longitudinal studies are essential to confirm sustained clinical benefits and competency outcomes. Rather than replacing educators, AI should function as an augmentative tool that enhances mentorship, objectivity, and scalability within dental curricula. As augmented reality, predictive analytics, digital twins, and large language models continue to evolve, the convergence of these technologies may transform dental education into an integrated, personalized, and globally accessible learning ecosystem. Strategic, evidence-based adoption will be critical to ensuring that AI-enhanced simulation fulfills its promise while maintaining educational integrity and patient-centered values.

REFERENCES

[1] Altafi H, Suresh S, Zareinia K. (2025). The potential of cloud-based AI-enabled platforms in healthcare education. *Int J Intell Robot Appl.* 9:683–693.

[2] Fang Q, Reynaldi R, Araminta AS, Kamal I, Saini P, Afshari FS, Tan SC, Yuan JC, Qomariyah NN, Sukotjo C. (2024). Artificial intelligence (AI)-driven dental education: Exploring the role of chatbots in a clinical learning environment. *The Journal of Prosthetic Dentistry.*

[3] El-Hakim M, Anthonappa R, Fawzy A. (2025). Artificial intelligence in Dental Education: A scoping review of applications, challenges, and gaps. *Dent J (Basel).* 13:384. Cited: in: : PMID: 41002657.

[4] Wei H, Dai Y, Yuan K, Li KY, Hung KF, Hu EM, Lee AH, Chang JW, Zhang C, Li X. (2025). AI-powered problem-and case-based learning in medical and dental education: a systematic review and meta-analysis. *International Dental Journal.* 75.

[5] Najeeb M, Islam S. (2025). Artificial intelligence (AI) in restorative dentistry: Current trends and future prospects. *BMC Oral Health.* 25:592. Cited: in PMID: 40251567.

[6] Revilla-León M, Gómez-Polo M, Vyas S, Barmak AB, Özcan M, Att W, Krishnamurthy VR. (2022). Artificial intelligence applications in restorative dentistry: A systematic review. *J Prosthet Dent.* 128:867–875. Cited: in: : PMID: 33840515.

[7] Setzer FC, Li J, Khan AA. (2024). The use of artificial intelligence in endodontics. *J Dent Res.* 103:853–862. Cited: in PMID: 38822561.

[8] Ourang SA, Sohrabniya F, Mohammad-Rahimi H, Dianat O, Aminoshariae A, Nagendrababu V, Dummer PMH, Duncan HF, Nosrat A. (2024). Artificial intelligence in endodontics: Fundamental principles, workflow, and tasks. *Int Endod J.* 57:1546–1565. Cited: in: : PMID: 39056554.

[9] Khan SF, Siddique A, Khan AM, Shetty B, Fazal I. (2024). Artificial intelligence in periodontology and implantology-a narrative review. *Journal of Medical Artificial Intelligence.* 7.

[10] Scott J, Biancardi AM, Jones O, Andrew D. (2023). Artificial intelligence in periodontology: A scoping review. *Dent J (Basel).* 11:43. Cited: in: : PMID: 36826188.

[11] Alshadidi AAF, Alshahrani AA, Aldosari LIN, Chaturvedi S, Saini RS, Hassan SAB, Cicciù M, Minervini G. (2023). Investigation on the application of artificial intelligence in prosthodontics. *Appl Sci (Basel).* 13:5004.

[12] Schwendicke F, Rahimi HM, Tichy A. (2025). Artificial intelligence in prosthodontics. *Dental Clinics.* 69:315–326.

[13] Alfaraj A, Nagai T, AlQallaf H, Lin W-S. (2024). Race to the moon or the bottom? Applications, performance, and ethical considerations of artificial intelligence in prosthodontics and implant dentistry. *Dent J (Basel).* 13:13. Cited: in: : PMID: 39851589.

[14] Panahi O, Eslamlou SF. Artificial intelligence in oral surgery: Enhancing diagnostics, treatment, and patient care. *J Clin Den & Oral Care.* 3.

[15] Miragall MF, Knoedler S, Kauke-Navarro M, Saadoun R, Grabenhorst A, Grill FD, Ritschl LM, Fichter AM, Safi A-F, Knoedler L. (2023). Face the future-artificial intelligence in oral and maxillofacial surgery. *J Clin Med.* 12:6843. Cited: in: : PMID: 37959310.

[16] Wong KF, Lam XY, Jiang Y, Yeung AW, Lin Y. (2023). Artificial intelligence in orthodontics and orthognathic surgery: a bibliometric analysis of the 100 most-cited articles. *Head & Face Medicine.* 19.

[17] Gracea RS, Winderickx N, Vanheers M, Hendrickx J, Preda F, Shujaat S, Cadenas de Llano-Pérula M, Jacobs R. (2025). Artificial intelligence for orthodontic diagnosis and treatment planning: A scoping review. *J Dent*. 152:105442. Cited: in: : PMID: 39505292.

[18] Vishwanathaiah S, Fageeh HN, Khanagar SB, Maganur PC. (2023). Artificial intelligence its uses and application in pediatric dentistry: A review. *Biomedicines*. 11:788. Cited: in: : PMID: 36979767.

[19] Ali M, Irfan M, Ali T, Wei CR, Akilimali A. (2025). Artificial intelligence in dental radiology: a narrative review. *Ann Med Surg (Lond)*. 87:2212–2217. Cited: in: : PMID: 40212156.

[20] Hung KF, Ai QYH, Leung YY, Yeung AWK. (2022). Potential and impact of artificial intelligence algorithms in dento-maxillofacial radiology. *Clin Oral Investig*. 26:5535–5555. Cited: in: : PMID: 35438326.

[21] Elnagar MH, Yadav S, Venugopalan SR, Lee MK, Oubaidin M, Rampa S, Allareddy V. (2024). ChatGPT and dental education: Opportunities and challenges. *Semin Orthod.* 30:401–404.

[22] Annamma LM, Varma SR, Abuttayem H, Prasad P, Azim SA, Odeh R, George BT, Nair C, Karobari MI. (2024). Current challenges in dental education-a scoping review. *BMC medical education*. 24.

[23] Rasouli S. (2025). Artificial Intelligence and Smart Technologies in Dental Education: Applications, Challenges, and Ethical Considerations. *Medical Education Bulletin.* 6:1051–1057.

[24] Islam NM, Laughter L, Sadid-Zadeh R, Smith C, Dolan TA, Crain G, Squarize CH. (2022). Adopting artificial intelligence in dental education: A model for academic leadership and innovation. *J Dent Educ*. 86:1545–1551. Cited: in: : PMID: 35781809.

Navigating Dental Education Trends and Transforming Dental Pedagogy – Abas and Srikant N (Eds)
 ISBN: 978-1-041-32674-8

Exploring Knowledge, Attitudes, and Practices Regarding Oral Prophylaxis Among Bank Employees in Dakshina Kannada: Implications for Dental Curriculum Development

Chanchal Gupta
Former Intern Manipal College of Dental Sciences Mangalore Manipal Academy of Higher Education, Manipal, Karnataka, India

Sangeeta Umesh Nayak
Department of Periodontology Manipal College of Dental Sciences Mangalore Manipal Academy of Higher Education, Manipal, Karnataka, India

Keshava Pai
Department of Psychiatry Kasturba Medical College Mangalore Manipal Academy of Higher Education, Manipal, Karnataka, India

Mranali K. Shetty and K. David
Department of Periodontology Manipal College of Dental Sciences Mangalore Manipal Academy of Higher Education, Manipal, Karnataka, India

ABSTRACT: **Background:** Oral health is a vital aspect of overall well-being, affecting dental function, social interactions, and quality of life. Despite its importance, it often receives less attention among non-healthcare professionals, such as bank employees. Education on proper oral hygiene and regular oral prophylaxis is crucial for preventing oral diseases and promoting comprehensive health. Bank employees face significant stress due to workload and erratic schedules, making it challenging to maintain oral hygiene.

Aim: This study aims to assess knowledge, attitudes, and practices (KAPs) related to oral prophylaxis among bank employees in Dakshina Kannada.

Materials and Methods: A pilot study was conducted among 40 bank employees from Dakshina Kannada using a structured questionnaire (via Google Forms) to assess their demographics, knowledge, attitudes, and practices related to oral prophylaxis.

Results: The participants demonstrated a fair understanding of oral prophylaxis but highlighted areas of misconception and uncertainty. Attitudes toward dental scaling were mixed, with concerns about discomfort, cost, and potential side effects influencing their willingness to recommend the procedure. Many respondents adhered to recommended practices post-scaling, but a notable percentage had not undergone the procedure.

Conclusion: This study underscores the need for tailored oral health education and the integration of community-oriented components into dental curricula. By leveraging the expertise of public health dentistry, dental institutions, and periodontists, dental professionals can engage effectively with diverse populations, address specific oral health needs, and improve overall oral hygiene practices, particularly among stressed and overworked professionals such as bank employees.

Keywords: Oral health, Oral prophylaxis, Scaling, Bleeding gums, Bank employees

1 INTRODUCTION

Oral health is a critical aspect of overall well-being, yet it often receives less attention, particularly among non-healthcare professionals. It impacts not only dental function but also social interactions and quality of life. Education on proper oral hygiene and regular oral prophylaxis is vital for preventing oral diseases and ensuring comprehensive health. [1] According to the World Health Organization (WHO), oral health is characterized by the absence of pain in the mouth and face, as well as the absence of oral and throat infections, sores, gum disease, tooth decay, tooth loss, and other issues that can hinder one's ability to bite, chew, smile, speak, and maintain psycho-social well-being. Oral health-related illness affects all human beings, irrespective of location, country, nationality, race, or color. It is the fourth most expensive disease to treat in developing countries. [2] Despite ongoing efforts worldwide, oral health continues to be undervalued or neglected. [3]

Current studies have demonstrated that role conflict puts bank workers, clerks, officers, accountants, and computer specialists under stress. Workers in banks typically have hectic schedules, erratic work habits, and various stress patterns and coping mechanisms. Workplace pressure, elevated client expectations, and a greater degree of

DOI: 10.1201/9781042016075-36

responsibility alter the workday's rhythm, making it difficult for employees to unwind. The prolonged working hours and high concentration required at the workplace make this group more vulnerable to changes in their regular dietary habits. [4,5]

Dental education plays a crucial role in advocating oral health awareness, not just among students but also within the broader community, including professions such as banking. Public health dentistry and dental institutions serve as the bridge between clinical education and community engagement, while periodontists provide specialized knowledge on the prevention and treatment of gum diseases, which is crucial for effective oral prophylaxis. [4,5]

Oral prophylaxis, which includes preventive measures such as professional cleaning and proper oral hygiene practices, is essential for maintaining oral health and preventing conditions such as periodontal disease. For bank employees, who are often under significant workload and stress due to their responsibilities in handling financial aspects, maintaining good oral health can be particularly challenging. Stress and long hours may lead to the neglect of personal health, including oral hygiene, increasing their susceptibility to dental problems. [4,5]

This study aimed to assess the knowledge, attitudes, and practices related to oral prophylaxis among bank employees in Dakshina Kannada, providing insights that could inform targeted health interventions. Understanding the KAP of oral prophylaxis in this demographic population can help design effective health education programs and increase awareness of oral prophylaxis among bank employees, underscoring the need for tailored educational strategies. By integrating community-oriented components into dental curricula and leveraging the expertise of public health dentistry, dental institutions, and periodontists, future dental professionals can be better equipped to engage with diverse populations and address their specific oral health needs.

The findings aim to guide the development of a dental curriculum that emphasizes community outreach, public health initiatives, periodontal care, and education, ultimately fostering improved oral health practices and outcomes, particularly among stressed and overworked professionals such as bank employees. This can reduce the risk of dental problems and promote better oral hygiene practices among working professionals.

2 METHODOLOGY

Ethical approval for the study was obtained from the Institutional Ethics and Review Board of Manipal College of Dental Sciences, Mangalore, India (Protocol no. 24027). A total of 40 bank employees were selected via convenience sampling for this pilot study, providing initial insights into this specific demographic. Permission was secured from the bank manager of the respective bank, and all participants provided informed consent through Google Forms.

Data were gathered using a structured questionnaire consisting of 22 questions divided into four sections:

(1) **Demographic Details:** This section recorded the participants' age, sex, and years of employment in the banking sector.
(2) **Knowledge of Oral Prophylaxis:** Six questions were asked to assess participants' understanding of the procedure, its benefits, recommended frequency, and factors contributing to the need for dental scaling.
(3) **Attitudes toward Oral Prophylaxis**: Seven questions evaluated attitudes toward the effectiveness and preventive value of dental scaling, the universality of its recommendation, perceived barriers, personal experiences, and the likelihood of recommending dental scaling.
(4) **Practices related to Oral Prophylaxis:** Six questions focused on participants' practices related to dental scaling, such as post-scaling dietary restrictions, adherence to oral hygiene routines, scheduling of follow-up appointments, frequency of tooth brushing, use of prescribed mouthwash, and compliance with aftercare instructions provided by the dentist.

The questionnaire was reviewed and validated by a subject expert to ensure clarity and relevance. The responses were analyzed via SPSS version 29.0.2.0 software, with both descriptive statistics and frequency distributions employed to summarize and interpret the data.

3 RESULTS

The majority of the respondents—25 years of age or older—are female (57.5%), and their average age is approximately 30 years. They have been in the banking industry for an average of six years, with 22.5% having worked there for ten years or more. Regarding oral prophylaxis, 47.5% of respondents correctly identified that dental scaling reduces plaque and tartar, and 62.5% knew what instruments are used in the process. However, 40% of respondents were unsure about the purpose of scaling, and 27.5% were unsure about the techniques utilized, indicating a significant level of ambiguity.

Furthermore, 72.5% of respondents reported that smoking, consuming sugary meals, and maintaining poor dental hygiene increase the need for scaling, and 67.5% acknowledged the importance of regular scaling to preserve oral health. Despite this, misconceptions remain: 30% would not recommend dental scaling as part of an oral hygiene routine, and 42.5% disagreed with its necessity.

With respect to attitudes, 49% believe that dental scaling improves oral health, while 72.5% consider it a crucial preventive measure against dental problems. Nevertheless, concerns about discomfort, cost, and potential side effects influence their willingness to undergo or recommend the procedure. In practice, 60% avoid eating for a few hours after scaling, and 65% brush twice a day post-procedure, but 35% never undergo scaling, indicating a need for increased awareness and education about the benefits and proper practices associated with dental scaling.

4 DISCUSSION

There is significant evidence to suggest that a person's job can have a large influence on their health and well-being [6]. Occupational stress can impose or stimulate habits like smoking and alcohol. This effect is complex and impacts many facets of health. An occupational disease is defined as a "negative change in health state directly arising from more or less prolonged exposure to dangerous substances or situations directly related to the individual's work". [7,8] In light of this, investigating how various professions affect general health is essential. Since the mouth is a primary portal through which many diseases enter the body, [9] the environmental risks connected to specific jobs can have a multifaceted effect on oral health.

Myths and misunderstandings about oral health and care have an awful impact on the general public's awareness, mindset, and behaviour while seeking medical/dental attention. Seeking dental care is significantly hampered by these beliefs. False perception of the people is found in regard to even the basic facts, such as believing that visiting the dentist is only essential when dental pain arises, and dental scaling makes the teeth loose and replacement of tooth/maintaining milk teeth in arch is not needed for permanent teeth alignment. In the present study the participants were more aware about oral health care. [10]

In contrast to findings from previous studies, [11] the knowledge and practice distribution pattern linked to dental care among participants in this study did not exhibit a significant association with age, gender, employment, or working experience. Furthermore, contrary to the results published by Ehizele et al. in 2012, the participants in this study demonstrated a satisfactory degree of knowledge and a positive attitude toward oral prophylaxis. [12] This unexpected finding may suggest the existence of additional contributing factors that have raised awareness among different populations, such as more widely available oral health education or broader public health campaigns.

5 CONCLUSION

Oral health education must be incorporated into the dental curriculum to meet the unique requirements of various community groups, including bank personnel. Dental schools can better equip practitioners to implement effective preventive measures and educational interventions by emphasizing oral prophylaxis and recognizing the particular obstacles faced by these professionals. The collaboration of public health dentistry, dental facilities, and periodontists can lead to better-informed and healthier communities, ultimately enhancing the overall impact of dental education. By addressing these needs through focused education and outreach, it is possible to significantly improve oral health outcomes and lessen the negative impact that stress and workload have on oral hygiene practices among groups similar to bank employees.

REFERENCES

[1] Tadin, A.; Poljak Guberina, R.; Domazet, J.; Gavic, L. (2022). Oral hygiene practices and oral health knowledge among students in split, croatia. *Healthcare* 10, 406. https://doi.org/10.3390/healthcare10020406

[2] Woldeyohannes D, Getachew D, Lemma S, Gelaye B (2017) Oral health related illness and associated factors among bank workers and teachers in addis ababa, Ethiopia: Cross-Sectional study. *Health Sci J.* Vol. 11 No. 6: 532 (7)

[3] Patanapu SK, Arelli N, Veeraboina N, Reddy KV, Dantala SN, Voruganti S. (2022). Assessment of oral health status and treatment needs among TSRTC employees in Hyderabad City, Telangana, India. *Int J Community Med Public Health* 9:1366–74.

[4] Chandra, M., Jayakumar, H., and Vanishree, N. (2009). Oral health status and treatment needs among bank employees in bangalore city, India. An Epidemiological Study. *Journal of Indian Association of Public Health Dentistry*, 7(14), 169. https://doi.org/10.4103/2319-5932.196297

[5] Yao, X., Dembe, A.E., Wickizer, T., and Lu, B. (2015). Does time pressure create barriers for people to receive preventive health services?. *Preventive medicine*, *74*, 55–58. https://doi.org/10.1016/j.ypmed.2015.03.008

[6] Patel F, Shourie V, Muglikar S. (2022). A cross-sectional study assessing the relation between stress and chronic periodontitis in state transport employees in the city of Pune. *Univ Res J Dent.* 2015;5:14–8.

[7] Zinser V, Irigoyen ME, Rivera G, Maupomé G, Sánchez-Pérez L, Velázquez C. (2008). Cigarette smoking and dental caries among professional truck drivers in Mexico. *Caries Res.* 42(4):255–62.

[8] Gambhir RS, Nirola A, Singh J, Sekhon T, Anand S.(2015). Periodontal health status of transport workers of a union territory in India: A cross-sectional study. *J Indian Soc Periodontol.* 19:312–6.

[9] Schour I, Sarnat BG. (1942). Oral manifestations of occupational origin. *J Am Med Assoc.* 120:1197–207.

[10] Khan AD, Ali M, Ajmal MA, Wazir FS, Ahmad A, Awais M, Kabir S. (2024). Prevalence of misconceptions and myths regarding oral health among medical and dental students in peshawar, Pakistan. *Cureus.* 16(1):e52800. doi: 10.7759/cureus.52800. PMID: 38389603.

[11] Amuh VO, Okojie OH, Ehizele AO. (2022). Dental care knowledge and practice of a group of health workers in Benin City, Nigeria. *Ann Med Health Sci Res* 2014;4:307–10.

[12] Ehizele AO, Azodo CC, Ehigiator O, Ezeja EB. (2012). Misconceptions about oral health among a group of Nigerian primary school teachers. *Nig Dent J* 2012;20:37–40.

Navigating Dental Education Trends and Transforming Dental Pedagogy – Abas and Srikant N (Eds)
© 2027 The Author(s), ISBN: 978-1-041-32674-8

Introducing Multiple Assessment in Skill Training Modules on the Skill "Anterior Nasal Packing"*

Sumit Sharma
Department of E.N.T., Dr. KNS Memorial Institute of Medical Sciences Barabanki

Adarshlata Singh
Department of Dermatology

Vaibhav Anjankar
Director SHER, Jawaharlal Nehru medical College, Datta Meghe institute of higher education and research, Wardha

ABSTRACT: Introduction: Introducing multiple assessment methods in skill training modules for anterior nasal packing aims to enhance proficiency and ensure comprehensive competency in this critical medical procedure. Anterior nasal packing, essential for managing epistaxis, requires precise technique and understanding of anatomical nuances.

Objectives: Primary objective is to introduce multiple assessments in skill module by Development of content validated module for anterior nasal packing skill for under graduates, Assessment of the learners after Didactic session on anterior nasal packing skill for under graduates, Assessment of the learners after practice session on anterior nasal packing skill for under graduates and Study of feedback from faculty and learner after certification

Methodology: Students were divided into 2 groups, one group was trained by teh conventional NMC method while other group was trained by Multiple assessment method.

Conclusion: The use of multiple assessments in skill training modules within a skill lab setting offers a robust framework for evaluating and enhancing student learning. While there are challenges in implementing diverse assessments, the benefits they bring in terms of holistic evaluation, enhanced learning, adaptability, and engagement are significant. By adhering to best practices such as clear objectives, balanced assessment plans, continuous feedback, instructor training, and student involvement, educators can maximize the effectiveness of multiple assessments.

Keywords: Anterior Nasal Packing, Skill Training, Multiple Assessment Method, Reflective Practice, OSCEs evaluation, Clinical Skills Development, Multi-Faceted Evaluation

1 INTRODUCTION

NMC introduced Competency based medical education in undergraduate medical education from 2019 onwards across India in which a medical student has to acquire a set of competencies in each subject to pass the examination to become an Indian medical graduate. Competencies have been graded in various categories based on the millers pyramid on Knows, Knows how, Shows, Shows how and perform. The later part of competencies (Shows, Shows how and perform) require the student to practice skills in the skill lab because of which NMC has made it mandatory for all medical college to develop skill labs based on guidelines provided by the NMC. Skills lab provides a safe training environment in which a learner can be observed and be provided with the feedback necessary to improve. It also allows the learner to do tasks repetitively under supervision till the desired level of competency is achieved. [1]

2 REVIEW OF LITERATURE

Simulation is a learning strategy used to teach students to get a glimpse of real life situations before they are exposed to them. [1] It also helps students to practice these skills under supervision in a structured manner and take supervised decisions in safe environments. [2] NMC insists on skill training to ensure the development of healthcare professionals and the delivery of high-quality medical care. Skill lab training of students helps students to develop confidence in developing good communication, right attitude, apply the latest techniques, and develop clinical thinking and ethical principles [3,4] .

*Note: This is a Masters in Health Professional Education Project of Dr. Sumit Sharma batch 2023 from Datta Meghe institute of higher education and research, Wardha

DOI: 10.1201/9781042016075-37

Technology, such as virtual reality and simulation-based training, enhances learning experiences, while interdisciplinary collaboration promotes teamwork and communication skills [5].

The basic principle of skill training in skill lab is supervised simulated training of the student under the guidance of a faculty with proper assessment and feedback. For the implementation of teh same NMC has asked all teh colleges to develop structured modules for each skill – the basic layout plan for the module development has been laid out by NMC [6].

Need: As per IMG the UG students has to learn competencies which he/she performed in the society after completing the programme. To accomplish these competencies systematic assessment of the various skills are required. For the same there is need of develop and validate of module having systematic analysis of particular skill.

PROBLEM: (as per PICO format)

P – Development of module having multiple assessment for the acquisition of Anterior Nasal Packing skill among the under graduate.

I – Modules developed by the Institute to teach Skill - Anterior Nasal Packing.

C – The outcome of the training sessions will be compared with the module with and without multiple assessments

O – Expected outcome is that students will have better Skill acquision in a shorter period of time.

2.1 *Aim of the study*

The Aim of the present study is to introduce multiple assessment (using various components of WPBA) in skill modules for teaching skill - Anterior Nasal Packing skill in skill lab.

2.2 *Objectives of the study*

Primary objective is to introduce multiple assessments in skill module by :

(1) Development of content validated module for anterior nasal packing skill for under graduates.
(2) Assessment of the learners after Didactic session on anterior nasal packing skill for under graduates
(3) Assessment of the learners after practice session on anterior nasal packing skill for under graduates
(4) Study of feedback from faculty and learner after certification

3 METHODOLOGY

(a) Students training will be conducted in small groups of 10 students each. Two groups will be made,
(b) One group will be trained using NMC skill module with single summative assessment and the other group will be trained with the module with multiple assessments described below:
(1) Assessment of the objectives derived for the module with respect to all aspects of skill training. Feedback to be taken from 2-3 faculty members regarding Objectives.
(2) Assessment of the students for the theoretical knowledge gained after PPT presentations and video demonstrations using – MCQ's (approximately 20) / Context based tests. (Evaluate Knows and Knows How component of the Skill)
(3) Formative Assessment of the students after training sessions using / Mini –Cex. Giving feedback to students using Sandwich method (in which positive feedback serves as a cushion to negative feedback)
(4) Summative assessment of the students using OSCE checklist.
(a) Giving feedback to students using Pendleton's Rules for Feedback.
(b) Both the groups will be given training with both the methods.
(c) Both the Groups will be evaluated with respect to

- Knowledge gained (Pr test & Post test after certification)
- Skill gained (Pre test & Post test after certification)
- OSCE scores of the two groups
- Time taken for certification

3.1 *Data Analysis*

Both qualitative and quantitative data analysis was done. Feedback analysis qualitative and assessment comparison T test and ANOVA

3.2 *Observations*

(1) Faculty members have expressed positive opinions on the new skill module. Faculty members (total 3 in number) agreed to the list of Objectives and Checklist made for the module as adequate and suggested that no

change is needed in them. They commend its practical approach and comprehensive content, which effectively enhances student engagement and skill acquisition. The module's interactive elements and real-world applications are particularly praised, making learning both enjoyable and impactful. Overall, the faculty believes this module significantly improves students‘ readiness for professional challenges, fostering critical thinking and practical problem-solving abilities essential for their skill acquisition.

Table 1. Details of the students participated in the study (MBBS 2021-22 batch).

Group A (n=25)		Group B (n=25)	
Male	11	Male	11
Female	14	Female	14

In the present study we had taken a total of 50 students divided equally in two groups – Group – A and Group B

Table 2. Average Pre-test scores of the two groups.

Group A (n=25)	Group B (n=25)
Max Marks: 100 75 (75 %)	Max Marks: 100 75 (75%)

Students of both the groups were made to give a Pre-test and students of both the groups scored 75% in an MCQ based test consisting of 20 questions.

Table 3. Average scores after PPT presentation and Video demonstration and Practice sessions (Only Group B).

Group B (n=25)	
Max Marks: 100	
PPT presentation(MCQ Based)	65%
Video demonstration(MCQ Based)	70%
Practice sessions (DOPS/ Mini-Cex)	75%

Students of Group B were made to give a Post-test following PPT presentation (MCQ Based), Video demonstration (MCQ Based) and after Practice sessions which was Mini-Cex based. Students of Group B scored 65%, 70% and 75% respectively.

Table 4. Number of attempts taken by the students for completing the skill as per OSCE checklist (Practice sessions).

Group A (n=25)	Group B (n=25)
4.5	2.5

Since students of Group B was not subjected to Post test after PPT presentation, Video demonstration and after Practice sessions the average number of attempts taken by them to complete the skill as per OSCE checklist was 4.5 as compared to Group B who were subjected to Post test after each stage who took on an average of 2.5 attempts to complete the skill as per OSCE checklist, which is a significant difference.

Table 5. Average scores after Post-test of both groups.

Group A (n=25)	Group B (n=25)
Max Marks: 100	Max Marks: 100
80 (80%)	95 (95%)

After the summative assessment students of both the groups were then subjected to a post test and average score of all the students in group A was 80% and that of Group B was 95% in an MCQ based evaluation.

4 DISCUSSION

In the realm of skill training, particularly within the confines of a skill lab, the implementation of multiple assessment strategies is pivotal. Multiple faculty feedback enhances skill acquisition by providing diverse perspectives and expertise, which enriches the learning experience (Hattie and Timperley, 2007) [8]. Different instructors can identify various strengths and weaknesses, offering comprehensive and nuanced guidance (Sadler, 1989). This varied feedback helps learners address specific areas for improvement, fostering a well-rounded skill set (Nicol and Macfarlane-Dick, 2006) [9]. Additionally, exposure to multiple viewpoints encourages critical thinking and adaptability, essential for mastering complex skills (Boud and Molloy, 2013). Consistent, multi-source feedback also reinforces learning through repetition and varied reinforcement, aiding in deeper understanding and retention (Shute, 2008).

Interactive elements in PPTs, such as embedded quizzes, polls, and discussion prompts, engage learners and promote active learning, which is crucial for skill acquisition (Clark and Mayer, 2016)[12].

Video demonstrations significantly enhance skill acquisition by providing a dynamic and multifaceted learning experience. They deliver visual and auditory stimuli that cater to diverse learning styles, making complex information more accessible and understandable (Mayer, 2009). Multiple Assessments have many benefits like they provide Holistic Evaluation (Black and Wiliam, 1998)[14]. Enhanced Learning, (Hattie and Timperley, 2007) Adaptability and Personalization (Tomlinson, 2001) and Increased Engagement: (Fredricks, Blumenfeld, and Paris, 2004) [15]

Formative assessments are designed to monitor student learning and provide continuous feedback. Hattie and Timperley (2007) [8] did a Meta-analysis of studies on feedback in educational settings and found that Effective feedback, a core component of formative assessments, enhances student learning significantly. Summative assessments evaluate student learning at the end of an instructional period. They provide a comprehensive measure of student competence and skill mastery.

Harlen and James (1997)[16] analyzed the role and effectiveness of summative assessments in education and found that while summative assessments are essential for evaluating overall competence; their effectiveness is enhanced when combined with formative assessments. They concluded that in skill labs, summative assessments should be complemented with formative assessments to ensure a well-rounded evaluation of student abilities. Brookhart (2010)[17] examined the higher-order thinking skills in summative assessments and found that Summative assessments that focus on higher-order thinking skills provide a more accurate measure of student capabilities and concluded that skill training modules should design summative assessments that challenge students to apply their skills in complex, real-world scenarios.

Performance-based assessments require students to demonstrate their skills in practical, real-life scenarios. Wiggins (1993)[18] evaluated performance-based assessment in education and found performance-based assessments are highly effective in measuring practical skills and application of knowledge and concluded that Skill labs should incorporate performance-based assessments to accurately evaluate student competence in real-world tasks. Gulikers et al. (2004)[19] did case studies on the use of performance-based assessments in vocational training and found that these assessments promote deeper learning and better preparation for professional practice and concluded that performance-based assessments in skill labs foster practical skill development, preparing students for future careers.

But at the same time Multiple Assessments has many Challenges in Implementing like Resource Intensive (Brookhart, 2010)[17] Consistency and Standardization (Sadler, 2005) Student Anxiety (Cassady and Johnson, 2002)[20] and Technical and Logistical Issues (McMillan, 2013).

5 CONCLUSION

The use of multiple assessments in skill training modules within a skill lab setting offers a robust framework for evaluating and enhancing student learning. While there are challenges in implementing diverse assessments, the benefits they bring in terms of holistic evaluation, enhanced learning, adaptability, and engagement are significant. By adhering to best practices such as clear objectives, balanced assessment plans, continuous feedback, instructor training, and student involvement, educators can maximize the effectiveness of multiple assessments. This comprehensive approach not only prepares students more effectively for real-world applications but also fosters a deeper, more engaged learning experience. This holistic approach not only prepares students more effectively for real-world applications but also fosters a deeper, more engaged learning experience. Implementing these best practices ensures that skill labs can maximize the potential of multiple assessments, leading to improved educational outcomes.

REFERENCES

[1] Moran V, Wunderlich R, Rubbelke C. (2018). Simulation in Nursing Education. *Simulation: Best Practices in Nursing Education*: Springer, Cham.

[2] Dearmon V, Graves RJ, Hayden S, *et al.* (2013). Effectiveness of simulation-based orientation of baccalaureate nursing students preparing for their first clinical experience. *J Nurs Educ*. 52:29–38.

[3] T.V. Horodova-Andreeva *et al.* How medical education require skill training and onsite education? *Aktual'nì problemi sučasnoï medi* Vol. 23, Iss: 2.2, pp 67–71
[4] Hashim R *et al.* Role of Skill Laboratory Training in Medical Education - Students' Perspective. *J Coll Physicians Surg Pak)-* Vol. 26, Iss: 3, pp 195–198
[5] Hayat K. (2023). Transforming medical education and training. *Pakistan Biomedical Journal.* pp 01
[6] NMC Skill module.
[7] Nair BR, Moonen-van Loon JM. (2022). Programmatic assessment – What are we waiting for? *Arch Med Health Sci*;10:154–6.
[8] Hattie, J., and Timperley, H. (2007). The Power of Feedback. *Review of Educational Research*, 77(1), 81–112.
[9] David J. Nicol and Debra Macfarlane-Dick (2006): Formative assessment and self-regulated learning: a model and seven principles of good feedback practice, *Studies in Higher Education*, 31:2, 199–218
[10] Gagne, R.M., Wager, W.W., Golas, K.C., Keller, J.M. and Russell, J.D. (2005) Principles of instructional design. *Performance Improvement*, 44, 44–46. https://doi.org/10.1002/pfi.4140440211
[11] Sweller, Ayres, and Kalyuga. (2011). Cognitive load theory, *LSIS*, volume 1
[12] Clark and Mayer, (2016). *e-Learning and the Science of Instruction*, https://doi.org/10.1002/9781119239086.fmatter
[13] Bandura A, (1986). Social Learning Theory, Science Education in Theory and Practice, An Introductory Guide to Learning Theory (pp.85–99), https://doi.org/10.1007/978-3-030-43620-9_7
[14] Black, P., and Wiliam, D. (1998). Assessment and classroom learning. *Assessment in Education: Principles, Policy and Practice*, 5 (1), 7–74.
[15] Fredricks, J.A., Blumenfeld, P.C., and Paris, A.H. (2004). School engagement: Potential of the concept, state of the evidence. *Review of Educational Research*, 74(1), 59–109.
[16] Harlen, W., and James, M. (1997). Assessment and learning: Differences and relationships between formative and summative assessment. *Assessment in Education: Principles, Policy and Practice*, 4(3), 365–379.
[17] Brookhart, S.M. (2010). How to Assess Higher-Order Thinking Skills in Your Classroom. ASCD.
[18] Wiggins, Grant. (1993). Assessing student performance: Exploring the purpose and limits of testing. *Jossey-Bass.*
[19] Gulikers, J.T.M., Bastiaens, T.J., and Kirschner, P.A. (2004). "A five-dimensional framework for authentic assessment." *Educational Technology Research and Development*, vol. 52, no. 3, pp. 67–86.
[20] Cassady, J.C., and Johnson, R.E. (2002). Cognitive test anxiety and academic performance. *Contemporary Educational Psychology*, 27(2), 270–295. https://doi.org/10.1006/ceps.2001.1094
[21] Guskey, Thomas R. (2003). "How classroom assessments improve learning." *Educational Leadership*, vol. 60, no. 5, pp. 6–11.
[22] Darling-Hammond, L., and Richardson, N. (2009). Research on teacher learning: Supporting the development of professional learning communities. *Yearbook of the National Society for the Study of Education*, 108(1), 31–56.

Navigating Dental Education Trends and Transforming Dental Pedagogy – Abas and Srikant N (Eds)
 ISBN: 978-1-041-32674-8

Student Evaluation of Problem-Based Learning in the Dental Curriculum: A Prospective Questionnaire Study

Nidhin Philip Jose, Asavari Desai Shetty, and Supriya Nambiar
Department of Orthodontics and Orthopedics, Manipal College of Dental Sciences Mangalore, Manipal Academy of Higher Education, Karnataka, Manipal, India

Lida Mary Nidhin Philip
Nitte (Deemed to be University), AB Shetty Memorial Institute of Dental Sciences (ABSMIDS), Department of Oral and Maxillofacial Surgery, Mangalore, India

Dhruv Ahuja
Department of Orthodontics and Dentofacial Orthopedics, Manav Rachna Dental College, Manav Rachna International Institute of Research and Studies, Faridabad, Haryana, India

1 INTRODUCTION

Student-centered forms of learning are rapidly replacing traditional ones in many parts of the world. Leading universities have already tailored their curricula to include active learning strategies. Of the various methods, problem-based learning has been widely studied and implemented. Problem-based learning is particularly important in the field of health sciences, as diagnosis and treatment planning are essentially problem-based approaches in which students link learned facts with the patient's symptoms to arrive at a suitable course of treatment.

Problem-based learning is an instructional approach centered on the active exploration of real-world problems. Unlike traditional learning methods that focus on passive information absorption, PBL engages students in problem-solving processes that mimic real-life scenarios. In PBL, learners are presented with complex, open-ended problems that require them to apply critical thinking, collaboration, and research skills to find viable solutions.

A hallmark of PBL is its encouragement of self-directed learning. Students must identify what they know, what they need to learn, and how to acquire it. They work in groups to investigate the problem, discuss potential solutions, and reflect on their learning journey. This approach helps develop subject-specific knowledge and essential skills, such as teamwork, communication, and adaptability.

In PBL, instructors act as facilitators rather than traditional lecturers. Their role is to guide students, offering support and resources when needed while allowing them to take ownership of the learning process.

There is an ongoing shift in the manner curriculum is delivered in dental colleges. More institutions are incorporating problem-based learning. There is growing evidence that students trained through problem-based learning can handle real-life clinical situations better than those trained solely through traditional teaching and learning methods.

1.1 *Aims*

This study aims to assess the skills, knowledge, motivation, and attitudes of students who were exposed to problem-based learning versus those exposed to traditional learning methods.

2 MATERIALS AND METHODS

The study was conducted after obtaining Institutional Ethics Committee approval. The sample consisted of 100 undergraduate students selected from different sections of the undergraduate program. The students were randomly selected using random.org's random number generator, based on their roll numbers.

DOI: 10.1201/9781042016075-38

The study's scope was explained, and informed consent was obtained from each student before recruitment.
Inclusion Criteria

(1) Undergraduate students who could understand and consent to the study
(2) Students trained in PBL and traditional modes of teaching-learning

The students were divided into 2 groups – Group A consisted of 3rd-year students who were exposed to traditional modes of learning, comprising lectures and group demonstrations. Group B – consisted of Interns exposed to problem-learning methods like one-on-one chair-side mentoring/training during internships and objective structured clinical training. The students in group A were exposed only to traditional modes of learning, whereas the students in group B were exposed to both traditional and problem-based learning.

To gauge students' skills, knowledge, and attitudes, a self-assessment model using structured questionnaires was used. The structured questionnaire was developed using inputs from the questionnaire developed by Chen et al [1] at Chang Gung University School of Medicine and the Course Evaluation Questionnaire (CEQ) by Ramsden [2].

A Five-point Likert Scale from 1 to 5, where 1 means 'definitely disagree', 2 means 'disagree', 3 means 'neutral', 4 means 'agree', and 5 means 'definitely agree' was used by the students to answer the questions.

2.1 *Statistical analysis*

Statistical analysis was carried out using independent t-tests. The SPSS software was used to perform the statistical analysis.

3 RESULTS

Based on the questionnaires completed and returned, the responses from both groups were tabulated and analyzed. Participants in group A who were exposed to traditional learning methods reported understanding the concept of problem-based learning; however, most showed only weak agreement. Most students felt that the course had not markedly improved their ability to analyze and solve problems or to think independently. They, however, felt that their peer interaction and interaction with other medical staff had improved. Most of the students also felt they were poorly motivated towards the subject. There was strong agreement among the students when asked whether they wanted the curriculum structured around a problem-based approach.

Participants in group B who were exposed to the problem-based learning approach strongly agreed that they understood it. Most students felt that the course helped them solve problems and sharpened their thinking skills. The participants agreed strongly that the course has improved their interaction with peers and their motivation to study the subject further. They agree strongly that more parts of the curriculum should be structured around a problem-based approach.

Three questions were scored significantly higher in group B than in group A. These were as follows-

Q- I have understood the concept of problem-based learning that is inculcated in the chair-side mentoring and objective structured clinical training imparted through case history discussions and OSCE

Q- The course has improved my communication skills

Q- I feel motivated to study the subject further, and the course has helped me foster a positive attitude toward the subject

Q- I would like more parts of the curriculum to be structured involving problem-based learning

The questions that scored differently in both groups but were not statistically significant included

Q- The course has improved my ability to analyze and search for problems

Q- I am more confident in solving the problems that I encounter in my day-to-day clinic

Q- I am encouraged to think independently and to learn on my own initiative

Q- The course has sharpened my thinking process

Q- The training imparted has helped improve my patient–doctor and doctor-nurse relationship

Q- The course has helped me to interact better with my peers

Q- My professional knowledge has improved following the training

Q- My clinical techniques have improved following the training

Q- This course has helped me to develop my problem-solving skills

Q- Teachers motivate us to do our best work

Q- The course has sharpened my analytical skills

Q- After the program, I feel confident handling unfamiliar problems

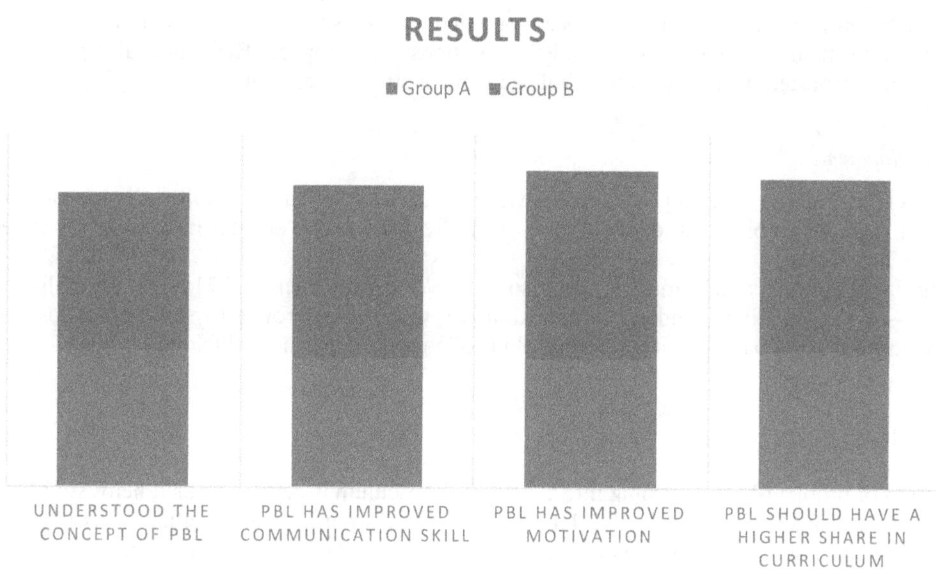

4 DISCUSSION

Problem-Based Learning (PBL) and traditional teaching are two distinct educational approaches with differing philosophies, structures, and outcomes. Understanding the key differences between them reveals how each method shapes learning experiences.

4.1 *Role of the teacher*

In traditional teaching, the teacher is the central figure, often acting as the primary source of knowledge. Lessons are typically delivered in a lecture-based format, with students expected to absorb information passively. The teacher's role is to provide facts, guide students through the content, and assess their understanding through tests or quizzes.

In contrast, PBL places the teacher in the role of a facilitator or guide. The teacher does not simply transmit information but helps students navigate problems, ask the right questions, and seek out resources. Instead of being the "sage on the stage," the teacher becomes the "guide on the side," encouraging student autonomy.

4.2 *Learning approach*

Traditional teaching tends to follow a structured, linear approach where knowledge is compartmentalized into subjects or units. Students learn content first, often through direct instruction, and may apply that knowledge in later exercises or tests. The focus is often on memorization and mastery of subject material.

PBL, on the other hand, is student-centered and inquiry-based. Students are presented with complex, real-world problems at the start of the learning process. They must actively engage in finding solutions, which involves researching, collaborating, and applying prior knowledge. Learning is often interdisciplinary and occurs in a more organic, self-directed manner.

4.3 *Knowledge application*

In traditional teaching, students may learn theory and content without necessarily applying it immediately to practical situations. Learning is often seen as preparation for future problem-solving, with application coming later through assignments, labs, or job-related tasks.

PBL involves the immediate application of knowledge. Students tackle real or simulated problems from the outset, requiring them to integrate and apply what they know as they learn. This method fosters a deeper understanding of concepts by showing students how what they are learning applies to real-world contexts.

4.4 *Assessment methods*

Traditional teaching often relies on standardized assessments such as exams, quizzes, and written assignments that evaluate a student's ability to recall information or demonstrate understanding of discrete topics.

In PBL, assessment is more dynamic and process-oriented. Students may be evaluated based on their problem-solving processes, teamwork, research skills, and the solutions they propose. Reflection and peer assessment are also commonly incorporated, fostering a more holistic view of student performance.

4.5 *Skills development*

Traditional teaching tends to focus on content knowledge, with less emphasis on soft skills such as collaboration, communication, and adaptability. Students often work individually, with success measured by academic performance and content mastery.

PBL emphasizes not only content mastery but also the development of critical 21st-century skills such as teamwork, problem-solving, creativity, and communication. By working in groups to solve problems, students gain practical experience that prepares them for real-world challenges and promotes lifelong learning.

5 CONCLUSION

The introduction of problem-based learning into the dental curriculum is beneficial, as it helps students think more critically and solve problems independently. The problem-based approach was perceived as improving student motivation and enhancing the learning experience compared to the traditional teaching method. While traditional teaching is effective for conveying large amounts of information and ensuring mastery of specific content, PBL fosters a more active, hands-on learning experience that promotes critical thinking, problem-solving, and collaboration. Both methods have their place in education, and blending elements of each can provide a well-rounded learning experience. There are challenges with shifting towards problem-based learning, but the benefits of doing so far outweigh the costs.

REFERENCES

[1] Yung-Chang Chen *et al.* (2002). Evaluation of problem-based learning education after clerkship at the Chang Gung University School of Medicine. *Chang Gung Med J*, 25:758–63

[2] Ramsden P. A performance indicator of teaching quality in higher education: The course experience questionnaire, *Studies in Higher education*, 16(2), 129–150

Navigating Dental Education Trends and Transforming Dental Pedagogy – Abas and Srikant N (Eds)
© 2027 The Author(s), ISBN: 978-1-041-32674-8

Unmasking the Hidden Danger: Educating Future Dentists on the Risk of E-Cigarettes

Mranali K. Shetty, Sangeeta Umesh Nayak, and K. David
Department of Periodontology, Manipal College of Dental Sciences Mangalore, Manipal Academy of Higher Education, Manipal, India

ABSTRACT: Unmasking the hidden danger: Educating future dentists on the risk of E cigarettes While smoking is widely recognized as detrimental to health, many health care students remain unaware of the dangers associated with e-cigarettes. Currently, vaping and E-cigarette use are highly popular, particularly among younger people. E-cigarette, often known as e-cigarettes, are battery-operated devices that vaporize liquids often contain nicotine, flavorings, and solvents. E- cigarettes Vaping is not safe, but is less dangerous than smoking, according to some data. Addiction to tobacco and nicotine has far more negative consequences for a person's health than positive consequences. Most health care students believe that e-cigarettes are safer than traditional cigarettes, are, and government agencies and educational institutions should emphasize the dangers of the individual constituents , present in e-cigarettes. By doing so,professional students can counsel patients about the harm caused by e-cigarettes and how to overcome their habits.

Keywords: E cigarettes, good health, smoking, dental curriculum

1 INTRODUCTION

Tobacco usage has negative impacts on general health, as well as on dental health/oral health. As an increasing number of modern tobacco and nicotine products are developed and marketed, tobacco use is becoming one of the world's greatest public health issues. Smoking cigarettes is the most common method for tobacco use [1]. In smoking, nicotine is the most addictive component, and smoked tobacco is available in various forms, such as cigarettes, cigars, pipes, bidis, and hookah. Smoking increases the risk for various diseases, including cancer, and teenagers use of "e-cigarettes," has skyrocketed.

Researchers are investigating the elements that contribute to the prevalence of vaping because of its rise. Social media and peer pressure are two such factors that affect smoking and vaping behaviour [2]. While it is widely recognized that smoking is detrimental to health, many health care students remain unaware of the dangers associated with E-cigarette.

2 E CIGARETTES AND THEIR COMPONENTS:

Currently, vaping and E-cigarette use are highly popular, particularly among younger people. E-cigarettes, often known as e-cigarettes, are battery-operated devices that vaporize liquids that often contain nicotine, which is extremely addictive and potentially detrimental to the growing brain, particularly in regions that govern behavior, mood, learning, attention [3]. Cartridges and e-liquids in e-cigarettes can contain various toxic compounds, including heavy metals such as nickel, tin, lead, and chromium, which may come from heating elements or other parts of the device. Additionally, the vapors produced by e-cigarettes can contain toxic and potentially cancer-causing chemicals such as formaldehyde, acetaldehyde, and acrolein. These substances can pose health risks, particularly with long-term or high-level exposure [4].

3 THE IMPACT OF E. CIGARETTES ON GENERAL AND ORAL HEALTH

According to the CDC, e-cigarettes are not safe and can have many adverse health effects. while being less dangerous than smoking, according to some data. Addiction to tobacco and nicotine has far more negative consequences for a person's health than positive consequences. Tobacco smoking is indeed linked to a significant number of health problems and early deaths. Smokers are at increased risk for various diseases, including lung cancer, chronic obstructive pulmonary disease (COPD), cardiovascular diseases, and other cancers [4]. Compared with nonsmokers, smokers are at increased risk for cardiovascular diseases. Tobacco use, whether smoked or

DOI: 10.1201/9781042016075-39

smokeless, is strongly linked to the development of oral squamous cell carcinoma (OSCC). It is associated with various mucosal lesions, including leukoplakia, smokeless tobacco keratosis at the site of tobacco placement, nicotinic stomatitis, smoker's melanosis, and erythroplakia. Additionally, smokers typically experience greater gingival recession, tooth loss, discoloration of tooth restorations and dentures and increased pocket depths than nonsmokers do [5]. The common cause of halitosis is smoking.

E-cigarette users presented a greater abundance of gram-negative bacteria such as *Porphyromonas* and *Veillonella* than did conventional cigarette smokers or individuals who had never smoked [2].

Organ damage, breathing issues, and addiction are additional possible risks associated with exposure to cigarettes. The American Lung Association states that while we still have much to discover about the long-term health impacts of e-cigarettes, they are worried that e-cigarettes may contribute to the emergence of a new wave of tobacco-related illnesses.

E-cigarette have gained popularity as an alternative to traditional tobacco smoking, but their long-term health effects and efficacy as a smoking cessation tool are still subjects of ongoing research. Tobacco smoking is indeed linked to a significant number of health problems and early deaths. Health care professionals' knowledge, attitudes and behaviors towards E-cigarette can influence how they advise patients on smoking cessation. Quitting smoking can greatly reduce these risks and improve overall health. Most health care students believe that e-cigarettes are safer than traditional cigarettes are. There appears to be variation in the proportion of E-cigarette users among different health colleges. A study by Alsanea S et.al. reported that, with the exception of medical students, there was no significant difference in the level of knowledge about e-cigarettes among students. Compared with dental students, medical students have notably higher levels of knowledge [6]. This may reflect differences in educational emphasis or exposure to information about E-cigarettes in their curricula [7].

4 DENTAL CARIES

Dental caries, also referred to as cavities or tooth decay, is influenced by several factors, including diet, oral hygiene, and lifestyle choices. Oral health can be significantly impacted by smoking. Nicotine and other chemicals in tobacco can disrupt the natural balance of bacteria in the mouth. This can promote the growth of harmful bacteria such as *Streptococcus mutans*, which is known to contribute to the development of caries. Smoking can reduce saliva production. A decrease in salivary flow can create a more favorable environment for bacteria that cause cavities. Reduced saliva flow, as seen with smoking or certain medical conditions, lowers the buffering effect, increasing the vulnerability of teeth to decay. Maintaining good oral hygiene, reducing sugary food intake, and avoiding tobacco products are important steps in preventing dental caries and promoting overall oral health [7].

5 GINGIVITIS

Some recent studies have reported that smokers exhibit less gingival inflammation [8] and less gingival bleeding than nonsmokers do, despite having similar or greater plaque levels, which is due mainly to vasoconstriction. The other changes observed are reduced gingival blood vessels with increased inflammation, decreased GCF flow, bleeding on probing, and decreased subgingival temperature.

6 PERIODONTAL DISEASE AND IMPLANTATION

Periodontal disease is multifactorial, and is influenced by a combination of genetic, environmental, and behavioral factors. Smoking exacerbates the prevalence and severity of periodontal damage, leading to greater pocket depth, attachment loss, bone loss, and tooth loss. The extent of these issues increases with the number of cigarettes smoked daily. Smokers face a greater risk of dental implant failure.

7 E CIGARETTES AND HEALING

Smokers do not respond well to periodontal therapy. Tobacco use has a significant effect on wound healing in the oral cavity, affecting various dental procedures and treatments, such as scaling and curettage, periodontal surgery, and tooth extraction.

7.1 *Factors contributing to impaired healing*

Reduced blood flow: Nicotine and other chemicals in tobacco cause vasoconstriction, which reduces blood flow to the tissues. Adequate blood flow is crucial for delivering the nutrients and oxygen necessary for healing.

Decreased collagen production: Smoking can reduce the synthesis of collagen, which is essential for tissue repair and regeneration.

PMNs, or neutrophils, are a type of white blood cell that is crucial for the immune response and for defending against infections. Studies have shown that smoking impairs PMN function, reducing their ability to effectively combat bacterial infections and contributing to wound healing.

8 SMOKING RESPONSE TO PERIODONTAL THERAPY

Nonsurgical - decreased clinical response to scaling and root planning

Surgical options include decreased reduction in probing depth, clinical attachment gain, and increased deterioration of the furcation after surgery.

Studies have revealed that e-cigarettes significantly hinder oral wound healing, as demonstrated by clinical and histological evidence. In addition to nicotine, e-cigarettes also include propylene glycol, glycerol, and flavorings that, when heated, can release a variety of toxins into oral tissues, slowing the healing process. There is a chance that mechanisms such as tissue hypoxia, the release of proinflammatory markers, elevated oxidative stress, improved apoptosis, keratinocyte migration inhibition, and surgical wound contamination are involved [9].

8.1 *Smoking cessation*

Quitting smoking is one of the most effective strategies for improving periodontal health and the success rate of dental implants. Smoking cessation can help reduce inflammation, improve blood flow, and enhance the healing process. when smokers maintain a good oral health and ceases smoking can have a longer survival rates with regards to implants. [10]

Overall, tackling smoking as a risk factor is essential for effectively managing periodontal disease and ensuring the success of dental implants. Encouraging patients to quit smoking and providing support for smoking cessation can significantly benefit their oral and overall health.

9 ROLE OF THE DENTAL CURRICULUM

The dentistry curriculum is essential in educating students about e-cigarettes and their negative effects. Dental schools may provide aspiring dentists with the knowledge they need to comprehend the possible risks associated with e-cigarette use, including nicotine addiction, oral health concerns, and other systemic health issues, by integrating thorough instruction on e-cigarettes into the curriculum. Through this instruction, dentistry students can become public health advocates and successfully advise their patients—particularly young people—pertaining to the risks related to e-cigarettes. Additionally, a well-informed dental profession may support larger public health campaigns by raising awareness and advocating for preventative measures that can lower e-cigarette use and encourage healthier lifestyle choices.

10 CONCLUSION

Addressing the misconceptions surrounding e-cigarettes and their health impacts is crucial. Health professional education programs should include comprehensive modules on the effects of smoking and e-cigarette use. This should cover not only the general health impacts but also specific issues related to oral and dental health. Patients should be provided with brochures or handouts that outline the risks associated with e-cigarettes, focusing on both general health and specific oral health concerns. Organize workshops and seminars in schools and universities to raise awareness about the dangers of e-cigarettes. Collaborate with schools, dental associations, and public health organizations to promote awareness and education about e cigarettes. Joint efforts can amplify the reach and impact of educational initiatives by guiding patients toward healthier choices and supporting smoking cessation by guiding patients toward healthier choices and supporting smoking cessation.

REFERENCES

[1] Teresa W. Wang, Andrea S. Gentzke, Melisa R. Creamer, Karen A. Cullen, Enver HolderHayes, Michael D. Sawdey, Gabriella M. Anic, David B. Portnoy, Sean Hu, David M. Homa, Ahmed Jamal, Linda J. Neff (2019): Tobacco product use and associated factors among middle and high school students in the united states, *MMWR Surveill Summ* 68

[2] Dazhe James Cao, Kim Aldy, Stephanie Hsu, Molly McGetrick, Guido Verbeck, Imesha De Silva, Sing-yi Feng (2020): Review of health consequences of E-cigarettes and the Outbreak of Electronic Cigarette, or Vaping, *Product Use-Associated Lung Injury*

[3] AlMuhaissen S, Mohammad H, Dabobash A, Nada MQ, Suleiman ZM. (2022). Prevalence, knowledge, and attitudes among health professions students toward the use of E-cigarettes. *Healthcare (Basel)*. 10(12):2420

[4] Cassio Luiz Coutinho Almeida -da-Silva, Harmony Matshik Dakafay, Kenji O Brien, Dallin Montierth, Nan Xiao and David M. (2021). Ojcius.Effects of electronic cigarette aerosol exposure on oral and systemic health. *Biomed J* 44(3):252–259

[5] R Holliday, B W Chaffee, N S Jakubovics, R Kist and P M Preshaw. (2021). E-cigarettes and Oral Health. *J Dent Res* 100(9):906–913.

[6] Alsanea S, Alrabiah Z, Samreen S, Syed W, Bin Khunayn RM, Al-Arifi NM, Alenazi M, Alghadeer S, Alhossan A, Alwhaibi A, Al-Arifi MN. (2022). Prevalence, knowledge and attitude toward electronic cigarette use among male health colleges students in Saudi Arabia-A cross-sectional study. *Front Public Health.* 10:827089.

[7] Sangeeta Gajendra, Scott Mcintosh, Sucharu Gosh. (2023). Effects of tobacco product use on oral health and the role of oral healthcare providers in cessation: A narrative review. *Tobacco Induced Diseases* 21:12.

[8] N W Johnson and C A Bain. (2000). Tobacco and oral disease. *British Dental Journal* 189,200–206.

[9] Majid, O.W. (2024). Preliminary evidence of impaired oral wound healing in e-cigarette users: a call for perioperative vaping cessation. *Evid Based Dent* **25**, 63–64.

[10] Madi M, Smith S, Alshehri S, Zakaria O, Almas K. (2023) Influence of Smoking on Periodontal and Implant Therapy: A Narrative Review. *International Journal of Environmental Research and Public Health.* 20(7):5368. https://doi.org/10.3390/ijerph20075368

Factors Influencing Delay in Biopsy Reporting: An Audit of Reporting Times and Associated Variables

K.P. Nandita and N. Srikant
Department of Oral Pathology and Microbiology, Manipal College of Dental Sciences Mangalore, Manipal Academy of Higher Education, Manipal, India

ABSTRACT: **Background:** Timely biopsy reporting is crucial for accurate diagnosis and patient management. However, various operational and procedural factors can lead to delays, impacting patient care. This study investigated the factors contributing to biopsy reporting delays, defined as more than 15 days for bone biopsies and 7 days for soft tissue biopsies.

Methods: A retrospective audit was conducted to assess the associations between operational factors and biopsy reporting delays. Chi-square tests were performed to identify significant associations, and binary logistic regression was used to determine predictors of delays. The variables analyzed included lesion classification, decalcification, third Saturday occurrence, faculty holidays, academic travel, and others.

Results: Chi-square analysis revealed significant associations between biopsy delays and lesion classification (χ^2 = 37.832, p < 0.001), decalcification (χ^2 = 5.201, p = 0.023), the presence of a third Saturday (χ^2 = 5.493, p = 0.019), faculty holidays (χ^2 = 4.303, p = 0.038), and travel for regular academics (χ^2 = 32.212, p < 0.001). Logistic regression identified the presence of a third Saturday as a significant predictor of delay (OR = 4.115, p = 0.009), increasing the likelihood of delay by four times. In contrast, travel for regular academics was associated with a significant reduction in delay likelihood (OR = 0.126, p < 0.001). Other factors, including decalcification, Sundays, national holidays, academic engagement, and faculty leave, did not show significant predictive value.

Conclusion: This study highlights specific operational factors, particularly the presence of a third Saturday and academic travel, that significantly influence biopsy reporting delays. Addressing these logistical challenges could increase the efficiency of biopsy processing and reporting, ultimately improving patient care outcomes.

Keywords: Turnaround time (TAT), Audit, Biopsy reporting

1 INTRODUCTION

Timely biopsy reporting is critical for accurate diagnosis and effective treatment planning. Delays in reporting can lead to prolonged patient anxiety and potential delays in treatment initiation. The turnaround time, or TAT, is the amount of time it takes for a laboratory to receive a sample, analyze it, and provide a final histopathological diagnosis. The mean turnaround time (TAT) of all the samples is usually 5–6 days. Reporting a specimen quickly and accurately can help clinicians create fast and effective treatment plans. Histopathology reports may be delayed because of various factors. Delays in the processing of samples can occur at various stages, including receiving the sample, processing, staining, decalcification and reporting. [1]

Studies have highlighted various factors influencing the turnaround time in histopathology labs. For example, the decalcification process for bone samples is time-consuming and can significantly extend the reporting time. [2]. Additionally, the requirement for special stains or immunohistochemical studies can delay the final diagnosis [3]. Secondary referrals to external laboratories for expert opinions or further testing also contribute to delays [4]. Furthermore, institutional factors such as the presence of examinations or conferences may affect the availability of pathologists and subsequently delay reporting [1].

This study investigated the factors associated with delays in biopsy reporting at a pathology department. Delays were defined as >15 days for bone biopsies and $\geq$ 7 days for soft tissue biopsies. The study analyzes the impact of lesion classification, operational factors, and academic engagements on reporting times via chi-square tests and binary logistic regression.

1.1 *Aims*

This study aims to explore the delay in reporting histopathological specimens in the Department of Oral Pathology and Microbiology at the Manipal College of Dental Sciences, Mangalore. By evaluating the cases from 2023–2024, the study classifies delays, identifies underlying reasons, and proposes solutions to improve turnaround times.

DOI: 10.1201/9781042016075-40

1.2 *Objectives*

(1) To evaluate the delay in reporting histopathological specimens.
(2) To classify the delays into less than 7 days and more than 7 days.
(3) To identify the reasons for delays.
(4) To propose solutions to minimize reporting delays.

2 MATERIALS AND METHODS

2.1 *Study design*

This was a retrospective audit.

2.2 *Study population*

Histopathological specimens were submitted to the Department of Oral Pathology and Microbiology, Manipal College of Dental Sciences, Mangalore, from January 2023 to December 2024, covering approximately 500 cases.

2.3 *Data collection*

Data will be collected from departmental records, including the following:

- Date of receipt of each sample.
- Date of reporting of each sample.
- Number of days taken for reporting.

The delays for soft tissue biopsy were classified as follows:

- Less than 7 days
- More than 7 days

The delays for bone biopsy were classified as follows:

- More than 15 days

The reasons for delays are categorized as follows:

(1) Decalcification process
(2) Requirement for special stains
(3) Secondary referral for expert opinion
(4) Examinations or conferences affecting the availability of pathologists

3 STATISTICAL ANALYSIS

The proportion of cases that are delayed is calculated, and the reasons for these delays are analyzed. Statistical analysis was performed by calculating percentages for delays and their respective reasons.

Table 1. Biopsy delay (>15 days for bone and >=7 days for soft tissues).

		N	Biopsy reporting delay (>15 days Bone and >=7 days soft tissue)				Chi square	P value
			Normal		Delayed			
			Count	Column N %	Count	Column N %		
Classification	Bones and Joints	3	2	1.70%	1	1.60%	28.932	0.002
	Bacterial Infection	6	5	4.20%	1	1.60%		
	Salivary Gland	13	13	11.00%	0	0.00%		
	Odontogenic Cyst	72	41	34.70%	31	48.40%		
	Epithelium/Connective tissue Neoplasm	54	39	33.10%	15	23.40%		

(*continued*)

Table 1. Continued

		N	Biopsy reporting delay (>15 days Bone and >=7 days soft tissue)				Chi square	P value
			Normal		Delayed			
			Count	Column N %	Count	Column N %		
	Skin	5	3	2.50%	2	3.10%		
	Odontogenic Tumor	5	5	4.20%	0	0.00%		
	Metabolic Disorder	3	1	0.80%	2	3.10%		
	Pulp and periapical lesion	11	7	5.90%	4	6.20%		
	Disease of Periodontium	7	0	0.00%	7	10.90%		
	Spread of Oral Infection	1	1	0.80%	0	0.00%		
	Physical Chemical Injuries	2	1	0.80%	1	1.60%		
Decalcification	No	152	104	88.10%	48	75.00%	5.201	0.023
	Yes	30	14	11.90%	16	25.00%		
Third Saturday	No	150	103	87.30%	47	73.40%	5.493	0.019
	Yes	32	15	12.70%	17	26.60%		
Sunday	No	61	39	33.10%	22	34.40%	0.033	0.857
	Yes	121	79	66.90%	42	65.60%		
National Holiday	No	164	108	91.50%	56	87.50%	0.754	0.385
	Yes	18	10	8.50%	8	12.50%		
Sessional exam/ Academic burden	No	179	117	99.20%	62	96.90%	1.328	0.249
	Yes	3	1	0.80%	2	3.10%		
Faculty Holiday (# of faculty on leave)	No	141	97	82.20%	44	68.80%	4.303	0.038
	Yes	41	21	17.80%	20	31.20%		
Travel for regular academics	No	57	20	16.90%	37	57.80%	32.212	<0.001
	Yes	125	98	83.10%	27	42.20%		

(1) **Classification of** lesions: Chi-square analysis revealed a significant association between the classification of lesions and biopsy reporting delays ($\chi^2 = 28.932$, p = 0.002). Specifically, the delay was most prominent in cases involving odontogenic cysts, with 48.4% of such cases experiencing delays, compared with 34.7% in the non-delayed group. In contrast, cases involving salivary glands and odontogenic tumors presented no delays in biopsy reporting, whereas cases involving periodontal disease presented a 10.9% delay.

(2) **Operational Factors**: Several operational factors were also found to significantly influence biopsy reporting delays:

- **Decalcification**: Patients requiring decalcification experienced a greater rate of delay (25.0%) than did those without decalcification (11.9%) ($\chi^2 = 5.201$, p = 0.023).
- **Third Saturday**: A significant association was found between reporting delays and cases processed after the third Saturday of the month, with a delay rate of 26.6% compared with 12.7% for nondelayed cases ($\chi^2 = 5.493$, p = 0.019).
- **Faculty Holiday**: Biopsies processed when faculty were on holiday had a higher delay rate (31.2%) than did those processed when no faculty were on leave (17.8%) ($\chi^2 = 4.303$, p = 0.038).
- **Travel for Regular Academics**: This factor was strongly associated with delays, as cases where faculty were traveling for academic purposes had a significantly higher delay rate (57.8%) than those where faculty were present (16.9%) ($\chi^2 = 32.212$, $p < 0.001$).

(3) **Nonsignificant Factors**: The analysis revealed that Sunday processing ($\chi^2 = 0.033$, p = 0.857), national holidays ($\chi^2 = 0.754$, p = 0.385), and academic engagement ($\chi^2 = 1.328$, p = 0.249) did not significantly impact biopsy reporting delays.

4 BINARY LOGISTIC REGRESSION RESULTS

Binary logistic regression analysis was conducted to identify factors associated with delays in biopsy reporting (defined as >15 days for bone biopsies and ≥ 7 days for soft tissue biopsies). The model included variables such as decalcification, third Saturday, Sunday, national holiday, academic engagement, faculty leave, travel for regular academics, and disease subclass. The results are interpreted as follows:

Significant Predictors:

(1) **Third Saturday**:

- The presence of a third Saturday was a significant predictor of biopsy reporting delay (B=1.415B = 1.415B=1.415, p = 0.009). The odds ratio (OR) of 4.115 indicates that the likelihood of a delay is approximately 4 times greater when a third Saturday is involved than when it is not (95% CI: 1.414–11.975).

(2) **Travel for Regular Academics**:

- Travel for regular academic activities was another significant predictor, but in this case, it was associated with a reduction in the likelihood of delay (B=−2.073B = -2.073B=−2.073, $p < 0.001$). The odds ratio of 0.126 suggests that when travel for academics is needed, the likelihood of a delay is reduced by nearly 88% (95% CI: 0.054–0.295).

Nonsignificant Predictors:

(1) **Decalcification**:

- Although the presence of decalcification tended to reduce the odds of a delay (B=−0.826B = -0.826B=−0.826), it was not statistically significant (p = 0.274). The odds ratio of 0.438 (95% CI: 0.100–1.922) suggests that decalcification may reduce the likelihood of delay, but this effect is not conclusive.

(2) **Sunday**:

- The effect of Sunday on reporting delays was not significant (B=0.087B = 0.087B=0.087, p = 0.850). The odds ratio of 1.091 (95% CI: 0.442–2.694) indicates a minimal and nonsignificant impact.

(3) **National Holiday**

- Similarly, national holidays did not have a significant effect on biopsy delays (B=0.698B = 0.698B=0.698, p = 0.309), with an odds ratio of 2.009 (95% CI: 0.524–7.708).

(4) **Academic Engagement**:

- Academic engagement tended to increase the likelihood of a delay (B=2.014B = 2.014B=2.014), but this difference was not statistically significant (p = 0.128). The odds ratio of 7.494 (95% CI: 0.560–100.305) suggests a potential but inconclusive increase in delay risk.

(5) **Faculty Leave**:

- Faculty leave did not significantly predict delays (B=0.475B = 0.475B=0.475, p = 0.313), with an odds ratio of 1.608 (95% CI: 0.639–4.043).

(6) **Developmental Disturbances**:

- The presence of developmental disturbances as a subclass of disease was marginally nonsignificant (B=1.374B = 1.374B=1.374, p = 0.052), with an odds ratio of 3.952 (95% CI: 0.990–15.776), suggesting a possible but inconclusive increase in delay likelihood.

The logistic regression model identified the third Saturday and travel for regular academic activities as significant predictors of biopsy reporting delays. Other factors, including decalcification, Sundays, national holidays, academic engagement, faculty leave, and the presence of developmental disturbances, did not significantly predict delays.

5 DISCUSSION

The audit of delays in reporting histopathological specimens reveals significant insights into the current workflow and its impact on turnaround times. This study investigated the factors contributing to biopsy reporting delays, defined as more than 15 days for bone biopsies and 7 days for soft tissue biopsies.

This discussion will focus on the pros and cons of the existing reporting system, a detailed analysis of the reasons for delays, and potential solutions to minimize these delays.

Pros:

5.1 *Thorough analysis and accuracy*

- Despite its delays, the current system allows for thorough analysis, particularly for complex cases. The additional time ensures that all necessary tests, such as special stains and immunohistochemical studies, are completed with precision, reducing the risk of diagnostic errors. [2].

5.2 *Consultation and expert opinions*

- The process of seeking secondary referrals for expert opinions can extend the reporting time but is crucial for ensuring diagnostic accuracy, especially in challenging or rare cases. [4].

5.3 *Cons*

5.3.1 *Delayed diagnosis and treatment*

- The most significant drawback of the current system is the delay in providing diagnosis and treatment, which can lead to prolonged anxiety and potentially adverse outcomes for patients. Delays in reporting are particularly concerning in cases where timely intervention is critical, such as in patients with malignant conditions.

5.3.2 *Operational inefficiencies*

- The audit identified several operational inefficiencies within the laboratory that contribute to delays. These include the time-intensive decalcification process for bone samples and the use of special stains, both of which significantly extend the reporting time [2,3]. The presence of institutional factors, such as academics, examinations, and academic conference holidays, especially third staurays, further exacerbates these delays by reducing the availability of pathologists during critical periods [1].

5.3.3 *Resource drain*

- Prolonged processing times can also lead to increased use of resources, both in terms of staff time and laboratory materials.

5.4 *Analysis of the reasons for delays*

5.4.1 *Decalcification process*

- The decalcification of bone samples is a major contributor to delays. Uematsu *et al.* (2018) reported that this process is inherently time-consuming, often requiring several days to complete depending on the specimen size and bone density [2].

5.4.2 *Special staining and immunohistochemistry*

- The requirement for special stains and immunohistochemical studies, as discussed by Shi *et al.* (1991), adds to the complexity and duration of the reporting process. These tests are essential for accurate diagnosis, particularly in cases where routine staining does not provide sufficient information [3].

5.4.3 *Secondary referrals*

- As noted by Randhawa (2009), secondary referrals to external laboratories or specialists, although crucial for complex cases, introduce additional delays due to the time required for external consultation [4].

5.4.4 *Institutional factors*

- Brown *et al.* (2003) highlighted the impact of academic conferences, holidays and examinations on the availability of pathologists, leading to further delays in the reporting process. During these periods, the workload is either redistributed among fewer pathologists or postponed, both of which contribute to extended turnaround times [1].

5.5 *Potential solutions for minimizing delays*

5.5.1 *Optimizing the decalcification process*

- Efforts should be made to optimize the decalcification process, such as by using more efficient decalcifying agents or automated systems that can reduce the time required for this step without compromising the quality of the sample.

5.5.2 *Streamlining special stains and immunohistochemistry*

- Implementing more efficient protocols for special stains and immunohistochemistry could help reduce delays. Like the use of microwave-assisted staining, as suggested by Shi *et al.* (1991), it could be adopted to expedite the process [3].

5.5.3 *Improving communication and coordination*

- Enhancing communication and coordination between primary laboratories and external consultants could reduce delays in secondary referrals. Establishing a fast-track system for urgent cases may also help minimize turnaround times.

5.5.4 *Managing institutional schedules*

- To mitigate the impact of institutional factors such as academic conferences, better scheduling and workload distribution could be implemented.

Implementing a combination of these strategies can significantly reduce delays in biopsy reporting, even in the presence of scheduled holidays and academic obligations.

(1) Advance scheduling
  - Solution: Schedule biopsies in advance, taking holidays and academic activities into account.

(2) Implement a Shift System or Extended Working Hours
  - Solution: Introduce a rotational shift system for lab staff, ensuring a continuous workflow even during holidays.

(3) Digital Pathology and Telepathology
  - Solution: Implement digital pathology systems to enable remote review and reporting. [5]

(4) Delegation and Task Shifting
  - Solution: Delegate preliminary tasks to technicians or junior pathologists.

(5) Temporary Staffing Solutions
  - Solution: Hire temporary staff during peak times to maintain workflow.

(6) Automation in Histopathology
  - Solution: Invest in automation to speed up biopsy processing[6].

(7) Prioritization of Cases
  - Solution: Establish a prioritization system for biopsy cases. [7]

(8) Cross-Training Staff
  - Solution: Cross-trained staff to handle multiple tasks during the biopsy process.

(9) Collaboration with External Laboratories
  - Solution: Partner with external laboratories to handle overflow cases.

(10) Artificial Intelligence (AI)
  - Solution: Integrate AI for preliminary analysis of biopsy slides. [8]

The study highlights that specific logistical factors, such as the presence of a third Saturday and faculty holidays, significantly impact biopsy reporting times. The findings underscore the importance of operational planning to mitigate delays, especially on third Saturday and during periods requiring faculty leave. Additionally, travel for regular academic activities appears to facilitate timely reporting, possibly due to enhanced scheduling efficiency. The abovementioned factors provide evidence-based support for each solution, demonstrating how various strategies can help mitigate delays in biopsy reporting due to holidays and academic burdens.

6 CONCLUSION

The audit of the histopathological reporting process highlights key areas where delays occur, particularly in the decalcification process, the use of special stains, secondary referrals, and institutional scheduling. While the current system has strengths in ensuring diagnostic accuracy, the identified delays necessitate targeted interventions to improve efficiency. Implementing the proposed solutions could lead to significant reductions in turnaround times, ultimately enhancing patient care.

REFERENCES

[1] Brown RW, Lamke KD, Hajdu SI, *et al.* (2003). Effect of academic conferences on laboratory turnaround time. *Am J Clin Pathol.* 119(1):104–108.

[2] Uematsu T, Kasami M, Yuen S, Uchida Y. (2018). The time-consuming decalcification process for bone specimens in histopathology. *Histopathology.* 72(1):123–130.

[3] Shi S-R, Key ME, Kalra KL. (1991). Antigen retrieval in formalin-fixed, paraffin-embedded tissues: an enhancement method for immunohistochemical staining based on microwave oven heating of tissue sections. *J Histochem Cytochem.* 39(6):741–748.

[4] Randhawa PS. (2009). Experience with secondary referral for expert opinion in histopathology. *Indian J Pathol Microbiol.* 52(1):37–39.

[5] Hanna, M.G., *et al.* (2020). "Implementation of digital pathology offers clinical and operational increase in efficiency and cost savings." *Archives of Pathology & Laboratory Medicine*, 144(11), 1306–1316. DOI: 10.5858/arpa.2019-0494-OA

[6] Hsieh, H.M., *et al.* (2020). "Automation in the histopathology laboratory: Current status and future prospects." *Journal of Pathology Informatics*, 11(1), 2. DOI: 10.4103/jpi.jpi_28_20

[7] Turner, B.R., and Childs, G. (2016). "Pathology prioritization schemes: A framework for optimizing laboratory services." *Journal of Clinical Pathology*, 69(12), 1027–1034. DOI: 10.1136/jclinpath-2016-203928

[8] Raciti, P., *et al.* (2020). "Predicting cancer outcomes with histopathological images using deep learning." *Nature Medicine*, 26(7), 943–948. DOI: 10.1038/s41591-020-0907-1

Navigating Dental Education Trends and Transforming Dental Pedagogy – Abas and Srikant N (Eds)
© 2027 The Author(s), ISBN: 978-1-041-32674-8

Role of Outcome-Based Education in Implementing Oral Cancer Screening Using Micronuclei Assay (Exfoliative Cytology) and Salivary MicroRNA as Screening Tools for Controlling Oral Cancer by Dental Students

Avinash B R
Department of Public Health Dentistry, Manipal College of Dental Sciences Mangalore, Manipal Academy of Higher Education, Karnataka, Manipal, India

Junaid Ahmed
Department of Oral Medicine and Radiology, Manipal College of Dental Sciences Mangalore, Manipal Academy of Higher Education, Karnataka, Manipal, India

Praveen Jodalli and Ramya Shenoy
Department of Public Health Dentistry, Manipal College of Dental Sciences Mangalore, Manipal Academy of Higher Education, Karnataka, Manipal, India

Nidhi Manaktala
Department of Oral Pathology and Microbiology, Manipal College of Dental Sciences Mangalore, Manipal Academy of Higher Education, Karnataka, Manipal, India

Suchitra Shenoy M
Department of Microbiology, Kasturba Medical College Mangalore, Manipal Academy of Higher Education, Karnataka, Manipal, India

1 INTRODUCTION

Oral cancer being a significant public health issue, it contributes to high mortality and morbidity rates. According to the World Health Organization (WHO), oral cancers account for approximately 3% of all cancer cases globally, with mortality rates approaching 50% in some regions [1]. The increasing prevalence of oral cancer, particularly in developing countries, necessitates effective early detection strategies to improve patient outcomes and reduce the burden of disease.

Early detection of oral cancer is critical, as it is often associated with better treatment outcomes and improved survival rates. Traditional screening methods, including visual examinations and biopsies, have limitations in sensitivity and specificity. Consequently, there is a growing interest in utilizing molecular and cytological techniques for early detection. The micronuclei assay, which analyzes exfoliated cells for chromosomal abnormalities, and microRNA profiling, which assesses specific RNA molecules associated with cancer, are promising tools for improving screening accuracy.

This paper explores the role of Outcome-Based Education (OBE) in equipping dental students with the necessary skills and knowledge to implement these screening tools effectively. By focusing on the desired outcomes of the learning process, OBE can enhance the competencies of dental students, enabling them to contribute significantly to oral cancer screening and prevention efforts.

2 BACKGROUND

2.1 *The burden of oral cancer*

Oral cancer is primarily associated with risk factors such as tobacco use, alcohol consumption, and human papillomavirus (HPV) infection. The incidence of oral cancer varies by region, with higher rates observed in South Asia and parts of Africa. In India, for example, oral cancer is one of the most common cancers, accounting for approximately 30% of all cancer cases [2]. The late-stage diagnosis of oral cancer is a significant concern, as many patients present with advanced disease, leading to poorer prognosis and higher treatment costs [3].

2.2 *The importance of early detection*

Early diagnosis is critical for improving survival rates in oral cancer patients. Studies have shown that the 5-year survival rate for patients diagnosed at an early stage can exceed 80%, while those diagnosed at advanced stages

DOI: 10.1201/9781042016075-41

have significantly lower survival rates [4]. However, many cases are diagnosed at advanced stages due to a lack of awareness and insufficient screening initiatives.

Traditional screening methods, including visual examinations and biopsies, have limitations in sensitivity and specificity. Visual examinations can miss early lesions, while biopsies are invasive and may not be feasible for routine screening. Consequently, there is a growing interest in utilizing molecular and cytological techniques for early detection.

2.3 *Innovative screening methods*

The micronuclei assay is a promising cytological technique that analyzes exfoliated cells for chromosomal abnormalities. Micronuclei are small, extra-nuclear bodies that form due to chromosomal fragmentation or failure of cytokinesis. The presence of micronuclei in exfoliated cells from the oral cavity has been associated with increased cancer risk [5]. This assay is non-invasive, making it suitable for routine screening.

MicroRNA profiling is another innovative approach that focuses on the expression levels of specific microRNAs linked to oral carcinogenesis. MicroRNAs are small, non-coding RNA molecules that regulate gene expression and have been implicated in various cancer pathways. Altered expression of specific microRNAs has been associated with the development and progression of oral cancer [6]. By assessing microRNA profiles in saliva or exfoliated cells, dental professionals can identify individuals at higher risk for developing oral cancer.

2.4 *Outcome-based education framework*

Outcome-Based Education is an educational strategy that focuses on the desired outcomes of the learning process. In the context of dental education, OBE emphasizes the development of competencies that students must achieve by the end of their training. This approach is particularly relevant for implementing oral cancer screening practices, as it encourages active learning and practical application of knowledge.

OBE is characterized by clearly defined learning outcomes, assessment methods aligned with those outcomes, and a focus on student-centered learning. In the context of dental education, OBE can enhance students' understanding of oral cancer, its risk factors, and the importance of early detection. By incorporating innovative screening methods into the curriculum, dental students can develop the skills necessary to implement these techniques effectively.

3 METHODS

3.1 *Curriculum development*

The curriculum for dental students will be designed to incorporate OBE principles, focusing on the competencies required for effective oral cancer screening. The curriculum will include theoretical knowledge about oral cancer epidemiology, risk factors, and the biological basis of the screening methods. Practical sessions will involve hands-on training in sample collection and analysis, as well as case studies to enhance critical thinking and decision-making skills.

Micronuclei Assay: This method involves collecting exfoliated cells from the oral cavity and staining them to identify micronuclei, which are indicative of genomic instability. Students will be trained in the collection, preparation, and analysis of samples, as well as interpreting results.

MicroRNA Profiling: This technique focuses on the expression levels of specific microRNAs that have been linked to oral carcinogenesis. Students will learn to collect saliva samples, perform RNA extraction, and utilize quantitative polymerase chain reaction (qPCR) for analysis.

Training Modules: The curriculum will include training modules that cover the following topics:

Epidemiology of Oral Cancer: Understanding the prevalence, risk factors, and demographics associated with oral cancer.

Screening Techniques: Detailed instruction on the micronuclei assay and microRNA profiling, including their biological basis, methodology, and interpretation of results.

Patient Communication: Training on how to effectively communicate the importance of oral cancer screening to patients, including addressing concerns and misconceptions.

Ethical Considerations: Discussing ethical issues related to cancer screening, including informed consent and the implications of false-positive and false-negative results.

3.2 *Implementation of screening tools*

The implementation of the micronuclei assay and microRNA profiling as screening tools will involve several key steps:

Sample Collection: Students will learn to collect exfoliated cells from the oral cavity using standardized techniques. This non-invasive procedure will be emphasized to encourage patient participation.

Laboratory Analysis: Students will be trained in laboratory techniques for analyzing samples. This includes staining techniques for the micronuclei assay and RNA extraction and qPCR for microRNA profiling.

Data Interpretation: Students will learn to interpret the results of their analyses, correlating findings with clinical implications. This will involve case studies and discussions to enhance critical thinking skills.

Community Engagement: Students will be encouraged to participate in community outreach programs to promote oral cancer screening awareness. This may include organizing screening camps, educational workshops, and collaborating with local health organizations.

3.3 *Assessment and evaluation*

To evaluate the effectiveness of the OBE curriculum, a multi-faceted assessment approach will be employed:

Knowledge Assessments: Pre- and post-training assessments will be conducted to measure students' knowledge gains regarding oral cancer and screening techniques.

Practical Skills Evaluation: Students will be assessed on their practical skills in sample collection and analysis through direct observation and competency checklists.

Attitude Surveys: Surveys will be administered to gauge students' attitudes towards oral cancer screening and their perceived role in promoting early detection.

Longitudinal Tracking: Following graduation, alumni will be tracked to assess their involvement in oral cancer screening initiatives and their impact on patient outcomes.

4 RESULTS

The implementation of OBE in dental education has shown promising results in enhancing students' competencies in oral cancer screening. Preliminary assessments indicate that students who underwent OBE-based training demonstrated improved knowledge and skills in utilizing the micronuclei assay and microRNA profiling for oral cancer detection.

4.1 *Knowledge gain*

Students exhibited a significant increase in understanding the molecular mechanisms of oral cancer and the importance of early detection. Pre-training assessments revealed that only 45% of students could accurately identify the risk factors associated with oral cancer. Post-training assessments indicated that this figure increased to 85%, demonstrating the effectiveness of the OBE curriculum in enhancing knowledge.

4.2 *Practical skills*

Hands-on training led to improved proficiency in sample collection and analysis. Students reported increased confidence in performing these procedures, with 90% of participants expressing a strong willingness to implement these screening techniques in their future practices. Observational assessments indicated that students successfully demonstrated the ability to collect samples and analyze them accurately.

4.3 *Attitudes towards screening*

The OBE approach fostered a positive attitude towards the importance of oral cancer screening. Surveys indicated that 95% of students recognized their role as future dental professionals in promoting early detection and patient education. This shift in attitude is crucial for encouraging the next generation of dental practitioners to prioritize oral cancer screening in their practices.

5 DISCUSSION

The integration of innovative screening tools into dental education through an Outcome-Based Education framework has the potential to transform oral cancer detection practices. The micronuclei assay and microRNA profiling offer complementary approaches to traditional screening methods, enhancing sensitivity and specificity in detecting early-stage oral cancers.

5.1 *Challenges and barriers*

Despite the advantages, several challenges remain in implementing these screening tools in dental education. These include the need for adequate training resources, the integration of new technologies into existing curricula, and ensuring that students are prepared to communicate the importance of screening to patients effectively. Additionally, there may be resistance from practitioners who are accustomed to traditional screening methods.

5.2 *Future directions*

Continued research is necessary to validate the effectiveness of these screening tools in diverse populations. Studies should focus on the sensitivity and specificity of the micronuclei assay and microRNA profiling in various demographic groups to ensure their applicability across different populations. Furthermore, collaboration between dental schools, healthcare providers, and public health organizations can facilitate the implementation of comprehensive oral cancer screening programs.

5.3 *Role of dental students*

Dental students are uniquely positioned to lead oral cancer screening initiatives within their communities. By equipping them with the necessary skills and knowledge, they can advocate for early detection and contribute to reducing the burden of oral cancer. Engaging students in community outreach programs not only enhances their learning experience but also fosters a sense of social responsibility.

5.4 *Implications for dental education*

The incorporation of OBE principles into dental education can enhance the overall quality of training programs. By focusing on competencies related to oral cancer screening, dental schools can produce graduates who are better prepared to address public health challenges. This approach aligns with the evolving role of dental professionals as integral members of the healthcare team, emphasizing their responsibility in promoting preventive care.

6 CONCLUSION

The role of Outcome-Based Education in implementing oral cancer screening using the micronuclei assay and microRNA profiling is critical for enhancing early detection efforts. By focusing on the desired outcomes of dental education, students can develop the competencies needed to utilize these innovative screening tools effectively. The integration of molecular and cytological techniques into dental curricula not only prepares students for their future roles as healthcare providers but also contributes to the broader goal of controlling oral cancer through early detection and intervention.

As the burden of oral cancer continues to rise, it is imperative that dental education evolves to meet these challenges. By adopting OBE principles and incorporating innovative screening methods, dental schools can empower the next generation of practitioners to make a meaningful impact on oral cancer prevention and control.

REFERENCES

[1] BMC Oral Health. (2023). Oral cancer screening knowledge and practices among dental professionals at the University of Toronto. *BMC Oral Health*, 23, 343. Retrieved from BMC.

[2] Cheung, L.C. *et al.* (2021). Risk-based oral cancer screening — lessons to be learnt. *Nature Reviews Clinical Oncology*. Retrieved from Nature.

[3] Ford, P.J., and Farah, C.S. (2013). Early detection and diagnosis of oral cancer: Strategies for improvement. *Oral Oncology*, 49(5), 383–390. Retrieved from ScienceDirect.

[4] Ghosh, S., and Sinha, A. (2023). The role of MicroRNAs in oral cancer: A review of current literature. *Oral Oncology*, 133, 105–112. doi:10.1016/j.oraloncology.2023.105112.

[5] Gupta, B., Johnson, N.W., Kumar, S., and Kumar, S. (2020). Oral cancer in India: A review of the current status and future directions. *Asian Pacific Journal of Cancer Prevention*, 21(4), 967–973. doi:10.31557/APJCP.2020.21.4.967.

[6] Sinha, A., and Ghosh, S. (2022). MicroRNA as a Biomarker for Oral Cancer: A Review. *Journal of Oral Pathology and Medicine*, 51(1), 5–12. doi:10.1111/jop.13182.

[7] Warnakulasuriya, S., and Kerr, A.R. (2021). Oral Cancer Screening: Past, Present, and Future. Journal of Dental Research. Retrieved from NCBI.

[8] Wong, T.Y., and Wong, S.Y. (2021). The role of dental professionals in oral cancer screening: A review. *Journal of the American Dental Association*, 152(4), 305–313. doi:10.1016/j.adaj.2021.01.016.

Navigating Dental Education Trends and Transforming Dental Pedagogy – Abas and Srikant N (Eds)
 ISBN: 978-1-041-32674-8

JIGPATH: A Puzzle-Based Approach to Mastering Oral Histopathology

Fahizah
Biomaterials and Research Centre, Yenepoya Dental College, Yenepoya Deemed to be University, Mangalore

Riaz Abdulla and Devika Jayarajan
Department of Oral Pathology and Microbiology, Yenepoya Dental College, Yenepoya Deemed to be University, Mangalore

ABSTRACT: Oral histopathology, a fundamental subject in dental education, is often challenging for students due to its complex nature and traditional teaching methods. This study aimed to assess the effectiveness of JigPath, an innovative jigsaw puzzle learning tool, in enhancing student engagement, understanding, and retention of histopathological concepts. Fifty-four third-year BDS students participated in this pilot study at a single institution. Students were first introduced to histopathological concepts through a 20-minute lecture and a hands-on session where they assembled JigPath puzzles. These puzzles, designed by laser printing from durable material, depicted key histological structures, encouraging active learning through physical interaction and collaboration. Qualitative feedback from students indicated a high level of engagement, with 87% agreeing that the puzzles made learning more interactive and engaging. Additionally, 94.4% reported improved visualization and understanding of histological features, while 92.6% acknowledged enhanced teamwork during the puzzle activity. Moreover, 96.3% of students desired more topics to be taught using similar puzzle-based methods. These findings suggest that JigPath puzzles can be an effective supplementary tool in dental education, promoting active learning and collaboration. Further research is recommended to explore the long-term impact of this approach on student performance.

Keywords: Oral histopathology, Jigsaw puzzles, Dental education, Interactive learning, Gamification

1 INTRODUCTION

Effective dental education is paramount in ensuring a competent and well-equipped healthcare workforce. While traditional didactic teaching methods have their place, they may not fully address the complex needs of modern medical students. This necessitates exploring innovative teaching strategies that foster more profound understanding, engage students in the learning process, and better prepare them for clinical practice.

The effectiveness of various pedagogical approaches in enhancing medical and dental education. Recent studies investigating diverse teaching methods, each offering unique advantages. The studies encompass a range of disciplines, including histology, oral pathology, cardiology, dentistry for special needs individuals, and cavity preparation [1]. The metaphor of "spirits of past, present, and future" connects historical figures and discoveries in histology with contemporary practice and future advancements. This approach aims to create a more engaging and enriching student learning experience, fostering knowledge acquisition and a deeper appreciation for the field's evolution.

Shifting the focus to a student-centred approach, the efficacy of pedagogy in an oral pathology course emphasizes student participation in teaching and learning, encouraging them to take ownership of their education. It evaluates whether this collaborative approach leads to improved student engagement, understanding of the subject matter, and overall performance in the course [2].

Using manipulatives, like a puzzle-based game approach, as a teaching tool for the cardiac cycle has enhanced student learning and retention compared to traditional lecture-based methods [3]. Previous studies used the Jigsaw technique, which involved dividing students into small groups. Each group focuses on a specific aspect of the topic and then shares its knowledge with the class. I analysed how this approach affects student collaboration, understanding of the subject matter, and overall learning outcomes in this crucial area of dentistry [4].

Another form of cooperative learning, Jigsaw-based learning, effectively teaches cavity preparation to dental students. This method involves student collaboration in small groups to learn different aspects of the task, fostering a deeper understanding and skill development [5].

This study's objective was to evaluate the effectiveness of histopathology jigsaw puzzles in improving student knowledge, retention, and engagement. By providing a hands-on and interactive learning experience, jigsaw puzzles can help students visualize complex structures, develop problem-solving skills, and reinforce key concepts.

Previous research has demonstrated the benefits of jigsaw puzzles in enhancing learning across various educational domains, including science and mathematics. While jigsaw puzzles have been shown to improve cognitive

DOI: 10.1201/9781042016075-42

function, problem-solving skills, and spatial reasoning, their application in dental education, particularly for histopathology, remains relatively unexplored. This study sought to address this gap by investigating the potential of jigsaw puzzles as a novel and engaging tool for enhancing oral histopathology learning. Specifically, we aimed to determine if jigsaw puzzles could improve students' understanding of histological structures, ability to identify and diagnose oral diseases, and overall satisfaction with the learning experience.

2 MATERIALS AND METHODS

2.1 *Methodology*

2.1.1 *JigPath puzzle fabrication*

The creation of JIGPATH puzzles involved a multi-step process. First, slides illustrating oral histopathology were hand-drawn. These designs were then digitized using advanced software and laser printing onto durable materials to produce robust and long-lasting puzzle pieces. This fabrication process ensured that the puzzles could withstand repeated use in a classroom setting (Figure 1).

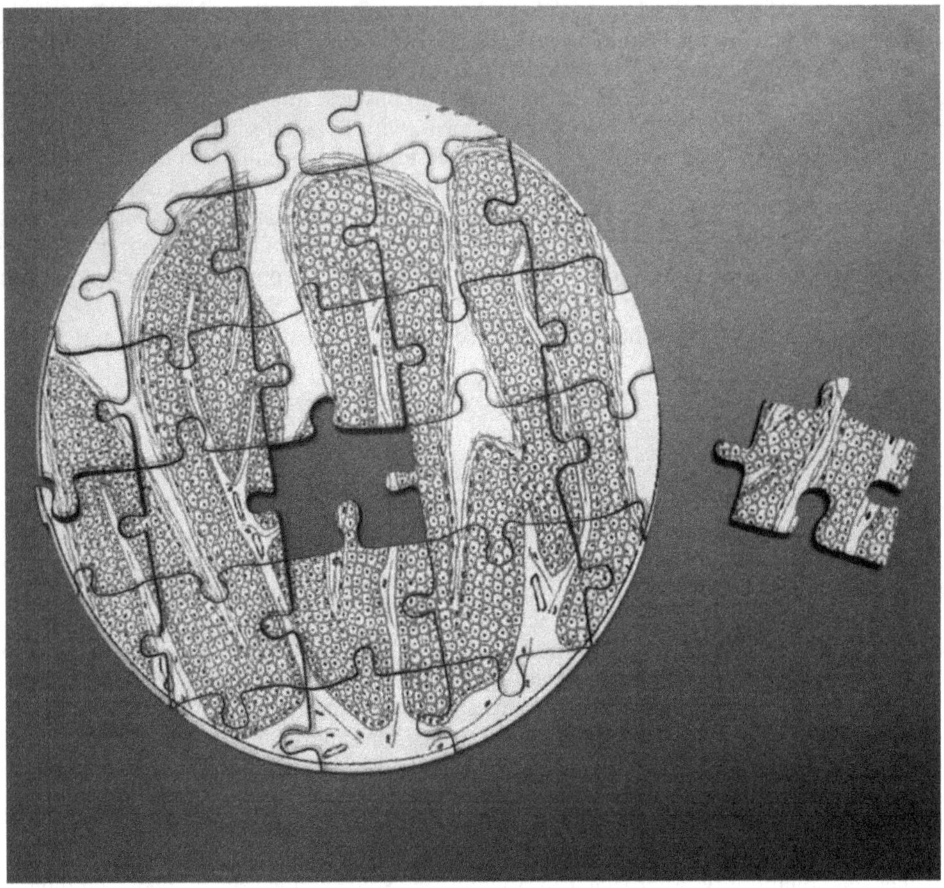

Figure 1. Fabrication of JIGPATH puzzle using durable material with printed histological details.

2.1.2 *Study design*

The study was a pilot project at a single dental institution, targeting third-year Bachelor of Dental Surgery (BDS) students. A sample size of 54 students was selected for the initial study. The sample size was calculated to assess the impact of JIGPATH puzzles on engagement, retention, and collaboration. Based on a confidence level of 95%, an effect size of 0.5 (medium), and a power of 0.80, a minimum of 50 participants was required. With a sample of 54 students, this pilot study was adequately powered for initial insights, though more extensive studies are recommended for broader validation.

2.1.3 *Inclusion and exclusion criteria*

Inclusion Criteria:

(1) Third-year Bachelor of Dental Surgery (BDS) students enrolled in a single institution.

(2) Students who have completed introductory coursework in histology and are familiar with basic histological concepts.
(3) Participants willing to attend both the lecture-based and puzzle-based learning sessions as part of the study.

Exclusion Criteria:

(1) Students who did not provide consent to participate in the study.
(2) Students with prior experience using puzzle-based learning tools in histology, to avoid potential bias.
(3) Students unable to attend all required sessions due to scheduling conflicts or other personal reasons.

2.1.4 *Teaching approach*

The study involved a two-part teaching approach. First, students received a 20-minute lecture on specific oral lesions, focusing on their histological features. This segment used traditional teaching methods, including slides of histology samples (Figures 2,3).

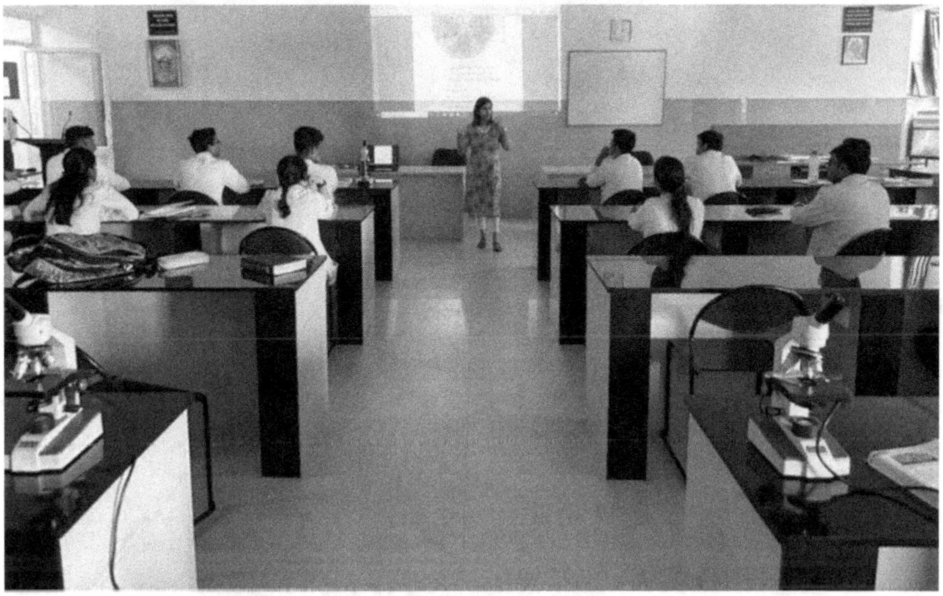

Figure 2. Lecture session introducing histology concepts to students.

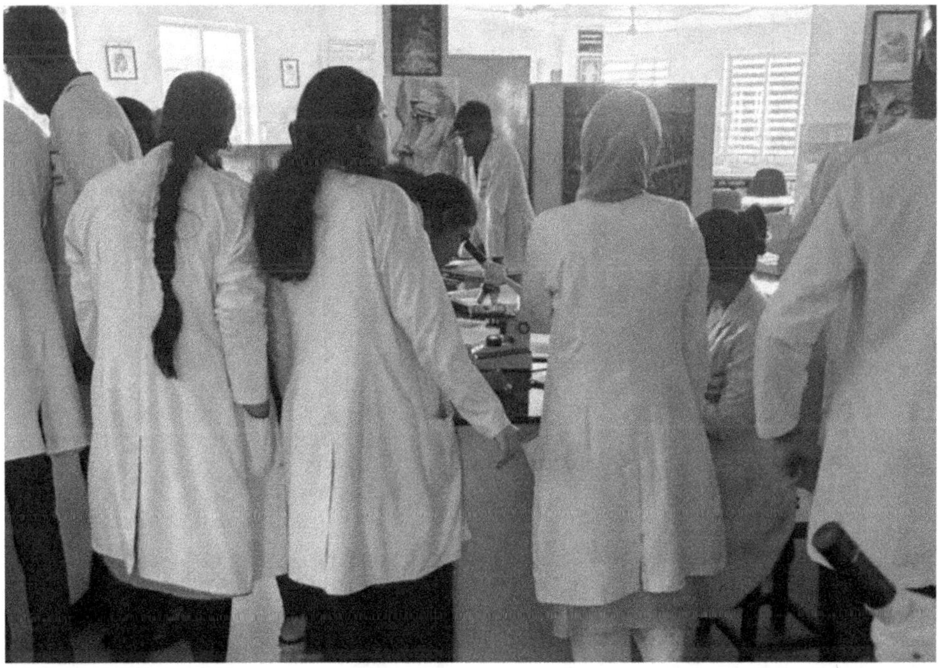

Figure 3. Students examining histology slides under the microscope.

After the lecture, the students participated in a hands-on session, where they were asked to assemble the JIGPATH puzzles. This activity was designed to reinforce the concepts presented during the lecture by providing a tactile and interactive learning experience (Figures 4,5).

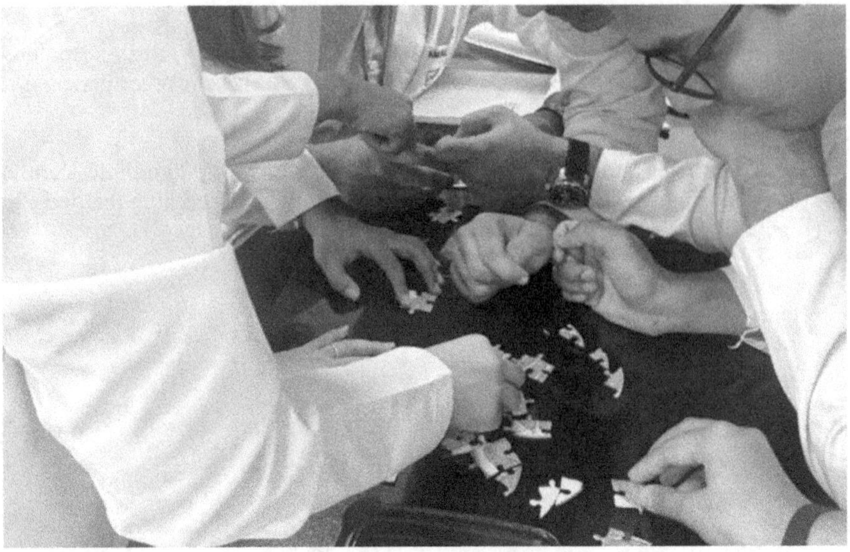

Figure 4. Students assembling JIGPATH puzzle pieces collaboratively.

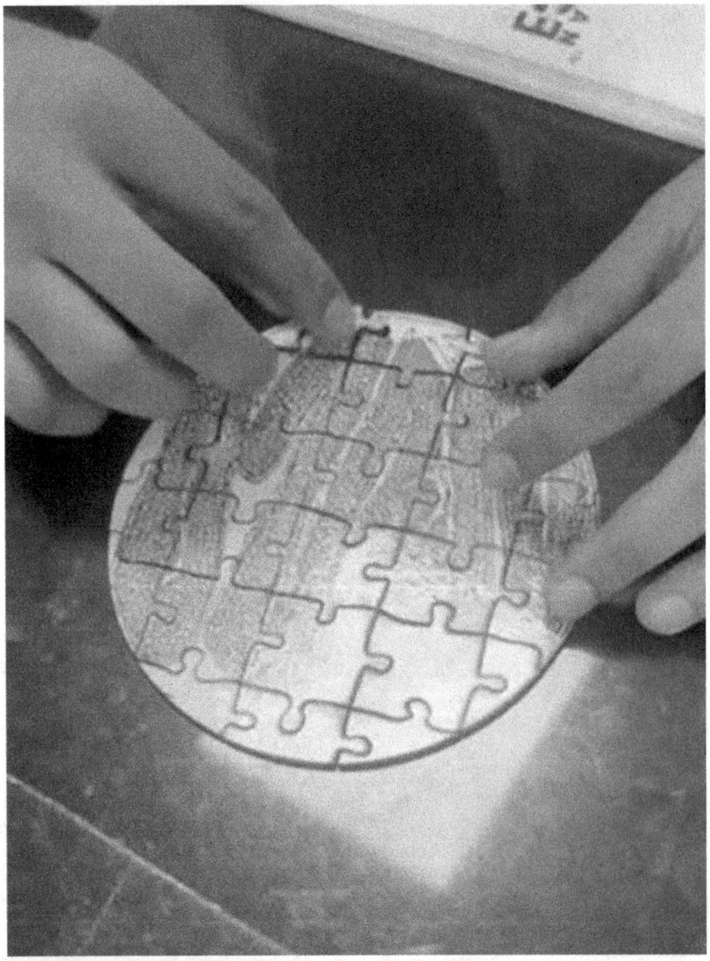

Figure 5. Completed JIGPATH puzzle showing a histological section.

2.1.5 *Feedback collection*

A qualitative survey was conducted among the students to gauge the effectiveness of JIGPATH. The survey focused on three key areas: student engagement and interaction, retention and understanding of histopathological concepts, and the impact on collaboration and teamwork. The results were analyzed to understand the students' perceptions and the overall success of the puzzle-based approach.

3 RESULTS

The survey results were overwhelmingly positive, with students reporting significant benefits from using JigPath (Table 1).

Table 1. Presents the percentage of student feedback across key areas, including engagement, understanding, retention, teamwork, and preferences for future puzzle-based learning methods. 1: Strongly agree, 2: Agree, 3: Neutral, 4: Disagree, 5: Strongly Disagree.

Objective	Feedback Questions	1	2	3	4	5
1 Enhancing Student Engagement and Interaction	JigPath learning tool made understanding histology slides more engaging.	44.4%	42.6%	9.3%		3.7%
	JigPath puzzle learning activity made learning histology more enjoyable.	66.7%	27.8%	3.7%		
2 Improving Retention and Understanding of Histological Concepts	JigPath helped me visualize the slides better and increased retentiveness about the histological features of the diseases.	33.3%	61.1%	3.7%		1.9%
	I found the JigPath puzzles an effective way to review complex histology slides.	48.1%	37%	13%		1.9%
	Physical interaction with the puzzles enhanced my understanding compared to traditional lecture-based learning.	50%	37%	11.1%		1.9%
3 Impact on Collaboration and Teamwork	JigPath puzzles encouraged me to work collaboratively with my peers.	53.7%	38.9%	5.6%		1.9%
	I would like to see more histology/pathology topics taught using puzzle-based learning methods.	57.4%	38.9%		1.9%	1.9%
	Overall, I found the JigPath learning tool to be a valuable addition to my education.	51.9%	40.7%	5.6%		1.9%

3.1 *Engagement and interaction*

The analysis of student feedback on the JigPath puzzle learning tool revealed strong engagement with the material. Precisely, 87% of students (calculated from 44.4% "Strongly Agree" and 42.6% "Agree") reported that the puzzles made histology slides more engaging and facilitated a better understanding of the material. Furthermore, 94.5% of students (a combination of 66.7% "Strongly Agree" and 27.8% "Agree") indicated that the learning experience was more enjoyable with JigPath puzzles compared to traditional lecture-based methods. This finding supports the increasing recognition of gamified learning as a practical approach for enhancing student motivation and engagement in educational settings (Graph 1).

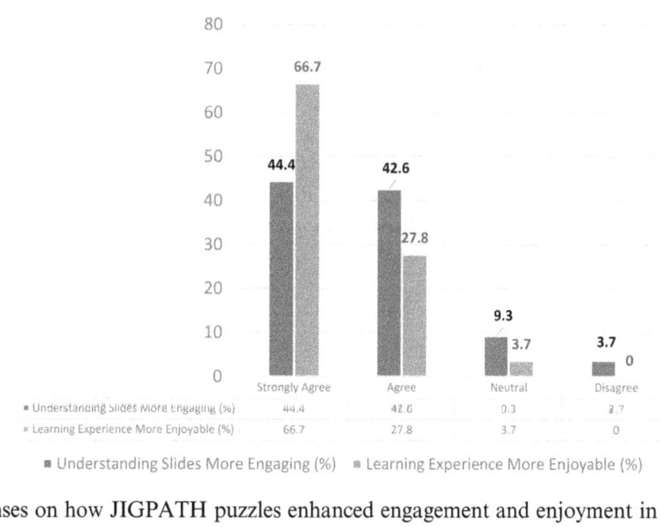

Graph 1. Student responses on how JIGPATH puzzles enhanced engagement and enjoyment in learning histology.

3.2 *Retention and understanding*

Analysis of student responses highlighted the effectiveness of JigPath puzzles in enhancing retention and understanding of histological features. Specifically, 94.4% of students (comprised of 33.3% "Strongly Agree" and 61.1% "Agree") reported that the puzzles significantly improved their ability to visualize and retain knowledge of histological structures. The physical assembly of puzzle pieces reinforced their understanding, as the interactive nature of this activity provided a memorable learning experience. Additionally, 85.1% of students (48.1% "Strongly Agree" and 37% "Agree") found the puzzles to be an effective tool for reviewing complex histology slides, indicating their utility in consolidating intricate material (Graph 2).

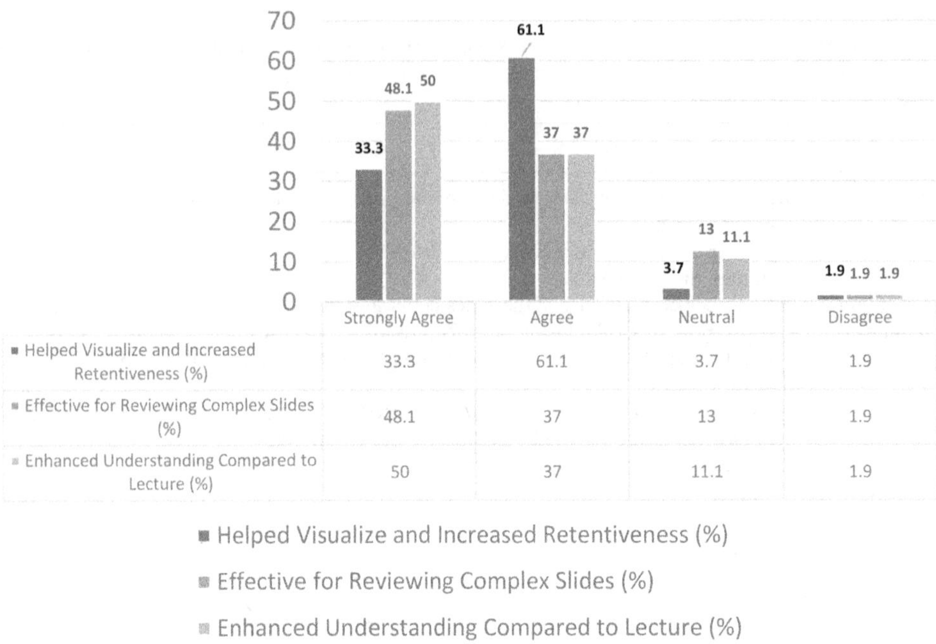

	Strongly Agree	Agree	Neutral	Disagree
Helped Visualize and Increased Retentiveness (%)	33.3	61.1	3.7	1.9
Effective for Reviewing Complex Slides (%)	48.1	37	13	1.9
Enhanced Understanding Compared to Lecture (%)	50	37	11.1	1.9

Graph 2. Student feedback on the effectiveness of JIGPATH puzzles in improving retention and comprehension of histological concepts.

Furthermore, 87% of students (50% "Strongly Agree" and 37% "Agree") expressed that the hands-on puzzle experience was more beneficial than traditional lecture-based methods for understanding complex concepts. Many students also noted improvements in spatial reasoning, an essential skill for interpreting microscopic tissue structures, underscoring the value of active learning in histology education.

3.3 *Collaboration and teamwork*

The JigPath puzzle demonstrated a positive impact on student collaboration. A substantial 92.6% of students (53.7% "Strongly Agree" and 38.9% "Agree") indicated that working with peers to assemble the puzzles improved their teamwork skills. The cooperative format of the puzzle-based learning activity fostered camaraderie and encouraged collaborative problem-solving among students (Graph 3).

In addition, 96.3% of students (57.4% "Strongly Agree" and 38.9% "Agree") expressed interest in seeing more histology and pathology topics taught using similar puzzle-based methods, highlighting the appeal and perceived value of this approach. Moreover, 92.6% of students (51.9% "Strongly Agree" and 40.7% "Agree") regarded JigPath puzzle as a valuable supplement to their educational experience, further underscoring the potential benefits of integrating gamified, collaborative learning tools in the curriculum.

4 DISCUSSION

The findings from this study contribute to the growing body of evidence suggesting that gamified learning and interactive educational tools can significantly enhance student engagement, retention, and collaboration in dental education. The JigPath puzzles allowed students to engage deeply with the subject material, transitioning from passive learning to an active, problem-solving approach.

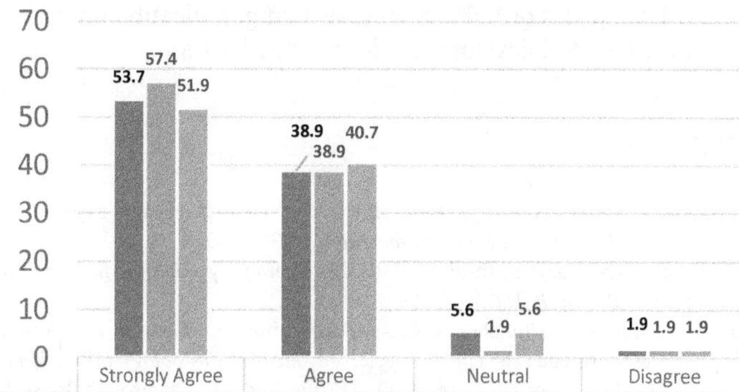

	Strongly Agree	Agree	Neutral	Disagree
Encouraged Collaboration with Peers (%)	53.7	38.9	5.6	1.9
Interest in More Puzzle-Based Topics (%)	57.4	38.9	1.9	1.9
Overall Valuable Educational Tool (%)	51.9	40.7	5.6	1.9

Encouraged Collaboration with Peers (%)
Interest in More Puzzle-Based Topics (%)
Overall Valuable Educational Tool (%)

Graph 3. Student perceptions of JIGPATH puzzles' impact on teamwork and collaborative learning in histology.

This study aligns with prior research on gamified medical and dental education learning. Gentry *et al.* (2019) conducted a systematic review of the effectiveness of gamification in medical education, finding that game-based approaches increased student motivation, engagement, and content retention [6]. Similarly, our study observed high levels of student engagement, with 87% reporting that JigPath puzzles enhanced their understanding and enjoyment of histology, reinforcing the benefits of interactive and enjoyable learning tools in medical education.

Additionally, using puzzle-based learning tools aligns with findings by Nazeer *et al.* (2018), who examined crossword puzzles in anatomy education and reported that these activities improve cognitive retention and recall through active engagement [7]. Our study similarly found that 94.4% of students felt that JigPath puzzles helped them visualize and retain histological features effectively. These findings suggest that puzzle-based learning can be a valuable adjunct to traditional methods, reinforcing memory and comprehension of complex concepts.

Furthermore, Appandraj *et al.* (2021) explored the impact of the Jigsaw method on student collaboration in clinical diagnostics and observed significant improvements in teamwork and communication skills [8]. This aligns with our results, where 92.6% of students indicated that JigPath encouraged collaborative problem-solving, fostering a sense of camaraderie. Both studies underscore the benefits of structured, cooperative learning activities in building interpersonal skills, which are essential for clinical practice.

These findings are also consistent with prior research on active learning approaches. Amir *et al.* [9,10] demonstrated that serious games, including jigsaw puzzles, significantly improve student knowledge, retention, and satisfaction in oral histology, supporting our observation that interactive learning experiences enhance motivation and comprehension. Bhandary *et al.* [11] further compared the effectiveness of Jigsaw and inquiry-based learning in dental education, concluding that both methods enhance student engagement and learning. Together, these studies highlight the role of gamified and collaborative tools in promoting active learning.

Finally, Gilani *et al.* [12] investigated crossword puzzles as a self-learning modality for dental students and found that such tools improve vocabulary, retention, and problem-solving skills. This suggests puzzle-based activities like JigPath effectively support independent learning and skill development.

One limitation of our study is the relatively small sample size. Further research with a larger sample would help to confirm these findings and allow for broader generalization. Additionally, future studies could explore the long-term impact of puzzle-based learning on student performance and clinical competencies, providing a more comprehensive view of its benefits in dental education.

5 CONCLUSION

The JigPath project demonstrates that puzzle-based learning can be a valuable complement to traditional lectures in dental education. By engaging students in a hands-on, interactive learning experience, the puzzles helped improve their retention and understanding of complex histopathological concepts. Additionally, the collaborative nature of the activity fostered teamwork among students, further enhancing their educational experience.

Given the positive feedback from students, it is recommended that dental schools consider incorporating more puzzle-based learning activities into their curricula, particularly in subjects that are traditionally difficult for students to grasp. The success of JigPath suggests that gamification holds excellent promise as a tool for improving knowledge retention and skill development in dental education.

REFERENCES

[1] Hortsch M. (2023). Histology as a paradigm for a science-based learning experience: Visits by histology education spirits of past, present, and future. *Anatomical Sciences Education.* 16(3):372–83.

[2] Sabari NS, Roslan NN, Yazid F, Ibrahim N. (2022). Peeragogy teaching method in oral pathology course. *Journal of International Dental and Medical Research.* 15(2):707–11.

[3] Marcondes FK, Moura MJ, Sanches A, Costa R, de Lima PO, Groppo FC, Amaral ME, Zeni P, Gaviao KC, Montrezor LH. (2015). A puzzle used to teach the cardiac cycle. *Advances in Physiology Education* 39(1):27–31.

[4] Suárez-Cunqueiro MM, Gándara-Lorenzo D, Mariño-Pérez R, Piñeiro-Abalo S, Pérez-López D, Tomás I. (2017). Cooperative learning in 'Special Needs in Dentistry' for undergraduate students using the Jigsaw approach. *European Journal of Dental Education.* 21(4):e64–71.

[5] Alabdulmunim AA, Alyahya Y, Gaikwad RN. (2022). Jigsaw-based cooperative learning for studying cavity preparation in dental undergraduate students of Saudi Arabia. *Journal of Pharmaceutical Negative Results.* 2789–93.

[6] Gentry SV, Gauthier A, Ehrstrom BL, Wortley D, Lilienthal A, Car LT, Dauwels-Okutsu S, Nikolaou CK, Zary N, Campbell J, Car J. (2019). Serious gaming and gamification education in health professions: systematic review. *Journal of Medical Internet Research.* 21(3):e12994.

[7] Nazeer M, Sultana R, Ahmed MM, Asad MR, Sami W, Hattiwale HR, Sreekanth T. (2018). Crossword puzzles as an active learning mode for student directed learning in anatomy teaching: Medical undergraduate perceptions. *International Journal of Medical Research & Health Sciences.* 2018;7(10):12–9.

[8] Appandraj S, Sivagamasundari V, Sakthivadivel V. (2021). Role of JIGSAW method of teaching in improving clinical diagnosis among final year medical students–A prospective observational study. *Asian Journal of Medical Sciences.* 12(12):44–9.

[9] Amir LR, Leonardy IC, Dewatmoko SN, Yanuar R, Suniarti DF, Idrus E, Sipiyaruk K, Puspitawati R. (2023). Serious game as oral histology learning strategy for undergraduate dental students; crossover randomized controlled trial. *BMC Oral Health.* 23 (1):585.

[10] Amir LR, Dewatmoko SN, Leonardy IC, Yanuar R, Suniarti DF, Idrus E, Sipiyaruk K, Puspitawati R, Wimardhani Y. (2024). Perceived enablers of and barriers to serious game as oral histology learning strategy for undergraduate dental students. *Dentistry Journal.* 2024 Sep;12(9):280.

[11] Bhandary M, Thimmaiah C, Shahid M, Shetty Y, Rao K A. Potential of active learning in dentistry: A comparative study of Jigsaw versus inquired-based learning. *Journal of Dental Education.*

[12] Gilani R, Niranjane P, Daigavane P, Bajaj P, Mankar N, Vishnani R. (2020). Crossword puzzle: An effective self-learning modality for dental undergraduates. *Journal of Datta Meghe Institute of Medical Sciences University.* 15(3):397–401.

 ISBN: 978-1-041-32674-8

Illuminating Minds and Expanding Scientific Horizons of Oral Health

Shruthi Shrikar Shenoy
SDM College of Dental Sciences and Hospital, A constituent unit of Shri Dharmasthala Manjunatheshwara University, Sattur, Dharwad, Karnataka

Deepthi Shetty
Department of Oral and Maxillofacial Surgery, SDM College of Dental Science and Hospital, A Constituent Unit of Shri Dharmasthala Manjunatheswara University, Sattur, Dharwad, Karnataka

Balram Naik
Department of Conservative Dentistry and Endodontics, SDM College of Dental Sciences and Hospital, A constituent unit of Shri Dharmasthala Manjunatheshwara University, Sattur, Dharwad, Karnataka

Niranjan Kumar
Department of Plastic & Reconstructive Surgery, SDM College of Medical Science & Hospital, A constituent unit of Shri Dharmasthala Manjunatheshwara University, Sattur, Dharwad

ABSTRACT: **Purpose:** Rapid advancements in technology are reshaping dental education and clinical practice, with both virtual reality (VR) and augmented reality (AR) emerging as revolutionary tools. These aids provide an immersive learning environment, allowing dental students and professionals to simulate real-world clinical procedures, thus enhancing their skill set without the risks associated with living patients. The primary objective of this review is to explore the impact of AR and VR in the field of dental education, providing AI-driven virtual patient simulators, hybrid AR-VR learning, and VR-based skill competitions.

Methods: A thorough review of the literature was carried out utilizing MEDLINE (via EBSCO), PubMed, Scopus, the Web of Science Core Collection (via Thomson Reuters) and the Cochrane Library (via Wiley). Studies were selected on the basis of their relevance to the application of AR and VR in dentistry, specifically their impact on clinical training and educational methodologies.

Results: These technologies deepen students' anatomical understanding and decision-making skills in a risk-free environment. VR also offers a novel method for teaching dental entrepreneurship, enabling students to explore business management scenarios and develop leadership skills.

Conclusion: VR and AR provide effective, risk-free platforms for dental education. Advanced specializations in fields such as oral oncology and dental sleep medicine, combined with global health initiatives, will equip future dentists with the skills and adaptability needed in a rapidly challenging and demanding profession.

Keywords: dental education, innovation, virtual and augmented reality, artificial intelligence, entrepreneurship

1 INTRODUCTION

The Sanskrit word Shastravistarah beautifully encapsulates our vision with Shastra meaning scriptural compendium and Vistarah meaning expansion [1,2]. Through this concept, we aim to broaden the horizons of the dental curriculum, incorporating the latest advancements and interdisciplinary approaches to create a more dynamic and effective learning experience [2,3]. Dental education is rapidly evolving, with advancements in technology and interdisciplinary approaches transforming how students learn and practice [1,3]. With increasing demands for innovation and efficiency in healthcare, especially after the COVID-19 crisis, emerging technologies such as augmented reality (AR) and virtual reality (VR) are becoming essential tools in modern dental training [4]. These tools not only create immersive learning environments but also enhance clinical skills and prepare students for leadership in dental entrepreneurship [3,4]. These immersive tools allow learners to visualize complex anatomical structures and simulate dental procedures in a risk-free environment [5].

With the increasing need for digital proficiency in healthcare, dental institutions are switching to these technologies to enhance both theoretical and practical training [6]. This review focuses on the role of AR and VR in the dental curriculum, highlighting their potential in clinical skill-building, their application in dental entrepreneurship, and their interdisciplinary benefits [4–7]. The aim is to analyze the literature on these technologies, identify current gaps, and propose areas for future research. In the context of dental education, there is evidence supporting the efficacy of AR and VR in creating interactive, student-centered learning experiences [8]. However, the specific

DOI: 10.1201/9781042016075-43

impact of these tools on long-term clinical performance and innovation in dental practice remains underexplored in our country [7–9].

A gap in the literature regarding dental entrepreneurship, tele dentistry, and sustainability in dentistry needs to be addressed in the curriculum, with a focus on virtual consultations, remote monitoring, and ethical aspects of digital patient care [3,10]. In the context of the literature, AR and VR have been recognized for their potential to transform various fields of healthcare [11]. However, there is limited research specifically focused on their application in dental education [12]. This review seeks to bridge this gap by synthesizing current research, identifying the benefits and limitations of these technologies, and providing insights for future advancements in the field [11–13].

2 METHODS

This review article was compiled via a systematic search of peer-reviewed articles and relevant literature available from multiple databases, including MEDLINE (via EBSCO), PubMed, Scopus, Web of Science Core Collection (via Thomson Reuters), Cochrane Library (via Wiley) and Google Scholar [13,14]. The search strategy employed Mesh keywords such as "Augmented Reality in oral health", "Virtual Reality in dental education", "Artificial Intelligence in dental training" and "Innovative dental education technologies" [15].

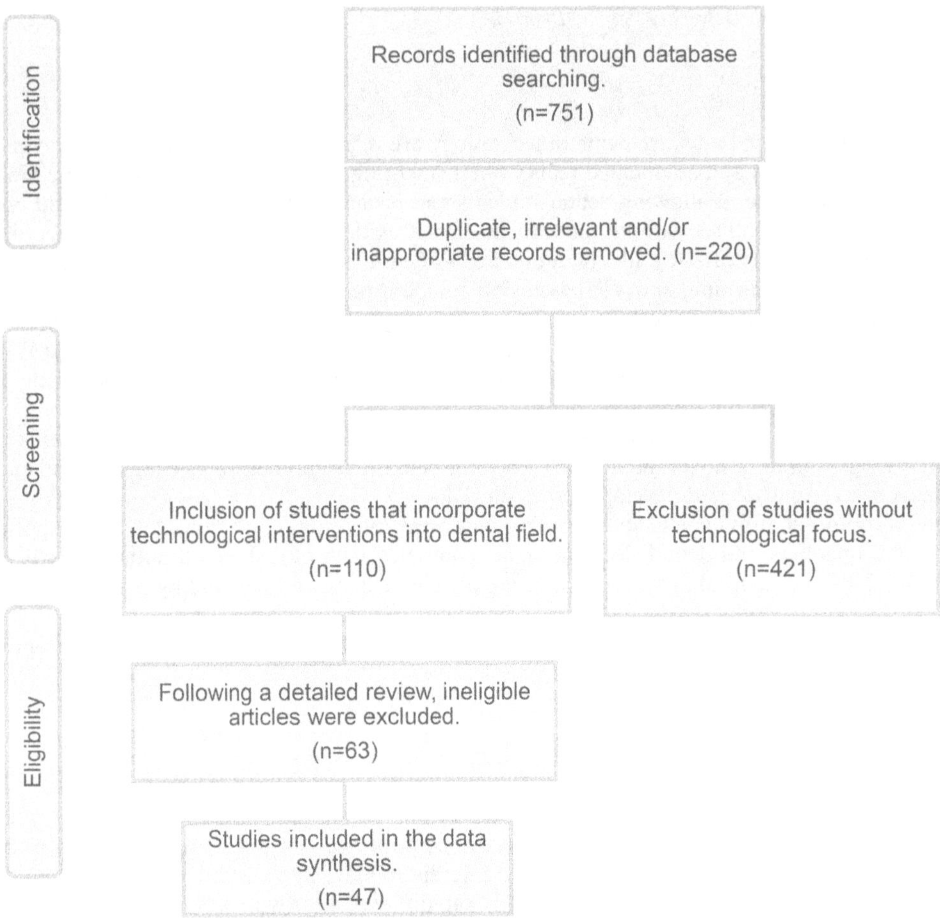

The keywords were modified to work with all of the previously stated databases [15]. While conducting our electronic search, we further searched for pertinent papers on the basis of the keywords found in the searched articles [14,15]. The bibliographies of the exposed full texts were manually searched for more research [16]. Studies that focused on the use of AR and VR in improving dental and entrepreneurial skills were included [17].

The results were collected from a single Mendeley library (Mendeley Desktop v1.19.6.) Duplicates were eliminated [18], [19] The exclusion criterion was articles that focused solely on nontechnical aspects of dental education or clinical practice without exploring technological interventions [19,20].

A total of 751 articles were initially identified across databases. After removing duplicates (approximately 220 articles), 531 unique articles were screened based on titles and abstracts. Of these, 110 articles met the initial inclusion criteria for full-text review. Following a detailed review, 47 studies were included in the final analysis.

3 RESULTS

The reviewed studies highlight a clear trend: VR and AR technologies not only are reshaping traditional dental education but also enable students to engage in more practical, hands-on learning from early in their training [18–21]. By simulating clinical scenarios and patient interactions, VR and AR help students build confidence and refine their decision-making skills before entering the clinical environment [1,22].

Key findings include the following:

(1) **Improved Learning Outcomes**: Compared with traditional methods, studies have revealed that students who use VR simulations have improved performance in understanding oral anatomy and mastering clinical procedures [22]. For example, VR simulations allow learners to manipulate 3D models of the jaw, teeth, and oral cavities, increasing their spatial awareness of complex anatomical regions [23].
(2) **Risk-Free Environment**: VR provides a platform for students to practice procedures in a virtual environment, reducing the risk associated with live patient interactions [11,24]. This is particularly valuable for high-risk procedures such as oral surgery [23,24].
(3) **Innovative Entrepreneurship in Dentistry**: AR-driven simulations enable students to develop leadership skills in dental entrepreneurship by exploring business management scenarios, helping them gain practical knowledge about running a dental practice [25,26]

Benefit	Description
Improved Learning Outcomes	Enhanced understanding of oral anatomy and clinical skills [22,23].
Risk-Free Environment	Allows practice of high-risk procedures without patient interaction [24].
Fostering Dental Entrepreneurship	AR-based scenarios help develop leadership and business management skills [25,26].

This comprehensive evaluation demonstrated that VR improved knowledge retention and dental manual skill development after brief training sessions [27]. Only a small number of studies have reported extended follow-up times and negligible variations among conventional and virtual groups [28].

Despite the growing adoption of technologies in dental education, gaps remain [27–29]. For example, more longitudinal studies are needed to determine the lasting impact of these technologies on clinical performance [30].

4 DISCUSSION

The integration of AR and VR in dental education represents a paradigm shift [31]. The evolving landscape of dental education necessitates the integration of cutting-edge technologies and interdisciplinary approaches to produce well-rounded, innovative professionals [32,33]. The significance of this topic is particularly highlighted after the COVID-19 pandemic, which has accentuated the need for a shift toward a virtual learning environment in healthcare education [34]. Traditional methods of teaching anatomy, clinical procedures, and practice management are augmented by these technologies, providing a more comprehensive learning experience [35]. Currently, there is a gap in the integration of advanced technologies such as AR, VR, and AI-driven patient simulators in the dental curriculum, which can bridge the disconnect between theoretical knowledge and hands-on clinical experience [36,37].

The potential of VR and AR in tele-dentistry and remote patient care remains an untraversed area, especially in light of the recent shift toward digital healthcare during the COVID-19 crisis [38,39]. A gap in the literature regarding dental entrepreneurship, tele dentistry, and sustainability in dentistry needs to be addressed in the curriculum, with a focus on virtual consultations, remote monitoring, and ethical aspects of digital patient care [40,41].

The ability to practice complex procedures in a virtual environment prepares students for real-world scenarios, reducing the learning curve during clinical practice [38–40]. The implications for the field of dentistry are vast [40]. With VR-based training, students can learn at their own pace, repeat procedures, and receive real-time feedback, all of which contribute to enhanced skill acquisition [39–41].

Furthermore, AR-based systems can help students visualize dental structures in three dimensions, improving spatial understanding and precision during surgery [38–41]. Alternatively, they could serve as an educational medium to foster comprehension of dental principles and offer secure and economical learning [42,43]. Various authors designate simulators and AR for different purposes [43,44]. Virtual technology appears to improve dental students‘ educational outcomes within the boundaries of this review [45]. They replicate real-world processes as closely as possible to enable further practice in a secure setting [43–45]. They may serve as a diagnostic tool for students with fine motor skill deficiencies, who are likely to have difficulty in preclinical exams [43–46].

However, the widespread adoption of these technologies faces several challenges [42]. Financial constraints and the need for technical infrastructure are significant barriers [40–42]. In addition, further investigations are needed to determine the lasting effects of VR and AR-based learning on clinical outcomes [43]. Furthermore, few studies have considered students' perceptions of the existence of VR simulators [44].

Larger sample sizes and longer duration clinical trials are needed for further research to validate the possible benefits of different virtual technologies on dental education results [17,18,44]. Information on several topics, such as long-term student follow-up and the impact of VR on clinical practices, is limited owing to the retrospective nature of our research, which incorporates data from published studies rather than from individuals [37,42]. While meta-analysis was not possible, the search method revealed an array of studies that addressed the goal of the systematic review. Instead, we used a descriptive approach to determine the successful outcome of virtual applications [13,43,44].

There are numerous facets of dental education and training that the dental profession needs to rethink [44]. The future of dentistry holds immense potential with the integration of avant-garde technologies [46], [47]. Robotics in dentistry, for example, could revolutionize precision in surgical procedures and enhance patient care. Further research should explore these possibilities, focusing on how to create more efficient, adoptable and personalizedsolutions [47].

Dentistry will never be a virtual profession, but dental education in the future can be "integrated," combining online and in-person instruction [47]. Future studies should focus on exploring how these technologies can support sustainable practices in dental care and whether they can be adapted for tele-dentistry, which is becoming an increasingly important area of study [45].

As dental training continues to evolve, the adoption of AR, VR and AI-driven patient simulators will be crucial in fostering innovative thinking, enhancing clinical skills, and equipping students with the tools necessary to meet the demands of modern oral healthcare [45–47].

5 CONCLUSION

To summarize, the inclusion of virtual reality (VR) and augmented reality (AR) in dental schools signifies a revolutionary change toward a more dynamic and engaging educational process. The COVID-19 crisis emphasized the importance of virtual communication and technology-driven models. These tools not only address the disconnect between academic and practical clinical experience but also educate the next generation of dental professionals to navigate complex clinical scenarios with greater confidence. By adopting these innovations, we can prepare future dental professionals to be better equipped to face the challenges of modern healthcare.

ACKNOWLEDGEMENTS

We would like to acknowledge SDM University for its support, resources and guidance throughout this research journey.

FUNDING

"The authors declare that no funds, grants, or other support was received during the preparation of this manuscript."

REFERENCES

[1] Dzyuba N, Jandu J, Yates J, Kushnerev E. (2022). Virtual and augmented reality in dental education: The good, the bad and the better. *Eur J Dent Educ.* doi: 10.1111/eje.12871. Epub ahead of print. PMID: 36336847.

[2] https://www.shabdkosh.com/search-dictionary?lc=hi&sl=hi&tl=en&e=%E0%A4%B6%E0%A4%BE%E0%A4%B8%E0%A5%8D%E0%A4%A4%E0%A5%8D%E0%A4%B0+%E0%A4%B5%E0%A4%BF%E0%A4%B8%E0%A5%8D%E0%A4%A4%E0%A4%B0%E0%A4%A3

[3] Jumlongkul, Arnon. (2023). Innovation and entrepreneurship in dental curriculum: from practice to creativity in the face of pandemic. *SN Applied Sciences.* 5. 10.1007/s42452-023-05566-7.

[4] Kwon HB, Park YS, Han JS. (2018). Augmented reality in dentistry: a current perspective. *Acta Odontol Scand.* 76(7):497–503.

[5] Moussa R, Alghazaly A, Althagafi N, Eshky R, Borzangy S. (2022). Effectiveness of virtual reality and interactive simulators on dental education outcomes: Systematic review. *Eur J Dent.* 16(1):14–31.

[6] Sharmin N, Chow AK. (2020). Augmented reality application to develop a learning tool for students: transforming cellphones into flashcards. *Healthc Inform Res.* 26(3):238–242.

[7] Joda T, Gallucci GO, Wismeijer D, Zitzmann NU. (2019). Augmented and virtual reality in dental medicine: A systematic review. *Comput Biol Med.* 108:93–100. doi: 10.1016/j.compbiomed.2019.03.012. Epub 2019 Mar 15. PMID: 31003184.

[8] Rhienmora P, Haddawy P, Khanal P, Suebnukarn S, Dailey MN. (2010). A virtual reality simulator for teaching and evaluating dental procedures. *Methods Inf Med.* 49(4):396–405. doi: 10.3414/ME9310. Epub 2010 Jun 22. PMID: 20582388.

[9] Huang TK, Yang CH, Hsieh YH, Wang JC, Hung CC. (2018). Augmented reality (AR) and virtual reality (VR) applied in dentistry. *Kaohsiung J Med Sci.* 34(4):243–248. doi: 10.1016/j.kjms.2018.01.009. PMID: 29655414.

[10] Amin M, Lai JY, Lindauer PA, McPherson K, Qari H. (2021). Should dental schools adopt teledentistry in their curricula? Two viewpoints. *J Dent Educ*. 85(7):1238–1244.

[11] Wu, Hsin-Kai; Lee, Silvia Wen-Yu; Chang, Hsin-Yi; Liang, Jyh-Chong. (2013). Current status, opportunities and challenges of augmented reality in education. *Computers & Education*. 62. 41–49. 10.1016/j.compedu.2012.10.024.

[12] Kwon H.B., Park Y.S., Han J.S. (2018). Augmented reality in dentistry: a current perspective. *Acta Odontol. Scand*. 76: pp. 497–503.

[13] Suebnukarn S, Haddawy P, Rhienmora P, Jittimanee P, Viratket P. (2010). Augmented kinematic feedback from haptic virtual reality for dental skill acquisition. *J Dent Educ*.;74(12):1357–66. PMID: 21123503.

[14] Alvitez-Temoche D, Silva H, Aguila ED, Mauricio F, Espinoza-Carhuancho F, Mayta-Tovalino F. (2024). Scientometric analysis of the world scientific production on augmented and virtual reality in dental education. *J Contemp Dent Pract*. 25(4):358–364. doi: 10.5005/jp-journals-10024-3675. PMID: 38956852.

[15] Kacmaz KS, Kaçmaz C. (2024). Bibliometric analysis of research in pediatrics related to virtual and augmented reality: A systematic review. *Curr Pediatr Rev*. 20(2):178–187. doi: 10.2174/1573396319666230214103103. PMID: 36786143.

[16] Bakr MM, Massey WL, Alexander H. (2015). Can virtual simulators replace traditional preclinical teaching methods: a students' perspective?. *Int. J. Dent. Oral Health*. 2(1).

[17] Buchanan JA. (2001). Use of simulation technology in dental education. *J Dent Educ*. 65(11):1225–31. PMID: 11765868.

[18] Lackey MA. (2004). One year's experience with virtual reality preclinical laboratory simulation at the University of Tennessee. *Int J Comput Dent*. 7(2):131–41. English, German. PMID: 15516091.

[19] LeBlanc VR, Urbankova A, Hadavi F, Lichtenthal RM. (2004). A preliminary study in using virtual reality to train dental students. *J Dent Educ*. 68(3):378–83. PMID: 15038639.

[20] Hu S, Lai BWP. (2022). Increasing empathy for children in dental students using virtual reality. *Int J Paediatr Dent*. 32(6):793–800. doi: 10.1111/ipd.12957. Epub 2022 May 5. PMID: 35146818.

[21] Alsufyani N, Alnamlah S, Mutaieb S, Alageel R, AlQarni M, Bukhari A, Alhajri M, AlSubaie A, Alabdulkarim M, Faden A. (2023). Virtual reality simulation of panoramic radiographic anatomy for dental students. *J Dent Educ*. 87(8):1200–1209. doi: 10. 1002/jdd.13240. Epub 2023 May 16. PMID: 37191982.

[22] Thurzo A, Urbanová W, Novák B, Czako L, Siebert T, Stano P, Mareková S, Fountoulaki G, Kosnáčová H, Varga I. (2022). Where is the artificial intelligence applied in dentistry? systematic review and literature analysis. *Healthcare (Basel)*. 10(7):1269. doi: 10.3390/healthcare10071269. PMID: 35885796; PMCID: PMC9320442.

[23] Iwanaga J, Loukas M, Dumont AS, Tubbs RS. (2021). A review of anatomy education during and after the COVID-19 pandemic: Revisiting traditional and modern methods to achieve future innovation. *Clin Anat*. 34(1):108–114. doi: 10.1002/ca.23655. Epub 2020 Aug 24. PMID: 32681805; PMCID: PMC7404762.

[24] Bjelovucic R, Bak J, Wolff J, Taneja P. (2023). Dental students' attitudes on cardiopulmonary resuscitation training via virtual reality: an exploratory study. *Br Dent J*. 235(8):607–612. doi: 10.1038/s41415-023-6388-2. Epub 2023 Oct 27. PMID: 37891299; PMCID: PMC10611567.

[25] Afrashtehfar KI, Yang JW, Al-Sammarraie A, Chen H, Saeed MH. (2021). Preclinical undergraduate students' perspectives on the adoption of virtual and augmented reality to their dental learning experience: A one-group pre- and posttest design protocol. *F1000Res*. 10.473. doi: 10.12688/f1000research.53059.2. PMID: 36703700; PMCID: PMC9837452.

[26] Haroon Z, Azad AA, Sharif M, Aslam A, Arshad K, Rafiq S. (2020). COVID-19 Era: Challenges and Solutions in Dental Education. *J Coll Physicians Surg Pak*.;30(10):129–131. doi: 10.29271/jcpsp.2020.supp2.129. PMID: 33115587.

[27] Rodrigues P, Nicolau F, Norte M, Zorzal E, Botelho J, Machado V, Proença L, Alves R, Zagalo C, Lopes DS, Mendes JJ. (2023). Preclinical dental students self-assessment of an improved operative dentistry virtual reality simulator with haptic feedback. *Sci Rep*. 13(1):2823. doi: 10.1038/s41598-023-29537-5. PMID: 36801901; PMCID: PMC9936106.

[28] Reymus M, Liebermann A, Diegritz C. (2020). Virtual reality: an effective tool for teaching root canal anatomy to undergraduate dental students - a preliminary study. *Int Endod J*. 53(11):1581–1587. doi: 10.1111/iej.13380. Epub 2020 Sep 2. PMID: 32750729.

[29] Towers A, Field J, Stokes C, Maddock S, Martin N. (2019). A scoping review of the use and application of virtual reality in preclinical dental education. *Br Dent J*. 226(5):358–366. doi: 10.1038/s41415-019-0041-0. PMID: 30850794.

[30] McAlpin E, Levine M, Brenner C, Opazo C, Bathini S, Choi SJV, Louisville M, Grandhi U. (2022). Evaluating the effectiveness of a virtual reality simulation for preclinical local anesthesia dental education. *Eur J Dent Educ*. doi: 10.1111/eje.12854. Epub ahead of print. PMID: 36107420.

[31] Algarni YA, Saini RS, Vaddamanu SK, Quadri SA, Gurumurthy V, Vyas R, Baba SM, Avetisyan A, Mosaddad SA, Heboyan A. (2024). The impact of virtual reality simulation on dental education: A systematic review of learning outcomes and student engagement. *J Dent Educ* doi: 10.1002/jdd.13619. Epub ahead of print. PMID: 38807268.

[32] Liebermann A, Erdelt K. (2020). Virtual education: Dental morphologies in a virtual teaching environment. *J Dent Educ*. 84 (10):1143–1150. doi: 10.1002/jdd.12235. Epub 2020 Jun 8. PMID: 32511757.

[33] Rhienmora P, Haddawy P, Khanal P, Suebnukarn S, Dailey MN. (2010). A virtual reality simulator for teaching and evaluating dental procedures. *Methods Inf Med*. 49(4):396–405. doi: 10.3414/ME9310. Epub 2010 Jun 22. PMID: 20582388.

[34] de Boer IR, Lagerweij MD, Wesselink PR, Vervoorn JM. (2019). The effect of variations in force feedback in a virtual reality environment on the performance and satisfaction of dental students. *Simul Healthc*;14(3):169–174. doi: 10.1097/SIH. 0000000000000370. PMID: 31116175.

[35] Gottlieb R, Lanning SK, Gunsolley JC, Buchanan JA. (2011). Faculty impressions of dental students' performance with and without virtual reality simulation. *J Dent Educ*. 75(11):1443–51. PMID: 22058393.

[36] Lackey MA. (2004). One year's experience with virtual reality preclinical laboratory simulation at the University of Tennessee. *Int J Comput Dent*. 7(2):131–41. English, German. PMID: 15516091.

[37] Imber S, Shapira G, Gordon M, Judes H, Metzger Z. (2003). A virtual reality dental simulator predicts performance in an operative dentistry manikin course. *Eur J Dent Educ*. 7(4):160–3. doi: 10.1034/j.1600-0579.2003.00299.x. PMID: 14753761.

[38] Wu HK, Lee SW, Chang H, Liang JC. (2013). Current status, opportunities and challenges of augmented reality in education. *Comput Educ* 62:41–49

[39] Deery C. (2020). The COVID-19 pandemic: Implications for dental education. *Evid Based Dent* 21(2):46–47. doi:10. 1038/s41432-020-0089-3.

[40] Farronato M, Maspero C, Lanteri V, *et al.* (2019). Current state of the art in the use of augmented reality in dentistry: a systematic review of the literature. *BMC Oral Health* 19(1):135

[41] Yoshida Y, Yamaguchi S, Kawamoto Y, Noborio H, Murakami S, Sohmura T. (2011). Development of a multilayered virtual tooth model for the haptic dental training system. *Dent Mater J* 30(1):1–6

[42] Huang T-K, Yang C-H, Hsieh Y-H, Wang J-C, Hung C-C. (2018). Augmented reality (AR) and virtual reality (VR) applied in dentistry. *Kaohsiung J Med Sci* 34(4):243–248

[43] Suebnukarn S, Rhienmora P, Haddawy P. (2012). The use of cone-beam computed tomography and virtual reality simulation for presurgical practice in endodontic microsurgery. *Int Endod J* 45(7):627–632

[44] Murbay S, Neelakantan P, Chang JWW, Yeung S. (2020). 'Evaluation of the introduction of a dental virtual simulator on the performance of undergraduate dental students in the preclinical operative dentistry course' *Eur J Dent Educ*;24(1):5–16

[45] Mirghani I, Mushtaq F, Allsop MJ, *et al.* (2018). Capturing differences in dental training using a virtual reality simulator. *Eur J Dent Educ* 22(1):67–71.

[46] Gottlieb R, Baechle MA, Janus C, Lanning SK. (2017). Predicting performance in technical preclinical dental courses via advanced simulation. *J Dent Educ* 81(1):101–109

[47] Nilsson TA, Hedman LR, Ahlqvist JB. (2011). Dental student skill retention eight months after simulator-supported training in oral radiology. *J Dent Educ* 2011;75(5):679–684

Navigating Dental Education Trends and Transforming Dental Pedagogy – Abas and Srikant N (Eds)
© 2027 The Author(s), ISBN: 978-1-041-32674-8

Digital Evolution in Dental Education: Cloud-Based Learning Tools

Shweta Yellapurkar, N Srikant, Karen Boaz, and KP Nandita
Department of Oral Pathology and Microbiology, Manipal College of Dental Sciences Mangalore Manipal Academy of Higher Education, Manipal, Karnataka, India

Amitha Junaita Lewis
Department of Oral Pathology and Microbiology, Manipal College of Dental Sciences Mangalore

Nidhi Manaktala
Department of Oral Pathology and Microbiology, Manipal College of Dental Sciences Mangalore Manipal Academy of Higher Education, Manipal, Karnataka, India

ABSTRACT: The COVID-19 pandemic has prompted a major change in dental education from traditionally structured, hands-on, in-person learning to remote education. This paper discusses the role of cloud-based learning tools in managing the disruption in education, especially in the Department of Oral Pathology and Microbiology at MCODS Mangalore. The geographical flexibility and accessibility of cloud technology enable students to access and engage with educational materials remotely. Initiatives such as a "Digital Museum" used 3D scans and peer learning through cloud-based platforms to provide students with alternating access to specimen demonstration and critical thinking with interactive platforms such as YouTube and Quick Response codes. Online collaborative platforms such as Google Docs, Kahoot!, and Mentimeter were used to promote active engagement activities in real-time with participation, and continuous feedback. Furthermore, video demonstrations in oral pathology were developed to complete practical exercises, such as tooth carving, and implemented with technologies in classes, such as using Microsoft Teams and the Virtual Learning Environment Brightspace. Instructor-prepared resources such as podcasts, webinars, and video multimedia tutorials were used to break complex topics into increments and promote critical thinking. Personal video-recorded lectures or tutorials were stored in the cloud, offering students on demand and asynchronous access for review. The application of online tools and cloud technology effectively combines in-person face to face learning to prepare students in a progressive learning environment and ongoing professions, while supporting self-directed, adaptive learning and lifelong learning precepts. Emerging artificial intelligence developments and cloud technology are expected to continue to enhance and personalize education and learning.

Keywords: Cloud-based learning, Online assessment, Virtual learning, COVID 19, Dentistry, Digital Evolution

1 INTRODUCTION

The dental field has a distinctive approach to education, particularly with respect to hands-on learning, setting it apart from other professions. With the sudden closure of educational institutions due to the COVID-19 outbreak, alternative learning methods have been incorporated to ensure that students continue their education and prevent the spread of the pandemic. [1] In the current age of technological advancements, adapting the dental curriculum to meet these changes is imperative. Ubiquitous learning tools allow for learning experiences that are personalized and tailored to individual needs, regardless of where one is located. These tools make accessing and interacting with authentic and digital learning resources easier. In higher education, a wide range of e-learning tools can be used ubiquitously. [2]

Several universities have utilized technologically advanced teaching methods, such as mobile and electronic teaching, for several years. These methods make use of computing and e-learning technology to increase the effectiveness of learning activities. This has remarkably changed the way in which students learn and interact with learning content in recent years. [2]

One such initiative could be the incorporation of cloud-based learning technologies into the educational system. It offers several crucial advantages to dental students, such as flexibility, access to a vast array of resources, and interactive learning opportunities. [3,4]

This article focuses on different cloud-based learning platforms used in our Department of Oral Pathology and Microbiology, MCODS Mangalore, and discusses how this platform can improve dental education by outlining its advantages, characteristics, and possible implementation approaches.

Our department has practiced several innovative and interactive methods of learning, but this time, we developed a variety of Cloud-based web learning options tailored to cater to the needs of dental students, offering enhanced flexibility and interactivity through cloud technologies to accommodate different learning preferences and requirements.

1.1 *Here are some key modalities*

(1) **Digital Museum**

Our department is committed to the diagnosis of oral diseases and the comprehensive education of students, encompassing the instruction of clinical and radiographic presentations of lesions, as well as the detailed characteristics of gross and cut sections of these lesions. With a diverse collection of specimens and a consistent influx of clinical material from various departments and private physicians, faculty members engage students in hands-on grossing and processing procedures to enhance their clinical orientation. The involvement of students in museum mounting activities has proven to be an effective pedagogical tool, allowing them to learn the techniques for orienting specimens for educational displays, an essential part of pathology education. [5,6]

We previously introduced an economical method for mounting samples, which was adopted in our department. [7] In this activity, students are supervised as they mount specimens, enabling them to visualize the samples in completed transparent jars and enabling them to appreciate the texture, surface, and orientation of the samples relative to normal anatomical structures. Following the mounting process, the samples are labeled, and the students are tasked with creating placards. These labels connect the gross features of the samples to clinical and microscopic features, which provides context regarding the disease process. This is consistent with the evidence-based best-practice approach to education in pathology, which recommends linking gross pathology to clinical and microscopic features to optimize understanding. [8]

In addition to typical museum mounting of samples, we have developed an innovative approach called **"The Digital Museum,"** for the purpose of individual tooth samples. It provides a structured approach for students studying the developmental disturbances of hard tissues from identification to 3D scanning to sharing knowledge.

During identification, students are tasked with identifying hard tissue developmental disturbances in the samples, such as microdontia, supernumerary teeth, dilacerations, and other disturbances, on the basis of the study of a textbook or reference and the collection of other characteristics of the disturbance. These specimens are mounted in small glass jars, while students further explore the internal anatomy of the teeth by taking their own radiographs, either via CBCT or plain radiography.

Once the internal anatomical features are identified and observed, a 3D scanner reads the fine detailed structure of the sample via data scans. Saved data scans are saved as Avi videos and uploaded along with videos on the institute's YouTube channel, embedding a QR code to the jar containing the sample. Successive batches of students can now participate in self-learning by scanning the QR code to view the specimen for the relevant understanding of the 3D video and viewing the specimen itself. [9,10] By doing so, we are attempting to promote learning about the knowledge gap, or what has been coined **"cloud-based peer learning" (CBPL).**

To further enhance the learning experience, we have an interactive digital museum website. This platform enables students and alumni to view specimens interactively, videos, 3D files, and CBCT scans, offering an immersive learning experience that deepens their understanding of pathology. Such initiatives not only make learning more engaging but also contribute to a growing repository of educational resources for the institute. For alumni, these specimens provide a legacy and a point of reflection during future visits, fostering a sense of nostalgia and continuity. [11]

(2) **Interactive *Learning Tools: (Podcasts)***

Audio podcasts have a broad range of opportunities for use in (higher) education. It can be a monolog, cohosted, an interview, story telling or a panel podcast. Choose a topic, a format that you feel needs constant revision for your students, who are active listeners. Complex topics are broken down into smaller, more manageable segments. Record it in a tool and publish the completed episode to a podcast hosting platform such as Analgia, WordPress, which is user friendly; create the RSS feed; and use email, social media, and your network to obtain the word out about your show. We created one such thing from our department, which was an enormous success. [12]

(3) ***Online Quizzes and Assessments (Google Docs and other online quizzing platforms)***

The faculty in our department more often uses Google Docs to create interactive tests, quizzes, and practice exams with multiple-choice questions and short answers. This allows students to gradually assess their understanding of the material they are studying. Instant feedback is provided by this platform.

Socrative, quizizz, and kahoot! are a few more online engaging quiz sites that offer an interactive method of evaluating student knowledge. Multiple-choice, open-ended, and image-based quizzes are customizable by teachers. Students can take part with their mobile devices, and real-time results display encourages competition while maintaining an educational atmosphere. The limitations of these platforms are that they are dependent mainly on internet access and possibly face difficulties with data collection. [13]

Online Quizzing Platforms:

- Kahoot! (https://kahoot.com/)
- Quizizz (https://quizizz.com/)
- Socrative (https://www.socrative.com/)
- Mentimeter (https://www.mentimeter.com/)

4 **Collaborative *Platforms (Webinars through teams)***

Another approach we adopted was to organize webinars and online workshops conducted by subject matter experts. These events offer students the chance to learn from professionals, participate in discussions, and engage in hands-on activities. This approach proved to be effective in fostering communication, resource sharing, and teamwork. It also includes channels for various topics, chats, video calls, file sharing, and seamless integration with other Microsoft 365 tools. Additionally, Google Meet was utilized for video conferencing, Google Drive was used for file storage, and Google Docs/Sheets/Slides were used for collaborative document creation.

Collaborative learning has become a cutting-edge pedagogical approach in recent years, particularly for students who are increasingly inclined to take notes and record class activities on electronic devices. Today's students, in contrast to those ten years ago, often use tablets that have touch screens so that they can take pictures, write them, and record audio notes. To create a more engaging learning environment, educators must incorporate generative AI technologies, such as the GPT, into their curricula as they continue to advance. For example, in a benign and connective tissue pathology review session, a teacher started a group project by having students access a shared Word document on their devices. The document was shown live on a screen and included a table that the students filled in together. The teacher facilitated the activity by intervening only when necessary. Upon completion of each section, relevant images were sourced from the internet and displayed live, allowing the teacher to guide students in identifying valid resources and critically analyzing information. This approach engages students by aligning with their digital habits and fosters active participation and critical thinking. By incorporating live internet searches and dynamic content, the method keeps students engaged through constantly changing visuals and collaborative group work, encouraging a proactive approach to learning. [14–16]

5 ***Carving demo,* viva *and discussion & chat rooms (teams meet and one drive mail)***

Preclinical dental education places a strong emphasis on developing fine motor skills. To help dental students improve their manual dexterity and fine motor skills, they are introduced to anatomical tooth carving. Numerous carving techniques exist, including geometric (block carving technique) and wax build-up. We first demonstrated the technique to them live. The limited number of laboratory hours and limited view field make it difficult and time-consuming to teach students proper instrumentation and to develop a thorough understanding of dental anatomical features through multiple practical laboratory demonstrations.

However, the pandemic-induced transition to remote learning environments highlights the value of virtual spaces in fostering group problem solving and peer learning. With physical classrooms transitioning to virtual formats, forums and chat rooms serve as essential conduits for maintaining academic continuity. These platforms facilitate not only the dissemination of information but also the social and cognitive processes that are integral to learning.

Consequently, our department faculty captured videos of teeth drawing and carving demonstrations, which were subsequently posted on the student platforms offered by Microsoft Teams and BrightSpace. These videos provided a comprehensive guide on the sequential process of carving and presented an overview of the tooth's anatomical structures to be carved. The instructors illustrated the anatomical properties of a model and highlighted the correct ways to use the carving tools. To guarantee precision, the faculty thoroughly examined the completed carved tooth from various perspectives to ensure the visibility of all the anatomical elements discussed in the videos and lectures. https://youtube.com/playlist?list=PLQELc_3QksjH-

A blended learning strategy was applied for the dental anatomy practical course, where each week, the students would receive a lecture on the anatomy and morphology of a specific tooth, which was echoed in the student laboratory session where there was a live demonstration of the same tooth. First, we teach students to manipulate carving instruments and learn basic skills before they attempt to replicate a model tooth made by the instructors. It was only after the students had been introduced to video demonstrations that they were asked to watch the videos before the laboratory to prepare for the lab experiment. Students would carve the model tooth alone before presenting it to the laboratory session for feedback to show that they engaged with the video materials.

For students who did not have proper equipment and/or broadband internet service, the college made computer labs available for viewing video demonstrations. Students were also offered the opportunity to watch videos the week they would practice the tooth in the laboratory and to keep practicing tooth carving and writing about it at home. "Wheeler's Dental Anatomy, Physiology, and Occlusion" by Stanley Nelson was also suggested as a reference. [17]

Formative assessment is a crucial component of the teaching and learning process, and assessment is a significant aspect of the educational system. Formative assessment occurs during the learning process and is used to evaluate learning. The online video voce was conducted via the Teams Meet or Google Meet videoconferencing app. [18]

This asynchronous nature of forums enabled students to reflect on and contribute to discussions at their own pace, while synchronous chat rooms supported real-time interaction with demonstrations of carving and immediate feedback and video-vocing of relevant topics.

6 **Implementation** ***of Mentored Learning (Teams)***

We also adopted a mentored learning approach through teams to facilitate continued education. The students were divided into six faculty members, with each group assigned specific topics for study. Following the independent study period, the students were required to submit assignments on their designated topics. These submissions were then rigorously evaluated by the faculty, with feedback provided to enhance the learning process. The final assignments were refined to ensure clarity and ease of memorization, promoting better retention of the material among the students.

7 **Multimedia*****Resources***

(a) Video Lectures (**Impartus®**)

Periodic lecture timetables for enrolled students are made, and the lecture time is allotted online for the lecture capture system. Real-time recording of lectures is performed and securely stored in the cloud, providing students with on-demand access to these files. This system offers the dual benefit of enabling students to review topics at their convenience and access recorded lectures if they are unable to attend live sessions.

(b) Interactive Tutorials and Animations **(BrightSpace)**

After each chapter, the students are provided with comprehensive learning materials relevant to the topics covered in class. These resources include interactive tutorials, animations, YouTube links, and research articles that elucidate concepts in dental pathology, disease processes, and treatment techniques. Additionally, multiple-choice questions (MCQs) and assignments are administered to evaluate the students' level of understanding. These educational tools are thoughtfully designed to foster knowledge acquisition through an engaging and creative learning process. LMS platforms, such as BrightSpace, Moodle, and Canvas, are increasingly implemented in dental institutes to cater to the diverse learning needs of students. These systems, whether commercial or custom-developed by institutions, provide a comprehensive environment for delivering educational content. LMS platforms are capable of incorporating various media, including audio, video, PowerPoint presentations, and PDF articles, to create an engaging learning experience. Additionally, they offer interactive tools such as quizzes, fill-in-the-blank exercises, and assignment submission portals, which enhance student engagement and assessment. [19]

(c) Access to Research and Journals (*IP Address*)

Research databases that give students access to scholarly journals published in reliable online venues, enabling them to interact with novel concepts or studies in their area of interest and broadening their understanding of developing issues related to dentistry science, innovation, and practice.

(d) YouTube-edtech:

Different teaching modalities encourage students to actively engage in critical thinking and foster a strong self-learning process. As a result, our students are inspired to pursue various entrepreneurial roles. Several of our students have even created YouTube study content, serving as a valuable resource for future dental students.

2 APPLICATION OF CLOUD-BASED LEARNING IN DENTAL EDUCATION

Cloud-based educational technologies are intended to help students become life-long learners. If students and teachers are to maximize these possibilities, they need proper training. Institutions should invest time in providing tutorials, training, and technical support to minimize problems transitioning into, and adopting, new educational technology. Choosing a cloud-based platform to use in an educational program requires a careful comparison of features, usability, appropriateness to the instructional content, support for media formats and interactive tools, and robustness of the security system. The successful adoption of cloud resources also requires educators to find a way to integrate online materials and in-person sessions and to ensure that students have a functional understanding of how to use cloud resources.

3 FUTURE RECOMMENDATIONS

Real-time advancements in cloud technologies and artificial intelligence will translate into new tools and pedagogies for enriching teaching and learning experiences in dental education, leading to more educational opportunities that are personalized and immersive. If access to all these cloud-based resources is increased, it provides opportunities for the so-called democratization of education and could reach students from isolated communities or usual suspect communities to improve global dental care.

4 CONCLUSION

Cloud-based educational technologies provide students with access to unlimited educational resources, tools and services to assist with learning at "the time it suits the student. Ultimately, students are assisted through these technologies to become independent learners, collaborators, and critical thinkers, which will improve their life-long learning dispositions.

REFERENCES

[1] Maatuk, A.M., Elberkawi, E.K., Aljawarneh, S. *et al.* (2022). The COVID-19 pandemic and E-learning: challenges and opportunities from the perspective of students and instructors. *J Comput High Educ*; 34, 21–38.

[2] Aljawarneh, S.A. (2020). Reviewing and exploring innovative ubiquitous learning tools in higher education. *J Comput High Educ.* 32, 57–73.

[3] Prasad, Prathibha, Gunasekaran, Lalithambigai, Khair, Al Moutassem B., Shetty, Raghavendra, Shetty, Naresh. (2024). WhatsApp as a tool in blended learning in dental education. *Journal of Pharmacy and Bioallied Sciences* 16(Suppl 2):p S1673–S1678, . DOI:10.4103/jpbs.jpbs_425_23

[4] Messina DM, MikhailSS, Messina MJ, Novopoltseva IA. (2022). Assessment of learning outcomes of first year dental students using an interactive Nearpod educational platform. *J Dent Educ.* 86:893–899

[5] Ajileye A, Adeyemi O. (2020). Museum techniques and practices in histopathology: A compendium. *J. Med. Lab. Sci.* 30:18–34.

[6] Shashidara R, Patil S, Rao RS, Scindiya E, Tryphena A. (2017). Grossing of oral pathologies-revisited. *J Contemp Dent Pract.* 18 (12):1213–1222.

[7] Natarajan, Srikant; Ranjan, Jyoti; Boaz, Karen. (2012). Museum mounting techniques: Revisited econo-mode. *Indian Journal of Pathology and Microbiology*. 55(2): 260–261.

[8] Parasakthi M. (2020). Scope and features of museum setup techniques in oral pathology. *JBPR [Internet].* [cited 2024Sep.8];9(5).

[9] Latiff, Amir, Din, Aisha, Bin Munshi, Muhammad Afif, Alashkham, Fatma. (2023). Adapting medical museums: Technology, education, and research. *Environment-Behavior Proceedings Journal.* 8. 197–204. 10.21834/e-bpj.v8i26.5171.

[10] Mahesh Kumar U, Vayugundla Venkata Sai Raj Kumar. (2019). Role of innovations in pathology museum in imparting knowledge among medical students – a hospital based prospective study. *International Journal of Contemporary Medical Research* 6(6):F39–F44.

[11] Zhang X, Hu J. (2022). A study on the learning experience of visitors of digital museums in STEAM education: From the perspective of visitors' visual evaluation. *Front Psychol.* 13:994693.

[12] Walmsley AD, Lambe CS, Perryer DG, Hill KB. (2009). Podcasts–an adjunct to the teaching of dentistry. *Br Dent J.* 206(3):157–160

[13] Pereira AC, Dias da Silva MA, Patel US, Tanday A, Hill KB, Walmsley AD. (2022). Using quizzes to provide an effective and more enjoyable dental education: A pilot study. *Eur J Dent Educ.* 26(2):404–408.

[14] Johnson, D.W., and Johnson, R.T. (2009). An educational psychology success story: Social interdependence theory and cooperative learning. *Educational Researcher* 38(5), 365–379.

[15] Laurillard, D. (2013). *Rethinking University Teaching: A Conversational Framework for the Effective Use of Learning Technologies.* Routledge.

[16] Schmidt, H.G., Wagener, S.L., Smeets, G.A., Keemink, L.M., and Van Der Molen, H.T. (2015). On the Use and Misuse of Lectures in Higher Education. *Health Professions Education.* 1(1):12–18.

[17] Alzer H, Ismail NH, Alsoleihat F. (2023). Blended learning with video demonstrations enhances dental students' achievements in tooth carving. *Adv Med Educ Pract.* 14:1425–1431.

[18] Kumar GNP, Urs ANR, Undi M, Bakkannavar SM. (2022). Online viva voce as a formative assessment method in forensic medicine during COVID-19 pandemic. *J Educ Health Promot.* 11:160

[19] Dabbagh, N. and Kitsantas, A., (2012). Personal learning environments, social media, and self-regulated learning: A natural formula for connecting formal and informal learning. *The internet and Higher Education*, 15(1),3–8.

Navigating Dental Education Trends and Transforming Dental Pedagogy – Abas and Srikant N (Eds)

The Rewards and Roadblocks of Competency-Based Dental Education

Sumita Upadhyay
Department of Pediatric and Preventive Dentistry, Kathmandu University School of Medical Sciences, Dhulikhel, Nepal

ABSTRACT: Competency-based education (CBE) has appeared as a transformative approach in dental education. This paradigm shift aims to produce graduates who are not only knowledgeable but also competent in the clinical skills required for professional practice. While there are marked benefits of CBE including a more personalized learning experience and preparing the dentists that are well-equipped to meet the evolving demands of dental care, several challenges go along with its implementation. Significant change in the educational philosophy, the resistance to change by the faculty and students, the need for extensive faculty development, the logistical complexities of assessment and curriculum design may be the roadblocks to be faced. To address these roadblocks a meticulous planning and a commitment to continuous improvement is required. This narrative review provides a balanced analysis of the advantages and challenges valuable for dental educators and administrators for implementing competency-based programs to develop well-rounded, competent, and confident dental graduates for the future.

Keywords: Competency - based education, dental education, curriculum development, faculty development, challenges

1 INTRODUCTION

The word "competency" in health professional education implies the behavior that is anticipated of self - dependent clinicians which involves acknowledging the skills and it's worth in combined response to the various clinical situations encountered. [1]

The competencies for general dentists given by the American Dental Education Association (ADEA) include critical thinking, professionalism, interpersonal and communication skills, health promotion, practice management and the use of informatics and patient care. [2] The assessments of competency levels the candidate from novice to expert. [3]

The traditional curriculum consists of the incremental delivery of content aimed at imparting knowledge and the learners are expected to retain it. In addition, it is teacher oriented and content focused and leads to more of the mechanical mode of learning with an overloaded curriculum. The system has been found to fail to provide students adequate exposure in critical thinking and decision making when they have to face circumstances in professional practice. [4]

Competency-based education (CBE) has a role of transforming the dental education scenario. The students acquire self-directed capabilities to apply the knowledge in clinical skills. On this basis, there has been a shift from teacher-centered conventional learning to student-centered learning. This paradigm shift aims to produce graduates who are not only knowledgeable but also competent in the clinical skills required for professional practice.

While there are marked benefits of CBE, including a more personalized learning experience and the preparation of dentists that are well - equipped to meet the evolving demands of dental care, several challenges accompany its implementation.

This narrative review aims to provide a balanced analysis of the advantages and challenges in implementing competency - based dental education evidenced in the literature.

2 METHODS

A literature search of PubMed and Google Scholar was performed via the following key terms: "competency-based education", "dental education", "curricular development", "faculty development", "challenges".

The search was bound to full-texts published from 2019 - 2024.

The inclusion criteria for selecting studies were as follows:

- Publications focused on competency-based education specifically in the field of dentistry.
- Studies and reviews that discussed the benefits, challenges, or implementation of Competency - based dental education (CBDE)

 DOI: 10.1201/9781042016075-45

The exclusion criteria were as follows:

- Literature that primarily addressed competency-based education in fields other than dentistry
- Studies published in languages other than English.
- Articles that lacked relevance to the topic

3 RESULTS

The search yielded a total of 180 articles. Based on the inclusion and exclusion criteria, 120 articles were excluded and a total of 20 articles which were highly relevant to the topic were selected for the narrative review.

The content of the review was divided into two parts:

3.1 *Rewards of competency - based dental education (CBDE)*

Personalized learning experience:

The effectiveness of conventional lecture classes has been questioned by educationists. CBE in contrast, incorporates flipped classrooms, which transfer the responsibility for learning from teachers to students. The students learn at their own pace and mode, gathering information from various resources, with teachers being the facilitator. Students are given flexibility in space and time, and they can evaluate their own learning. They are being closely observed, and timely feedback is given by the teacher. [5,6]

Another education method in CBE is scaffolding, where the educator with cautious planning gradually lowers the support for the content, methods and learning strategy for the students to make them competent. There is no pressure for the student for the time they take. [7,8]

Assessment for learning:

With CBE, there is a transfer of focus from "assessment of learning" to "assessment for learning". The students can reflect their performance with self-assessment and are encouraged to fill the gaps to develop the skills. Both the teachers and students become collectively responsible for the assessment. Entrustable professional activities (EPAs) and Workplace-based assessments (WBAs) are based on actual "doing" of the top level of Miller's pyramid has been considered the judicious method of professional competence appraisal. [9,10]

Enhanced clinical preparedness:

Graduates whose education was competency based were more qualified in communication and critical assessment than those who opted for conventional learning. [11,12]

3.2 *Roadblocks*

Difficulty in adoption:

Concerns of incomplete adoption have been reported, possibly because the construct of competency - based education is understood inconsistently, leading to varying levels of adoption across institutions and universities, differing acceptance among administrative authorities, faculty, and students, disparities in applying to various educational specialities, and a wide range of perceptions regarding its impact or benefits. [13,14]

Resource implementation:

CBDE demands major changes in organizational and faculty roles to promote curriculum change and assessment. [15,16] The process also presents a significant logistical challenge. For the transformation from traditional education to CBE, well adoption of teaching techniques is imperative. [17]

Challenges in assessment:

There are questions regarding authenticity for the assessment of CBE. [13] The assessing tool; portfolios, focus on evaluating an individual's 'performance' rather than their 'competence' or overall ability to perform. When the activities are measured against rubrics or checklists, learners may reach the required threshold without being fully motivated to develop true competence. This undermines the core rationale of CBE. [4]

4 DISCUSSION

The benefits of CBDE, particularly in enhancing clinical preparedness are significant and align with the evolving needs of the dental profession. The focus on real-world competencies ensures the graduates to be efficient technically and capable of critical thinking and overcoming the challenges in clinical practice. Personalized learning pathways also allow students to achieve mastery at their own pace, potentially leading to more confident and competent practitioners.

The transition from traditional education to CBE will inevitably impact stakeholders, especially those directly associated with the educational system, such as the institution, faculty, students, and boards responsible for designing and implementation of the curriculum. The rationale for CBDE should be effectively conveyed to them through professional development programs for successful implementation. These programs or modules can be supported by dental education regulatory authorities, made partially mandatory, or incentivized to encourage participation. [4]

A blueprint of the curriculum must be formed that includes all the components, competencies, learning objectives and pedagogical approaches including assessments. [11]

The dental schools in Canada rely on the competencies established by the Association of Canadian Faculties of Dentistry (ACFD). It comprises forty-seven competences for the graduates. [18–20] Additionally, many professional organizations utilize the Can-MEDS framework to recognize the key competencies in the students,. [21] However, the curriculum content should be based on community needs. [22]

Teachers must adopt the position of facilitators and get acquainted with teaching strategies that effectively support learners in achieving the desired learning objectives. The technique of assessments should be carefully developed or selected to measure the desired competencies accurately. Research have shown positive correlation of clinical requirements completed by students with their competence. So, to produce competent graduates, some clinical quota should go along with the competency assessments. [23] Additionally, the competency of teachers is just as crucial as that of students. [24]

After the implementation of the curriculum, it should be evaluated regularly. Considering the educational requirements with the changing era, there is also need for incorporating Artificial Intelligence (AI) into the curriculum. [25]

To strengthen the dental education in India and to meet the international standards, the Dental Council of India has also processed the transformation to CBDE in the country. India comprises the highest number of dental schools among south Asian countries. A positive outcome from this crucial step may inspire neighboring countries to take similar actions. [26]

5 CONCLUSION

The rewards of CBDE particularly in producing well-prepared, lifelong learners who are equipped to respond the challenges of modern dentistry outweigh the roadblocks, provided that institutions are willing to commit to the necessary changes. Policy makers, administrators and facilitators should adopt the best approach to develop competent graduates for the best health care delivery in the country.

REFERENCES

[1] Chambers DW, Gerrow JD. (1994). Manual for developing and formatting competency statements. *J Dent Educ*.1994;58:361–6.

[2] American Dental Education Association Competencies for the new general dentist. *J Dent Educ* 2008;72:823–826.

[3] Dreyfus S, Dreyfus H. (1980). A five-stage model of the mental activities involved in directed skill acquisition. *California University Berkeley Operations Research Center [monograph on the Internet]*; 1980. Available from: https://apps.dtic.mil/dtic/tr/fulltext/u2/a084551.pdf. (accessed on 29 March 2019).

[4] Khanna R, Mehrotra D. (2019). The roadmap for quality improvement from traditional through competency based (CBE) toward outcome-based education (OBE) in dentistry. *J Oral Biol Craniofac Res*. 9(2):139–142.

[5] https://flippedlearning.org/wp%20content/uploads/2016/07/FLIP_handout_FNL_Web.pdf.

[6] Anitha KV, Prakash PSG. (2023). "Competency-based dental education": An upcoming learning approach. "Competency-based dental education": An upcoming learning approach. *J Interdiscip Dentistry*. 2023;13:51–2.

[7] https://www.buffalo.edu/catt/teach/develop/build/scaffolding.html#:~:text=Scaffo

[8] Hurtubise, L., Hall, E., Sheridan, L., and Han, H. (2015). The flipped classroom in medical education: engaging students to build competency. *J Med Educ Curric Dev*. 2: 35

[9] Tonni I, Gadbury-Amyot CC, Govaerts M, Ten Cate O, Davis J, Garcia LT, Valachovic RW. (2020). ADEA-ADEE Shaping the Future of Dental Education III: Assessment in competency-based dental education: Ways forward. *J Dent Educ*. 4 (1):97–104.

[10] Wolcott MD, Mason MR, Broome AM, Tittemore AJ, De Rossi SS, Quinonez RB. (2020). Faculty perspectives of an entrustable professional activity (EPA) framework in predoctoral dental education. *J Dent Educ*. 84(9):955–963.

[11] Yip HK, Smales RJ. (2000). Review of competency-based education in dentistry. *Br Dent J*. 189(6):324–6.

[12] Deogade SC, Naitam D. (2016). Discipline-based versus competency-based education in dentistry. *European Journal of Pharmaceutical and Medical Research*. 3(1):269–272.

[13] Licari FW, Chambers DW. (2008). Some paradoxes in competency-based dental education. *J Dent Educ*. 72(1):8–18.

[14] Koshy E, Nair KC, Annamma LM, Gurumurthy V. (2024). "Competency based dental education - A narrative review". *Acta Sci Dent Sci*. 8(8):74–83.

[15] Briggs CL, Patston PA, Knight GW, Alexander L, Norman N (2013). Fitting form to function: reorganization of faculty roles for a new dental curriculum and its governance. *J Dent Educ*. 7(1):4–16.

[16] Hunt RJ, Bushong M. (2010). ADEA CCI vision focuses on preparing graduates for discoveries of the future. *J Dent Educ*. 74 (8):819823.

[17] Maart RD, Adam RZ, Frantz JM. (2023). Strategies to implement competencies as it relates to a competency framework in a dental undergraduate curriculum: A systematic review. *Eur J Dent Educ*. 27(3):746–755.

[18] Whitney EM, Walton JN, Aleksejuniene J, Schönwetter DJ. (2015). Graduating dental students' views of competency statements: Importance, confidence, and time trends from 2008 to 2012. *J Dent Educ.*79:322–30.

[19] Gerrow JD, Murphy HJ, Boyd MA. (2006). Competencies for the beginning dental practitioner in Canada: A validity survey. *J Dent Educ.* 70:1076–80.

[20] Frank JR, Danoff D. (2007). The CanMEDS initiative: Implementing an outcomes-based framework of physician competencies. *Med Teach.* 29:642–7.

[21] Ghafoor, Sarah and Junaid Sarfraz Khan. (2019). "Outcome-based Dental Education and Identification of Practice Gaps; A Narrative Review." *J Pak Dent Assoc.* 28(1):41–46.

[22] Lagali-Jirge V. (2015). Need for paradigm shift in Indian dental education: A case for change toward competency-based education. *J Ind Acad Oral Med Radiol.* 27(2):230–236.

[23] Marchan, S.M., Coldero, L.G. and Smith, W.A. (2023). An evaluation of the relationship between clinical requirements and tests of competence in a competency-based curriculum in dentistry. *BMC Med Educ* 23: 585.

[24] Chuenjitwongsa S, Oliver RG, Bullock AD. (2018). Competence, competency-based education, and undergraduate dental education: a discussion paper. *Eur J Dent Educ.* 22(1):1–8.

[25] Busch F, Hoffmann L, Truhn D, Ortiz-Prado E, Makowski MR, Bressem KK, Adams LC; (2024). COMFORT Consortium. Global cross-sectional student survey on AI in medical, dental, and veterinary education and practice at 192 faculties. *BMC Med Educ.* ;24(1):1066.

[26] Deshpande AN, Mathur VP, Lele GS, Nirmal L, Saha S, Muthu MS, Marwah N, Khanna R, Anandakrishna L. (2024). Identifying needs and preparing for curriculum changes in indian dental education. *Int J Clin Pediatr Dent* 17(7):842–850.

 ISBN: 978-1-041-32674-8

Integration of Oral and Overall Healthcare by Enhancing Competencies Among Health Professionals for Improved Primary Prevention: An Interprofessional and Collaborative Approach

Supriya Nambiar
Department of Orthodontics & Dentofacial Orthopedics, Manipal College of Dental Sciences Mangalore, Manipal Academy of Higher Education, Manipal, India

Soumendra Sahoo
MMMC, Melaka Manipal, Malaysia, Manipal Academy of Higher Education, Manipal

Ciraj A.M
Melaka Manipal Medical College Manipal, MFILIPE Manipal, Manipal Academy of Higher Education, Manipal, India

Asavari Desai
Department of Orthodontics & Dentofacial Orthopedics, Manipal College of Dental Sciences Mangalore, Manipal Academy of Higher Education, Manipal, India

Anupama Nayak
Department of Paedodontics, Manipal College of Dental Sciences Mangalore, Manipal Academy of Higher Education, Manipal, India

Mithun Pai
Department of Public Health Dentistry, Manipal College of Dental Sciences Mangalore, Manipal Academy of Higher Education, Manipal, India

Nanditha Sujir
Department of Oral Medicine & Radiology, Manipal College of Dental Sciences Mangalore, Manipal Academy of Higher Education, Manipal, India

ABSTRACT: **Introduction:** Health professions Education and practice has always been in silos. Increased collaboration among healthcare workers helps to reduce disease burden **Aim**: Assess the knowledge and attitude about oral health, oral and systemic link among healthcare learners **Methods:** The project comprised of a needs assessment survey among medical practitioners of a tertiary hospital in India. An objective assessment of an interprofessional group of healthcare learners was done. Teaching modules designed by AIIMS, CDER was used as educational tool. **Results**: Medical practitioners had sound knowledge regarding oral health but had inadequate knowledge about oral–systemic link and 98% felt interprofessional education in healthcare is the need of the hour. Pre and post educational module assessment of the interprofessional learner groups showed that social work group had the least knowledge and medical students had the highest that was statistically Significant with a p value of <0.001. **Conclusion**: The needs based survey elicited great enthusiasm for interprofessional collaboration from medical practitioners even terming it as the need of the hour for bridging the gap between oral and systemic health. Oral Health awareness was the least among the social work students compared to nursing students and Medical students.

Keywords: Health professional, Oral-systemic health link, Interprofessional collaboration

1 INTRODUCTION

Oral health is integral to general health and can restrict activities in school, at work and at home, causing loss of productive hours. Moreover, there is diminished quality of life due to psychosocial impact of these diseases. The strong correlation between most oral diseases and noncommunicable systemic diseases is due to the common risk factors. Many general disease conditions also have oral manifestations. There are several barriers to oral healthcare like, a lack of acknowledgement of the importance of oral health, perception of oral health as independent and secondary to general health, no access to an oral health provider due to geographic distance, dental treatment is unaffordable and quality of dental treatment is varied. Singh et al. [1] suggested integrating oral health into general health so that it becomes more acceptable to the community, thereby addressing oral care inequality in India. But, grass-root level health workers and doctors do not have adequate knowledge about oral hygiene and prevention of

 DOI: 10.1201/9781042016075-46

oro-dental problems [2]. Kothia et al [3] have summarized the need for National Oral Health Policy involving oral health promotion through prevention, narrowing the rural-urban gap, organizing a data recording system, quality dental education; and definite budget allocation for oral health as seen in developed countries. This was initiated in India through the National Oral Health Program to provide integrated, comprehensive oral healthcare in existing facilities with the main objective of integrating oral health promotion and preventive services with general healthcare system at various levels of the primary healthcare system. The Directorate General of Health Services and Ministry of Health & Family Welfare, Government of India launched this primary preventive oral health care program focused on primary prevention, which is most cost effective, appropriate and desirable. [4] It is therefore, essential that to combat oral diseases, preventive approach including health education and promotion be given prime importance. The need of the hour is to develop an accessible, low-cost, sustainable primary preventive program using the existing health infrastructure and resources. Thus for this purpose, oral health education of the health workers ,school teachers and public is the main strategy and awareness generation is the major component of the oral health. But with the present scenario of healthcare professionals confined to their silos, Medical professionals continue to be taught and practice in a "medical" way, nurses in a "caring" way, and dentists and dental hygienists in a "dental" way, with an absolute lack of communication between these healthcare professionals [5].

The role that a healthcare professional can play in bridging the divide between oral and systemic health, depends on , his/her own knowledge about oral disease and its effect on general health, his attitude towards an interprofessional practice to improve patient health. The importance of sound oral health for better function, esthetics and psychological wellbeing, should be stressed by the medical and other healthcare professionals. This calls for an integrated educational environment for health care learners. Therefore the aim of this study was to assess change in knowledge and attitudes towards primary prevention in oral & systemic health care using a collaborative and interprofessional approach among healthcare learners.

2 MATERIALS AND METHODS

This was a cross-sectional study done over a period of 18months from October 2018 to January 2020 as part of an Interprofessional project of FAIMER Fellowship . Permission was obtained from the concerned authorities and Ethical clearance (protocol no :18128) was obtained from the institutional review board. List of medical faculty were obtained from the University website. The sample size was calculated based on total of 200 medical practitioners at our tertiary hospital at Mangalore. With confidence level of 95% and design effect 1, sample size was estimated to be around 90 participants. Considering 10% nonresponse rates 80 was taken as final sample size for the needs assessment. Prior to the start of the educational module, a needs assessment survey regarding the project was undertaken among the medical fraternity .This was done using a validated google form questionnaire distributed as email among 80 medical doctors from Mangalore with more than 2 years of post-specialty work experience. A pretested anonymous google form questionnaire was mailed to each participant and were individually asked to voluntarily complete and acknowledge the submission. Majority of the filled questionnaires were obtained back immediately. Those faculties who failed to respond, a 1-week time was given, and questionnaires were then mailed a second time. It was designed in English, was validated externally as well as internally, and modifications were then made accordingly before the final questionnaire was administered. A pilot study was conducted on 10 subjects selected randomly, to pretest the method and pilot study subjects were not included in the main study. For reliability of the questionnaire, a questionnaire was mailed twice to the respondents, 1-week apart and the co-efficient of reliability were calculated. Questionnaire had three parts. One consisted demographic information such as age, gender and years of experience in practice. Part two assessed their knowledge regarding preventive oral health care. Twenty statements regarding prevention of early childhood caries, periodontal diseases, oral cancer, malocclusion, and dental visit assessed the respondent's knowledge of prevention. Part three assessed attitudes of medical practitioners toward interprofessional collaborative primary preventive oral health care.. After the needs assessment survey ,an inter professional sample of 119 healthcarelearners were decided upon which comprised of 36 medical students from KMC, Mangalore, 44 Nursing students from Indira Hospital ,Mangalore, and 39 Social work students from Roshni Nilaya, Mangalore. Teaching modules and pre and post questionnaires were designed such that a health care learner will be able to understand the basic problem, correlate it with systemic health and refer to a dental setup. Modules used for oral health care awareness was designed on the National Oral Health Mission modules obtained from CDER ,AIIMS, New Delhi with key areas of focus. The key areas of focus were Early child hood caries & Dental Caries ,Gingival & Periodontal problems, Crowding, peri-oral procumbency & Jaw discrepancies , Eruption &Shedding schedule-basic description , Habits Assessment and Counselling, Identification of precancerous lesions, Demonstration of oral hygiene measures. Resource persons with relevant professional background was recruited from the dental institution with emphasis on the faculty specialty. An objective assessment of the inter professional team was done using a internally and externally validated questionnaire prior to the educational module. After the Teaching module session, the participants were subjected to the same questionnaire for the post test. During this post test session, the participants were reassessed for their knowledge level on oral health. Descriptive statistics included means and standard deviation of the respondent's knowledge and attitude scores.

3 RESULTS

The participants in the needs assessment phase presented with a mean age of 38.6 years. Of 59 participants, 60 % were males and 40 % females. Knowledge of preventive dental care in expectant mothers and neonates with relation to caries was the most accurate except for the timing of oral health check during pregnancy . When comparing overall knowledge of preventive dental care, there was not much statistically significant differences found for knowledge related to prevention of caries, periodontal diseases, habits, and malocclusion. Positive attitudes were expressed by almost all the respondents who felt interprofessional collaboration as essential (5.1%), need of the hour (6.8%), and valuable (12%) to the community. There was only a single negative attitude indicating that collaboration is not a good idea.(1.7%).

The Awareness lectures with pre & posttest shows that among the medical Students the difference between the pre and post scores was around 3.306 which was statistically significant with a p value of 0.004.The Nursing students showed higher post score with a difference of 10.7 which was statistically significant with a p value of <0.001. The Social Service students on comparison had a higher post score with a difference of 17.718 which was statistically significant with a p value of <0.001. Comparison of the three groups showed that social work students group has the highest differential value of 17.72 and medical students has the least value of -3.31. This difference is statistically Significant with a p value of <0.001. Posthoc Tukey tests comparing Nursing and Medical students showed a mean difference of 14.0 which is statistically significant with a p value of <0.001. Comparing nursing and social work students groups showed a mean difference of -7.013* that is statistically significant with a p value of <0.001. Comparing medical and social work student groups showed a mean difference of -21.024* that is statistically significant with a p value of <0.001.(Table 1)

Table 1. Comparison of the differences between post- and pre-values among the three groups via one-way ANOVA with Tukey's post hoc test.

	Difference between pre & post assessment			
Groups	N	Mean	Sd	F value
Nursing	44	10.7	6.515	91.543
Medical	36	3.31	6.351	
Social work	39	17.72	7.56	
Total	119	8.76	10.871	

Dependent variable		Difference between pre & post		
(I)group	(J)group	Mean diff	Std Error	P value
Nursing	Medical	14.010*	1.535	<0.001
	Socialwork	-7.013*	1.502	<0.001
Medical	Social work	-21.024*	1.578	<0.001

4 DISCUSSION

This study was undertaken to emphasize the importance of Interprofessional collaboration in primary preventive oral health care .The study subjects were selected from a pool of medical students ,nursing students and social work students because Anganavadi workers , ASHA workers and school teachers have been the personnel of interest in projects undertaken by the National oral health awareness project. Datta A and Datta [6] conducted a study on "Nutritional counselling in prevention of caries – a team approach" and they concluded that a collaborative effort is mandatory for the successful implementation of nutritional counseling in pediatric medical and dental settings as it is time to think and act together. Folayan MO et al [7] ,concluded that there is a significant role of mothers in promoting adoption of caries risk preventive measures by children and maternal oral health behavior is the most significant factor that had effect on the oral health behavior of children aged .They also emphasized the important role of mothers in helping children develop good oral health practices. This led to the assumption that the best method to impart training to the mothers are through the medical and allied health personnel with whom they interact most. So, training for medical and allied health personnel were undertaken. The major strength of the project methodology was that this training was imparted to an interprofessional group of health workers which helps them to open up to more possibilities regarding patients overall health care rather than being restricted to their silos. The needs based survey that was undertaken was to understand the response of the medical professionals towards interprofessional collaboration in primary preventive oral healthcare which can help in bridging the gap between oral health and systemic health. This elicited great enthusiasm from medical practitioners, some even terming it as the need of the hour. Oral Health awareness was the least among the social work students compared to nursing students and Medical students which can be attributed to the greater knowledge from the curriculum that is available for the medical and nursing students unlike the social service students. The extent of application of this knowledge in every day patient care is questionable and will have to be assessed in a case based Inter professional scenario.

Medical professionals are the key personnel who can play a very important role in improving overall health of patients because of their knowledge as well as their clinical day to day experience. [8,9] They encounter a lot of oral health problems among patients during their practice such as tooth ache, swelling in oral cavity, bleeding gums, various white and red patches, which, on regular examination of the oral cavity can be identified at the initial stages and thereby leads to an early referral. Dental conditions like caries and gingival problems are quite insidious in nature, often with no pain or overt symptoms and, if left untreated, will continue to destroy both gum tissue and the underlying bone. This condition poses a threat to overall health too or can be a manifestation of a systemic problem. Overall, the medical practitioners in this study showed positive attitudes towards interprofessional collaboration in oral and systemic health care, terming it as being essential, useful, and valuable. This is a positive indication that they too envisage a greater interprofessional interaction in oral systemic healthcare. As practice was not included in the study, prevention-oriented knowledge and attitudes found may not, however, translate to participant's everyday professional activity.

5 CONCLUSION

From the current study it can be concluded that the medical professionals possess a very good level of awareness regarding the impact of oral diseases on general health, but that is not translated to a routine oral checkup during medical examination. For better overall patient health, an interprofessional team-based care is the most promising answer. But to attain the objective of IPP in healthcare, one has to begin with interprofessional education. The findings of this study highlight the need for integrating systemic and oral healthcare utilizing a more collaborative and interprofessional mode of education of healthcare learners, so that patients will benefit from this transfer of knowledge and also will lead to increased referrals to the dental setup.

REFERENCES

[1] Singh, S. *et al.* (2015). Oral health inequality and barriers to oral healthcare in India. *European Journal of Dental Treatment and Research*, 4, 242–245.

[2] Ramya K, Prasad KVV *et al*, (2011). "Public oral primary preventive measures: An Indian perspective", *Journal of International Oral Health*, October, 2011,Volume 3; Issue 5.

[3] Kothia, N.R. *et al.* (2015). Assessment of the status of National Oral Health Policy in India. Int. *Journal of Health Policy Management*, 4, 575–581.

[4] Kharbanda .O.P, Dhingra.K;" (2017). Oral health inequality in India: Perspectives and solutions "[*Nature India Special Issue: Oral Health Inequalities and Health Systems in Asia-Pacific*] https://doi.org/10.1038/nindia.2017.29 Published online 20 March 2017.

[5] Valachovic.W.R;" (2019). Integrating oral and overall health care: Building a foundation for interprofessional education and collaborative practice. *Journal of Dental Education*, Volume 83, Number 2 Supplement.

[6] Ankush Datta, and Geetika Datta, (2014). "Nutritional counseling in prevention of caries – A team approach." *International Journal of Dental Sciences and Research*, vol. 2, no. 6B: 31–33. doi:10.12691/ijdsr-2-6B-9.

[7] M.O Folayan, Kikelomo A, *et al.*, (2015). Prevalence, and early childhood caries risk indicators in preschool children in suburban Nigeria, *BMC Oral Health*. 2015; 15: 72. Published online 2015 Jun 30. doi: 10.1186/s12903-015-0058-y

[8] Jorge Hernn Ramirez; Roger Arce; Adolfo Contreras, (2010). Why Must Physicians Know about Oral Diseases? *Teaching and Learning in Medicine*, 2010; 22(2): 148–55

[9] Atchison.K.A *et al.* Integrating oral health and primary care in the changing health care landscape", *NC Medicaljournal.com, NCMJ* vol. 78, no. 6.

Navigating Dental Education Trends and Transforming Dental Pedagogy – Abas and Srikant N (Eds)
© 2027 The Author(s), ISBN: 978-1-041-32674-8

Evaluating the Impact of Team-Based Learning Versus Didactic Methods on Long-Term Performance and Student Satisfaction in Dental Education

Vaishali K, Karishma Jagadeesh, and Vibha Shetty
Faculty of Dental Sciences, Ramaiah University of Applied Sciences, Bengaluru

ABSTRACT: Advanced online instructions have partially replaced traditional didactic lectures in education. This study compares the effects of online and offline team-based learning (TBL) and didactic methods on long-term assessment results and student satisfaction.

Objective:
To compare

(1) Long-term evaluation results comparing didactic and TBL approaches
(2) Student satisfaction with didactic and TBL delivery, both offline and online
(3) Student satisfaction using didactic and TBL approaches

Methods:
The topics of dental materials were divided into didactic and TBL approaches. For TBL, nine subgroups of six to seven dental students, comprising groups of sixty first-year and sixty second-year UG students learning the subject of dental materials, were randomly assigned. Three days before the session, a voice-over PowerPoint presentation was sent. The individual readiness assurance test (iRAT) and the team readiness assurance test (tRAT) were administered to the students. Following the evaluation, the facilitator reiterated important points and assigned application-based issues or debate-focused conversation to each subgroup. A more challenging posttest was given to each student individually. Test results and feedback were gathered via Google forms. Long-term evaluation was carried out at the end of the year.

Results:
Long-term evaluation scores were greater with topics taught with TBL than didactic. However, students preferred didactic over TBL approaches, expressing greater satisfaction with offline modes for both.

Conclusion:
Although the didactic approach was still the technique of choice for the students, they admitted that TBL enhanced their critical thinking, reasoning, teamwork and presentation confidence. The changing nature of education and its effects on student outcomes are highlighted in this study.

Keywords: Team-Based learning, Didactic, Online and Offline teaching

1 INTRODUCTION

In Indian dental education, students study dental materials extensively in the first two years, focusing on their composition, chemical processes, applications, and limitations. Traditionally, a didactic approach has been used, relying heavily on rote memorization. This method often fails to engage students, making it difficult for them to understand and apply the material clinically. Studies have shown that students in both dental hygienist and dental hygienist programs struggle with exams on dental materials due to a lack of emphasis on self-directed learning and critical thinking [1]. Moreover, traditional teaching methods do not effectively foster essential skills such as teamwork and communication.

Student-centered learning approaches, such as team-based learning (TBL), offer a more interactive and engaging alternative. TBL emphasizes preparation before class and collaborative group work, which can enhance critical thinking and application skills. TBL has been effectively used in various clinical education settings, including prosthodontics and oral pathology [2–4]. It has been shown to be comparable to case-based learning (CBL) and the flipped-classroom model [5].

The COVID-19 pandemic accelerated the shift to online education, making virtual learning environments commonplace. This transition necessitated adapting traditional teaching methods to online formats. TBL, with its inherent flexibility, adapts well to online platforms such as MS teams. This study aims to compare the effects of online and offline Team-Based Learning (TBL) and Didactic methods on long-term assessment results and student satisfaction.

DOI: 10.1201/9781042016075-47

1.1 *Objective:*

To compare

(1) Long-term evaluation results comparing didactic and TBL approaches
(2) Student satisfaction with didactic and TBL delivery, both offline and online
(3) Student satisfaction using didactic and TBL approaches

2 MATERIALS AND METHODS

2.1 *Research design*

This longitudinal comparative study evaluated students' satisfaction and performance via TBL versus traditional didactic methods, comparing both online and offline delivery.

2.2 *Ethical approval*

The study was approved by the Health Professions Education Unit and the ethical committee of Ramaiah University of Applied Sciences.

2.3 *Sampling and participants*

The study involved 120 students from the first and second years of dental education, with 60 students from each year. All the participants were new to the TBL approach. The topics related to dental materials were divided into TBL and traditional didactic methods. Three authors, who served as facilitators, were involved in the preparation, administration, and evaluation of the study.

2.4 *Team-based learning (TBL)*

(1) Preclass Preparation:
- The students received a voice-over PowerPoint presentation and video clips (5–8 minutes) on dental materials three days before the session.
- These materials were shared via email and WhatsApp to support self-directed learning.

(2) In-class schedule:
- **Individual Readiness Assurance Test (iRAT):** This test was conducted via Google Forms with 10 multiple-choice questions. To assess cognitive learning of individual student through pre-class preparation from study material provided.
- **Team Readiness Assurance Test (tRAT):** The class of 60 was randomly divided into 9 teams of 6–7 members. The teams were decided on ad hoc basis without prior assessment of individual scores, as these students were new to the topic of Dental Materials. Teams answered the same questions with group discussions and submitted a single response. To assess the effectiveness of team learning and team activity in collectively answering the same assessment, using the same pre learning material sent. The intention was to convey to the students the advantages of peer discussion and learning.
- **Facilitator discussion:** The facilitator reviewed the iRAT and tRAT answers with clarification on the topics. This was followed by the facilitator presenting the salient points of the reading material to reinforce the subject and give the students an opportunity to clarify any uncertainties on the topic.
- **Application-Based Questions and Discussion:** Facilitators presented 3-4 application-based questions, which students discussed in teams and presented their answers. Teams were evaluated in terms of the breadth and quality of their answers, teamwork, and speed.
- **Individual Posttest:** Students completed a more challenging posttest to assess higher-level understanding and retention.

(3) Postclass feedback: Feedback data were collected via Google Forms to gauge student satisfaction with the class.

2.5 *Didactic teaching method*

Topics not covered by TBL were taught via traditional didactic methods. These sessions involved a PowerPoint presentation by the faculty, which focused on the composition, chemistry, uses, advantages, disadvantages, and clinical applications of the dental materials. Students attended these lectures without prior preparation and took notes during class. Feedback was collected through Google Forms.

Online vs. offline formats:

- **Online Format:** Due to the COVID-19 pandemic, classes were delivered online via MS teams for both TBL and didactic methods. The breakout room feature in MS teams was used for team discussions.
- **Offline Format:** In-person classes were organized with physical team spaces and writing boards for collaborative activities.

Postclass feedback survey:
A survey was conducted to assess student experiences with both didactic and TBL methods in online and offline formats. The survey was divided into three phases:

- Preparation for the Class
- Understanding and Retention in the Class
- Perception of the Class

Responses were rated on a 5-point Likert scale ranging from strongly agree (5) to strongly disagree (1).
Long-term assessment:
To assess the long-term impact of team-based learning (TBL) versus didactic methods, students' year-to-end exam scores were analyzed on questions from both methods.

3 RESULTS

(1) Long-term assessment: Long-term evaluation results comparing didactic and TBL approaches revealed significantly higher scores for topics taught with TBL than for those taught with didactic approaches. TBL not only enhances the understanding and application of material in the short term but also contributes to better long-term retention and recall.

On the basis of the feedback from 104 out of 120 students who completed the survey on teaching methods, several key insights have emerged regarding didactic and team-based learning (TBL) approaches in both online and offline formats:

(2) Preference for Offline Classes: Students expressed a clear preference for offline classes over online classes. They found offline settings to be more conducive to teacher–student and peer interactions. This face-to-face engagement facilitated better participation, respect for different viewpoints, and overall teamwork.

(3) Didactic vs. TBL methods:

- Didactic Method: Students favored the didactic approach over TBL in both online and offline formats. They reported that the traditional lecture-based method provided a clearer understanding and better grasp of the finer details of the subject matter.
- TBL Method: While TBL has advantages, such as improved peer interaction and application-based learning, which increase the understanding of material, students note some challenges. The longer duration of TBL sessions was found to be tiring, and discussions were occasionally dominated by more articulate students, which could impact the overall effectiveness of group activities.

Despite its drawbacks, TBL was appreciated for fostering teamwork and increasing confidence in presentations. The method's focus on practical application of knowledge and peer collaboration was recognized as valuable in enhancing students' learning experiences.

4 DISCUSSION

In Indian dental education, the study of dental materials is crucial but often challenging due to the theoretical nature of the subject and limited clinical exposure. Traditional didactic methods, which focus on rote learning, fail to engage students and often result in poor retention and application of knowledge [6].

TBL was introduced to address these issues by encouraging self-directed learning and active participation. Compared with traditional didactic methods, TBL significantly improved student engagement, understanding, and retention; similar results were reported in studies conducted by Hattie J. *et al.* and Burgess A. *et al.*. [7,8]. The ability to discuss and apply concepts in teams enhanced critical thinking and application skills.

The shift to online learning due to the COVID-19 pandemic revealed both opportunities and challenges. The online TBL maintained its effectiveness but faced issues such as reduced interaction and distractions. Offline TBL sessions were preferred by students because of better interaction and engagement, although they required more logistical planning.

The long-term assessment results indicate that topics taught via the team-based learning (TBL) approach yield higher retention rates than those taught via the didactic method do. While the didactic method may offer clearer immediate understanding and a more straightforward delivery of content, the TBL method appears to be more effective in helping students retain and recall information over a longer period. This underscores the value of TBL in promoting deeper learning and sustained engagement with the subject matter.

The preference for traditional didactic methods in both online and offline formats highlights the need to balance familiar teaching styles with innovative methods such as TBL. Students may need time to adapt to more active learning approaches, which can be more demanding than passive lecture-based methods.

5 CONCLUSION

TBL offers a valuable alternative to traditional didactic methods by fostering teamwork, communication, and the application of knowledge. It provides significant benefits in enhancing student engagement and understanding. However, the TBL needs to be adapted to shorter, more focused modules to accommodate shorter attention spans. Despite the advantages of online learning, offline teaching methods still have significant benefits in terms of interaction and engagement. Future studies should explore these methods further and consider integrating TBL more effectively into dental education. Limitations of this study include the sample size and lack of a control group, which may affect the generalizability of the results. Further research could involve larger sample sizes and diverse educational contexts to validate these findings.

ACKNOWLEDGMENT

This was a nonfunded study conducted in the Faculty of Dental Sciences, Ramaiah University of Applied Sciences, Bengaluru, Karnataka, India.

All changes made have been highlighted in this document.

All the reviewers' comments have been acknowledged.

Thank you.

REFERENCES

[1] Gali S, Shetty V, Murthy NS, Marimuthu P. (2015). Bridging the gap in 1st year dental material curriculum: A 3 year randomized cross over trial. *The Journal of Indian Prosthodontic Society*. 15(3):244–9.

[2] Echeto L. (2016). Removable partial denture components and applications: a team-based learning module. *MedEdPORTAL*. 12:10408.

[3] Haley CM, Brown B, Koerber A, Nicholas CL, Belcher A. (2020) Comparing case-based with team-based learning: dental students' satisfaction, level of learning, and resources needed. *Journal of dental education*. 84(4):486–94.

[4] Hayama R, Okura K, Oshima M, Hosoki M, Suzuki Y, Miyagi M, Inoue M, Rodis OM, Matsuka Y. Comparison between flipped classroom and team-based learning in a prosthodontic class at Tokushima University.

[5] Nishigawa K, Omoto K, Hayama R, Okura K, Tajima T, Suzuki Y, Hosoki M, Shigemoto S, Ueda M, Rodis OM, Matsuka Y. (2017). Comparison between flipped classroom and team-based learning in fixed prosthodontic education. *Journal of Prosthodontic Research*. 61(2):217–22.

[6] Zachry AH, Nash BH, Nolen A. (2017). Traditional lectures and team-based learning in an occupational therapy program: A survey of student perceptions. *The Open Journal of Occupational Therapy*. 5(2):6.1–10

[7] Hattie J, Timperley H. (2007). The power of feedback. *Review of Educational Research*. 77(1):81–112.

[8] Burgess A, Mellis C. (2015). Feedback and assessment for clinical placements: achieving the right balance. *Advances in Medical Education and Practice*. 373–81.

 ISBN: 978-1-041-32674-8

Edutainment in Dental Education Trends and Practices: A Review

Mithun Pai BH
Associate Professor, Department of Public Health Dentistry, Manipal College of Dental Sciences Mangalore, Manipal Academy of Higher Education, Manipal, Karnataka, India

Shweta Yellapurkar
Associate Professor, Department of Oral pathology and Microbiology, Manipal College of Dental Sciences Mangalore, Manipal Academy of Higher Education, Manipal, Karnataka, India

ABSTRACT: The neologism for the two most significant elements of childhood—education and entertainment—is edutainment. Its etymology can be traced back to the great Walt Disney, who created a series of health-based programs for the neighbourhood dentist Tommy Tucker's Tooth. Education is a crucial component of health promotion, but it often seems to fall on deaf years because dental education can be rather dull and repetitive.

Methods:

An integrated, comprehensive search was carried out in the following databases: PUBMED and Scopus. Two independent reviewers performed the searches to identify the primary studies. The P.V.O. framework (P = Population, V = Variable, and O = Outcome) was used to develop the research question. After the determination of the databases to be utilised, articles were gathered via descriptors or keywords.

Results:

The review revealed that only four articles were found in the literature for the given keywords with the necessary inclusion and exclusion criteria.

Conclusion:

The review highlights only two studies from the literature that provided insights into the use of edutainment in dental education. The review also highlights the minimal use of edutainment in the dental curriculum.

Keywords: Dental education, Edutainment, curriculum, review

The neologism for the two most significant elements of childhood—education and entertainment—is edutainment. Its etymology can be traced back to the great Walt Disney, who created a series of health-based programs for the neighbourhood dentist Tommy Tucker's Tooth. Later, when filming for the National Geographic Society, *sociologists* Marshal McLuhan and actor B. Heyman *popularised* the term. Education has been applied in many spheres of life, but it *has been* especially successful in promoting health and helping drug addicts get well. In fact, the idea of edutainment was deemed so successful that many businesses, including technical management firms, adopted it as a means of employee training. Gerald Lesser, a Harvard psychologist and educator who pioneered edutainment, created the children's television program "Sesame Street," which aimed at integrating multiculturalism with learning [1] [2].

Education is a crucial component of health promotion, but it often seems to fall on deaf years because dental education can be rather dull and repetitive. Therefore, to capture the interest of the students, more recent and interesting models of dental teaching tools must be provided. A new trend in education called "SERIOUS GAMES FOR HEALTH" uses games to train and instruct people in a variety of fields, including the military, business, education, and patient care, among others [3]. These games have been used in rehabilitation and to promote healthy habits, benefiting patients and professionals alike. They are also valuable partners in health education, training, and simulation.

In the current technological age, a tool that can be easily integrated into education is entertainment education or edutainment. This technology, when used as a medium of instruction, promotes active learning, which holds the key to increasing students' interest, motivation, and active engagement in learning. Puzzles, video games, mime, animation, and other activities that surprise and delight students while they are learning can all be considered forms of educational entertainment. On the basis of communication and multimedia technology, multimedia provides alternatives that are both educational and enjoyable. One of its most important functions is the translation of narrative activities into visual representations. The use of a variety of media, including text, design, graphics, images, audio, video, and animation, to better communicate a message is known as multimedia [3,4].

A novel substitute for conventional education is edutainment. It can be separated on the basis of the intent and substance of each part and can be further classified as:

 DOI: 10.1201/9781042016075-48

1) Edutainment, or informal education, enhances consumers' life control. Usually, conversation or story formats are used to present it.
2) Experience-based education (skill education). Typically, experiences such as simulations (virtual mobility) are used to demonstrate it.

Edutainment can be classified according to the target group:

1) Motivation-oriented (individuals with similar interests, irrespective of age, current degree of expertise, etc.).
2) Age-oriented [5].

Maintaining a balance between instruction and entertainment is a difficulty when creating edutainment content. The implementation of educational materials that are neither arduous nor overly engaging is a desirable goal [5].

1 METHODS

An integrated, comprehensive search was carried out in the following databases: PUBMED and Scopus. Two independent reviewers performed the searches to identify the primary studies. The searches were carried out in August 2024, with an initial time limit of the last 10 years.

The P.V.O. framework (P = population, V = variable, and O = outcome) was used to develop the research question, which was "Edutainment that is aimed at education in the dental curriculum?" After the determination of the databases to be utilised, articles were gathered via descriptors or keywords. Making this choice is necessary to have access to documents related to the subject of study.

The factor used to choose which studies to include was their relevance to the research issue, which was assessed by looking at the study's title, descriptors, and abstract. The following factors were then used to define the inclusion criteria: a) design: methodology where edutainment was used as the teaching medium; b) target population: dental students; and c) language: English.

The exclusion criteria included (1) papers from editorial reviews and literature reviews that involved developing or applying the material for a purpose other than teaching and (2) protocols of observational or intervention studies.

The studies were chosen and assessed via two filters during this procedure. The selection of pertinent publications functioned as the first filter.

2 RESULTS

The review revealed that only four articles were found in the literature for the given keywords with the necessary inclusion and exclusion criteria. The following are the articles.

Authors	Title	Year	Journal
Demirjian A; David B;	Learning medical and dental sciences through interactive multimedia [6].	1995	Medinfo. MEDINFO
Harikiran AG; Vadavi D; Shruti T;	Beta Testing an Oral Health Edutainment Card Game Among 12-13-Year-Old Children in Bangalore, India [7].	2017	Games for health journal
Mehrotra P;	Edutainment in dental curriculum-A systematic review [4].	2020	Journal of Oral Biology and Craniofacial Research
Pamungkas A C; Suharsini M S; Rizal M F;	Enhancing Cognitive Comprehension of Dental Health Education Using Mobile Apps in Down Syndrome Children [8].	2024	Journal of International Dental and Medical Research

3 DISCUSSION

A curriculum is a vital part of the educational process that not only helps students achieve their educational goals but also helps teachers form a blueprint of what is included in the process, such as a list of subjects, learning tools, class time, lesson plans, and assessment methods. A curriculum can be considered the "core" of any educational program. With the government implementing new policies for education, the importance of the curriculum has increased many-fold. The way our society has changed has made the curriculum a dynamic process that needs to be looked into and revamped and sometimes overhauled at regular intervals.

Edutainment involves providing education amalgamated with invention, learning and fun for not only students but also teachers and educators. This didactic tool shifts learning from teacher centric system to a student-centric system and motivates students to actively engage in the learning process. This may also help students overcome apprehension and boredom, thus improving their overall understanding of the process.

The following review was conducted to understand edutainment in the field of dental education. The field of dentistry has accomplished much from its inception, and the dental curriculum has developed from its focus being teacher centric to student focal. The review has been an eye opener, as searches revealed that very few articles are published in the field of edutainment in the dental curriculum. The field of dentistry, with its various specialties, would be an ideal field of study for edutainment. An array of developments can be made in the same way.

The scope for edutainment in the field of dentistry is unlimited. The articles above are a mixture of experimental studies and reviews that have utilised edutainment in various aspects of education, with the exception of the study conducted by Harikiran et al. [7] in Bangalore, which explored the development of a card game aimed at allowing children to take proper care of their oral health, which is part of oral health promotion rather than curriculum implementation.

In 1995, Demirjian and David [6] discussed the use of edutainment in the fields of medicine and dentistry. The study revealed new resources that are used to instruct and learn about a range of medical areas, especially dentistry and dermatology. Numerous educational software programs have been created, covering diverse facets of the discipline: skin cancer, dental development, temporomandibular joint, and masticatory muscles.

In 2020, Mehrotra P [4] conducted a systematic review on the use of gaming, animation and miming as edutainment tools in the dental curriculum and discussed their usage and limitations. The study examined one article that used animation as a stand-alone tactic and one that used it to augment traditional lectures. All the publications stressed that animation should be used only as an additional teaching tool, not as a substitute for traditional teaching methods.

A clinical study by Pamungkas A Cin 2024 [8] evaluated the effectiveness of educational mobile apps in promoting oral health knowledge and daily practices among a sample of 34 children with Down syndrome accompanied by their mothers. They also detailed the use and feasibility of the apps.

4 CONCLUSION

The review highlights only two studies from the literature that provided insights into the use of edutainment in dental education. The review also sheds light on the minimal use of edutainment in the dental curriculum. A bright and exciting future is ahead for edutainment, a very promising auxiliary teaching and learning tool. Surprisingly, the concept has been found to be less useful in the field of clinical dentistry, when used along with virtual reality, it might have a major effect on learning in dentistry.

REFERENCES

[1] Michael B. *the animated man A life of walt disney. first.* University of California Press;

[2] Corona F, Cozzarelli C, Palumbo C. Information Technology and Edutainment : Education and Entertainment. 2013;(December 2015).

[3] Rahmani N, Davoodabadi F, Noormohammadi R, Karamitanha F, Nourian A. Using Edutainments in Teaching Orthodontic Lateral Cephalometric and Dental Cast Analysis. *J Med Educ.* 2023;22(1):1–8.

[4] Mehrotra P. Edutainment in dental curriculum-A systematic review. *J Oral Biol Craniofacial Res.* 2020 Oct 1;10(4):417–21.

[5] Walldén S, Soronen A. Edutainment: From television and computers to digital television. Univ Tampere Hypermedia Lab. 2004;(May):72.

[6] Demirjian A, David B. Learning medical and dental sciences through interactive multimedia. *Medinfo.* 1995 Jan 1;8 Pt 2:1705–1705.

[7] Harikiran AG, Vadavi D, Shruti T. Beta Testing an Oral Health Edutainment Card Game Among 12–13-Year-Old Children in Bangalore, India. https://home.liebertpub.com/g4h. 2017 Dec 1;6(6):334–42.

[8] Pamungkas AC, Suharsini MS, Rizal MF. Enhancing Cognitive Comprehension of Dental Health Education Using Mobile Apps in Down Syndrome Children. *J Int Dent Med Res.* 2024;17(2):578–82.

Navigating Dental Education Trends and Transforming Dental Pedagogy – Abas and Srikant N (Eds)
© 2027 The Author(s), ISBN: 978-1-041-32674-8

Incorporating Digital Technology into Teaching Curriculum in Orthodontic Postgraduate Education: A Review of Benefits and Drawbacks

Shravan Shetty
Department of Orthodontics and Dentofacial Orthopedics, Manipal College of Dental Sciences Mangalore, Manipal Academy of Higher Education, Manipal, Karnataka, India

ABSTRACT: **Objective:** This review examined the integration of digital technology into orthodontic postgraduate education and compared its effectiveness with that of traditional teaching methods. Outcome-based education (OBE), learning management systems (LMSs), and massive open online courses (MOOCs) were examined, highlighting their impact on educational outcomes and clinical preparedness. **Significance of the Review and Contribution to the Field:** The findings underscore how digital technologies, such as three-dimensional imaging, computer-aided designing, and virtual reality, have transformed orthodontic education by enhancing learning flexibility, precision in treatment planning, and alignment with contemporary clinical practices. The incorporation of OBE frameworks and LMS platforms facilitates the effective tracking of educational outcomes and personalized learning experiences. Interactive platforms further contribute by increasing student engagement and providing diverse assessment tools. **Highlights of key trends, patterns, and gaps in the literature:** A comprehensive literature search was conducted across four major databases (PubMed, Scopus, Web of Science, and Google Scholar) from January 2000 to June 2024. The review identifies a consistent trend toward the adoption of digital tools to supplement and, in some cases, replace traditional teaching methods. Patterns show improved student performance and satisfaction associated with blended learning approaches. However, gaps in the literature remain, particularly regarding long-term outcomes and potential overreliance on technology in the educational setting. **Conclusion:** A balanced approach that integrates traditional and digital methods may provide a comprehensive educational experience. Future research should focus on establishing best practice guidelines and ensuring equitable access to digital technology for advancing orthodontic postgraduate education.

Keywords: Digital Technology, Outcome assessment, Computer-Assisted Instruction

1 INTRODUCTION

Digital technology has increasingly influenced orthodontic postgraduate education, offering innovative methods to enhance traditional learning practices. The integration of tools such as three-dimensional (3D) imaging, computer-aided design (CAD), 3D printing and virtual reality (VR) represents a significant shift in educational paradigms [1,2]. These digital tools facilitate a deeper understanding of complex orthodontic concepts and provide hands-on experience, which can be particularly beneficial in orthodontics, where visual and spatial understanding is crucial [3,4].

This review aims to examine the effectiveness of incorporating these digital tools into orthodontic curricula, comparing them with traditional teaching methods. It also explores outcome-based education (OBE) frameworks, learning management systems (LMSs), and massive open online courses (MOOCs) [5–7]. The significance of this review lies in its ability to shed light on how digital technologies can enhance learning experiences and clinical outcomes in orthodontics. Prior studies have shown that digital tools can improve precision and engagement, yet concerns about their long-term effectiveness and potential overreliance persist [8]. This review addresses these issues and contributes to the ongoing discourse on optimizing digital integration in orthodontic education.

2 METHODS

2.2 *Search Strategy and Criteria*

A comprehensive search was conducted via PubMed, Scopus, Web of Science, and Google Scholar. The search covered publications from January 2000 to June 2024, focusing on keywords such as "digital technology in orthodontics," "outcome-based education in orthodontics," "learning management systems" and "interactive teaching platforms".

2.3 *Inclusion and Exclusion Criteria*

The review included peer-reviewed articles, conference proceedings, and book chapters published in English. Eligible studies addressed digital technology, including 3D diagnosis, 3D printing in orthodontic postgraduate education, comparisons between traditional and digital methods, or evaluations of specific digital tools. Nonpeer-reviewed articles and those lacking methodological rigor were excluded. Studies that provided empirical data on the effectiveness of digital tools compared with traditional methods were prioritized.

3 RESULTS

The search yielded 1,500 studies. After applying the inclusion and exclusion criteria, 30 studies were included in the final analysis. These studies provide a broad perspective on the trends, benefits, and challenges associated with digital technology in orthodontic education.

Sl no	Author, Year	Aim of the Study	Study Type and Technology Accessed	Results	Conclusion	Strength and Limitation
1	Koolivand H, et al. (2024)	Compare the effectiveness of virtual reality-based education vs conventional teaching in dental education	Systematic review; Virtual Reality (VR)	VR-based education may improve student engagement but lacks definitive evidence of superior learning outcomes	VR education is a promising adjunct to traditional methods but needs further research for conclusive benefits	Strength: Comprehensive review of available studies; Limitation: Limited high-quality studies in the area
2	Alhamed FJ, et al. (2023)	Assess pre-doctoral dental students' education, knowledge, attitudes, and behavior regarding CAD/CAM	National survey; CAD/CAM technology	Students had moderate knowledge and positive attitudes but variable behavior toward CAD/CAM use	Incorporating CAD/CAM into the curriculum can enhance students' readiness for digital dentistry	Strength: Large sample size; Limitation: Self-reported data may introduce bias
3	Sytek L, et al. (2021)	Compare orthodontic residents' performance and attitudes using 2D, 3D, and VR surgical simulation methods	Comparative study; 2D, 3D, VR simulations	VR simulations improved spatial understanding and confidence in residents compared to 2D methods	VR offers a more immersive learning experience, potentially leading to better surgical outcomes	Strength: Direct comparison of different modalities; Limitation: Limited to short-term performance
4	Sipiyaruk K, et al. (2023)	Explore the role of technology-enhanced simulation-based learning in orthodontic education	Scoping review; Simulation technology	Technology-enhanced learning can supplement traditional education, improving skill acquisition	Simulation-based learning is effective but requires integration with conventional methods for comprehensive education	Strength: Wide scope covering various technologies; Limitation: Lack of standardized outcome measures
5	Ehlinger C, et al. (2023)	Review the use of entrustable professional activities (EPAs) in dental education	Scoping review; EPA framework	EPAs are increasingly used to assess competence but require better implementation strategies	EPAs could standardize competency assessment but need clearer guidelines for use in dental education	Strength: Addresses a gap in assessment methods; Limitation: Variability in EPA definitions across studies
6	Farhadi Z, et al. (2024)	Assess the need for MOOCs in medical school curriculum from the perspective of instructors and students	Need assessment study; MOOCs	Both students and instructors recognize the potential of MOOCs but identify challenges in integration	MOOCs can enhance medical education if properly integrated into the existing curriculum	Strength: Dual perspective (instructors and students); Limitation: Context-specific findings may not be generalizable
7	Al-Nuaimi MN, et al. (2022)	Evaluate the use of learning management systems (LMS) during the COVID-19 pandemic	Theoretical model evaluation; LMS	LMS usage increased significantly, but effectiveness varied depending on user proficiency	LMS are vital for remote learning but require ongoing support and training for effective use	Strength: Timely study during the pandemic; Limitation: Theoretical model may not capture all practical challenges
8	Grissinger M. (2019)	Understand human over-reliance on technology in healthcare settings	Observational study; Technology in healthcare	Over-reliance on technology can lead to errors and reduced critical thinking	Balancing technology use with human judgment is essential in healthcare	Strength: Highlights a critical issue in healthcare; Limitation: Observational nature limits causality
9	Furqon M, et al. (2023)	Examine the impact of LMS usage on students' learning outcomes	Empirical study; LMS	LMS usage positively correlates with improved learning outcomes, particularly in resource-rich environments	LMS can enhance learning, but success depends on resource availability and user engagement	Strength: Quantitative data on LMS effectiveness; Limitation: Context-specific results may not apply universally
10	Al Mansoori A, et al. (2023)	Review technology-enhanced learning using LMS and VR goggles	Critical review; LMS, VR goggles	Technology can enhance learning, but integration challenges and accessibility issues remain	LMS and VR are valuable tools but require careful implementation to be effective	Strength: Covers emerging technologies in education; Limitation: Lack of empirical data in the review

Figure 1. Summary of Key Findings from Reviewed Studies.

11	Sezer B, et al. (2019)	Develop and validate a scale for LMS acceptance	Scale validation study; LMS	The scale was found to be valid and reliable for measuring LMS acceptance among students	The validated scale can be used to assess LMS adoption and guide improvements	Strength: Rigorous validation process; Limitation: Limited to one educational context
12	Barsaoui M, et al. (2021)	Investigate the effectiveness of Socrative as a tool for increasing student learning	Intervention study; Socrative (LMS)	Socrative usage improved engagement and understanding in students	Socrative is an effective tool for enhancing learning in interactive settings	Strength: Demonstrated effectiveness of a specific tool; Limitation: Small sample size limits generalizability
13	Reese D, et al. (2021)	Evaluate the Coursera MOOC 'Take the Lead on Healthcare Quality Improvement'	Evaluation study: MOOC	Participants reported improved knowledge and skills in healthcare quality improvement	MOOCs like Coursera can effectively supplement traditional healthcare education	Strength: Focus on a specific, practical MOOC; Limitation: Self-reported data may introduce bias
14	Stoilov L, et al. (2024)	Compare the efficacy of virtual preparation simulators vs. traditional preparations on phantom heads	Comparative study; Virtual preparation simulators	Virtual simulators provided comparable or better results in certain aspects of preparation	Virtual simulators are a viable alternative to traditional methods in dental education	Strength: Direct comparison with traditional methods; Limitation: Specific to dental preparation, may not generalize to other skills
15	San Diego JP, et al. (2022)	Compare haptic vs. phantom head dental chair simulators in teaching clinical skills	Cluster-randomized trial; Haptic simulators, Phantom head simulators	Haptic simulators were found to be as effective as traditional methods for teaching cavity preparation	Haptic technology offers a new avenue for teaching clinical skills in dentistry	Strength: Randomized controlled design; Limitation: Limited to cavity preparation, broader applications need testing
16	Plessas A. (2017)	Assess whether computerized VR simulation can replace conventional phantom heads in preclinical dentistry	Comparative study; VR simulation	VR simulations showed potential but were not sufficient to fully replace traditional methods	VR can supplement but not yet replace traditional dental education methods	Strength: Early exploration of VR in dentistry; Limitation: Limited scope and small sample size
17	Monaghesh E, et al. (2023)	Review the application of virtual reality in dental implants	Systematic review; VR in dental implants	VR is increasingly used for planning and training in dental implants but lacks comprehensive validation	VR offers significant potential for dental implantology, though further research is needed	Strength: Focus on a niche application of VR; Limitation: Early-stage technology with limited long-term data
18	Øvrebø LJ, et al. (2022)	Evaluate assessment methods and tools for critical care nursing students in clinical placements	Integrative review; Clinical assessment tools	A variety of tools are used, with varying effectiveness and acceptance among educators	A standardized approach to assessment in critical care nursing is needed	Strength: Comprehensive review of assessment tools; Limitation: Lack of consensus on best practices
19	Gosak L, et al. (2021)	Systematically review digital tools used in behavior change support education for health and other students	Systematic review; Digital tools for behavior change	Digital tools can support behavior change education, but effectiveness varies widely	Digital tools are useful adjuncts in education, requiring careful selection and implementation	Strength: Broad scope covering multiple tools; Limitation: Heterogeneity of tools and outcomes complicates conclusions
20	Raghunathan K, et al. (2023)	Baseline evaluation of nursing students' informatics competency for digital health practice	Descriptive exploratory study; Digital health tools	Nursing students showed varying levels of informatics competency, highlighting the need for better training	Improved training in digital health is crucial for preparing nursing students for modern practice	Strength: Addresses a critical area in nursing education; Limitation: Descriptive nature limits depth of analysis

Figure 1. (Continued)

3.1 *Enhanced Learning Flexibility and Engagement*

Digital tools, such as LMS platforms, enable asynchronous learning, allowing students to access course materials at their convenience and engage in interactive assessments that reinforce knowledge retention [9–11]. Interactive platforms such as Socrative and Coursera have been shown to increase student engagement by offering diverse assessment tools and fostering active participation [12,13]. These platforms also support peer interaction and collaborative learning, which are essential for developing critical thinking and problem-solving skills in orthodontics.

3.2 *Improved precision in treatment planning*

The use of 3D imaging for diagnosis, CAD for planning tooth movements and customizing orthodontic appliances, and three-dimensional printing technologies has significantly improved the precision of treatment planning and

21	Nagarajappa A, et al. (2024)	Explore current practices and future directions in simulation in medical education	Review article; Simulation technology	Simulation is widely used, but integration and standardization remain challenges	Simulation will continue to play a crucial role in medical education, but needs better integration	Strength: Overview of current and future trends; Limitation: Broad focus may lack depth in specific areas
22	Feenstra TM, et al. (2023)	Review digital tools used to train surgical skills, and conduct a meta-analysis	Systematic review and meta-analysis; Digital tools for surgical training	Digital tools are effective for surgical training, particularly in enhancing skill acquisition	Digital tools can enhance surgical training, but should complement, not replace, traditional methods	Strength: Meta-analysis provides strong evidence; Limitation: Variability in study quality and outcomes
23	Pandey R, et al. (2024)	Discuss the advancements in orthodontics through digital innovation	Review article; Digital tools in orthodontics	Digital tools are transforming orthodontic practice, with benefits in efficiency and patient outcomes	Digital innovation is revolutionizing orthodontics, though challenges remain in widespread adoption	Strength: Focus on a rapidly evolving field; Limitation: Limited empirical data on long-term outcomes
24	Cunha TMAD, et al. (2021)	Review orthodontic digital workflow and its clinical applications	Review article; Digital workflow in orthodontics	The digital workflow improves efficiency and accuracy in orthodontic practice	Digital workflow is becoming essential in modern orthodontic practice	Strength: Practical focus on workflow; Limitation: Limited discussion of implementation challenges
25	Naik N, et al. (2022)	Discuss legal and ethical considerations in AI in healthcare	Review article; AI in healthcare	AI presents significant legal and ethical challenges that need addressing before widespread adoption	Addressing legal and ethical concerns is crucial for the responsible use of AI in healthcare	Strength: Comprehensive review of critical issues; Limitation: Theoretical discussion may lack practical applicability
26	Radwan HA, et al. (2023)	Investigate perceptions, practices, and challenges of digital technologies in dentistry in Saudi Arabia	Survey study; Digital technologies in dentistry	Dentists are adopting digital technologies, but face challenges in training and infrastructure	Digital technology adoption in dentistry is growing, but more support is needed for effective use	Strength: Region-specific insights; Limitation: Limited generalizability beyond the study context
27	Jahangiri L, et al. (2020)	Explore the integration of digital dentistry in high-volume dental institutions	Observational study; Digital dentistry	Digital dentistry integration faces challenges, particularly in scaling and training	Successful integration of digital dentistry requires significant investment in training and infrastructure	Strength: Focus on practical challenges in large institutions; Limitation: Limited to high-volume settings
28	Soltanimehr E, et al. (2019)	Compare virtual vs. traditional education in dental radiographic interpretation	Comparative study; Virtual education tools	Virtual education was as effective as traditional methods for teaching radiographic interpretation	Virtual tools can supplement traditional education, but may not fully replace it	Strength: Focus on a specific skill; Limitation: Small sample size limits broader applicability
29	Hakami Z. (2021)	Compare virtual and traditional learning methods for orthodontic knowledge and skills	Quasi-experimental study; Virtual learning tools	Virtual learning was found to be effective, but not superior to traditional methods	Virtual learning is a viable alternative, but needs to be used alongside traditional methods	Strength: Direct comparison of learning methods; Limitation: Quasi-experimental design limits causality
30	Schenck A. (2024)	Examine the relationship between technology and critical thinking in South Korean EFL learners	Empirical study; Technology in education	Technology use was positively correlated with improved critical thinking skills	Technology can enhance critical thinking, but must be integrated thoughtfully into education	Strength: Focus on critical thinking, a key educational outcome; Limitation: Cultural context may limit generalizability

Figure 1. (Continued)

the realism of clinical simulations [1,2,14]. These tools allow students to visualize complex anatomical structures and practice preclinical and clinical procedures in a controlled environment, thereby enhancing their clinical skills [15–17].

3.3 *Alignment with Contemporary Clinical Practices*

Digital technologies ensure that orthodontic education aligns with current clinical practices, equipping students with up-to-date skills and knowledge. This alignment is crucial for meeting the demands of modern orthodontic practice and preparing students for the evolving landscape of clinical care. The integration of these digital tools during postgraduate education will help students learn about recent advances during their tenure and reduce their reliance on external laboratories for additional training in the future. The ability to integrate digital tools into treatment planning and execution prepares students for real-world scenarios and enhances their clinical competency [18–22].

3.4 *Challenges and drawbacks*

Despite their numerous benefits, the integration of digital technologies presents challenges, including high costs, potential overreliance, ethical issues and the need for continuous technical support [23–27]. Addressing these challenges is essential for optimizing the use of digital tools in education and maintaining a balanced approach that combines digital and traditional methods. Institutions must also consider the accessibility of technology and the potential need for faculty training to effectively implement and utilize these tools.

4 DISCUSSION

The integration of digital technology into orthodontic postgraduate education offers substantial benefits, including enhanced learning flexibility, increased student engagement, and improved precision in treatment planning [12–17]. Digital tools align educational practices with contemporary clinical demands, ensuring that students are well prepared for modern orthodontic practice. However, challenges such as high implementation costs and potential overreliance on technology must be addressed [23,27]. While digital tools can significantly enhance learning experiences, they should complement rather than replace traditional teaching methods [28,29]. A balanced approach that combines both digital and traditional methods is essential for providing a comprehensive educational experience. The review identifies gaps in the literature, particularly regarding the long-term outcomes of digital technology use and the risks of overreliance [25,26,30]. Future research should focus on these areas, establishing best practice guidelines for effective digital tool integration in orthodontic education. Efforts should also be made to ensure equitable access to digital technologies, especially in resource-limited settings. Figure 1 shows a summary of the key findings from the reviewed studies.

5 CONCLUSION

This review highlights the transformative impact of digital technology on orthodontic postgraduate education, including benefits such as enhanced learning flexibility, engagement, and precision in treatment planning. A balanced approach that integrates digital and traditional methods is recommended to optimize educational outcomes.

REFERENCES

[1] Koolivand H, Shooreshi MM, Safari-Faramani R, Borji M, Mansoory MS, Moradpoor H, Bahrami M, Azizi SM. Comparison of the effectiveness of virtual reality-based education and conventional teaching methods in dental education: a systematic review. *BMC Med Educ.* 2024 Jan 3;24(1):8.

[2] Alhamed FJ, Neiva GF, Bak SY, Karl E, Inglehart MR. Predoctoral dental students' computer-aided design/computer-aided manufacturing-related education, knowledge, attitudes and behavior: A national survey. *J Dent Educ.* 2023 Apr;87(4):562–571.

[3] Sytek L, Inglehart MR, Ramaswamy V, Aronovich S, Edwards S, Kim-Berman H. Comparisons of orthodontic residents' performance and attitudes using 2D, 3D, and virtual reality surgical simulation methods. *J Dent Educ.* 2021 Aug;85(8):1415–1426.

[4] Sipiyaruk K, Kaewsirirat P, Santiwong P. Technology-enhanced simulationbased learning in orthodontic education: A scoping review. *Dental Press J Orthod.* 2023 Jul 17;28(3):e2321354.

[5] Ehlinger C, Fernandez N, Strub M. Entrustable professional activities in dental education: a scoping review. *Br Dent J.* 2023 Feb;234(3):171–176.

[6] Farhadi Z, Rezaei E, Bazrafkan L, Amini M, Sanaiey NZ, Barati-Boldaji R, Mehrabi M. Need assessment of medical school curriculum for MOOCs: perspectives of instructors and students of Shiraz University of Medical Sciences. *BMC Med Educ.* 2024 Feb 13;24(1):141

[7] Al-Nuaimi MN, Sawafi OSA, Malik SI, Al-Emran M, Selim YF. Evaluating the actual use of learning management systems during the covid-19 pandemic: an integrated theoretical model. *Interactive Learning Environments* 2022; 31:6905–30.

[8] Grissinger M. Understanding Human Over-Reliance on Technology. *P T.* 2019 Jun;44(6):320–375.

[9] Furqon M, Sinaga P, Liliasari L, Riza LS. The Impact of Learning Management System (LMS) Usage on Students. *TEM Journal* 2023:1082–9.

[10] Al Mansoori A, Hamdan A, Harraf A, Buallay A, Arora P, Alsabatin H. Technology enhanced learning through learning management system and virtual reality googles: a critical review. In: Hamdan A, Harraf A, Buallay A, Arora P, Alsabatin H, editors. *From Industry 4.0 to Industry 5.0.* Cham: Springer; 2023. p. 470.

[11] Sezer B, Yilmaz R. Learning management system acceptance scale (LMSAS): a validity and reliability study. *Australas J Educ Technol.* 2019;35(3):15–30.

[12] Barsaoui M, Riahi H. Socrative as a tool for increasing students learning. *Tunis Med.* 2021 Avril;99(4):399–403.

[13] Reese D, Dolansky MA, Moore SM, Bolden H, Singh MK. Quality improvement education innovation: evaluation of Coursera MOOC 'Take the Lead on Healthcare Quality Improvement'. *J Res Nurs.* 2021 Mar;26(1-2):62–78.

[14] Stoilov L, Stephan F, Stark H, Enkling N, Kraus D, Stoilov M. Efficacy of Virtual Preparation Simulators Compared to Traditional Preparations on Phantom Heads. *Dent J (Basel).* 2024 Aug 14;12(8):259.

[15] San Diego J.P., Newton T.J., Sagoo A.K., Aston T.A., Banerjee A., Quinn B.F.A., Cox M.J. Learning Clinical Skills Using Haptic vs. Phantom Head Dental Chair Simulators in Removal of Artificial Caries: Cluster-Randomized Trials with Two Cohorts' Cavity Preparation. *Dent. J.* 2022;10:198.

[16] Plessas A. Computerized Virtual Reality Simulation in Preclinical Dentistry: Can a Computerized Simulator Replace the Conventional Phantom Heads and Human Instruction? Simul. *Healthc.* 2017;12:332–338.

[17] Monaghesh E, Negahdari R, Samad-Soltani T. Application of virtual reality in dental implants: a systematic review. *BMC Oral Health.* 2023 Aug 28;23(1):603.

[18] Øvrebø LJ, Dyrstad DN, Hansen BS. Assessment methods and tools to evaluate postgraduate critical care nursing students' competence in clinical placement. An integrative review. *Nurse Educ Pract.* 2022 Jan;58:103258.

[19] Gosak L, Štiglic G, Budler LC, Félix IB, Braam K, Fijačko N, Guerreiro MP, Lorber M. Digital Tools in Behavior Change Support Education in Health and Other Students: A Systematic Review. *Healthcare (Basel).* 2021 Dec 21;10(1):1.

[20] Raghunathan K, McKenna L, Peddle M. Baseline evaluation of nursing students' informatics competency for digital health practice: A descriptive exploratory study. *Digit Health.* 2023 May; 9:20552076231179051.

[21] Nagarajappa A, Kaur S. Simulation in contemporary medical education: Current practices and the way forward. *Indian J Anaesth.* 2024 Jan;68(1):17–23.

[22] Feenstra TM, van der Storm SL, Barsom EZ, Bonjer JH, Nieveen van Dijkum EJM, Schijven MP. Which, how, and what? Using digital tools to train surgical skills; a systematic review and meta-analysis. *Surg Open Sci.* 2023 Oct 4;16:100–110.

[23] Pandey R, Kamble R, Kanani H. Revolutionizing Smiles: Advancing Orthodontics Through Digital Innovation. *Cureus.* 2024 Jul 8;16(7):e64086.

[24] Cunha TMAD, Barbosa IDS, Palma KK. Orthodontic digital workflow: devices and clinical applications. *Dental Press J Orthod.* 2021 Dec 15;26(6):e21 spe6.

[25] Naik N, Hameed BMZ, Shetty DK, Swain D, Shah M, Paul R, Aggarwal K, Ibrahim S, Patil V, Smriti K, Shetty S, Rai BP, Chlosta P, Somani BK. Legal and Ethical Consideration in Artificial Intelligence in Healthcare: Who Takes Responsibility? *Front Surg.* 2022 Mar 14;9:862322.

[26] Radwan HA, Alsharif AT, Alsharif MT, Aloufi MR, Alshammari BS. Digital technologies in dentistry in Saudi Arabia: Perceptions, practices and challenges. *Digital Health* 2023;9.

[27] Jahangiri L, Akiva G, Lakhia S, *et al.* Understanding the complexities of digital dentistry integration in high-volume dental institutions. *Br Dent J.* 2020;229:166–168.

[28] Soltanimehr E, Bahrampour E, Imani MM, Rahimi F, Almasi B, Moattari M. Effect of virtual versus traditional education on theoretical knowledge and reporting skills of dental students in radiographic interpretation of bony lesions of the jaw. *BMC Med Educ.* 2019 Jun 25;19(1):233.

[29] Hakami Z. Comparison between Virtual and Traditional Learning Methods for Orthodontic Knowledge and Skills in Dental Students: A Quasi-Experimental Study. *Healthcare (Basel).* 2021 Aug 24;9(9):1092.

[30] Schenck A. Examining Relationships between Technology and Critical Thinking: A Study of South Korean EFL Learners. *Education Sciences* 2024;14:652.

Navigating Dental Education Trends and Transforming Dental Pedagogy – Abas and Srikant N (Eds)
 ISBN: 978-1-041-32674-8

Role of Gatekeepers in Suicide Prevention Among Medical and Dental Students

Amoli Singh

Department of Orthodontics and Dentofacial Orthopedics, Manipal College of Dental Science Mangalore, Manipal Academy of Higher Education, Manipal, Karnataka, India

Ann Sales

Department of Prosthodontics and Crown and Bridge, Manipal College of Dental Science Mangalore, Manipal Academy of Higher Education, Manipal, Karnataka, India

ABSTRACT: Suicide is a critical public health issue, and medical and dental students are at heightened risk due to academic pressures, emotional exhaustion, and fear of professional repercussions, all of which contribute to mental health challenges. Gatekeeper training programs have emerged as a prominent strategy for suicide prevention, equipping peers, faculty, and health professionals with the skills to identify, support, and refer students in crisis. This scoping review explores the effectiveness of gatekeeper training in suicide prevention within medical and dental school environments, drawing from a variety of studies that focus on both specialized student populations and broader university settings. A review of the literature from PubMed, PsycINFO, and Google Scholar was conducted, with a focus on studies published within the last 15 years. The evidence suggests that gatekeeper training improves the ability to identify at-risk students and increases confidence in intervention skills. Key outcomes include enhanced referral behaviors, sustained mental health awareness, and a reduction in stigma related to seeking mental health support. However, challenges remain regarding the long-term sustainability of gatekeeper skills and the need for continuous training reinforcement. In conclusion, gatekeeper training programs are valuable interventions for suicide prevention in medical and dental schools. These programs foster early identification of students in distress and promote a culture of mental health awareness. Future research should focus on developing standardized evaluation measures and integrating modern resources, such as telehealth, to extend the impact of gatekeeper programs. Additionally, institutional support is essential for reducing stigma and encouraging help-seeking behaviors among students.

Keywords: Gatekeeper training, suicide prevention, mental health, students, college counseling

1 INTRODUCTION

Suicide is a significant global public health concern, and one population that is particularly vulnerable to mental health issues is medical and dental students. These students face unique and immense pressures in their educational and professional lives, which increase their risk of mental health disorders, including anxiety, depression, and suicidal ideation. The demanding academic workload, pressure to succeed, and emotional exhaustion contribute to higher stress levels in medical and dental students than in other student populations. Research consistently shows that these students experience elevated rates of anxiety, depression, and suicidal thoughts. [1,2]

Despite the alarming prevalence of mental health issues, many students refrain from seeking help due to stigma surrounding mental health, fear of professional repercussions, and the belief that they should be able to cope with these stressors independently. This creates a critical gap in mental health support within academic environments. To bridge this gap, gatekeeper training programs have emerged as a key strategy in suicide prevention, particularly among high-risk groups such as medical and dental students. [3]

Gatekeepers, such as peers, faculty members, and campus health professionals, are trained to recognize early signs of mental distress, suicidal ideation, and crisis. They are equipped to provide immediate support and refer students to mental health services. [4] These programs aim to increase the capacity of individuals within educational institutions to act as first responders, ensuring that students in crisis receive help before reaching a breaking point. Gatekeeper programs have been shown to improve early identification and intervention in various educational settings, making them an essential safety net for medical and dental students. [4,5]

This scoping review aims to explore the effectiveness of gatekeeper training in preventing suicide among medical and dental students. By reviewing studies focused on these populations, as well as research from broader university contexts, this review seeks to provide a comprehensive overview of how gatekeeper programs function in academic environments and their potential for long-term impact.

DOI: 10.1201/9781042016075-50

2 METHODS

This scoping review followed a systematic approach to identify studies related to gatekeeper training for suicide prevention in medical and dental education. Article search was carried out in PubMed, PsycINFO, and Google Scholar for articles published within the last 15 years (2009-2024) using keywords such as "gatekeeper training," "suicide prevention," "mental health," "medical students," and "dental students." The search initially yielded 47 studies.

2.1 *Screening Process*

Out of the 47 studies retrieved, 25 articles were selected for a full-text review based on relevance to the topic and title and abstract screening. The inclusion criteria consisted of (1) studies focusing on gatekeeper training or suicide prevention within educational settings, particularly medical and dental schools, (2) studies published in peer-reviewed journals, and (3) studies with measurable outcomes related to intervention effectiveness.

2.2 *Exclusion Criteria*

The exclusion criteria consisted of (1) focused solely on clinical training without a mental health intervention component, (2) were opinion pieces or case studies without empirical data, or (3) did not specify educational settings.

3 RESULTS

In total, 8 articles were included in this review after meeting all inclusion criteria, with 17 studies excluded due to unrelated focus or lack of outcome measures. The review included randomized controlled trials, systematic reviews, and evaluation studies, with a focus on medical and dental student populations. Both specialized research on these student groups and broader university-based studies were considered to draw meaningful comparisons and insights. [6,7]

The studies reviewed highlight the effectiveness of gatekeeper programs in identifying and addressing mental health concerns. Below is a summary of key findings from studies focused on both medical and dental students and the general student population.

Study	Population	Study Design	Intervention	Key Findings/Outcomes
Bolton SL. (2020)	Medical students	Randomized Controlled Trial	Gatekeeper training for suicide intervention	Improved identification of at-risk students; increased confidence in intervention skills posttraining. [1]
Orovecz JJ. (2020)	University students (various disciplines)	Evaluation study	University-based gatekeeper training	Positive changes in knowledge, attitudes, and behaviors regarding suicide prevention posttraining. [2]
Wyman PA et al. (2008)	Secondary school staff	Randomized Controlled Trial	Gatekeeper program for school staff	Significant increase in staff's ability to identify at-risk students, lasting effect for over a year. [3]
Reiff M et al. (2019)	College students	Development and Evaluation	"I CARE" campus gatekeeper program	Enhanced mental health awareness and support for students in distress; improved referral behaviors. [4]
Holmes G et al. (2021)	Mixed populations (long-term review)	Systematic Review	Long-term efficacy of gatekeeper training	Sustained knowledge retention and improved intervention skills; highlighted the need for continuous reinforcement of training. [5]
Johnson LA, Parsons ME. (2012)	Adolescent school population	Implementation evaluation	Gatekeeper program for school nurses	Increased confidence in intervening with students showing signs of suicide risk. [6]
Curric Dev, (2021)	Healthcare professionals, including medical staff	Workshop-based training	Gatekeeper training in suicide prevention	Effective in equipping healthcare professionals to recognize, support, and refer at-risk students. [7]
Nomura K (2020)	University students and other sectors	Systematic Review	Gatekeeper programs across various sectors	National-level support increased implementation; highlighted need for more standardized outcome measures. [8]

4 DISCUSSION

The reviewed studies provide compelling evidence of the critical role that gatekeepers play in suicide prevention within medical and dental schools. Gatekeeper programs address the gap in early intervention by empowering individuals in educational environments to identify students in mental distress and guide them toward appropriate help. These programs not only increase the likelihood of timely interventions but also contribute to shifting institutional cultures toward greater mental health awareness.

The effectiveness of gatekeeper programs has consistently been highlighted across various studies. Training equips gatekeepers with the ability to identify behavioral and emotional signs of distress, which may not always be immediately apparent. For instance, subtle changes in mood, behavior, or academic performance often precede crises. Gatekeeper training provides individuals with tools such as active listening, empathy, and mental health literacy, enabling them to offer immediate support and guide students toward mental health services. [1,2,5] A study by Bolton [1] demonstrated that medical students trained in suicide interventions had a significantly increased ability to identify at-risk peers and greater confidence in their ability to intervene. This is crucial in high-pressure academic settings such as medical and dental schools, where students might hesitate to seek professional help due to stigma or concerns over confidentiality [2,3]. The findings from Orovecz's [2] evaluation of university-based gatekeeper training similarly emphasized positive behavioral and attitudinal changes, highlighting the broad applicability of these interventions. Furthermore, the broader evidence, such as that provided by the "I CARE" program [4], points to improvements not only in recognition and intervention but also in a shift in referral behaviors, where gatekeepers feel more empowered to encourage students to seek professional help. This improvement in referral behavior is particularly important because, in many cases, students experiencing distress may not recognize the severity of their situation or might be reluctant to seek help owing to fear of judgment.

While the immediate outcomes of gatekeeper training are well-documented, long-term sustainability remains a critical area for improvement. Several studies, such as those by Holmes et al. [5] and Nomura et al. [8], emphasize the importance of the continuous reinforcement of skills acquired through gatekeeper training. Holmes's systematic review [5] indicated that while gatekeepers retain basic knowledge and intervention skills shortly after training, the effects can diminish over time, particularly in environments where they are not frequently called upon to intervene. This finding suggests that, in the high-stress environment of medical and dental schools, regular refresher training sessions may be required to maintain the effectiveness of gatekeepers. Implementing follow-up programs or booster sessions could help ensure that gatekeepers continue to feel confident in their ability to identify and intervene in mental health crises. The Japan national-level review [8] further underscored the need for standardized outcome measures, as varying definitions of success and effectiveness make it difficult to compare results across studies and programs. Long-term evaluations should consider not only the retention of knowledge and skills but also the ability of gatekeepers to adapt to evolving mental health challenges. For example, as telemedicine and online mental health resources become more prevalent, future training programs should incorporate these tools to extend the reach and effectiveness of gatekeepers. This would allow gatekeepers to make more informed referrals, connecting students with a wider range of mental health services. [6,8]

Beyond training individuals, gatekeeper programs contribute to fostering a more supportive academic environment. Creating a culture that promotes mental health awareness is essential, especially in professional environments where students may perceive that seeking help could jeopardize their careers. In medical and dental schools, where students are often hesitant to display vulnerability, gatekeeper programs help reduce the stigma associated with mental health issues by normalizing conversations around emotional wellbeing. [7] The Advanced C.A.R.E program demonstrated how integrating mental health literacy and empathy into healthcare training environments creates a more supportive atmosphere. When gatekeepers are not only trained to intervene but also encouraged to promote mental health as part of their professional responsibilities, it becomes easier for students to seek help without fear of being stigmatized. This approach is particularly relevant in fields such as medicine and dentistry, where the pressure to appear competent and resilient can discourage individuals from acknowledging mental health struggles. Gatekeeper programs also serve as a bridge between students and mental health services, helping students overcome the barriers to seeking help. By establishing trust and reducing the stigma associated with mental health problems, gatekeepers can encourage students to access the necessary support sooner, thereby preventing the escalation of mental health issues into suicidal ideation or attempts [3,5]. This creates a more proactive, rather than reactive, approach to mental health care within educational institutions.

Despite the successes of gatekeeper programs, challenges remain. One of the key challenges is ensuring that the gatekeepers themselves are adequately supported. While these individuals are trained to assist others, they may also experience burnout, particularly in high-stress environments such as medical and dental schools. Institutions must ensure that gatekeepers have access to their own support networks, as well as opportunities for debriefing and self-care after difficult interventions [6]. Another challenge lies in integrating gatekeeper programs seamlessly into the academic environment. In some institutions, students and faculty may resist these programs because of time constraints or concerns over academic priorities. To overcome this, academic institutions must work to embed gatekeeper training into the broader curriculum, ensuring that mental health support is viewed as an integral part of student and faculty wellbeing. [5,7]

5 CONCLUSION

Gatekeeper programs are an essential component of suicide prevention strategies in medical and dental schools, helping to bridge the gap between distressed students and mental health services. These programs enhance the ability of gatekeepers to identify early signs of distress, provide emotional support, and refer students to appropriate resources. However, challenges such as sustaining long-term efficacy, reducing stigma, and ensuring adequate institutional support must be addressed for these programs to reach their full potential.

To further improve gatekeeper training, future research should focus on the development of standardized metrics to evaluate effectiveness, longitudinal studies to assess long-term outcomes, and the incorporation of modern mental health resources such as telehealth platforms. Additionally, institutions must prioritize fostering a supportive culture that encourages early help-seeking behavior, which ultimately enhances the mental wellbeing of students and reduces the risk of suicide.

REFERENCES

[1] Bolton SL, Gunnell D, Turecki G. Gatekeeper training for suicide intervention in medical students: A randomized controlled trial. *J Affect Disord.* 2020;276:252–259.

[2] Orovecz JJ. *Evaluating the impact of a university-based gatekeeper training on student attitudes, knowledge, and behaviors toward suicide prevention [master's thesis].* University of Florida; 2020.

[3] Wyman PA, Brown CH, LoMurray M, Schmeelk-Cone K, Petrova M, Yu Q, *et al.* An outcome evaluation of the Sources of Strength suicide prevention program delivered by adolescent peer leaders in high schools. *Am J Public Health.* 2010;100(9):1653–1661.

[4] Reiff M, Toro PA, Carrico AW. I CARE: A campus-wide gatekeeper training program for suicide prevention. *J Am Coll Health.* 2019;67(6):545–552.

[5] Holmes G, Clacy A, Hermens DF, Lagopoulos J. The long-term efficacy of gatekeeper training in suicide prevention: A systematic review. *Arch Suicide Res.* 2021;25(1):177–207.

[6] Johnson LA, Parsons ME. School nurses as gatekeepers: Implementing a school-based suicide prevention program for adolescents. *J School Health.* 2012;82(7):293–299.

[7] Advanced C.A.R.E. Program. Gatekeeper training for healthcare professionals: Results from a workshop-based intervention in suicide prevention. *J Med Educ Curric Dev.* 2021;8:238–245.

[8] Nomura K, Inoue S, Yamanouchi Y. A review of national-level gatekeeper training in Japan: Implications for suicide prevention. *J Public Health Policy.* 2020;41(3):123–131.

Navigating Dental Education Trends and Transforming Dental Pedagogy – Abas and Srikant N (Eds)
© 2027 The Author(s), ISBN: 978-1-041-32674-8

Preparing Dental Students for Career Success: As Part of the Curriculum

Yashodhara Hazra and Arathi Rao
Pediatric and Preventive Dentistry, Manipal College of Dental Sciences Mangalore, Manipal Academy of Higher Education, Manipal, Karnataka, India

Ramya Shenoy
Public Health Dentistry, Manipal College of Dental Sciences Mangalore, Manipal Academy of Higher Education, Manipal, Karnataka, India

ABSTRACT: Stress is a common experience that affects individuals at different stages of life. In academic settings, stress has been linked to impaired performance and mental health issues, including anxiety, depression, and substance misuse. Among dental students, stress is particularly prevalent due to the demanding curriculum, technique-sensitive procedures, and patient care responsibilities. Studies indicate that stress levels are especially high among final-year students, interns, and postgraduate dental students.

In this context, tools like the Job Seeking Self-Efficacy Scale (JSS), Perceived Stress Scale (PSS), and Dental Environmental Stress (DES) Questionnaire help assess stress levels and identify key stressors.

Addressing the mental health challenges associated with job-seeking and employment stress among dental graduates is crucial. Educational institutions should implement measures such as personalized career counseling, stress management workshops, skill development programs, and psychological support services. Additionally, updating university curricula and providing relevant training can better prepare students for the demands of the labor market. By adopting these strategies, institutions can improve students' well-being and facilitate a smoother transition from education to professional practice.

Keywords: academics, dental students, dental education, stress, unemployment, job-seeking

1 BACKGROUND

Everyone experiences stress at different stages of life. It is the body's response to change, which can be either positive—motivating and encouraging peak performance—or negative—leading to anxiety and reduced productivity. Both desirable and undesirable events can trigger stress, which may arise from mental or physical sources. People react to stress in different ways, and the intensity of their [1]

Stress has reportedly been shown to negatively impact students' academic performance. Reduced productivity in daily tasks and professional obligations, such as a decreased desire to learn, are a few consequences of stress. [1] Additional consequences of stress include psychological issues, which can negatively impact mental health.

2 STRESS AMONG DENTAL STUDENTS

Numerous studies have documented the pressures that students encounter during their academic journeys. [2–6] The results indicate that stress is related to training and the amount of coursework, particularly for those who provide patient care. Distress has been found to be very common among dentistry students. [2–5] Stress among dental students can stem from the demands of patient care and the rigorous, highly technique-sensitive curriculum. Higher stress levels are reported among final-year students, interns (junior residents), and postgraduate students. [5,7] After completing their dental education, these students enter a very competitive workforce. Stress can have an impact on a new dentistry graduate's ability to find employment or their choice of career. [5]

Upon entering the workforce, healthcare providers often encounter many problems. These challenges may develop throughout the shift from student to practitioner. At the undergraduate level, students also start to identify specific levels of difficulty in their future careers. Given the uncommon possibility that a dentist may decide to change careers after starting their practice, it is imperative that students in the dental sector understand the difficulties they may face in their future careers. It seems that anxiety about one's future profession throughout one's dental school is a widespread problem. [8] Another expected source of stress is the rapid expansion of dental schools in India, leading to an influx of newly graduated dentists entering the workforce. [9,10]

Education and employment play vital roles in determining people's futures and advancing the growth and development of a country. The problem of unemployment is a silent plague. Underemployment and unemployment have a negative influence on many facets of human functioning and lower an individual's mental health. [8,11]

In India, the field of dentistry has grown dramatically in recent years. Notably, both the number of dental colleges and the number of individuals entering the field have significantly increased during the past 15 years. However, the likely decline in dental jobs in the coming years due to oversupply and market saturation remain major issues for both professionals and the general public. [12] The dental curriculum is regarded as difficult, stressful, and complex, requiring a wide range of social, clinical, and intellectual abilities related to patient management. Dental students experience high levels of stress during training, which may be related to the extensive curriculum, extremely technique-sensitive procedures, and patient and time management. This stress may lead to increased mental health issues such as anxiety, depression, and substance misuse, as well as reduced work productivity, ultimately resulting in burnout.. Cooper et al., reported that, among all healthcare professions, dentistry was the most stressful. [13,14]

3 METHODS TO ASSESS STRESS

The Job-Seeking Self Efficacy Scale, Perceived Stress Scale and Dental Environment Stress Questionnaire (DES) are some of the scales that can be used to assess stress.

3.1 *The job-seeking self efficacy scale [15] (Table 1)*

The Job Seeking Self-Efficacy (JSS) questionnaire is a 12-item tool designed to measure an individual's confidence in job-seeking situations. Participants rate their confidence on a scale from 1 (not at all confident) to 7 (very confident). Developed by Wright and Cullen (2002), the JSS scale was first field-tested by Strauser et al. It has been evaluated in four studies, demonstrating that the 12-item JSS is unidimensional with high internal consistency. The scale shows strong psychometric properties, with Cronbach's alpha values of 0.93 and 0.96, indicating high reliability. Additionally, evidence supports its construct and concurrent validity. Correlation analysis has shown that higher JSS scores are associated with lower perceived overall stress levels.[15]

3.2 *Perceived stress scale (Table 2) [16]*

The Perceived Stress Scale (PSS) is a 10-item measure where responses range from 0 to 4 (0 = Never, 1 = Almost Never, 2 = Sometimes, 3 = Fairly Often, 4 = Very Often), with reverse scoring applied to positively worded items (4, 5, 7, and 8). The PSS evaluates how individuals perceive situations in their lives as stressful, with higher scores indicating greater perceived stress, which may suggest difficulty in coping and vulnerability to burnout. The scale is

Table 1. Describes the 12 point job seeking ability questions. [15]

Sl. No.	Questions
1.	How confident are you requesting a job application form?
2.	How confident are you completing a job application form?
3.	How confident are you producing a CV (curriculum vitae)?
4.	How confident are you travelling to the interview?
5.	How confident are you in your interview skills generally?
6.	How confident are you in your physical self- presentation at the interview?
7.	How confident are you in your oral self-presentation at the interview?
8.	How confident are you about meeting new people?
9.	How confident are you about contributing to a meeting or discussion?
10.	How confident are you about working with a team?
11.	How confident are you working by yourself?
12.	When it comes to your career progression, how confident would you say you are?

Table 2. Describes the 10 point Perceived Stress Scale. [16]

Sl. No.	Questions
1.	In the last month, how often have you been upset because of something that happened unexpectedly?
2.	In the last month, how often have you felt that you were unable to control the important things in your life?
3.	In the last month, how often have you felt nervous and stressed?
4.	In the last month, how often have you felt confident about your ability to handle your personal problems?
5.	In the last month, how often have you felt that things were going your way?
6.	In the last month, how often have you found that you could not cope with all the things that you had to do?
7.	In the last month, how often have you been able to control irritations in your life?
8.	In the last month, how often have you felt that you were on top of things?
9.	In the last month, how often have you been angered because of things that happened that were outside of your control?
10.	In the last month, how often have you felt difficulties were piling up so high that you could not overcome them?

Table 3. Describes the 12 point Dental Environment Stress Questionnaire (DES). [19]

Sl. No.	Questions
1.	Amount of assigned classwork
2.	Lack of cooperation by patients in their home care
3.	Difficulty of classwork
4.	Responsibilities of comprehensive patient care
5.	Competition for grades
6.	Patients being late or not showing for their appointments
7.	Examination and grades
8.	Difficulty in learning clinical procedures
9.	Atmosphere created by clinical faculty
10.	Relations with members of the opposite sex
11.	Receiving criticism about work
12.	Difficulty in learning precision manual skills

designed to measure the extent to which respondents feel their lives are unpredictable, uncontrollable, and overloaded. It has been validated for use with students and shows good reliability, with Cronbach's alpha values of 0.78 and 0.71, respectively. [16–18]

3.3 *Dental Environment Stress Questionnaire (DES) [19] (Table 3)*

The Dental Environmental Stress (DES) Questionnaire is a 12-item tool used to assess stressors experienced during predoctoral dental training. Each item is rated on a four-point scale: 1 = Not Stressful, 2 = Slightly Stressful, 3 = Moderately Stressful, and 4 = Very Stressful, with an additional "Not Applicable" option.

It is necessary to conduct additional studies to examine coping strategies and interventions designed to target the particular stressors that dental professionals face during their training and transition. [6]

Career counseling services are necessary for dental students since they often lack sufficient knowledge regarding postgraduate courses, available jobs, and hiring and placement procedures. In a similar vein, students view guest speaker events favorably because they provide students with first-hand experience with real-world learning and because guest speakers offer insights into the practical side of the field through personal stories and job recommendations. Career fairs serve the same purposes, helping students network with industry leaders, better understanding their career goals, and increasing their chances of landing a job. Consequently, to guarantee that students are as prepared as possible for the workforce, dental institutions should create career counseling programs, host career fairs, and schedule guest speaker engagements. University curricula need to be updated, and additional training opportunities provided to equip graduates with the skills required to meet labor market demands.[8]

4 CONCLUSION

High levels of stress can lead to burnout, which leads to reduced work efficiency, depression anxiety and various other health concerns. As teachers we need to understand the implications of job-seeking stress and its disastrous effects on mental health and address the increasing problem of unemployment among dental graduates and postgraduates. The following can be included as part of the curriculum to address job seeking/employment stress:

(1) Personalized career counseling
(2) Conducting stress management workshops that include mindfulness practices, time management skills and coping strategies.
(3) Providing them with networking opportunities through alumni and industry mentorship
(4) Skill development programs such as communication, negotiation and presentation skills
(5) Additional professional development opportunities
(6) Psychological and emotional support through counseling services and peer support groups.

By implementing these practical applications, educational institutions can effectively support students experiencing increased job-seeking stress, helping them navigate the transition from education to employment more successfully and promoting their overall well-being.

REFERENCES

[1] Saad Alshamrani A, A. Alshalan T. (2021). Stress among dental students: brief review and messages to all related. *Oral Heal Dent Stud.* 2(1):1–6.

[2] Gorter R, Freeman R, Hammen S, Murtomaa H, Blinkhorn A, Humphris G. (2008). Psychological stress and health in undergraduate dental students: Fifth year outcomes compared with first year baseline results from five European dental schools. *Eur J Dent Educ.* 12(2):61–8.
[3] Humphris G, Blinkhorn A, Freeman R, Gorter R, Hoad-Reddick G, Murtomaa H, *et al.* (2002). Psychological stress in undergraduate dental students: Baseline results from seven European dental schools. *Eur J Dent Educ.* 6(1):22–9.
[4] Elani HW, Bedos C, Allison PJ. (2013). Sources of Stress in Canadian Dental Students: A Prospective Mixed Methods Study. *J Dent Educ.* 77(11):1488–97.
[5] Pau AKH, Croucher R. (2003). Emotional intelligence and perceived stress in dental undergraduates. *J Dent Educ.* 67(9):1023–8.
[6] Tangade PS, Mathur A, Gupta R, Chaudhary S. (2011). Assessment of stress level among dental school students: An indian outlook. *Dent Res J* 8(2):95–101.
[7] Juneja R, Sikka N, Kumar V, Chahal S, Arora M, Middha M, *et al.* (2021). Factors causing stress in postgraduate dental students during COVID-19 pandemic: A cross-sectional survey. *Dent Res J.* 18(1):92.
[8] Fita S, Alshuraim F, Almulhim A, Alhumaid J, Alhareky M, Nazir M. (2020). Possible future career challenges and associated factors among dental students and interns. *Int J Dent.* 9730125. https://doi.org/10.1155/2020/9730125.
[9] Mohan M, Ravindran TKS. (2019). Unemployment and vulnerable financial situation among recent dental graduates of Kerala, India - Results from a cross-sectional study. *J Glob Oral Heal.* 1(1):49–57.
[10] Mohan M, Ravindran TKS. (2018). Failure of policy initiatives in regulating health professional education: the case of dental education in india. *J Health Manag.* 20(4):486–97.
[11] Kumar Dixit J, Tiwari P, Kumar Gupta S, Singh P, Gupta H. (2011). Educated unemployed: A challenge before sustainable education. sustainable manufacturing – *Proc. of the International Conference on Sustainable Manufacturing: Issues, Trends and Practices (ICSM – 2011)*, BITS, Pilani, India, 2011;November 10–12,
[12] Jaiswal AK, Srinivas P, Suresh S. (2014). Dental manpower in India: Changing trends since 1920. *Int Dent J* 64(4):213–8.
[13] Harikiran AG, Srinagesh J, Nagesh KS, Sajudeen N. (2012). Perceived sources of stress amongst final year dental under graduate students in a dental teaching institution at Bangalore, India: A cross sectional study. *Indian J Dent Res.* 23(3):331–6.
[14] Cooper CL, Rout U, Faragher B. (1989). Mental health, job satisfaction, and job stress among general practitioners. *Br Med J.* 298 (6670):366–70.
[15] Strauser DR, Berven NL. (2006). Construction and field testing of the Job Seeking Self-Efficacy Scale. *Rehabil Couns Bull.* 49 (4):207–18.
[16] Cohen S, Kamarck T, Mermelstein R. (1983). A global measure of perceived stress. *J Health Soc Behav.* 24(4):385–96.
[17] Chan S.F., La Greca A.M. (2013). Perceived Stress Scale (PSS). In: Gellman M.D., Turner J.R. (eds) *Encyclopedia of Behavioral Medicine*. Springer, New York.
[18] Anwer S, Manzar MD, Alghadir AH, Salahuddin M, Abdul Hameed U. (2020). psychometric analysis of the perceived stress scale among healthy university students. *Neuropsychiatric Disease and Treatment.* 16:2389–2396.
[19] Elani HW, Allison PJ, Kumar AR, Mancini L, Lambrou A, Bedos C. (2014). A systematic review of stress in dental students. *Journal of Dental Education.* 78: 226–42.

Navigating Dental Education Trends and Transforming Dental Pedagogy – Abas and Srikant N (Eds)

Simulation, the Practice of Perfecting Clinical Skills in Teaching: A Narrative Review

Jefferson Prince and Premalatha Shetty

Department of Oral and Maxillofacial Surgery, Manipal College of Dental Science Mangalore, Manipal Academy of Higher Education, Manipal, India

ABSTRACT: The training of oral and maxillofacial residents has traditionally been the Halstedian teaching model. However, as technology and patient awareness increases, the training of a young maxillofacial surgeon must also include other simulation-related models in addition to didactic lectures to increase competency. The simulation models also reduce the learning curve required for trainees and make them more competent in performing the various procedures that the specialty encompasses. Simulation models have been increasingly used, ranging from low-fidelity to medium- and high-fidelity models, virtual reality (VR), and the increasing use of artificial intelligence (AI) in training procedural scenarios. The increased use of simulation in training and assessing trainees has developed into an essential tool. Using simulation enables both the proficiency of the trainee and enhances patient safety, which was previously dependent solely on the resident's clinical experience.

Keywords: Simulation, Maxillofacial training, Manikin, Virtual Reality, Healthcare

1 INTRODUCTION

Any surgeon needs skill and expertise in their specialty; a good surgeon is never born but trained. Oral and maxillofacial surgery involves complex surgeries, resections, and reconstructions of the facial skeleton and soft tissues that can be mastered only with experience. Teaching surgical skills to trainees is one of the most crucial tasks for teachers/trainers in the field of maxillofacial surgery. Nevertheless, young trainees may be prone to more mistakes and need more skills that require time and practice to develop. This learning curve may compromise patient care, even when performed under the direct supervision of trainers, as trainees also need to develop dexterity and acclimatization to instrument usage.

Simulation technologies have emerged in transforming and enhancing surgical skills training in oral and maxillofacial surgery. Synthesizing current research and empirical evidence underscores the advantages of simulation in offering a controlled environment for trainees to practice and refine complex surgical techniques. The benefits include accelerated learning curves, error management, and the opportunity for practice without patient risk. [1] This paper explores the growing importance of simulation-based education for improving surgical proficiency and patient outcomes and reviews the current simulation practices.

2 METHODOLOGY

A search was made in PubMed, Scopus, and Embase databases using the keywords simulation, simulation-based training, resident training, dental education, oral and maxillofacial surgery education, training module, manikins, virtual reality in oral and maxillofacial surgery, augmented reality in oral and maxillofacial surgery.

The investigators identified the articles from the databases and then screened the abstract and the whole article to see if it was relevant. Articles related to surgical simulations, hospital care, and treatment, manikins for maxillofacial or head and neck surgeries, surgery residency training programs, and dental training related to surgeries were screened and selected. Articles on maxillofacial education that did not have simulations as the scope of their article were excluded from the study. Studies on simulations apart from surgeries or other procedures related to oral and maxillofacial training were excluded from the study. An initial search among the databases showed 343 articles. The articles were screened for relevance, and 22 articles were selected. After excluding the duplicate articles, 12 were identified and used for the study. The data from the articles were grouped according to the purpose they served in the oral and maxillofacial training program.

3 DISCUSSION

3.1 *Simulation*

Simulation and simulation manikins aid the resident surgeon in practicing and reproducing various treatments and their management in a risk-free environment without causing any harm to the patient. [2] Simulation training

DOI: 10.1201/9781042016075-52

originated in the Link Trainer and was used for flight simulation by trainee pilots. From there, it evolved into nursing and medical training programs. [3] Simulation in healthcare and resident training involves the recreation of real-life scenarios, and treatment procedures to improve healthcare services' safety, effectiveness, and efficiency. [4]

Simulation helps make tailor-made educational tools designed to fit the program and course objectives and helps residents gain experience with uncommon treatment and procedures. [5] Simulation makes the learner and not the patient the focus of education. As such, the errors that occur can be made into ways of teaching by overseeing experts. [5] Simulation plays an important role in evaluation of nontechnical and cognitive skills, the acquisition of which is necessary to attain procedural mastery. [6] Simulation training is crucial for maxillofacial surgical training for the following reasons.

3.2 *Risk-free learning environment*

Maxillofacial surgery involves complex anatomy, including delicate structures of the body, nerves and blood vessels, where mistakes can have significant consequences. Surgeons can make mistakes in simulations and learn from them without causing harm, enhancing their learning experience. Especially in acute life-threatening events, recognition and treatment based on simulation models, along with case discussions, aid in improving and meeting learning requirements. [2] Simulation aids in better error tolerance with young trainees. The Halstead model for surgical training, which is "see one, do one, and teach one," might have aided in the surgical training for the past century but also had the surgeons practicing on actual patients, even if doing so under an expert overseeing the procedures. With advances in medicine and technology, these need to be superseded through simulation, thereby flattening the curve for an experience that the trainee needs and delivering a better quality of care for the patients.

Medical errors are among the leading causes of death worldwide. The percentage of errors is higher in the procedures involved with trainees than among those that did not involve trainees. The most prevalent contributing factors include errors in judgment, teamwork breakdowns, and a lack of technical competence. [7] These can be substantially reduced via simulations, thereby contributing to better quality of care for patients.

3.3 *Development of complex skills*

Maxillofacial surgery requires high levels of precision and dexterity. Simulation enables repetitive practice of techniques such as suturing, bone manipulation, and implant placement. Advanced surgical simulations can mimic real-life scenarios, helping trainees improve hand™eye coordination and spatial awareness in a controlled setting. This improvement was observed in the study by Lund *et al.* [8] They demonstrated a virtual patient and compared it with a simulation-based system for a mandibular third molar with tactile feedback. They reported a high improvement in the simulator with tactile feedback and suggested its inclusion in the curriculum. The tangible outcomes of interest in using simulation are complication rates and operating room (OR) efficiency. [6]

3.4 *Repetition and mastery*

Trainees can perform the same procedure repeatedly to refine their technique. This repetition helps master complex procedures, which may not be possible with live patients owing to limited availability or ethical concerns. Simulators often provide immediate feedback, allowing for continuous improvements in techniques, decision-making, and skill acquisition. [6] Assessments can also be made for specific skills via simulation training [6], outcome-based education, and competency-based education, which ensure that trainees become competent at the end of their training, for which the simulators aid immensely.

3.5 *Exposure to rare and complex cases*

Trainees can experience a wide range of cases, including rare or complicated surgeries, which they might not frequently encounter in actual practice. This experience broadens their exposure and prepares them for various clinical situations.

Simulations can recreate high-pressure scenarios, helping trainees develop the ability to stay calm and make sound decisions under stress. It can also aid in specific educational goals using the trainer, which the learner can perform without harming the patient. [5]

3.6 *Interdisciplinary collaboration*

Many maxillofacial procedures involve collaboration with other specialists, such as anesthesiologists and nurses. Simulation provides a platform for training in team-based care, enhancing communication and teamwork during surgeries. Simulations can mimic the entire operating room workflow, helping trainees understand and optimize their role in the surgical team or emergencies, thus improving performance. Simulation-based training would be a valuable supplement to clinical training. [6,9] It also aids in good transfer of skills from simulation to the actual clinical operating environment, increasing patient satisfaction, decreasing morbidity, and reducing the time required of teaching required intraoperatively. [9]

3.7 *Innovative techniques and technologies*

Simulation allows trainees to become familiar with new surgical techniques and cutting-edge technologies, such as computer-assisted surgery, robotic systems, or 3D printing, without the pressure of operating on live patients. Simulation training is a safe, effective, and comprehensive method for preparing maxillofacial surgeons because of the complexities and challenges of real-world surgical practice. [10]

Simulation in health care is on the verge of becoming the standard in education and training and becoming the standard in health care education. [3] From various manikins to complex simulators and virtual reality, simulators aid in training surgical residents in which patient safety and resident training can go hand in hand.

3.8 *Current simulation practices*

For modern trainees, doing more is more important than learning more. With a renewed focus on patient safety, innovation in teaching is vital for the future of oral and maxillofacial surgery training.

Animal and cadaver laboratories are the first examples of using simulation in surgical training. The advantages of these methods are the high validity of anatomical structures, good haptics, and good tissue quality. [6] Previously, human cadavers, animal cadavers, and live animals were used for surgical demonstrations and training. [4] However, changing values, ethics, and regulations around the use of animals and cadaveric tissue have resulted in increased expenses and access. However, residency training programs, of late, have begun to offer their trainees exposure to simulation, simulation laboratories, low- and high-fidelity box trainers, computerized virtual reality, and 3D printing. [6,11] More recently, augmented reality, which uses the superimposition of a 3D real environment specific to individual patients, has aided in augmenting planning and training for maxillofacial surgical procedures. [12] Virtual patients, task trainers, high-fidelity manikins, virtual reality, and augmented reality are the forms of simulation currently available and are in development for maxillofacial resident training programs.

4 CONCLUSION

Practice makes a man perfect. This dictum goes even more in regard to the maxillofacial surgeon, which encompasses a variety of treatment care and procedures. These require practice, experience, and expertise to become proficient and monitor learning for an extended period, as each branch of its specialty demands. Simulation in different forms and methods is the way to make dental professionals proficient in their field while taking care of the patient's best interests in the treatment provided. Simulation practices, therefore, take a maxillofacial surgeon more toward the perfection that the specialty demands, and the patient requires.

REFERENCES

[1] Robert RC, Patel CM. Oral Surgery Patient Safety Concepts in Anesthesia. (2018). *Oral Maxillofac Surg Clin North Am* 30 (2):183–193.

[2] Kalsi AS, Higham H, McKnight M, Dariwal DK. (2013). Simulation training for dental foundation in oral and maxillofacial surgery-A new benchmark. *Br Dent J* 215(11):571–576.

[3] Aebersold M. (2016). The history of simulation and its impact on the future. *AACN Adv Crit Care* 27(1):56–61.

[4] Busaidy KF. (2019). Advances in surgical training using simulation. *Oral Maxillofac Surg Clin North Am* 31(4):621–626.

[5] Coffey-Zern S, Calvi RMD, Vorrasi JS, Meara DJ. (2015). Incorporating simulation into oral and maxillofacial surgery residency education and training: christiana care's method. *Journal of Oral and Maxillofacial Surgery* 73(7):1244–1245.

[6] Kim-Fine S, Brennand EA. (2016). Surgical Simulation and competency. *Obstet Gynecol Clin North Am* 43(3):575–590.

[7] Singh H, Thomas EJ, Petersen LA, Studdert DM. (2007). Medical Errors Involving Trainees A Study of Closed Malpractice Claims From 5 Insurers. *Arch Intern Med* 167(19):2030–2036.

[8] Lund B, Fors U, Sejersen R, Sallnäs E-L, Rosén A. (2011). Student perception of two different simulation techniques in oral and maxillofacial surgery undergraduate training. *BMC Med Educ* (11):82.

[9] Ahmed N, McVicar IH, Mitchell DA. (2019). Simulation-based training in maxillofacial surgery: are we going to be left behind? *British Journal of Oral and Maxillofacial Surgery* 57(1):67–71.

[10] Grall P, Ferri J, Nicot R. (2021). Surgical training 2.0: A systematic approach reviewing the literature focusing on oral maxillofacial surgery – Part I. *J Stomatol Oral Maxillofac Surg* 122(4):411–422.

[11] Fuller JC, Justicz NS, Kim J, Cheney M, Castrillon R, Hadlock T. (2019). A facial plastic and reconstructive surgery training module using surgical simulation for capacity building. *J Surg Educ* 76(1):274–280.

[12] Ayoub A, Pulijala Y. (2019). The application of virtual reality and augmented reality in Oral & Maxillofacial Surgery. *BMC Oral Health* 19(1).

Navigating Dental Education Trends and Transforming Dental Pedagogy – Abas and Srikant N (Eds)
© 2027 The Author(s), ISBN: 978-1-041-32674-8

Trends in the Occurrence of Oral Pathologies: Is Our Curriculum Up to Date?

Amitha J Lewis and Srikant N
Department of Oral Pathology and Microbiology, Manipal College of Dental Sciences Mangalore, Manipal Academy of Higher Education, Manipal, India

Nandita Sujir and Karen Boaz
Department of Oral Medicine and Radiology, Manipal College of Dental Sciences Mangalore, Manipal Academy of Higher Education, Manipal, India

Nandita K.P.
Department of Oral Pathology and Microbiology, Manipal College of Dental Sciences Mangalore, Manipal Academy of Higher Education, Manipal, India

Ceena Denny
Department of Oral Medicine and Radiology, Manipal College of Dental Sciences Mangalore, Manipal Academy of Higher Education, Manipal, India

Nidhi Manaktala and Shweta Y.
Department of Oral Pathology and Microbiology, Manipal College of Dental Sciences Mangalore, Manipal Academy of Higher Education, Manipal, India

ABSTRACT: **Introduction:** Oral pathology is a critical component of dental education and focuses on diagnosing diseases affecting the oral cavity. Understanding the demographics and gathering region-specific data of these oral diseases is essential to address health concerns effectively. Healthcare institutions have the social responsibility to maintain a dynamic curriculum by adapting their teaching requirements to address the evolving prevalence of diseases within the community they serve.

Aim: This study aims to evaluate the prevalence of certain oral pathologies and correlate it with the weight given under the current educational curriculum for undergraduate students.

Materials and Methods: Data regarding the clinical information and histopathological diagnosis of oral biopsies obtained from 2014 to 2024 were categorized and analyzed. The oral pathology undergraduate syllabus was reviewed and compared with the prevalence of head and neck pathologies to identify whether the topics were given adequate weight in the curriculum.

Results: Odontogenic cysts and malignant epithelial neoplasms constituted approximately 16.8% and 16.4%, respectively, of the total lesions observed over a period of ten years. A comparison of the lesions with the time allocated for teaching revealed that skin lesions accounted for 122 cases, with 6 hours dedicated to teaching these cases, resulting in an average time of 0.5 hours per lesion. Similarly, 145 cases of salivary gland lesions were observed, with 5 teaching hours allocated, with an average of 0.5 hours per lesion.

Conclusion: The findings of this research show the need to continuously update the curriculum to match with the current trends in the occurrence of oral lesions. Most of the commonly occurring pathologies are well represented in the curriculum yet minor changes keeping in mind the wide variety of lesions encountered can be considered.

Keywords: oral pathology, curriculum, head and neck lesions, prevalence

1 INTRODUCTION

Understanding the demographics and prevalence of oral diseases across different regions and populations is crucial for developing effective public health strategies and ensuring that clinical practice is relevant to the populations we serve. The changing dynamics of the epidemiology of oral diseases can be attributed to geographic influences, evolutionary changes and lifestyles. Evolutionary processes are altering human susceptibility to specific oral diseases. Changes in diet, genetics and the ever-changing microbial system impact the incidence and severity of various oral diseases, including oral cancers. [1,2]

Oral pathology is a critical component of dental education, which focuses on diagnosing and managing diseases affecting the oral cavity. The knowledge of the prevalence of a particular disease helps us understand its distribution across different age groups and identify populations at risk for a particular disease. It is essential that we gather accurate data specific to our own population to address these health concerns effectively. [2], [3]

 DOI: 10.1201/9781042016075-53

Understanding the prevalence of various conditions can also help tailor educational programs to ensure comprehensive training for undergraduate dental students. [4] For curriculum delivery, we often rely on textbooks authored by foreign experts. While these resources are invaluable, they often describe various diseases, their etiologies and clinical features that are more prevalent in their regions, which may not reflect the common occurrences within our population. In addition to the differences observed across countries, India's diverse population, with its wide range of habits, cultural practices, and etiquette, plays a significant role in influencing disease processes, which need to be thoroughly addressed and taught. Consequently, this can lead to a mismatch between the knowledge imparted to students and the actual clinical scenarios they encounter in practice.

The evolving patterns of disease prevalence highlight the need to prioritize those commonly occurring lesions in our curriculum. [4] Therefore, it is imperative to reassess and adapt the curriculum to better suit the Indian context. By incorporating region-specific data and focusing on the oral diseases most prevalent within our communities, we can ensure that our education system produces clinicians who are better equipped to meet the needs of the population they serve. Thus, this study aims to survey the head and neck biopsy cases received over a period of ten years to determine the commonly occurring pathologies and assess the adequacy of their coverage in the undergraduate curriculum.

2 MATERIALS AND METHODS

This cross-sectional study was conducted in the Department of Oral Pathology and Microbiology, MCODS, Mangalore, after obtaining clearance from the Institutional Ethics Committee

Data collection: The data for the study was obtained from head and neck biopsy cases received by the Department of Oral Pathology and Microbiology from 2014–2024. The data regarding the histopathological diagnosis and the clinical information were retrieved from the archives of the Department and transferred to Excel format. Data regarding age, sex, site of the lesion and histopathological diagnosis were included. At every stage, anonymity of the patient's details was maintained. Biopsies for which the diagnosis was not conclusive and repeat biopsies of previously diagnosed lesions were excluded from the study.

For ease of analysis, the data obtained were organized into major categories: odontogenic lesions, oral potentially malignant disorders, salivary gland neoplasms, malignant epithelial neoplasms, malignant connective tissue neoplasms, benign connective tissue neoplasms, diseases of bone and diseases of the skin. The number and frequency of each of these cases were evaluated over a period of ten years.

Syllabus evaluation for curriculum review: The current undergraduate curriculum was reviewed, and the topics covered were listed. The time allocated to teaching each type of pathology was documented.

Correlation

A comparison of the prevalence of common head and neck cases with the time devoted to teaching them in the curriculum was carried out to identify any gaps where common pathologies may not be sufficiently covered.

3 RESULTS

The research findings indicate a correlation between the number of histopathological cases encountered in the Department of Oral Pathology and Microbiology and the hours allocated for teaching these lesions in the BDS curriculum in India.

For lesions categorized as "absolutely needed," such as those related to the **skin**, **salivary gland**, **pulp and periapical lesions**; **potentially malignant disorders**; and **odontogenic cysts**, a considerable number of cases have been observed in the department. For example, **skin lesions** accounted for 122 cases, with 6 hours dedicated to teaching them, resulting in an average time of 0.5 hours per lesion. Similarly, 145 cases of **salivary gland lesions** were observed, with 6 teaching hours allocated, with an average of 0.5 hours per lesion.

Lesions such as **odontogenic tumors** and **bone lesions** are also marked as "Absolutely needed," and while their case numbers are lower (36 and 21, respectively), they receive more teaching hours (6 hours each), indicating more time devoted per lesion (0.75 hours). Notably, **benign connective tissue neoplasms** have a high case count (104), with 7 hours allocated to teaching, with an average of 0.15 hours per lesion.

According to the Dental Council of India (DCI) syllabus, the number of lesions to be taught under each category is as follows: For Skin, 10 lesions are to be taught, including conditions such as Lichen Planus, Lupus Erythematosus, and Pemphigus. Under salivary glands, 11 lesions, such as sialolithiasis and pleomorphic adenoma, are covered. The pulp and periapical lesions included 6 lesions, such as pulp inflammation and osteomyelitis. Potentially malignant disorders encompass 4 lesions, including leukoplakia and oral precancer. For odontogenic tumors, 5 lesions, such as ameloblastoma, are highlighted. Odontogenic cysts cover 5 lesions, including dentigerous and radicular cysts. Malignant Epithelial Neoplasms and malignant connective tissue neoplasms require the teaching of 4 and 6 lesions, respectively, including basal cell carcinoma and fibrosarcoma. The bone conditions included 8 lesions, such as fibrous dysplasia and osteogenesis imperfecta. Finally, benign epithelial neoplasms (e.g., papilloma) have 3 lesions, whereas benign connective tissue neoplasms (e.g., fibroma) have 7 lesions.

Table 1. Detailed breakdown of the weightage given to histopathological analysis across different types of lesions.

	Count	Hours Taught	Number of lesions Taught	Number of lesions seen in within the categories	Number of Lesions to be taught as per DCI syllabus	Average time per lesion
Skin	122	6	13	12	10	0.5
Salivary gland	145	5	11	10	11	0.5
Pulp and periapical Lesions	96	4	11	13	6	0.307692
Potentially malignant disorder	149	4	4	12	4	0.333333
Odontogenic tumour	36	6	12	8	5	0.75
Odontogenic cyst	297	6	8	17	5	0.352941
Malignant epithelial Neoplasm	299	3	4	6	4	0.5
Malignant connective tissue Neoplasm	6	2	10	6	6	0.333333
Bone	21	6	14	8	8	0.75
Benign epithelial Neoplasm	15	1	3	4	3	0.25
Benign connective tissue neoplasm	104	7	20	20	7	0.15

However, in our department, we are observing a wider variety of cases in each category than is being taught. For example, in the skin category, 12 lesions were observed, and in the pulp and periapical lesions, 13 lesions were identified, with similar increases across other categories, such as potentially malignant disorders, where 12 lesions were identified. To adapt to this, the faculty in our institution are proactively updating the curriculum to include descriptions of these additional lesions. We believe that all dental colleges should adopt a similar approach, ensuring that the curriculum remains dynamic and up to date. This should be a continuous process that involves collaboration with the community and seeking feedback from individuals in society to ensure that the curriculum reflects real-world trends in dental health.

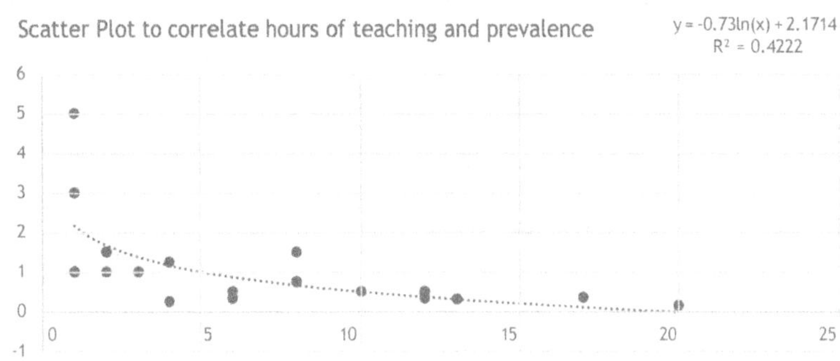

5 DISCUSSION

The present study assessed the various histopathological cases reported by the Department of Oral Pathology from 2014-2024 and classified these oral diseases into major categories. This was further compared with the number of hours dedicated to teaching each of these diseases in the present curriculum. Most of the studies focus on a particular disease or group of diseases instead of the entire spectrum. Studying this disease spectrum over a ten-year period provides us with valuable inputs regarding region-specific trends in the prevalence of oral diseases, which can in turn provide invaluable inputs if our curriculum is in line with disease trends. [5] Table 1 presents a detailed breakdown of the weightage given to histopathological analysis across different types of lesions. By analyzing the number of lesions, hours taught, and the number of lesions included in the curriculum and the average time spent per lesion, we can make observations regarding the adequacy and alignment of the syllabus with clinical practice.

5.1 *Lesion frequency and curriculum focus*

- **Odontogenic Cysts and Malignant Epithelial Neoplasms:** These two categories stand out with the highest counts, 297 and 299, respectively. Despite this high frequency, the hours allotted for malignant epithelial neoplasms (3 hours) is lower than the 6 hours dedicated to odontogenic cysts. Given that both lesions are frequently encountered in clinical practice, particularly in regions where oral cancer rates are high, this raises concerns about whether sufficient time is dedicated to malignant neoplasms. These lesions carry significant diagnostic and treatment implications and potentially warrant more in-depth coverage.

- **Benign Connective Tissue Neoplasms:** Despite having a moderate count of 104, a relatively high number of lesions are taught (20), yet only 7 hours are allocated, resulting in a low average time per lesion (0.15 hours). This suggests a possible imbalance between the number of conditions included and the time spent on each, potentially compromising the depth of understanding.
- **Potentially Malignant Disorders:** With 149 cases and only 4 hours dedicated to teaching, the time per lesion (0.33 hours) might be insufficient. Given the clinical significance of early detection and management, there is a need for increased emphasis on these lesions in the curriculum.

One of the core reasons to base the syllabus on the frequency of conditions is to align academic learning with clinical realities. For example, oral cancer, mucosal lesions, and periodontal diseases occur with high frequency, especially in certain populations, such as those in India, where tobacco use is prevalent. By prioritizing these conditions, the syllabus would better reflect the disease burden faced by healthcare professionals. Teaching time and emphasis should be allocated proportionally to the frequency and clinical significance of these conditions. This does not mean excluding rare pathologies altogether but prioritizing those that students are most likely to encounter. For example, more time could be devoted to the diagnosis and management of oral squamous cell carcinoma (OSCC), leucoplakia, and oral potentially malignant disorders (OPMDs), given their increasing prevalence in many regions of the world. [5–7]

While some oral diseases may be common, others may have a significant impact on patients' overall health. [6]

Allen [7] noted that the commonness of a disease alone should not be the basis for curriculum design. Darling et al. [8], in agreement with Odell et al. [9], suggested that dental students should learn topics that have a significant impact on patient morbidity and mortality. For example, melanoma, though not very common and not limited to the oral cavity alone, can be life threatening to patients. Thus, sufficient knowledge of such neoplasms is a requirement when designing the curriculum. Darling et al. suggested a third criterion, namely, the uniqueness of a condition or disease. There are many such oral diseases that may not be well known by other professionals, such as odontogenic tumours and cysts, periodontal diseases, etc., so the onus of identifying such diseases lies primarily on the dentist. Therefore, thorough knowledge of such oral diseases is required in the curriculum.

The limitation of the study is that it included only the cases that we received in the institution and though we did receive a wide variety of cases the trends may vary across different regions.

6 CONCLUSION

Oral pathology as a subject need not be as challenging and understated as it is perceived. By introspecting what we want to teach and how we want to teach and what exactly it is that we want our students to learn, we can gain tremendous improvement in the students' understanding of the subject.

The curriculum can be adjusted to match regional needs by emphasizing common illnesses and taking demographic-specific elements into account, which will eventually improve patient treatment. A well-rounded education will be ensured by striking a balance between this and understanding of uncommon conditions, and regular changes to the syllabus will help keep it current over time.

REFERENCES

[1] Saluja TS, Singh IP, Creanga AG, Khurana S. (2023). A retrospective analysis of trends in oral and maxillofacial pathology lesions: An Institutional Archival study. *Int J Health Environ Res* 1:60–64.

[2] Mendez M, Carrard VC, Haas AN, *et al.* (2012). A 10-year study of specimens submitted to oral pathology laboratory analysis: lesion occurrence and demographic features. *Braz Oral Res.* 26(3):235–241.

[3] Monteiro LS, Albuquerque R, Paiva A, de la Peña-Moral J, Amaral JB, Lopes CA. (2017). A comparative analysis of oral and maxillofacial pathology over a 16-year period, in the north of Portugal. *Int Dent J.* 67(1):38–45.

[4] Hussain M, Khan Z, Qazi SR. (2019). Curriculum modification based on local disease prevalence: A study from Pakistan. *Medical Education*, 53(7):656–662.

[5] Sofizadeh N, Bjerkehagen B, Solheim T, Sapkota D, Søland TM. (2023). The spectrum and frequency of histopathological diagnosis of oral diseases in Oslo: Implications to oral pathology syllabus. *Eur J Dent Educ.* 27(2):325–331.

[6] Kragelund C, Reibel J, Hietanen J, *et al.* (2012). Scandinavian fellowship for oral pathology and oral medicine: Guidelines for oral pathology and oral medicine in the dental curriculum. *Eur J Dent Educ.* 16(4):246–253.

[7] Allen CM. (1996). Oral and maxillofacial pathology: what should we teach and how should we teach it?. *Oral Surg Oral Med Oral Pathol Oral Radiol Endod.* 82(3):235. doi:10.1016/s1079-2104(96)80341-6

[8] Darling MR, Daley TD. (2006). Oral pathology in the dental curriculum: a guide on what to teach. *J Dent Educ.* 70(4):355–360.

[9] Odell EW, Farthing PM, High A, *et al.* (2004). British society for oral and maxillofacial pathology, UK: minimum curriculum in oral pathology. *Eur J Dent Educ.* 2004;8(4):177–184.

Navigating Dental Education Trends and Transforming Dental Pedagogy – Abas and Srikant N (Eds)
 ISBN: 978-1-041-32674-8

'Lab on a Chip' as an Objective Endodontic Prognostic Tool in Evidence-Based Dental Education

Bettina Ashwini Vergis

Department of Conservative Dentistry & Endodontics, Srinivas Institute of Dental Sciences, Srinivas Nagar, Mukka, Surathkal, Mangaluru, Karnataka

ABSTRACT: Lab-on-a-chip (LOC) technology in endodontics is a potential tool to increase diagnostic precision in treating endodontic disease while enabling tailored treatment protocols. LOC integrates multiple laboratory functions onto a single microchip, allowing real-time analysis and point-of-care diagnostics in endodontic procedures. One significant application of LOC in endodontics is in bacterial detection within the root canal system. LOC devices can identify specific pathogens or bacterial biofilms in infected canals, allowing clinicians to adapt specific antimicrobial treatments on the basis of the individual microbial profile. This real-time feedback can increase the effectiveness of disinfection procedures before obturation. LOC and microfluidic systems are quite sensitive and can detect low concentrations of bacteria. This is crucial for identifying *E. faecalis*, which may be present in low numbers in some clinical samples. Another application of LOC could be to identify individual biomarkers such as MMPs and cytokines to enable decision-making in vital pulp treatment. The incorporation of Lab-on-a-Chip (LOC) technology into dental education could significantly increase the objective predictability of endodontic treatment. By introducing students to LOC technology, they can learn to analyze biological markers and bacterial profiles, improving their diagnostic and clinical decision-making skills. LOC technology could be incorporated into dental research programs, encouraging students to explore innovations in diagnostics and biomarker identification. This integration could equip future dental professionals to provide precision-based endodontic therapy.

Keywords: biomarker, biosensor, lab-on-a-chip (LOC), pulpitis, endodontics

1 INTRODUCTION

Pulpal inflammation is a result of the complex interplay between the microbiota and the host immune response, along with genotypic and environmental influences. In-depth analysis of inflammatory biomarkers and molecular mechanisms involved in pulpal inflammation and apical periodontitis provides insight for clinicians regarding the formulation of evidence-based specific treatment strategies and the assessment of healing in response to these strategies. [1] Quantitative methods, such as enzyme-linked immunosorbent assay (ELISA), western blot analysis, reverse transcription quantitative polymerase chain reaction (RT-qPCR), radioimmunoassay and enzyme assays have been employed to study pulpal biomarkers sampled via pulpal tissue, dentinal fluid, GCF and blood. [2] In terms of microbiological detection in endodontic samples, conventional culture techniques have become almost obsolete and paved the way for newer molecular methods such as polymerase chain reaction (PCR) and gene sequencing. [3] However, none of the above methods can be adopted in point- of-care settings and their drawbacks include the need for complex expensive equipment, inconsistency in results due to technique sensitivity, specialized expertise and training needed for sample preparation and data analysis. [4]

2 MATERIALS AND METHODS

The transition from Sample-to-Lab to Lab-to-Sample: progression pathway to Lab-on-a Chip

Advancements in biotechnology have paved the way for the development of biosensors and microelectromechanical systems (MEMS). Biosensors are primarily devices used to assess biomarkers in point-of-care settings (chairside). [5] While there are various simple chairside biomarker assays such as lateral flow immunoassays and rapid fluorescence tests, biosensors overcome the inherent disadvantages of the former tests as they recognize the biological analytes sent to reader devices through electrical signals. [6,7] Biosensor systems have been miniaturized in the form of MEMS via microfluidics and micro total analysis systems with reduced requirements for reagents and detection times. [8]

DOI: 10.1201/9781042016075-54

Multiple technologies have been further combined on an integrated chip in the form of lab-on-a-chip (LOC) devices. Thus Lab-on-a-chip (LOC) systems constitute a subset of MEMS, resulting in the miniaturization and integration of laboratory functions on a single chip. [9] The collected data can be sent to a detector via wireless transfer for readout as well as qualitative and quantitative measurements.

The primary advantages of Lab-on-a-Chip include the following: the requirement of minute sample and reagent volume, minimum turnaround time, automation of complex workflows, portability and multiplexing capacity.

3 DISCUSSION

3.1 *Applications of Lab-on-a-Chip: exploring potential in the detection and monitoring of systemic conditions and oral diseases*

Lab-on-a-chip technology has been used for the qualitative detection, quantification and monitoring of bacteria, viruses, cytokines, hormones and metabolites, glucose monitoring, and even detection of chronic kidney disease and cancer. [9] Field-effect transistor sensors have enabled rapid detection of ions, molecules, oligonucleotides and proteins. [10] LOCs have been explored as wearable devices to enable constant monitoring of pathological processes to provide enhanced diagnostics, telemedicine provision and even artificial intelligence(AI)-assisted personalized management. [1] Biosensors integrated in mouthguards have been used to detect and monitor metabolite levels in saliva. [11] Furthermore, graphene-based nanobiosensors have been used for adhering to the enamel surface or marginal gingiva to detect oral microorganisms at a singular level. [12]

3.2 *Lab-on-a-Chip: possibilities in endodontic diagnosis, treatment, education and research*

The development of LOC based technologies enables the bypass of external laboratory-based analyses as it provides the necessary metabolic, immunological or microbiological information that can aid in diagnosis and clinical decision making and serve as a prognostic marker. [6] For example: objective detection and quantification of pulpal inflammatory biomarkers such as MMP-9, IL-8, substance P, and neurokinin A, at the chairside level via LOC devices could serve as quick and objective prognostic markers for vital pulp therapy , as their levels are known to be increased in patients with symptomatic pulpitis. [2] They carry out a variety of laboratory functions, such as sample manipulation and biomarker detection , displaying sensitivity comparable to that of conventional metabolite analysis methods such as mass spectrometry (MS), nuclear magnetic resonance (NMR), and chromatography methods. [9]

The microfluidic systems involved in lab-on-a-chip technology require microlitres to nanolitres of the sample, making it extremely sensitive to low concentrations of bacteria compared with other biochemical tests. These devices also ensure quick and streamlined microbial detection, high-level precision in molecular diagnostics with regard to detection of pulpal and periapical inflammatory biomarkers. Moreover, these devices could aid in monitoring of the efficacy of canal disinfection measures prior to obturation. [4] This could further lead to the development of targeted endodontic treatment strategies in various endodontic case scenarios. Additionally, in situations of atypical tooth pain / persistent idiopathic dentoalveolar pain (PIDAP), the deployment of LOC devices could be performed to demonstrate the absence of inflammatory mediators around the tooth. This could aid in preventing the misdiagnosis of atypical tooth pain as pulpally related; thus avoiding false treatment. [6]

All these advantageous features of Lab-on-a chip devices serve well in dental educational set-ups by improving objectivity in diagnosis rather than making arbitrary judgements. By introducing students to LOC technology, they can learn to analyze biological markers and bacterial profiles, improving their diagnostic and clinical decision-making skills. LOC technology could be incorporated into dental research programs, encouraging students to explore innovations in diagnostics and biomarker identification.The devices also aid in strategizing pulpal treatments and endodontic disinfection modalities which address the specific cause of pulpal disease or inflammation. Finally , since the features of the laboratory are now available at the point-of-care settings via lab-on-a-chip devices , it makes it easier to be employed in daily dental practice for dental students.

3.3 *Challenges*

The microchannels in microfluidic devices are prone to clogging, which can be mitigated by inbuilt filters. Since the LOC devices require very little sample,a small variation in quantity could have a drastic impact on the results. Moreover, micromanufacturing such devices is expensive, and requires specialized manpower and technology, thus making commercialization unfeasible.

3.4 *Suggestions for Research*

The development of these devices in clinical settings in dental institutions requires an amalgamation of research and technology. There is a wide range of scope for research in terms of

(a) Identifying pulpitis-specific biomarkers that distinguish between reversible and irreversible pulpitis.
(b) Development of efficient microfluidic devices with the help of 3D printing.
(c) Enabling sampling of pulpal/ dentinal fluid with reduced contaminants with the help of devices such as micropipettes.
(d) The use of magnetic nanoparticles to aid in enhancing the flow of the sample in devices with an enhanced signal-to-noise ratio.
(e) Machine learning uses artificial intelligence to aid in the identification and real-time monitoring of molecular inflammatory and anti-inflammatory mediators in dental medicine. [13]

4 CONCLUSION

Chairside point-of-care (POC) diagnostics have been widely explored in the biomedical arena for prompt and precise diagnosis of diseases as well as assessment of disease progression, healing and prognosis. The use of LOC microfluidics in dentistry offers new avenues for the objective identification of pulpal inflammation and microbiological, immune and genomic factors associated with endodontic disease. Although faced with various challenges such as intricate production processes, complex operating mechanisms, and commercialization barriers, Lab-on-a-chip offers strong potential for providing precision medicine and evidence-based pulp therapy. The need of the hour is to find ways to translate these devices into clinically adoptable diagnostic and prognostic tools.

REFERENCES

[1] Steigmann L, Maekawa S, Sima C, Travan S, Wang CW, Giannobile WV. (2020). Biosensor and lab-on-a-chip biomarker-identifying technologies for oral and periodontal diseases. *Front Pharmacol.* 11:588480. doi: 10.3389/fphar.2020.588480. PMID: 33343358; PMCID: PMC7748088.

[2] Kaur B, Kobayashi Y, Cugini C, Shimizu E. (2021). A mini review: The potential biomarkers for non-invasive diagnosis of pulpal inflammation. *Front Dent Med.* 2:718445. doi: 10.3389/fdmed.2021.718445. Epub 2021 Dec 19. PMID: 38947881; PMCID: PMC11212789

[3] Nóbrega LM, Montagner F, Ribeiro AC, Mayer MA, Gomes BP. (2016). Bacterial diversity of symptomatic primary endodontic infection by clonal analysis. 30(1):e103. https://doi.org/10.1590/1807-3107BOR-2016.vol30.0103. PMID: 27737357.Braz Oral Res

[4] Ardila CM, Jiménez-Arbeláez GA, Vivares-Builes AM. (2023). The potential clinical applications of a microfluidic lab-on-a-chip for the identification and antibiotic susceptibility testing of *enterococcus faecalis*-associated endodontic infections: A systematic review. *Dent J (Basel)*. 12(1):5. doi: 10.3390/dj12010005. PMID: 38248213; PMCID: PMC10814515.

[5] Mascini M, Tombelli S. (2008). Biosensors for biomarkers in medical diagnostics. *Biomarkers. Nov*;13(7):637–57. doi: 10.1080/13547500802645905. PMID: 19061054.

[6] Zehnder M, Belibasakis GN. A critical analysis of research methods to study clinical molecular biomarkers in Endodontic research. *Int Endod J.* 55 Suppl 1(Suppl 1):37–45. doi:10.1111/iej.13647. Epub 2021 Oct 31. PMID: 34655496; PMCID: PMC9298367.

[7] Kim J, Campbell AS, de Ávila BE, Wang J. (2019). Wearable biosensors for healthcare monitoring. *Nat Biotechnol.* 37(4):389–406. doi: 10.1038/s41587-019-0045-y. Epub 2019 Feb 25. PMID: 30804534; PMCID: PMC8183422.

[8] Seker E, Sung JH, Shuler ML, Yarmush ML. (2011). Solving medical problems with BioMEMS. *IEEE Pulse.* 2(6):51–9. doi: 10.1109/MPUL.2011.942928. PMID: 22147069; PMCID: PMC4490689.

[9] Haji Mohammadi, Melika and Mulder, Sterre and Khashayar, Patricia and Kalbasi, Alireza and Azimzadeh, Mostafa and Aref, Amir. (2021). Saliva Lab-on-a-chip Biosensors: Recent novel ideas and applications in disease detection. *Microchemical Journal.* 168. 106506. 10.1016/j.microc.2021.106506.

[10] Kaisti M. (2017). Detection principles of biological and chemical FET sensors. *Biosens Bioelectron.* 98:437–448. doi: 10.1016/j.bios.2017.07.010. Epub 2017 Jul 5. PMID: 28711826.

[11] Kim J, Imani S, de Araujo WR, Warchall J, Valdés-Ramírez G, Paixão TR, Mercier PP, Wang J. (2015). Wearable salivary uric acid mouthguard biosensor with integrated wireless electronics. *Biosens Bioelectron.* 74:1061–8. doi: 10.1016/j.bios.2015.07.039. Epub 2015 Aug 1. PMID: 26276541; PMCID: PMC4718709

[12] Mannoor MS, Tao H, Clayton JD, Sengupta A, Kaplan DL, Naik RR, Verma N, Omenetto FG, McAlpine MC. (2012). Graphene-based wireless bacteria detection on tooth enamel. *Nat Commun.* 3:763. doi: 10.1038/ncomms1767. Erratum in: Nat Commun. 2013;4:1900. PMID: 22453836.

[13] Bianchi J, de Oliveira Ruellas AC, Gonçalves JR, Paniagua B, Prieto JC, Styner M, Li T, Zhu H, Sugai J, Giannobile W, Benavides E, Soki F, Yatabe M, Ashman L, Walker D, Soroushmehr R, Najarian K, Cevidanes LHS. (2020). Osteoarthritis of the Temporomandibular Joint can be diagnosed earlier using biomarkers and machine learning. *Sci Rep.* 10(1):8012. doi: 10.1038/s41598-020-64942-0. PMID: 32415284; PMCID: PMC7228972.

 ISBN: 978-1-041-32674-8

The Use of Activity Trackers and Self-Reported Anthropometric Measures Among Dental Students

Kalyana C Pentapati and Jaya-Snehitha Kuntamukkala
Department of Public Health Dentistry, Manipal College of Dental Sciences, Manipal Academy of Higher Education, Manipal, Karnataka, India

Abhinav N Tadikonda
Department of Public Health Dentistry, Sri Sai College of Dental Surgery, Vikarabad, Telangana, India

Vidya S Muliya
Department of Conservative Dentistry and Endodontics, Manipal College of Dental Sciences, Manipal Academy of Higher Education, Manipal, Karnataka, India

Nanditha K Mysore
Department of Prosthodontics, JSS Dental College & Hospital, JSS Academy of Higher Education & Research, Mysuru, Karnataka, India

ABSTRACT: Objective: We aimed to evaluate the use of wearable activity trackers among dental students. To examine the relationship between socio-demographic factors (age, sex, year of study) and BMI with the use of activity trackers.

Materials and methods: An online survey was conducted among undergraduate dental students of various dental colleges in India. The survey form was circulated through WhatsApp from August to September 2023. It had information on age, sex, height, weight, current year of study in dentistry and the use of activity tracker (yes/no), if yes, what was the average step count in the last one week.

Results: A total of 575 responded to the survey form of which females were 78.1% (n=449). The mean age of the students was 22.05 (SD: 1.5). Forty percent of the students were from preclinical years. Only a quarter of the students (24.5%) have reported that they are using activity trackers. The use of activity tracker was significantly higher among males (p=0.001 and among overweight and obese students (P=0.003).

Conclusion: The use of activity trackers among dental students is low. Among the students who used activity trackers, obese and overweight students were significantly more than others.

1 INTRODUCTION

Students pursuing dentistry are subjected to vigorous training in medical and dental subjects due to the complex dental curriculum, especially in India. It is extremely strenuous and induces fatigue with very little leisure time due to the extensive training and assessments within the stipulated timeframe. [1] Due to the nature of training, which involves long static procedures, the premature onset of musculoskeletal problems has been reported in previous studies [2,3]. Previous studies have reported stress [4–6] and burnout [7] among dental students, which decreases their overall quality of life and productivity. Owing to the lack of physical activity, increased weight gain, coupled with fatigue, can also be a significant problem. Prolonged static postures and lack of physical activity can result in weak core muscles which may lead to strain on the musculoskeletal system and leading to improper posture.

Physical activity in the past has been recorded by a variety of instruments like self-reported questionnaires, anthropometric measures, wearable activity trackers etc, all of which have advantages and limitations. Owing to the problems associated with lack of physical activity, wearable fitness trackers are gaining attention and acceptance. Wearable activity trackers offer numerous advantages like ease of use, comfort, rapid and real time self-assessment, monitor trends and the availability of this data on different mobile applications and devices, passive assessment of multiple parameters. However, it has limitations like user compliance and motivation, cost, recurrent expenditure, need for charging, some activities may need to be selected by the user in order to monitor the physical activity, validity of the instrument. In view of the above, there is a need to understand the acceptance of wearable activity trackers among dental students and its associated factors.

We aimed to evaluate the use of wearable activity trackers among dental students. To examine the relationships between sociodemographic factors (age, sex, year of study) and BMI with the use of activity trackers (proxy measure of physical activity). Null hypothesis was that there would be no significant differences with the use of activity trackers and socio-demographic factors (age, sex, year of study) and BMI.

Studies have evaluated the physical activity of dentists [8–10] and dental students [11] and the physical activity and stress of dental students [12], physical activity and obesity with academic performance [13]. Studies have not

DOI: 10.1201/9781042016075-55

been conducted on the use of activity trackers among dental students or their relationships with sociodemographic factors (age, sex, year of study) and BMI.

2 MATERIALS AND METHODS

An online survey was conducted among undergraduate dental students from various dental colleges in India. The survey form was circulated through WhatsApp from August to September 2023. The protocol was approved by the institutional ethics committee (IEC2: 199/2023). The survey form could be accessed only after the respondents provide informed consent. Students who were pursuing dentistry for atleast one year were included. Students not willing to participate and who were unaware of their weight and height were excluded. The data included information on age, sex, height, weight, current year of study in dentistry and the use of an activity tracker (yes/no); if yes, what was the average step count in the last week? Body mass index was calculated using the formula Weight in Kg divided by Height in metres squared. BMI was categorized as underweight (<18.5), healthy weight (18.5- <25), overweight (25 - <30) and obesity ($\geq$ 30) as per the CDC guidelines (https://www.cdc.gov/bmi/adult-calculator/bmi-categories.html).

The sample size was calculated on the basis of a prevalence of 60% [14], a power of 95% and 5% precision, and a design effect of 1.5. A total of 554 responses were obtained, which was increased to 582 to account for incomplete responses. Convenient sampling was used to collect data owing to the nature of the study design.

2.1 *Statistical analysis*

All the analysis was done using SPSS version 25. A p-value of <0.05 was considered statistically significant. Categorical variables were compared using Chi-square test. Binary Logistic regression analysis was done to evaluate the role of significant predictors for track band usage.

3 RESULTS

A total of 575 undergraduate dental students were included, 78.1% of whom were female (n=449). The mean age of the students was 22.05 years (SD: 1.5). Forty percent of the students were in their preclinical years. Only a quarter of the students (24.5%) reported that they were using activity trackers. The use of an activity tracker was significantly greater among males (p=0.001) and among overweight and obese students (P=0.003) (Table 1). The average step count among those used as activity trackers was 7503.06 (SD: 3251.62; median: 7600). A binary logistic regression analysis was performed to evaluate the significant predictors of track band usage. It was seen that the males compared to females (OR: 2.04) and obese/overweight compared to normal/underweight students (2.05) preferred track band usage. Adjusted analysis also showed similar trend with slight decrease in the OR (Table 2).

Table 1. The use of activity trackers and their relationships with sociodemographic factors (age, sex, year of study) and BMI.

		Do you use Fitness or Track Band to track your physical activity?				
		No		Yes		
		N	%	N	%	P value
Sex	Male	81	64.3%	45	35.7%	0.001
	Female	353	78.6%	96	21.4%	
Age	<22	274	77.2%	81	22.8%	0.227
	>22	160	72.7%	60	27.3%	
Year of study	Preclinical	180	78.3%	50	21.7%	0.205
	Clinical	254	73.6%	91	26.4%	
BMI	Underweight	59	84.3%	11	15.7%	0.003
	Normal	267	78.5%	73	21.5%	
	Overweight	81	66.4%	41	33.6%	
	Obese	27	62.8%	16	37.2%	

Table 2. Binary logistic regression to evaluate the significant predictors for the use of activity trackers.

	Crude			Adjusted		
	P-value	OR	95% CI	P-value	OR	95% CI
Sex	0.001	2.04	1.33-3.14	0.003	1.92	1.24-2.96
BMI	<0.001	2.05	1.37-3.06	0.001	1.94	1.29-2.92

4 DISCUSSION

Wearable activity trackers have gained substantial acceptance among general population and was reported to be popular trend. In view of the growing acceptance, interest, and relevance in public health, these activity trackers are becoming increasingly relevant in monitoring physical activity and well-being [15,16]. Owing to this background, we aimed to evaluate the acceptance of wearable activity trackers and its associated factors among dental students.

The overall use and acceptance of activity trackers among dental students is low. During dental treatment, it is often required to remove accessories like jewellery and watches to maintain universal precautions. This might be the reason for which the acceptance of wearable activity trackers might be low among dental students. Also, concepts like wearability, appearance, display, interaction, modeling and data measurement and presentation are known to influence the acceptance of these wearable activity trackers. [17–19] Clawson *et al.* opined that monitoring of Health should not be limited to a specific subset of users and technology should be developed for diverse users with support over time [20]. Research has shown that acceptance to wearable activity trackers was influenced by many social, cognitive and psychological factors [21–23].

Among the students who used activity trackers, males, overweight and obese students were more. The limited use of activity trackers among females might be attributed to the bulky nature, non-aesthetic appeal or cultural factors (bangle usage). The direct comparisons of the findings were not possible as there were no studies that were conducted on the use of activity trackers and associated factors among dental students.

Wearing of activity trackers among dental students needs to be encouraged. Newer devices have multitude of applications that will help students to monitor physical activity via step counts, reminders during prolonged sedentary activities, hydration, monitoring of sleep, heart rate, oxygen saturation, calorie consumption etc. However, the reliability of these applications must be established. Nevertheless, these devices can be used for non-medical applications to maintain good-health and well-being aligning to the sustainable developmental goals and simultaneously monitor physical activity. A previous study showed that individuals with higher physical activity measured by wearable technology showed lower mortality rates highlighting the scope for personalised prevention among the dental students [24].

Self-reported nature of the study is one of the limitations of the study. Temporal association between the use of activity trackers and obesity cannot be established owing to the cross-sectional study design. Due to the nature of the study, convenience sampling was considered, and design effect was implemented to overcome the clustering.

5 LIMITATIONS

The self-reported nature of the study is one of the limitations of the study. A temporal association between the use of activity trackers and obesity cannot be established owing to the cross-sectional study design. Owing to the nature of the study, convenience sampling was considered, and a design effect was implemented to overcome clustering.

6 CONCLUSION

The use of activity trackers among dental students is low. Among the students who used activity trackers, obese and overweight students were significantly more than others. Owing to the sedentary nature of the profession, students can be encouraged to use activity trackers and stay physically active. Future studies can be conducted on the role of activity trackers and physical activity among the dental students.

ACKNOWLEDGMENTS

We thank all the participants in the study.

Acknowledgments of funding sources, institutions, or individuals who contributed to the research: None

REFERENCES

[1] Dental Council of India. *BDS Course Regulations [Internet]*. 2007 [cited 2022 Jan 4]. Available from: https://dciindia.gov.in/Rule_Regulation/Revised_BDS_Course_Regulation_2007.pdf

[2] Chenna D, Madi M, Kumar M, Kumar V, Chopperla S, Tadikonda A, *et al.* (2023). Meta-analysis of the prevalence of Carpal Tunnel Syndrome (CTS) among dental health care personnel. *F1000Research*. 12:251.

[3] Chenna D, Pentapati KC, Kumar M, Madi M, Siddiq H. (2022). Prevalence of musculoskeletal disorders among dental healthcare providers: A systematic review and meta-analysis. *F1000Research* 111062 [Internet]. [cited 2022 Sep 20];11:1062. Available from: https://f1000research.com/articles/11-1062

[4] Basudan S, Binanzan N, Alhassan A. (2017). Depression, anxiety and stress in dental students. *Int J Med Educ* [Internet]. [cited 2023 Sep 13];8:179–86. Available from: /pmc/articles/PMC5457790/

[5] Sekhon TS, Grewal S, Gambhir RS, Sharma S. (2015). Perceived sources of stress among dental college students: An Indian perspective. *Eur J Gen Dent [Internet]*. [cited 2023 Sep 13];4(03):121–6. Available from: www.ejgd.org

[6] Jowkar Z, Masoumi M, Mahmoodian H. (2020). Psychological stress and stressors among clinical dental students at shiraz school of dentistry, Iran. *Adv Med Educ Pract* [Internet]. [cited 2023 Sep 13];11:113–20. Available from: https://www.dovepress.com/psychological-stress-and-stressors-among-clinical-dental-students-at-s-peer-reviewed-fulltext-article-AMEP

[7] Kumar YS, Pentapati KC, Methayil AC, Darsh A. (2018). Burnout syndrome and associated factors among dental students. *Indian J Public Heal Res Dev* [Internet]. [cited 2023 Sep 13];9(8):63–7. Available from: https://researcher.manipal.edu/en/publications/burnout-syndrome-and-associated-factors-among-dental-students

[8] Bonu S, Pachava S, Bommireddy V, Ravoori S. (2019). Physical activity among dentists in neo-capital area of a South Indian State: A cross-sectional study. *J Indian Assoc Public Heal Dent [Internet]*. [cited 2023 Sep 14];17(2):152. Available from: https://journals.lww.com/aphd/pages/default.aspx/article.asp?issn=2319-5932;year=2019;volume=17;issue=2;spage=152;epage=156;aulast=Bonu

[9] Srilatha A, Doshi D, Reddy Mp, Kulkarni S, Reddy Bs, Reddy S. Physical activity among dental health professionals in Hyderabad City: A questionnaire survey. *Dent Res J (Isfahan) [Internet]*. 2016 Nov 1 [cited 2023 Sep 14];13(6):544. Available from: https://pubmed.ncbi.nlm.nih.gov/28182058/

[10] Singh A, Purohit B. (2012). Physical activity, sedentary lifestyle, and obesity among indian dental professionals. *J Phys Act Heal [Internet]*. [cited 2023 Sep 14];9(4):563–70. Available from: https://pubmed.ncbi.nlm.nih.gov/21946026/

[11] AL-Mhanna SB, Wan Ghazali WS, Mohamed M, Mohamed RN, Mirza MB, Basheer SN, *et al.* (2022). The Impact of COVID-19 on physical activity patterns of dental students: A multinational survey. *Healthc [Internet]*. [cited 2023 Sep 14];10(11):2140. Available from: https://www.mdpi.com/2227-9032/10/11/2140/htm

[12] Hou Y, Mei G, Liu Y, Xu W. (2020). Physical fitness with regular lifestyle is positively related to academic performance among chinese medical and dental students. *Biomed Res Int [Internet]*. 2020 Jan 17 [cited 2023 Sep 14];2020:1–10. Available from: https://pubmed.ncbi.nlm.nih.gov/32016116/

[13] Kuntamukkala JS, Pentapati KC, Tadikonda AN, Muliya VS, Mysore NK, Tadikonda GK. Relationship of obesity and physical activity with academic performance among Indian dental students. *Acta Biomed.* 2024 Jan 1;95(1):e2024058.

[14] Ardila CM, Gómez-Restrepo ÁM. (2021). Relationship between physical activity, academic achievement, gender, and learning styles in students of a Latin American dental school: A cross-sectional study. *J Educ Health Promot* [Internet]. [cited 2023 Sep 14];10(1):149. Available from: https://pubmed.ncbi.nlm.nih.gov/34222524/

[15] Shei RJ, Holder IG, Oumsang AS, Paris BA, Paris HL. (2022). Wearable activity trackers–advanced technology or advanced marketing? [Internet]. Vol. 122, *European Journal of Applied Physiology*. [cited 2024 Sep 20]. p. 1975–90. Available from: https://pubmed.ncbi.nlm.nih.gov/35445837/

[16] Thompson WR. (2023). Worldwide Survey of Fitness Trends for 2023. *ACSM's Heal Fit J [Internet]*. [cited 2024 Sep 20];27 (1):9–18. Available from: https://journals.lww.com/acsm-healthfitness/fulltext/2023/01000/worldwide_survey_of_fitness_trends_for_2023.6.aspx

[17] Kim DJ, Lee Y, Rho S, Lim YK. (2016). Design opportunities in three stages of relationship development between users and self-tracking devices. In: *Conference on Human Factors in Computing Systems - Proceedings [Internet]*. Association for Computing Machinery; 2016 [cited 2024 Sep 20]. p. 699–703. Available from: https://dl.acm.org/doi/10.1145/2858036.2858148

[18] Meyer J, Fortmann J, Wasmann M, Heuten W. (2015). Making lifelogging usable: Design guidelines for activity trackers. In: *Lecture Notes in Computer Science* (including subseries Lecture Notes in Artificial Intelligence and Lecture Notes in Bioinformatics) [Internet]. Springer, Cham; [cited 2024 Sep 20]. p. 323–34. Available from: https://link.springer.com/chapter/10.1007/978-3-319-14442-9_39

[19] Shin G, Jarrahi MH, Fei Y, Karami A, Gafinowitz N, Byun A, *et al.* (2019). Wearable activity trackers, accuracy, adoption, acceptance and health impact: A systematic literature review. Vol. 93, *Journal of Biomedical Informatics*. Academic Press; p. 103153.

[20] Clawson J, Pater JA, Miller AD, Mynatt ED, Mamykina L. (2015). No longer wearing: Investigating the abandonment of personal health-Tracking technologies on craigslist. In: *UbiComp 2015 - Proceedings of the 2015 ACM International Joint Conference on Pervasive and Ubiquitous Computing [Internet]*. Association for Computing Machinery, Inc; [cited 2024 Sep 20]. p. 647–58. Available from: https://dl.acm.org/doi/10.1145/2750858.2807554

[21] Butryn ML, Arigo D, Raggio GA, Colasanti M, Forman EM. (2016). Enhancing physical activity promotion in midlife women with technology-based self-monitoring and social connectivity: A pilot study. *J Health Psychol.* 21(8):1548–55.

[22] Arigo D. (2015). Promoting physical activity among women using wearable technology and online social connectivity: a feasibility study. *Heal Psychol Behav Med [Internet]*. 2015 Jan [cited 2024 Sep 20];3(1):391–409. Available from: https://www.tandfonline.com/action/journalInformation?journalCode=rhpb20

[23] Karapanos E, Gouveia R, Hassenzahl M, Forlizzi J. (2016). Wellbeing in the Making: Peoples' Experiences with Wearable Activity Trackers. *Psychol Well Being.* 6(1).

[24] Strain T, Wijndaele K, Dempsey PC, Sharp SJ, Pearce M, Jeon J, *et al.* (2020). Wearable-device-measured physical activity and future health risk. *Nat Med [Internet]*. [cited 2024 Sep 20];26(9):1385–91. Available from: https://pubmed.ncbi.nlm.nih.gov/32807930/

Navigating Dental Education Trends and Transforming Dental Pedagogy – Abas and Srikant N (Eds)
© 2027 The Author(s), ISBN: 978-1-041-32674-8

Assessment of the Interprofessional Professionalism of Undergraduate Dental Students and Medical Students in a Teaching Hospital: A Cross-Sectional Study

Swet Nisha
Department of Periodontology, Haldia Institute of Dental Sciences and Research, Haldia, West Bengal

Debanjan Das
Department of Conservative Dentistry and Endodontics, Haldia Institute of Dental Sciences and Research, Haldia, West Bengal

Pratibha Shashikumar
Department of Periodontology, J.S.S. Dental College & Hospital, JSS Academy of Higher Education & Research, Mysuru, Karnataka

ABSTRACT: **Objective:** Interprofessional professionalism is an essential component of teamwork and collaborative practice. Our educational curriculum should be student centered, and evaluation should focus on promoting interprofessional education. The present study was designed to assess the interprofessional professionalism among medical and dental students working together for better oral health outcomes in a tertiary hospital. Interprofessional professionalism assessment (IPA) tool questionnaire given by Frost *et al.* was used for the assessment. **Materials & Methods:** This cross-sectional study was conducted at a tertiary teaching Institute, West Bengal from 2022-2023. The interprofessional professionalism performance of dental and medical students as team members was calculated. Data were expressed as descriptive (mean and standard deviation) .**Results:** The interprofessional professionalism of the students working as a team was scored as 1.36 ± 0.17 out of 5 ($f=0.32$, $p=0.413$). **Conclusion:** Interprofessional professionalism needs to be strengthened between medical and dental students. Team members need to be motivated toward collaborative practice.

Keywords: Interprofessional education, Interprofessional professionalism, professionalism, medical students, dental students

1 INTRODUCTION

Interprofessional professionalism (IPP) introduces the concepts of professionalism, teamwork and collaborative practice. It is one of the subsets of professionalism and shares principles of mutual respect and values. [1] IPP focuses on collaboration, which is multidimensional in nature. Team-based health care outcomes require that IPP competencies be fulfilled. [2] Roles and responsibilities should be shared among team members. The quality of oral care can be improved by practising IPP. Managing interprofessional conflicts, encouraging collaboration and enhancing communication requires cooperation, and IPP can play a crucial role in developing these skills. [3] Patient safety in dentistry is of prime importance, and utmost care should be taken when we consider interprofessional collaboration. [4] IPP demands commitment, understanding the responsibilities and roles of team members, mutual respect and the development of a feeling of togetherness. [5] The success of interprofessional teams demands constructive criticism, communication and a healthy working environment. [6] Oral health care is essential, and dental students should be aware of their roles and responsibilities along with medical students in early referrals and in the management of medically compromised and emergency cases.

The need for IPP for successful interprofessional practice cannot be understated. Frost *et al.* developed the IPP assessment tool, which has been widely used in interprofessional practice and assessment. [7] Dental education is still emerging in terms of development related to interprofessional practice in India. [8] Core competencies in dental education still need refinement in terms of interprofessional education and practice. The student-centered approach requires the development of IPP from the initial exposure to practical classes. IPP among team members needs time, and with practice, we can acquire this soft skill. Promoting interprofessional education and building collaborative practices can initiate safe and healthy environments for IPP. [9]

Formative assessment requires active learner engagement and timely feedback, and IPP can help foster interprofessional education. [10] The categorical classification of IPP assessment tools helps cover overall interprofessional aspects. The present study aimed to assess the interprofessional professionalism behaviors of undergraduate medical and dental students at a teaching institute. The present o study was designed to assess the interprofessional professionalism aspects among undergraduate medical and dental students at a teaching institute.

DOI: 10.1201/9781042016075-56

2 MATERIALS AND METHODS

2.1 *Study location*

This was a cross-sectional study conducted in the Department of Periodontology from February 2023 to March 2024 at the Haldia Institute of Dental Sciences and Research, Haldia, West Bengal, India.

2.2 *Study participants*

Medical students and first, second, third, and final dental students and interns participated in this study. A total of 834 students participated in this study. Written informed consent was taken from each participant and the study was carried out in accordance with Helinski guidelines and registered under Institutional ethical Committee (HIDSAR/ETHICS/2022/034A).

2.3 *Assessment*

In the present study, we have used Interprofessional Professionalism assessment (IPA) tool given by Frost *et al.* to assess the Interprofessional professionalism behavior of students. The scale was 26 items which were tailored to 18 items and was validated in Indian context. So, broadly four domains were included after validation:

(1) Altruism and caring included 4 items,
(2) Excellence included 5 items,
(3) Respect had 4 items and
(4) Communication 5 items.
Response format has a five point scale:
1 = Poor, 2= Fair, 3=Good,4= Very Good, and 5= Excellent.
Scoring criteria:
All the domains were assessed for each participant. The mean scores were between 1-5. Poor score: 1-2,
Weak score: 2.1-3,
Moderate score: 3.1-4, and
Strong score: 4.1-5.

Two independent evaluators introduced the basic principles of IPA to the participants. The evaluators explained the modified IPA items and training sessions and observed the participants' professional behavior on two different occasions.

The IPA validation was assessed for its use in Indian context. The original questionnaire given by Frost *et al.* was modified with only the four relevant domains considered. Content validity index values of each item was greater than 0.81 and all items in each domain were retained. Reliability was assessed by internal consistency (0.912) and reproducibility (ICC =0.783).

2.4 *Statistical analysis*

A normality test was performed to examine the data distribution, the Kolmogorov™Smirnov normality test was performed, and p=0.08 was obtained, suggesting that the data were normally distributed. Descriptive data are expressed as frequencies, percentages, means and standard deviations. A t test was used to compare the scores according to sex (male or female). Tukey's HSD post hoc test was used. $p<0.05$ was considered significant. The data were analyzed via the Statistical Package for Social Sciences (SPSS) 22.

3 RESULTS

The participants' demographic details are listed in Table 1. No experiences with interprofessional professionalism education were reported by 756 participants (90.6%).

Table 1. Demographic characteristics of the participants.

Medical Students	N	Dental Students	N
First year	88	First year	83
Second year	86	Second year	82
Third year	92	Third year	79
Final year	89	Final year	84
Interns	95	Interns	85
Total	421		413
Gender			
Male	223		287
Female	198		126

The scores of Interprofessional professionalism of team members were 1.36±0.17 of 5 (1.03-3.12). In the excellence domain the scores of the team members was noted as lowest(Table 2). Statistical significant gender difference was not seen among the team members in relation to interprofessional professionalism scores (p= 0.074), and professions (p= 0.365). The overall mean score of medical students was 1.60±0.08 and of dental students 1.56±0.12. No significant difference was seen between the scores of two groups (p = 0.214) and years of undergraduate program (p= 0.621).

Table 2. The interprofessional professionalism scores of the participants.

Domain	Undergraduate students	1st year	2nd year	3rd year	4th year	Intern	Mean SD	F	p value
Communication	Medical	1.24	1.43	1.12	1.33	1.54	1.32 ± 0.35	0.44	0.543
	Dental	1.35	1.33	1.65	1.34	1.56			
Respect	Medical	1.46	1.23	1.87	1.72	1.57	1.57 ± 0.75	0.82	0.413
	Dental	1.65	1.56	1.38	1.47	1.46			
Altruism	Medical	1.12	1.22	1.18	1.20	1.32	1.20 ±0.54	1.82	0.152
	Dental	1.14	1.16	1.44	1.36	1.15			
Excellence	Medical	1.03	1.05	1.23	1.34	1.03	1.13 ±0.44	1.04	0.145
	Dental	1.04	1.43	1.54	1.05	1.09			

4 DISCUSSION

Interprofessional professionalism is an emerging concept with a vision to encourage professionalism in terms of interprofessional education and practice. This will lead to safe working environment, enhance healthcare related outcomes and foster interprofessional values and practice among team members. Interprofessional Professionalism tool kit by Frost *et al.* measures the IPP and it is a good initiative and practice to measure IPP among team members. The tool kit is easy to understand and analyze. We had validated the tool and the challenges we faced were initially in understanding the domains though the scoring criteria were easy to apprehend.

Further, we decided to include only dental and medical students for IPP behavior assessment as we had antenatal oral health care project initiative by IPE team going on during this study and only these students were involved and approachable for assessment.

There lies a need to foster IPP among interprofessional team members and results from our study shows that for practicing IPE, IPP needs to be developed among team members. The rationale to develop IPP should be clearly explained and activities to enhance professionalism should be suggested and practiced.

Keshmiri *et al.* conducted Interprofessional professionalism(IPP) assessments in operating units for surgical residents and workers and reported that Interprofessional professionalism behavior was poor among residents and that there was a need for a structured curriculum to enhance Interprofessional professionalism. [11] We found similar results of poor IPP behavior among team members involved in IPE for oral health care. Hosseinpour *et al.* recognized interprofessional professionalism as a critical element of team-based care. [12] We also strongly recommend and suggest capacity building on IPP for all team members involved in Interprofessional education and practice. Khossravi *et al.* suggested the need for interprofessional case-based learning to promote Interprofessional professionalism. [13] We propose our future research will focus on interventions to promote IPP behavior and method of assessments .Rothdiener *et al.* suggested active participation in the development of communication and the management of cases. [14] This is essential for developing IPP among team members and activities to enhance communication can help in understanding the challenges and strategies to overcome. Similar results were obtained in our study; communication among medical and dental students in terms of Interprofessional Professionalism was poor, and the need for active participation was recommended by team members for oral health care. Keshmiri *et al.*, in their qualitative study, depicted Interprofessional professionalism as a motivating force in collaboration. [15] This study highlighted the voice of team members and gave suggestions for improvement and interventions. Though the results from this study cannot be generalised but we can take suggestions in our set up to improvise the IPP practice. Guraya *et al.* studied the climate associated with IPP among medical students, and the results revealed that a standard, universal programme is required for building IPP. [16] This multicentre studied gave an idea about various perspectives of IPP and we should provide safe working environment for team members. Sur *et al.* suggested that empathic care is needed in Interprofessional education (IPE). In our study, we found that students lacking empathy as team members and activities to promote empathy are beneficial in building IPP competencies. [17] Atwa *et al.*, in their cross-sectional study on medical, dentistry, and pharmacy students, suggested an online IP course for ethics and professionalism. [18] We didn't planned any online sessions and all the activities and questionnaire were collected offline.

Understanding the domains of IPP is essential for interprofessional education among students. Building core competencies requires proper planning, teamwork and implementation of programs for 1st-year students and

[12] Hosseinpour A, Keshmiri F, Jambarsang S, Jabinian F, Shiryazdi SM. (2022). The effect of interprofessional education on interprofessional professionalism behaviors of the surgical team members. *BMC Nurs.* 21(1):239.

[13] Khossravi J, Parandeh A, Vafadar Z. (2019). Effectiveness of educational workshop based on interprofessional approach in changing health science students' attitudes toward interprofessional learning and collaboration. *Educ Strat.* 12(4):125–33.

[14] Rothdiener M, Griewatz J, Meder A, Dall'Acqua A, Obertacke U, Kirschniak A, *et al.* (2020). Surgeons' participation in the development of collaboration and management competencies in undergraduate medical education. *PLoS ONE.* 15(6): e0233400.

[15] Keshmiri F. (2022). Exploring the experiences of the team members in the interprofessional socialization process for becoming an interprofessional Collaborator. *BMC Nurs.* 21(1):366.

[16] Guraya SY, Sulaiman N, Guraya SS, *et al.* (2021). Understanding the climate of medical professionalism among university students; a multicenter study. *Innovations in Education and Teaching International.* 58(3):351–60.

[17] Sur D. (2021). Interprofessional intentional empathy centered care (IP-IECC) in healthcare practice: a grounded theory study. *J Interprof Care.* 35(2):175–84

[18] Atwa H, Farghaly A, Badawi JT, Malik LF and Abdelnasser A. (2024). Evaluation of an online interprofessional course on ethics and professionalism: experience of medical, dental, and pharmacy students. *Front. Educ.*8:1338321

[19] Abdelaziz A, Mansour T, Alkhadragy R, Abdel Nasser A, and Hasnain M. (2021). Challenges to interprofessional education: will e-learning be the magical stick? *Adv. Med. Educ. Pract.* 12, 329–336.

[20] Berger-Estilita J, Chiang H, Stricker D, Fuchs A, Greif R, and McAleer S. (2020). Attitudes of medical students toward interprofessional education: a mixed-methods study. *PLoS One* 15:e0240835. doi: 10.1371/journal.pone.0240835

[21] Adamson K, Loomis C, Cadell S, Verweel LC. (2018). Interprofessional empathy: A four-stage model for a new understanding of teamwork. *J Interprof Care.* 32(6):752–61.

 ISBN: 978-1-041-32674-8

Bridging Theory and Practice: Assessing the Benefits and Challenges of Early Clinical Exposure in Dental Education

Jochima Eudora Cota and Nairica Rebello
Department of Oral and Maxillofacial Pathology, Goa Dental College and Hospital

ABSTRACT: Early clinical exposure (ECE) has emerged as a crucial element in dental education and is designed to bridge the gap between theoretical knowledge and practical application. By introducing students to clinical environments early in their training, ECE enhances critical thinking, decision-making, and hands-on skills. This review evaluated the impact of ECE on dental students' learning outcomes, clinical competence, and professional growth. A literature review revealed that ECE significantly improved students' manual dexterity, confidence, and understanding of clinical procedures. It also helps reduce anxiety and fosters better communication skills. Studies have shown that students exposed to clinical practice earlier perform better in practical evaluations and are more prepared for patient care. Peer-assisted learning within ECE programs also improves knowledge retention and promotes collaborative learning. Despite these benefits, challenges remain in integrating ECE into curricula without overwhelming students or compromising patient safety. Future research should focus on refining ECE approaches, balancing traditional and virtual learning tools, and assessing long-term impacts on professional development. Overall, ECE is vital for producing competent, confident dental professionals equipped to handle the complexities of patient care.

Keywords: Early Clinical Exposure, Dental Education, Peer assisted learning, Curriculum

1 INTRODUCTION

Early clinical exposure (ECE) has become a critical aspect of dental education aimed at integrating theoretical knowledge with practical experience from the early stages of training. It fosters a holistic learning experience by integrating preclinical knowledge with real-world scenarios, promoting critical thinking and decision-making. Research shows that students exposed to clinical environments early tend to demonstrate greater confidence and preparedness when handling patients in later years. [1] This review seeks to evaluate the impact of ECE on dental students' learning outcomes, clinical skills, and professional development. It highlights key trends, gaps, and areas for improvement in the literature.

2 METHODS

To ensure a comprehensive review, manuscript indexed in PubMed and Google scholar that focused on early clinical exposure in dentistry were selected. A retrospective review of the relevant literature was conducted to assess the impact of ECE in dental education. The keywords used for the search were "early clinical exposure," "dental education," "clinical skills," "patient contact," and "dental students". The inclusion criteria for selecting the articles were that they should be written in English, peer-reviewed, and provide insights into the dynamics, opportunities, and challenges of ECE in dental education. These studies were analyzed to identify key findings related to the effectiveness of ECE, including changes in student learning outcomes, skills development, and attitudes toward clinical practice.

3 RESULTS

The reviewed studies consistently demonstrated that ECE positively influences student learning and clinical performance (Table 1). Maheshwari *et al.* [2] reported that ECE improved students' understanding of prosthetic concepts, manual dexterity, and confidence when they transitioned to clinical work. Students exposed early to clinical cases performed better in practical evaluations than those without early exposure. Additionally, student feedback indicated that ECE helped bridge the gap between theory and practice, enhancing students' readiness for clinical responsibilities. Shigli *et al.* [3] demonstrated that students who participated in ECE scored significantly higher in clinical examinations and demonstrated greater proficiency in patient management than did the control

 DOI: 10.1201/9781042016075-57

group. The study further highlighted that early clinical exposure reduced students' anxiety, improved their communication skills, and enhanced their overall preparedness for future clinical rotations. Harish *et al.* [4] investigated the role of ECE as an adjunct teaching-learning tool in the dental discipline. They reported that integrating ECE into the curriculum positively impacted students' understanding of clinical procedures, leading to more efficient learning of theoretical concepts. The authors reported increased motivation among students to engage with clinical content early in their training, contributing to a deeper understanding of dental procedures and patient care. Obrez *et al.* [5] examined the implementation of a clinically oriented complete denture program for second-year dental students. The study revealed that ECE in prosthodontics allows students to grasp complex clinical procedures earlier, significantly improving their clinical competencies and readiness for patient interactions. Students with ECE outperformed those with traditional programs in terms of clinical reasoning, decision-making, and practical application. Ali *et al.* [6] reported that students had greater enthusiasm for clinical work, improved confidence in dealing with patients, and an enhanced ability to apply theoretical knowledge to real-world situations. Hande *et al.* [7] revealed that, compared with traditional learning methods, peer-assisted ECE led to better retention of knowledge and skills. The students appreciated the collaborative learning environment, which allowed them to engage more actively in clinical practice and learn from peers. The study emphasized the importance of peer mentorship in building confidence and competence in early clinical scenarios.

Table 1. Summary of key findings from reviewed studies.

Study	Key Findings	Impact on ECE
Maheshwari *et al.* (2024)	Improved manual dexterity and clinical confidence in prosthodontics	Bridging the gap between theory and practice
Hande *et al.* (2023)	Enhanced knowledge retention through peer-assisted learning	Emphasis on collaborative learning and peer mentorship
Shigli *et al.* (2017)	Higher clinical exam scores and reduced anxiety in students with early exposure	Increased proficiency in patient management
Harish *et al.* (2022)	Positive impact on understanding clinical procedures and patient care	Deeper engagement with clinical content
Obrez *et al.* (2009)	Early exposure to denture programs improved clinical reasoning and skills	Improved readiness for patient interactions in prosthodontics
Ali *et al.* (2017)	Greater enthusiasm for clinical work and application of theoretical knowledge	Enhanced learning experience and patient communication skills

4 DISCUSSION

ECE programs take various forms, such as shadowing, clinical immersion, and community-based clinical experiences. ECE can be implemented in the classroom, hospital and community set up. The student can be passive observer, active observer, passive participant and active participant. As a passive observer the student can view minor procedures in the outpatient department and the operation theatre. Log books and journals can be maintained as an active observer. Simulation based demonstrations can be done under passive participation whereas, as an active participant the student can assist a resident in performing the procedure. These programs aim to give students direct patient interaction and opportunities to observe and engage in clinical care, all under the guidance of experienced clinicians. [8] A review of these studies provides a clear consensus that early clinical exposure plays a pivotal role in shaping dental students' educational experiences. Across different dental disciplines, ECE has substantially improved students' clinical confidence, manual dexterity, and practical application of theoretical knowledge.

Maheshwari *et al.* [2] and Obrez *et al.* [5] reported significant gains in clinical competency among students introduced to early clinical work, particularly in prosthodontics. The ability to link theoretical concepts with practical applications at an early stage facilitates smoother transitions into advanced clinical work. Additionally, peer-assisted ECE, as highlighted by Hande *et al.*, [7] offers an innovative approach to learning by leveraging peer support to reinforce skills and knowledge retention.

Shigli *et al.* [3] and Harish *et al.* [4] both emphasized that ECE reduces anxiety and improves preparedness, with students demonstrating enhanced performance in clinical assessments. The reduction in anxiety, particularly, is a crucial finding, as clinical environments often induce stress in students during the transition from the classroom to patient care. By familiarizing students with clinical settings early on, ECE fosters a sense of comfort and confidence.

Although the benefits of ECE are clear, the reviewed literature also identifies challenges and areas for future research. For example, Verma [9] suggested that while ECE improves technical and critical thinking skills, integrating it effectively into curricula without overwhelming students or compromising patient safety remains a challenge. A major challenge in implementing ECE is to evaluate its effectiveness. Future research should focus on optimizing the balance between academic learning and clinical exposure, exploring the long-term impacts of ECE on professional development, and assessing its effectiveness by using questionnaires, tests, viva voce and OSPE/OSCE across diverse educational settings. The integration of virtual and conventional methods, as highlighted by Hande *et al.* [7] suggests that while technology can supplement learning, it should not replace hands-on clinical experiences. The combination of virtual tools with actual clinical practice provides a more comprehensive learning experience.

Innovations in pedagogy from ECE in dental education focus on bridging the gap between theoretical learning and practical application. ECE introduces students to clinical environments early in their training, enhancing manual dexterity, critical thinking, and decision-making skills. This early hands-on exposure builds clinical competence and boosts confidence in handling real-world patient care. Additionally, ECE helps reduce the anxiety typically associated with transitioning from the classroom to clinical settings, allowing students to feel more comfortable and prepared. Didactic lectures can be modified by case demonstrations, laboratory report interpretation. ECE's holistic approach to learning, which combines theory, practice, and technology, equips students with the skills and confidence needed for complex patient care.

5 CONCLUSION

The role of early clinical exposure in dental education is undeniably valuable, as evidenced by the improvements in clinical confidence, knowledge retention, and practical skills observed across multiple studies. ECE enables students to bridge the gap between theoretical learning and hands-on practice, preparing them for the complexities of patient care. The positive effects of ECE, particularly in reducing anxiety and improving clinical competence, highlight its significance in modern dental curricula.

Future research should aim to refine ECE programs, ensuring a balanced approach that supports student learning without overwhelming them. Additionally, exploring interdisciplinary approaches and integrating technological tools such as virtual simulations may further enhance the benefits of ECE, creating well-rounded dental professionals equipped for the demands of clinical practice.

ACKNOWLEDGMENT

None

REFERENCES

[1] Tayade MC, Latti RG. (2021). Effectiveness of early clinical exposure in medical education: Settings and scientific theories - Review. *J Educ Health Promot*. 10:117.

[2] Maheshwari K, Shigli K, Tiwari B, *et al.* (2024). Introduction and effectiveness of early clinical exposure among dental students in preclinical prosthodontics. *Cureus*. 16(8)

[3] Shigli K, Nayak SS, Sankeshwari B, *et al.* (2017). Effectiveness of an early clinical exposure module on the performance of second year dental students: a randomized controlled study. *Ann Med Health Sci Res*. 7:236–241.

[4] Harish HA, Panchbhai A, Gawande MN *et al.* (2022). Early clinical exposure: An adjunct teaching–learning tool in dental discipline. *J Datta Meghe Inst Med Sci Univ*. 17(4):877–80.

[5] Obrez A, Lee DJ, Organ-Boshes A, *et al.* (2009). A clinically oriented complete denture program for second-year dental students. *J Dent Educ*. 73(10):1194–201.

[6] Ali K, Zahra D, McColl E, *et al.* (2018). Impact of early clinical exposure on the learning experience of undergraduate dental students. *Eur J Dent Educ*. 22(1)

[7] Hande AH, Zade PR, Gawande MN, *et al.* (2023). Impact of peer-assisted early clinical exposure on learning in dental students. *J Datta Meghe Inst Med Sci Univ*. 18:475–80.

[8] Ingale MH, Tayade MC, Bhamare S. (2023). Early clinical exposure: Dynamics, opportunities, and challenges in modern medical education. *J Educ Health Promot*. 12:295.

[9] Verma M. (2016). Early clinical exposure: New paradigm in medical and dental education. *Contemp Clin Dent*. 7(3):287–8.

Navigating Dental Education Trends and Transforming Dental Pedagogy – Abas and Srikant N (Eds)
 ISBN: 978-1-041-32674-8

Enhancing Learning Outcomes: A Review of the Presentation-Assimilation-Discussion Paradigm in Dental Education

Nairica Rebello and Jochima Eudora Cota
Department of Oral and Maxillofacial Pathology, Goa Dental College and Hospital, Bambolim, Goa

ABSTRACT: Objective: The 'presentation-assimilation-discussion' (PAD) paradigm is a structured approach practiced in educational and research institutions to enhance comprehension and critical engagement among students. This review was undertaken with the objective of identifying the application of this technique to dental education.

Significance of the review and contribution to the field: The PAD model has been reported to effectively facilitate knowledge acquisition and retention across various disciplines.

Key trends, patterns, and gaps in the literature: Studies emphasize that clear, structured presentations significantly impact the understanding of a topic, with visual aids and concise summaries being imperative for effective delivery. Active learning techniques, such as interactive exercises and reflective questioning, play crucial roles in enhancing the assimilation process and consequently improve the retention and application of new concepts. Guided discussions improve understanding and spark intellectual curiosity. There is a paucity of studies exploring the application of this model to the life sciences.

Conclusion and future scope: The PAD paradigm is supported by evidence as a robust framework for promoting effective learning and critical thinking. Further research is recommended to explore the application of PAD in different educational fields and its potential impact on long-term knowledge retention and skill development.

Keywords: active learning, dental education, flipped classroom, PAD paradigm

1 INTRODUCTION

The Presentation-Assimilation-Discussion (PAD) paradigm is a novel innovative approach to teaching methodology. [1] This model, which emphasizes a structured sequence of presenting material, assimilating information, and discussing concepts, aims to enhance student engagement and learning outcomes. [2] The application of this model has been evaluated across several disciplines, including the social sciences. However, its application in dental education is largely unexplored. This review was undertaken with the objective of providing an overview of the PAD paradigm, identifying its effectiveness and limitations, and analyzing its application in dental education.

2 METHODS

A literature search was conducted using PubMed as the database. To ensure a comprehensive review, manuscripts indexed in PubMed and MEDLINE were selected. The search was conducted using keywords such as "PAD paradigm," "presentation-assimilation-discussion," "flipped classroom," and "problem-based learning." Non-peer-reviewed sources, studies not primarily focused on instructional methodologies and studies not written in English were excluded.

Database searches were performed in PubMed and MEDLINE, combining keywords and applying filters to refine the results to educational methodologies and instructional strategies. Relevant articles were reviewed for their description of the PAD model, its implementation, and outcomes.

3 RESULTS

The PAD paradigm has been successfully applied in various educational settings, including dental and medical education. A summary of the results obtained in this review is presented in Table 1. Studies conducted by Johnson *et al.* [1] and Ali & Syed [2] have reported its effectiveness in enhancing student comprehension and retention in histology. Cheng *et al.* [3] and Sharma *et al.* [4] reported that integrating PAD with flipped classroom models can improve student engagement. The flipped classroom approach, when combined with PAD, facilitates more interactive and student-centered learning environments. Lim & Chen. [5] and Owen *et al.* [6] have discussed the

DOI: 10.1201/9781042016075-58

application of PAD to problem-based learning scenarios, thus demonstrating its ability to foster critical thinking and collaborative problem-solving skills among students. Zhai *et al.* [7] evaluated the effectiveness of this technique in the context of oral pathology and concluded that, in comparison with traditional teaching techniques, it improved teaching outcomes in oral pathology. Despite its benefits, the PAD paradigm is fraught with obstacles such as resistance to change and difficulties in implementation. Sinouvassane & Nalini. [8] and Mortensen & Nicholson. [9] identified challenges in implementing PAD, such as resistance to newer teaching methods from students and faculty and the need for additional resources and training.

Table 1. Summary of the application of PAD in dental education.

Study	Area of focus	Findings
Johnson et al	Histology learning strategies	Enhanced learning through structured learning phases
Ali & Syed	Oral histology	Improved student performed through PAD
Cheng et al	Flipped classroom and PAD	Positive impact on learning attitudes and mastery
Sharma et al	Implementation of flipped classroom	Increased engagement and participation
Sinouvassane & Nalini	Perception of flipped classroom	Challenges in adoption and resistance
Zhai et al	PAD in oral pathology	Improved teaching outcomes

4 DISCUSSION

The PAD model was proposed as a novel teaching method in 2014 by Professor Xuexin Zhang of Fudan University, Shanghai, China. [7] The PAD paradigm has emerged as a progressive instructional approach designed to enhance learning by structuring educational activities into three sequential phases: presentation of new material by the educator, assimilation of information by the students, and discussion between the educator and students to reinforce and deepen understanding. [7] It is further subdivided into in-class PAD, which focuses on discussion immediately following the lecture, and cross-class PAD, which provides students with additional time for assimilation prior to discussion. This review of the PAD paradigm reveals that while it shows promise in enhancing educational outcomes, its effectiveness can be influenced by variability in the self-learning teaching environment. [2] By structuring lessons into the presentation, assimilation, and discussion phases, PAD aims to promote deeper understanding and student engagement, which is crucial in dynamic fields such as dental education. [7] Dental education is constantly evolving, which could be attributed in part to the development of novel treatment strategies on the basis of improved understanding of pathology. The PAD model could prove beneficial for encouraging students to 'think-outside-the-box' when practicing routine dental procedures to improve treatment outcomes. The integration of PAD with other innovative methods, such as flipped classrooms, appears to increase its benefits, suggesting a synergistic effect. [3,4] The model's emphasis on active participation and structured discussion is particularly valuable in developing practical skills and in-depth understanding in dental students. [5] However, the challenges highlighted, such as the need for educator training and potential resistance, underscore the complexity of implementing new teaching strategies.

Educational institutions should consider adopting the PAD model in conjunction with other innovations in teaching methodology to maximize its effectiveness.

On the basis of the available literature, we identified several shortcomings that could affect the implementation of this model. The implementation of PAD can be resource intensive, requiring significant time and effort from both educators and students. The model's success heavily relies on students' ability level of understanding of a subject, which can vary widely. Instructors may encounter resistance and struggle with integrating PAD into preexisting rigid curricula. Additionally, the success of PAD depends on the quality of discussion and assimilation activities, which can be challenging to manage effectively in large classes. Thus, it is necessary to incorporate it in a gradual manner to enable seamless integration.

Future research should focus on longitudinal studies that assess the long-term impacts of PAD on student learning outcomes and professional development. The long-term effects of the PAD model and its application across various subjects and educational levels should be explored. Additionally, comparative research should be undertaken to evaluate PAD against other pedagogical models in various educational contexts. Practical applications may involve creating training programs for educators and developing specific resources to support the adoption of PAD in diverse educational settings.

5 CONCLUSION

The PAD paradigm offers a valuable framework for enhancing dental education by structuring learning into presentation, assimilation, and discussion phases. The integration of PAD with other modern teaching methods, such as flipped classrooms, can further improve learning outcomes. Despite its benefits, challenges such as resistance to change and the need for educator training must be addressed. Future research should explore the long-term benefits and shortcomings of PAD and develop strategies to optimize its implementation in various educational settings.

ACKNOWLEDGMENTS

None.

REFERENCES

[1] Johnson S, Purkiss J, Holaday L, Selvig D, Hortsch M. (2015). Learning histology—Dental and medical students' study strategies. *Eur J Dent Educ.* 19(2):65–73.
[2] Ali SAA, Syed S. (2020). Teaching and learning strategies of oral histology among dental students. *Int J Morphol.* 38(3):634–639.
[3] Cheng X, Lee KKH, Chang EY, Yang X. (2017). The "flipped classroom" approach: stimulating positive learning attitudes and improving mastery of histology among medical students. *Anat Sci Educ.* 10(4):317–327.
[4] Sharma N, Lau CS, Doherty I, Harbutt D. (2015). How we flipped the medical classroom. *Med Teach.* 37(4):327–330.
[5] Lim LP, Chen AY. (1999). Challenges and relevance of problem-based learning in dental education. *Eur J Dent Educ.* 3(1):20–26.
[6] Owen C, Ryall MA, Corrigan G. (2007) Case-based learning: developing patient- and student-centered learning. *Med Educ.* 41 (5):508–509.
[7] Zhai J, Dai L, Peng C, Dong B, Jia Y, Yang C. (2022) Application of the presentation-assimilation-discussion class in oral pathology teaching. *J Dent Educ.* 86(1):4–11.
[8] Sinouvassane D, Nalini A. (2016) Perception of flipped classroom model among year one and year three health science students. *Int J Inf Educ Technol.* 2016;6(3):215–218.
[9] Mortensen CJ, Nicholson AM. (2015) The flipped classroom stimulates greater learning and is a modern 21st century approach to teaching today's undergraduates. *J Anim Sci.* 93(7):3722–3731.

 ISBN: 978-1-041-32674-8

Zooming into Precision: Power of Magnification in Dental Education

Bridhi Jalan and Karthik Shetty
Department of Conservative Dentistry and Endodontics, Manipal College of Dental Sciences Mangalore, Manipal Academy of Higher Education, Karnataka, Manipal, India

ABSTRACT: **Aim** - The main aim of this review is to focus on the role of magnification in dental education, enhancing clinical skills, learning outcomes and ergonomics. **Method** - A comprehensive literature search had been conducted in Medline (PubMed). Studies or papers published in the last 10years were included. Studies with access to full text and discussing the role of magnification tools (e.g. dental loupes and dental operating microscope) on learning outcomes, skill development, ergonomics and visual acuity were included. **Result** - Magnification improves both the dentist's and patient's experience by enhancing vision and comfort, while preventing musculoskeletal issues common in dentistry. Further research and institutional efforts are needed to fully understand and implement ergonomics in dental practice, especially for students. **Conclusion** - Magnification tools in dentistry improve skills, ergonomics, and confidence, but challenges like cost, learning curve, and long-term research must be addressed for broader adoption.

Keywords: microscopy, magnifying glass, lenses, manual dexterity, musculoskeletal disease, dental education

1 INTRODUCTION

Magnification has become an indispensable tool in modern dental education, significantly enhancing the precision and quality of dental care. By using devices such as dental loupes and operating microscope, students can observe the fine anatomical details of the oral cavity more clearly, allowing for improved accuracy in diagnosis and treatment. This heightened visual acuity enables better execution of complex procedures, such as restorative dentistry, endodontics and microsurgery. Furthermore, magnification aids in developing proper ergonomics, helping students maintain optimal posture during clinical practice, which can prevent long-term musculoskeletal issues.

Dental curriculum that use magnification tools improve students' hand dexterity and encourage critical thinking because they force them to pay attention to smaller details that they might otherwise miss. By including magnification in the curriculum, dental educators may make sure that future dental professionals are prepared to fulfil the ever-increasing standards for accuracy in patient treatment. In the end, this results in better patient outcomes, increased treatment success rates, and the growth of a workforce in the dentistry field that is more knowledgeable and meticulous. This review's main objective is to highlight how magnification improves clinical skills, learning objectives, and ergonomics in dental education.

2 METHODOLOGY

A thorough search of the literature had been done on Medline (PubMed). "Microscopy, magnifying glass, lenses, manual dexterity, musculoskeletal disease, dental education," as well as a combination of the terms, were utilized. The last ten years' worth of studies or articles were covered. Included were studies with full text accessibility that addressed the effects of magnification instruments (such as dental loupes and operating microscopes) on learning objectives, skill development, ergonomics, and visual acuity. Non-peer reviewed papers and those that did not concentrate on the educational side of magnification were not accepted. Because of the nature of this evaluation, no formal evidence-based quality assessment was carried out, and additional limits were only placed on the search to confine it to the English language.

3 RESULTS

Magnification has several benefits, it will soon surpass regular dental care as the standard. Clinical dentistry can be challenging to practice, regardless of expertise, but having good vision and being comfortable at the chairside improves the clinical experience for the patient and the dentist. By supporting the lumber region and maintaining the lower back's natural curve, one can avoid the musculoskeletal problems that are frequent in dentistry by

 DOI: 10.1201/9781042016075-59

utilizing magnifying equipment. Furthermore, the operator doesn't have to stoop to have a better view; instead, they may see a clearer image closer to them. To completely understand the role of ergonomics in dentistry, more research is necessary. Institutional interventions for ergonomic practice and execution are beneficial to the students.

4 DISCUSSION

The field of dentistry requires a lot of physical and visual skills. Dentists can see minute details that may be invisible to the unaided eye because of the limitations of human vision by using magnification. Carr and Murgel in a study, concluded that fine details cannot be distinguished by the unassisted eye at a distance of less than 0.2 mm. Magnification, on the other hand, makes it easier to see such details. The literature consistently demonstrates the positive impact of magnification tools such as dental loupes and operating microscopes on improving clinical precision, student competence, and ergonomics in dental education. The enhanced visual acuity provided by these tools allows students to perform tasks with greater accuracy, particularly in intricate procedures like endodontics and restorative dentistry. Importantly, the use of magnification improves manual dexterity and procedural outcomes, contributing to the overall skill development of dental students. Furthermore, the ergonomic benefits of magnification, including the prevention of neck and back strain, are significant, as musculoskeletal problems are common in dentistry.

The findings from the literature have several implications for dental education. First, given its established advantages, magnification ought to be used more frequently in graduate and undergraduate education. From the outset of students' instruction, the early introduction of loupes can facilitate the development of skills and encourage good ergonomic practices. Long-term magnification use may also lower the risk of occupational injuries, which is a major concern for dental professionals, while simultaneously improving clinical performance. Research indicates that the use of magnification improves accuracy in endodontics and cavity preparation, with students exhibiting increased confidence and clinical accuracy. Dental loupes are the more convenient option for everyday chores since they are portable and easy to use, even if operating microscopes provide greater magnification for complex operations.

Introduction of magnifying tools (eg. Dental loupes and operating microscope) in undergraduate will aid students in –

- Localization of demineralization of enamel tissue.
- Locating and removing outdated restorations with the least amount of disruption.
- Examining the edges of cavities and any residual carious tissue.
- Determining fissures and cracks in enamel.
- Monitoring the regulated application of liner and the sectional matrix adjustments.
- Class III cavities with little invasive pretreatment.
- Assessment of the restorations' marginal gaps.
- Voids or contaminants in materials used in restoration.
- Excess composite material removal.
- Handling minor, unintentional pulp chamber openings without causing mechanical harm to the pulp.

The enhanced vision and illumination in postgraduate curriculum will facilitate the following:

- Identifying small cracks and cavities
- Conservative access opening; unclear anatomical identification
- Handling canal sclerosis
- Verifying the cleanliness of the canal before obturation
- Define and eliminate pulp stones
- Handling dental resorption and perforations
- Finding the broken post, silver point, and separated instrument
- Smaller osteotomy, endodontic microsurgery, retro-preparation, and retro-fill. Magnified evaluation of the resected surface.

Magnification has countless benefits. More than just supplying the necessary equipment, integrating magnification into dentistry curriculum also calls for appropriate training, support, and careful planning on how to introduce magnification in order to maximize ergonomics and learning results. Standardizing its application across programs offers the chance to guarantee uniform skill development.

Several gaps identified in the literature highlight key areas for future research:

- Long-term Impact on Clinical Performance and Ergonomics: Although studies with short durations have demonstrated promising results, longer term studies are required to ascertain the long-term consequences of utilizing magnification on clinical performance, retention of skills, and ergonomic health throughout the course of a dentist's career.

- Cost-Effectiveness: Further investigation is required to determine whether including magnifying instruments in dental education is financially advantageous. Research could look at the cost-effectiveness for organizations and students as well as the possible return on investment in terms of better clinical results and fewer musculoskeletal injuries.
- Standardization of Magnification in Dental Curricula: Studies assessing the most effective ways to include magnification into dental education, including the optimum times and methods to do so, are required to ensure the greatest possible benefit. Research could also examine how standardizing the use of magnification affects career development and student results.
- Objective Measures of Skill Enhancement: To quantify the direct effects of magnification on skill learning, future research should include objective metrics such as error rates, clinical outcomes, and procedural efficiency.

5 CONCLUSION

The literature consistently supports the benefits of magnification tools, particularly dental loupes and microscopes, that help improve clinical skills, enhancing ergonomics, and boosting student confidence in dental education. For wider usage, nevertheless, issues including upfront costs, learning curves, and gaps in long-term research must be resolved. It is advised that more research be done to standardize magnification training, evaluate its long-term effects on clinical performance, and explore its cost-effectiveness in dental curricula.

REFERENCES

[1] Low JF, Dom TN, Baharin SA. (2018). Magnification in endodontics: A review of its application and acceptance among dental practitioners. *European Journal of Dentistry*. 12(04):610–6.

[2] Maret D, Peters OA, Delrieu J, Gaillac S, Ducreux P, Houze-Cerfon CH, Geeraerts T, Diemer F. (2024). The dental microscope in endodontic education: A feasibility study of a distance learning course. *Australian Endodontic Journal.*

[3] Ramesh A, Junxi Guo A, Patel HJ, Huang J, Huang CC, de Mello-Neto JM, Rodrigues Amaral R. (2024). The impact of magnification on undergraduate dental students‘ performance during cavity preparations: A systematic review. *Journal of Dental Education.*

[4] Plessas A, Bernardes Delgado M. (2018). The role of ergonomic saddle seats and magnification loupes in the prevention of musculoskeletal disorders. A systematic review. *International Journal of Dental Hygiene*. 16(4):430–40.

[5] Bud MG, Pop OD, Cîmpean S. (2023). Benefits of using magnification in dental specialties-a narrative review. *Medicine and Pharmacy Reports*. 96(3):254.

[6] Wajngarten D, Botta AC, Garcia PP. (2021). Magnification loupes in dentistry: A qualitative study of dental students' perspectives. *European Journal of Dental Education*. 25(2):305–9.

[7] Prishita DS, Mandlik J, Sharma A, Majumder H. (2022). Role of magnification in conservative dentistry and endodonTICS. *Journal of Pharmaceutical Negative Results* 6369–77.

[8] Perrin P, Ramseyer ST, Eichenberger M, Lussi A. (2014). Visual acuity of dentists in their respective clinical conditions. *Clinical oral investigations*. 18:2055–8.

[9] Garcia PP, Gottardello AC, Wajngarten D, Presoto CD, Campos JA. (2017). Ergonomics in dentistry: experiences of the practice by dental students. *European Journal of Dental Education*. 2017 Aug;21(3):175–9.

[10] Pazos JM, Wajngarten D, Dovigo LN, Garcia PP. (2020). Implementing magnification during pre-clinical training: effects on procedure quality and working posture. *European Journal of Dental Education*. 24(3):425–32.

[11] Narula K, Kundabala M, Shetty N, Shenoy R. (2015). Evaluation of tooth preparations for Class II cavities using magnification loupes among dental interns and final year BDS students in preclinical laboratory. *Journal of Conservative Dentistry and Endodontics*. 18(4):284–7.

[12] Dable RA, Wasnik PB, Yeshwante BJ, Musani SI, Patil AK, Nagmode SN. (2014). Postural assessment of students evaluating the need of ergonomic seat and magnification in dentistry. *The Journal of Indian Prosthodontic Society*. 14:51–8.

[13] Wajngarten D, Pazos JM, Menegazzo VP, Novo JP, Garcia PP. (2021). Magnification effect on fine motor skills of dental students. *PLoS One*. 16(11):e0259768

Navigating Dental Education Trends and Transforming Dental Pedagogy – Abas and Srikant N (Eds)
© 2027 The Author(s), ISBN: 978-1-041-32674-8

Three-Dimensional Dilemmas: Navigating the Dichotomy of 3D Printing

Tejaswini Shetty and Roma M
Department of Conservative dentistry and Endodontics, Manipal College of Dental Sciences, Mangalore, Manipal Academy of Higher Education, Mangalore, Karnataka, India

ABSTRACT: The integration of 3D printing technology in conservative dentistry and endodontics is reshaping treatment methodologies and enhancing patient outcomes. This review article aims to analyze the current applications, benefits, and limitations of 3D printing in these domains. A comprehensive literature search was conducted using databases such as PubMed, Scopus, and Web of Science, focusing on studies published over the last ten years that examine the utilization of 3D printing in dental practices.

The outcomes show that the accuracy of endodontic treatments and dental restorations is much increased by 3D printing. Surgical guidance, personalized endodontic devices, and patient-specific dental models are a few notable applications. These developments result in better procedural safety, shorter chair times, and better treatment planning. Furthermore, the capacity to produce accurate duplicates of intricate anatomical features improves patient education and enables more effective preoperative evaluations.

Despite the benefits, there are still issues, such as the requirement for dental practitioners to have proper training, material constraints, and expensive starting expenditures. In order to fully realize the potential of the technology, the assessment emphasizes how critical it is to address these challenges.

In conclusion, 3D printing represents a pivotal advancement in conservative dentistry and endodontics, offering enhanced customization and efficiency. Continued research and innovation are essential to refine materials and expand the scope of 3D printing applications in clinical practice, ultimately leading to improved patient care and outcomes in dentistry.

1 INTRODUCTION

The emergence of additive manufacturing, or 3D printing, has transformed a number of industries, including engineering, the arts, and medicine. This cutting-edge technology in dentistry is drastically changing established procedures, especially in conservative dentistry and endodontics. The potential benefits of producing intricate, precise, and highly customized dental restorations and equipment include improved patient satisfaction, improved clinical results, and streamlined workflow procedures.

The objective of this article is to methodically assess the applications of 3D printing in conservative dentistry and endodontics.

Examine the Applications: Identify and categorize the various applications of 3D printing in conservative dentistry (e.g., crowns, veneers, and inlays) and endodontics (e.g., root canal guides and custom instruments).

Analyse Clinical Outcomes: Assess the accuracy, durability, and overall clinical efficacy of 3D-printed restorations and devices compared to traditional techniques.

Identify Challenges: Highlight the limitations and barriers to the widespread adoption of 3D printing technologies in dental practices.

Suggest Future Directions: Propose areas for further research and development to enhance the integration of 3D printing in dentistry.

The creation of restorations and endodontic instruments using traditional procedures can take a long time, which frequently resulting in delay in patient treatment. To overcome these issues, 3D printing provides a potential solution for speedy restorations and treatment strategies improving efficiency of dental office's overall productivity.

Moreover, a growing corpus of research is highlighting the benefits of 3D printing, including better fit, less wasteful material use, and better patient outcomes. Nevertheless, despite these developments, there are still shortcomings in the standardization of materials and procedures as well as the long-term assessment of therapeutic effectiveness. This article will offer a thorough analysis of the available research, clarifying the advantages and difficulties of 3D printing in dentistry and opening the door for further research and application of this technology.

DOI: 10.1201/9781042016075-60

2 METHODOLOGY

2.1 *Search strategy*

2.1.1 *Databases and information sources*

A systematic search was conducted across various databases to ensure comprehensive coverage of the relevant literature including Google Scholar, Scopus, Web of Science, PubMed. The following search terms and phrases were used to capture relevant studies:

- "3D printing in conservative dentistry"
- "3D printers endodontics"
- "Additive manufacturing dental restorations"
- "3D printed dental crowns"
- "Endodontic applications of 3D printing"
- "3D printing dental composites"
- "3D printed root canal models"

Boolean operators (AND, OR) were employed to refine and focus the search results.

2.1.2 *Inclusion and exclusion criteria*

Inclusion Criteria:

- Peer-reviewed articles, clinical studies, and reviews published between 2013 and 2023.
- Studies that specifically address the use of 3D printing in conservative dentistry and endodontics.
- Articles that report on applications, techniques, clinical outcomes, or advancements.
- English-language publications.

Exclusion Criteria:

- Non-English articles.
- Studies unrelated to conservative dentistry or endodontics.
- Articles focusing solely on non-dental applications of 3D printing.

3 RESULTS

The review of the literature on 3D printing in conservative dentistry and endodontics yielded several key findings:

(1) **Applications in Conservative Dentistry:**
   - **Restorations**: 3D printing is increasingly used to fabricate dental restorations, including crowns, bridges, inlays, onlays, and veneers. Customization allows for a precise fit, reducing adjustment times and enhancing aesthetic outcomes.
   - **Materials**: Common materials employed include resin composites and ceramics, with ongoing research focused on developing new materials that offer improved mechanical properties and biocompatibility.

(2) **Applications in Endodontics**:
   - **Root Canal Guides**: 3D-printed guides significantly enhance the accuracy of root canal procedures, allowing for precise access and canal navigation.
   - **Custom Instruments**: The technology enables the production of custom endodontic instruments tailored to specific patient anatomy, improving treatment efficacy.

(3) **Accuracy and Clinical Outcomes**:
   - Numerous studies reported that 3D-printed restorations achieve a high level of accuracy, with many demonstrating superior fit compared to conventional methods. Clinical outcomes, including patient satisfaction and restoration longevity, are generally favourable, although more long-term data is needed.

(4) **Efficiency and Cost-Effectiveness**:
   - While the initial investment in 3D printing technology can be substantial, the potential for reduced labour costs, material waste, and quicker turnaround times presents significant advantages. Many practitioners noted improvements in operational efficiency.

(5) **Challenges and Limitations**:
   - **Material Limitations**: Current 3D printing materials may not fully replicate the mechanical properties of traditional dental materials, posing challenges for their use in high-stress applications.
   - **Technical Expertise**: Effective implementation of 3D printing requires specialized training and knowledge, which can hinder widespread adoption.
   - **Regulatory Concerns**: A lack of standardized regulations for 3D-printed dental products presents challenges for clinicians regarding safety and efficacy.

4 DISCUSSION

The literature research on 3D printing in endodontics and conservative dentistry has brought to light important technological developments and applications, as well as noteworthy obstacles and gaps that need to be filled. The results show that 3D printing has many advantages, such as better patient satisfaction, shorter chair times, and more accuracy in instruments and restorations. These benefits point to a paradigm change in dental operations and establish 3D printing as a useful instrument in contemporary dental practice.

There is a clear trend in the literature toward the use of 3D printing in endodontics and conservative dentistry. Research shows that 3D-printed restorations are frequently more accurate than those made using conventional techniques, which can result in better fit and longer-lasting outcomes. Moreover, the capacity to tailor restorations to each patient's unique anatomy solves a persistent problem in dentistry: obtaining the best possible fit and aesthetics. The development of customized root canal guides has demonstrated potential to improve procedural outcomes in endodontics, highlighting the technology's potential to improve clinical efficacy.

Notwithstanding the encouraging results, a number of restrictions were mentioned. Concerns are raised over their long-term durability in high-stress conditions because to their dependency on certain materials that might not be able to reproduce the mechanical qualities of conventional dental materials. Furthermore, widespread adoption is hampered by the requirement for specialized training and technological competence, especially in practices with low funding.

These discoveries have significant ramifications for the dentistry community. Enhancing patient care, lowering expenses over time, and increasing efficiency are all possible outcomes of integrating 3D printing into clinical procedures. Dental clinics could anticipate higher-quality patient care as more dental professionals get acquainted with 3D printing technology. Moreover, the continued creation of materials specifically designed for dental applications may be able to overcome current constraints and increase the use of 3D printing in difficult situations.

Areas for Future Research

Based on the review, several areas for future research can be identified:

Long-Term Clinical Studies: Comprehensive longitudinal studies that evaluate the long-term performance, resilience, and clinical outcomes of 3D-printed devices and restorations are desperately needed. Such studies would yield priceless information for professionals thinking about utilizing these technologies.

Material Development: Enhancing mechanical strength, aesthetic quality, and biocompatibility should be the main goals of research.

Standardization and Best Practices: It is crucial to do research to provide standardized procedures for 3D printing in dentistry. To guarantee consistent outcomes across various practices, this entails creating criteria for material selection, printing settings, and post-processing procedures.

Cost-Effectiveness Analysis: More thorough cost-benefit evaluations that contrast 3D printing with traditional techniques are required. Dental professionals could use this research to guide their investment decisions in 3D printing technology.

Training and Education: To fully realize the advantages of 3D printing technology and guarantee its appropriate application, it will be crucial to investigate efficient training courses for dental professionals.

5 CONCLUSION

Although research now available suggests that 3D printing will have a big impact on endodontics and conservative dentistry, overcoming the gaps and difficulties found will be necessary to fully realize the technology's promise. The dental industry may take advantage of 3D printing's benefits to enhance patient care and results by encouraging additional research and cooperation between manufacturers, researchers, and practitioners.

REFERENCES

[1] Dobroś K, Hajto-Bryk J, Zarzecka J. (2022). The 3D printed teeth models intended for hands-on practice in conservative dentistry. *Folia Medica Cracoviensia*. 29–41.

[2] Dobroś K, Hajto-Bryk J, Zarzecka J. (2023). Application of 3D-printed teeth models in teaching dentistry students: a scoping review. *European Journal of Dental Education*. 27(1):126–34.

[3] Reymus M, Fotiadou C, Kessler A, Heck K, Hickel R, Diegritz C. (2019). 3D printed replicas for endodontic education. *International Endodontic Journal*. 52(1):123–30.

[4] Huth KC, Borkowski L, Liebermann A, Berlinghoff F, Hickel R, Schwendicke F, Reymus M. (2024). Comparing accuracy in guided endodontics: Dynamic real-time navigation, static guides, and manual approaches for access cavity preparation–an in vitro study using 3D printed teeth. *Clinical Oral Investigations*. 28(4):212.

[5] Pasha S, Saleem A, Bilal M. (2023). Evaluation of internal adaptation and marginal fit of onlays fabricated using computer-aided design (CAD)-computer-aided manufacturing (CAM) and three-dimensional printing techniques: An in vitro study. *Cureus*. 15(6).

 ISBN: 978-1-041-32674-8

Techno Verse Era of Bioinformatics: A New Frontier in Dentistry

Haritma Nigam
Department of Oral Medicine and Radiology, Teerthanker Mahaveer Dental College and Research Centre, Moradabad

ABSTRACT: Current technology has made everything easier for us and has dramatically changed the way we live our daily lives. A relatively use of information science to biological problems is the focus of a new field called bioinformatics.

Bioinformatics has advanced and supported health research and raised it to a new level. Bioinformatics helps to promote dentistry research by the awareness of fundamental processes and its underlying causes related to some oral diseases. It can also help with personalised cancer treatment and early prediction, which can help with accurate cancer treatment and early detection. Additionally, bioinformatics offers image analysis for CT, MRI, and X-ray images and aids in the creation of patient care databases.

leading to increased diagnostic skills. A subsect of bioinformatics called "salivanomics" works with the saliva knowledge base to enable global data exploration of saliva. Genetic therapy and personalized medicine research can vary from the integration of bioinformatics with artificial intelligence and machine learning.

This paper provides insight into the bioinformatics tools and its application in dentistry.

Keywords: Bioinformatics, Cancer, Genetic therapy, Salivanomics, Technology

1 INTRODUCTION

The use of information science to address biological issues is the focus of the new field of bioinformatics. [1] One of its primary focus is on gathering, saving, retrieving, and evaluating data from databases. It has significantly accelerated healthcare research over the past ten years. Understanding the underlying pathways and mechanisms underlying some oral diseases is one way that bioinformatics may support dentistry research. Pharmaceutical companies are increasingly using bioinformatics in drug design, which shortens the time needed to create new medications. Additionally, it can help with the creation of patient care databases, and it can enhance diagnosis by processing CT and X-ray images.

Currently, bioinformatics is an emerging and rapidly evolving field that has wide implications in the biomedical research disciplines. The results from biomedical informatics research have started to modify dental medicine in a very profound way. [2] This discipline is a source of a steady stream of large and complex genomic data that can serve as evidence for evidence-based dental practices. Recently, biomedical informatics has been studied in connection with dental issues, and new terms such as "oral genomics" have been coined and used widely.

The Human Genome Project and development of high throughput technologies have led to the generation of large quantities of data. The increasing demand to understand, analyze and interpret these data has given rise to a new field of science: bioinformatics. [1]

Thus, bioinformatics can be described as a new field that solves biological problems by integrating biology, computer science, and mathematics. This multidisciplinary field necessitates a thorough comprehension of statistics, algorithms, and biological systems. The principles of machine learning, artificial intelligence, and neural networks are increasingly included in bioinformatics to analyse biological data and produce insightful findings. One Clinicians' capacity for diagnosis and treatment has been significantly enhanced by the power of computation and analysis applied to clinical data. [2]

Henceforth, seeing it as an emerging and rapidly evolving field, this manuscript provides insight into the basic concept of bioinformatics and its implications in dentistry. The discipline of bioinformatics involves many computational tools and methods that are aimed at managing, analyzing, and manipulating enormous amounts of biological data.

Bioinformatics is a *"research, development or application of computational tools for expanding the use of biological, behavioral or health data to acquire, store, organize or visualize such data". - National Institutes of Health (NIH)* [3]

2 HISTORY

Bioinformatics, a field that combines biology, computer science, and data analysis, has its roots in pioneering contributions from researchers like Dr. Robert Ledley and Dr. Margaret Okaley. The Human Genome Project,

 DOI: 10.1201/9781042016075-61

declared a success in 2000, marked a significant milestone in understanding human genetics and the application of bioinformatics for large-scale biological data analysis. [4]

3 GOALS

There are three main goals:

Data organization involves systematically arranging data for easy access, management, and analysis. Data analysis uses statistical, computational, or qualitative methods to identify patterns and generate insights, while data interpretation addresses research questions or business problems. [5]

4 COMPONENTS

The two subfields of bioinformatics are the creation of databases and computational tools and the use of these tools and databases to produce biological knowledge for a better understanding of living systems (Figure 1). Each of these two subfields complements the other. Writing software for structural, functional, and sequence analysis as well as creating and maintaining biological databases are all included in the tool development process. [1]

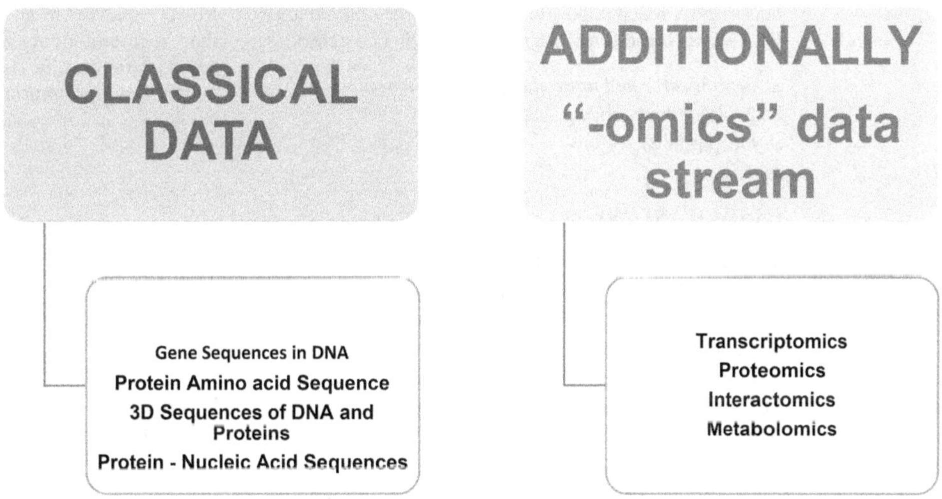

Figure 1. Components of bioinformatics.

5 TOOLS & TECHNIQUES

Numerous databases and tools are available to help with conducting research in the life sciences. These resources and datasets serve as the foundation for new studies in proteomics and genetics. Tools and databases in a certain field of life science can be categorised as follows based on analysis [7]:

Table 1. Tools and techniques of bioinformatics.

S NO.	TOOLS & TECHNIQUES:	BACKGROUND	ROLE
A	DATABASE	Collections of biological data that are used for data organisation and storage in a way that facilitates *easy retrieval* of information. **PRIMARY RAW:** • Contains original and unprocessed biological data. **INCLUDES:** Nucleotide or Protein sequences, Molecular structures. **EXAMPLES: NCBI, EMBL**	To retrieve, update, and query data

(*continued*)

Table 1. Continued

S NO.	TOOLS & TECHNIQUES:	BACKGROUND	ROLE
		• **SECONDARY/CURATED:** Databases derived from primary databases • Computationally processed information **INCLUDES:** Predict the structure and function of proteins expression **EXAMPLES: Swissprot, Prosite**	
B	SEQUENCE ALIGNMENT	Comparison of residues between sequences. Usually, displayed as rows in a matrix. The sequences may be nucleotide sequences (DNAs or RNAs) or amino acid sequences (Proteins). **METHODS:** **GLOBAL:** All along the length, the same length and alignment must be achieved. **LOCAL:** When the lengths of the sequences to be compared differ significantly.	Aligning the unknown sequence with one or more known sequences to predict the data.
C	INTERPRETATION	Without taking into account every potential consequence, a heuristic approach (algorithm) calculates the optimal answer. **BLASTA: (Basic Local Alignment Search Too ability)** • Search ***rarer and more significant sequences*** • ***Multiple*** best-scoring Alignments • Output is ***larger*** • ***Faster*** **FASTA (FAST-All):** • (Is an extension of "**FAST-P**"for proteins • and "FAST-N" for nucleotides • ***Only one*** alignment from one sequence • ***Slower*** • Output is ***less***	Representation of the entire data. If two sequences in an alignment share a common ancestor, Gaps can be understood as indels and mis-matches as point mutations. (that is, *insertion or deletion mutations.*
D	PHYLOGENETIC ANALYSIS	Study of the evolutionary relationships of species. **METHODS:** (1) Nested Clade (2) Bootstrap Method (3) Unrooted Tree (4) Rooted tree	In turn directs the development of the suitable vaccination.
E	PROTEIN STRUCTURE	Predicting a protein's secondary and tertiary structures from its basic structure by inferring its three-dimensional structure from its amino acid sequence.	Vital to the development of medica-tions and vaccines
F	METABOLIC PATHWAY	Enzymes catalyse a network of connected chemical events that work together to produce or break down one or a few metabolites. **Tool: KEGG: Kyoto Encyclopedia of Genes and Genomes.** Web site: http://www.genome.jp/kegg/.	In Studying Biological system

6 APPLICATIONS IN DENTISTRY

(1) MICROARRAY TECHNOLOGY: *Background: Oncomine* is a cancer microarray database that systematically analyzes data. The oral brush biopsy sample is analysed using computer-assisted image analysis, or OralCDx®. [7,8] Role: Determine how normal and malignant cells express different genes. A premalignant tumour progressing to a blatantly malignant state. Once the gene responsible for a specific disease is discovered, drug research targets can be determined.

Advantages:

✓ Less time-consuming and its Cost-effective.

(2) DATABASES FOR PATIENT CARE: Background: Information about the patient's diagnosis, treatments, and medication prescription is stored online. Role: A customised, well-designed hospital database that gathers current data from the patient who is visiting in no time. [7,9]

Advantages: Patient safety; patient satisfaction; and the ability to share information among hospitals. Therefore, helping with billing and documentation cuts down on paperwork and clerical workers.

(3) RADIOGENOMICS:
Background: Disease patterns and correlations can be found by computational analysis of medical pictures. The technique of breaking up a single image into smaller pieces or segments is known as image segmentation. Image registration: This procedure enables proper image alignment. Role: Supplying pertinent data for improved treatments and remedies. Benefits include being extremely accurate, saving time and effort, and being less costly. [7,9]

(4) **SALIVAOMICS BASE OF INFORMATION: Background:** It was the first website devoted to studies on salivary omics. In microbiome research, the Salivaomics Knowledge Base (SKB; http://www.skb.ucla.edu/) serves as a web resource, management system, and data repository. [7,9] It has three layers as following:
Data layer: Sources of data are kept Ontology layer: Nodes in controlled vocabularies are mapped to data items from these data sources. **Interface layer:** Enables browsing, submission, and query.
Role: It comprehends the data required to explore the biology, diagnostic potentials, pharmaco-proteomics and pharmaco-genomics of human saliva.

(5) **FORENSIC SCIENCE:**

Background: Based on biological samples, forensic DNA has emerged as a biologically reliable evidence method. DNA testing methods include thin-film transistor biosensors and DNA microarray sequencing. All living things have microsatellites in their genomes. Enabling genome mapping,forensic DNA has become a biologically valid evidence tool based on biological samples. [10]

Role: Person identification including age and gender

STR system (short tandem repeat): A minute blood sample is needed has incorporated in DNA identification technique for criminal analysis. [10]

ADVANTAGES [10,11]:

✓ 1. Analyze Large Data
✓ 2. Expensive Wet Labs not Required
✓ 3. Repetition of the same research many times
✓ 4. Time savings

DISADVANTES:

✓ 1. Reliability of the Stored Data
✓ 2. Costly to Hold Databases
✓ 3. Searching Databases can sometimes become time consuming

7 CONCLUSION

High-throughput techniques and data generation in dental sciences could revolutionize research. Bioinformatics could study genome-based clinical data, transforming current practices in diagnostics, therapeutics, and prognostics of oral diseases and disorders and that will definitely be a spark in our field of dentistry.

REFERENCES

[1] Lesk A. (2014). *Introduction to Bioinformatics*, 4th Edition. Oxford University Press.

[2] *Burket's Oral Medicine,Michael Glick and Greenberg*,Wiley Blackwell, 12th Edition.

[3] *National Institute of Health*, website https://commonfund.nih.gov/bioinformatics, [last accessed : 22, Oct, 2017].

[4] Jeff Gauthier *et al.*, (2019). *Briefings in Bioinformatics*, 20(6):1981–1996.

[5] J.M.S. Rana and K. S. (2012). *Vaisla- Introduction to Bioinformatics Bioinformatics- Tools and Applications*, 2012 Edition; Uttarakhand State Biotechnology Department (Ministry of Science & Technology and Biotechnology), Government of Uttarakhand.

[6] Ghatole K. (2020). Bioinformatics: A new arsenal in dental sciences. *International Journal of Applied Dental Sciences*. 6(3): 610–614. doi: 10.22271/oral.2020.v6.i3i.1015

[7] Saxena M, Srivastava S, Dular MS. (2024). Bioinformatics: A New Tool in Dentistry. *Eur J Med Health Res*, 2(1):83–90.

[8] Church GM, Gilbert W. (1984). Genomic sequencing. *Proc Natl Acad Sci U S A*. 81(7):1991–5. doi: 10.1073/pnas.81.7.1991.

[9] Liu L, Li Y, Li S, Hu N, He Y, Pong R, Lin D, Lu L, Law M. (2012). Comparison of next-generation sequencing systems. *J Biomed Biotechnol*. 2012:251364. doi: 10.1155/2012/251364

[10] Chowdhury B, Garai G. (2017). A review on multiple sequence alignment from the perspective of genetic algorithm. *Genomics. ct*;109(5–6):419–431. doi: 10.1016/j.ygeno.2017.06.007

Incorporation of Digital Dentistry in Undergraduate Teaching Curriculum

Vighnesh M and Karthik Shetty
Department of Conservative Dentistry and Endodontics, Manipal College of Dental Sciences, Mangalore, Manipal Academy of Higher Education, Mangalore, Karnataka, India

ABSTRACT: **Aim-** The main aim of this review is to explore and evaluate the role of digital dentistry in the undergraduate teaching curriculum. **Methods-** Keywords such as "digital dentistry," "artificial Intelligence in dentistry," "undergraduate dental education," "CAD/CAM," and "3D printing in dentistry" were used to conduct a thorough search. We used databases from PubMed, ScienceDirect, Scopus, Web of Science, and Google Scholar. Studies that addressed the integration of digital dentistry into the curriculum and that were written in English, peerreviewed, published within the previous ten years, and contained original research, reviews, case studies, or conference papers were included. **Results-** With the widespread adoption of CAD/CAM systems, 3D printers, intraoral scanners and digital radiography by dental schools, learning outcomes have improved for students, especially in terms of comprehension and competency with digital tools. It has been shown that providing students with practical experience with these technologies is crucial to increasing their self-esteem and competency. However, obstacles such as exorbitant prices, inadequate teacher preparation, and restricted equipment availability impede wider adoption. Furthermore, different institutions' student exposure to digital dentistry is uneven because of the absence of established guidelines for its integration. **Conclusion-** Enhancing student competency and coordinating education with clinical procedures are two benefits of integrating digital dentistry into undergraduate education. Effective integration requires addressing issues such as high costs, faculty training, and standardization. To guarantee equitable education, future research should concentrate on long-term results, faculty development, and financial viability.

Keywords: dental education, digital dentistry, Artificial Intelligence, CAD/CAM, 3D Printing, intra oral scanners, digital radiography

1 INTRODUCTION

The incorporation of digital technologies into dental curricula has commenced worldwide, with heterogeneous levels of adoption influenced by institutional infrastructure, resource availability, and educational demands.[1] One of the principal challenges in digital dental education is the necessity for continual adaptation to rapid technological advancements and their effective translation into clinical dental practice.[2][3]

Providing students with practical experience with state-of-the-art digital tools such as artificial intelligence (AI), CAD/CAM systems, 3D printing, and digital radiography, it also fosters clinical competency. Additionally, the curriculum promotes creativity and inquiry, motivating students to investigate novel approaches and avenues for investigation in the field of digital dentistry.[4][5]

Schlenz *et al.* demonstrated improved student understanding and performance with digital impression systems compared to conventional techniques.[6] Kavadella *et al.* in his study showed that virtual learning environments and digital simulations enhanced preclinical skill acquisition.[7] Zitzmann *et al.* highlighted the role of digital workflows and CAD/CAM training in preparing students for contemporary clinical practice.[8][9]

In this context, the present study evaluates the integration of digital technologies in clinical dental education and proposes a structured framework to enhance competency-based training.

2 METHODOLOGY

This methodology describes a meticulous way to review the literature on the incorporation of digital dentistry into dental education at the undergraduate level. Keywords such as "digital dentistry," "Artificial Intelligence in dentistry," "undergraduate dental education," "CAD/CAM," and "3D printing in dentistry" were used to conduct a thorough search. We used databases from PubMed, ScienceDirect, Scopus, Web of Science, and Google Scholar. Studies that addressed the integration of digital dentistry into the curriculum and those that were written in English, peer-reviewed, published within the previous ten years, and contained original research, reviews, case studies, or conference papers were included. The excluded articles were duplicates, non-peer reviewed, older than ten years,

 DOI: 10.1201/9781042016075-62

and unrelated to undergraduate education. To highlight important themes, difficulties, results, and best practices for incorporating digital technologies into dental curricula, a summary of the chosen studies was created.

3 RESULTS

Several significant conclusions and trends in the incorporation of digital dentistry into undergraduate education were made clear by the review. With the widespread adoption of CAD/CAM systems and 3D printers by dental schools, learning outcomes have improved for students, especially in terms of comprehension and competency with digital tools. It has been shown that providing students with practical experience with these technologies is crucial to increasing their self-esteem and competency. However, obstacles such as exorbitant prices, inadequate faculty training, and restricted equipment availability impede wider adoption. Furthermore, different institutions' student exposure to digital dentistry is uneven because of the absence of established guidelines for its integration.

The adoption of an interdisciplinary approach that integrates digital tools across various specialties, the growing emphasis on digital proficiency as a critical skill, and the increased emphasis on research and innovation are some of the key trends. However, there are still gaps, especially in terms of faculty preparation, resource availability, and the requirement for lengthy research on the effects of teaching digital dentistry. To guarantee fair learning opportunities and long-term integration of digital technologies into dental curricula, these gaps be filled.

4 DISCUSSION

An extensive summary of the state of digital dentistry integration into undergraduate dental education is given by the reviewed literature. Digital technology integration is becoming more common in the curriculum, according to the analysis, which has important ramifications for dental education and practice. To maximize this integration, there are a number of important issues and gaps that are brought to light by the results.[2][10]

A brief overview of how dental education has evolved to include digital technologies can highlight the significance of this paradigm shift in both teaching and clinical preparation. Over the past two decades, dental curricula have progressively incorporated a range of digital tools and instructional methods to better align student competence with modern clinical practice.[2] Early digital adoption focused on web-based learning, e-learning platforms, and basic digital radiography to support theoretical knowledge delivery and access to learning resources. As technology advanced, dental schools began integrating simulation technologies, intraoral scanners, digital surface mapping, and computer aided design/computer aided manufacturing (CAD/CAM) into preclinical and clinical training, enabling students to develop both cognitive and psychomotor skills in a more interactive and objective environment.[2][11] These innovations aim to improve diagnostic accuracy, procedural efficiency, and student readiness for technology rich practice settings. However, the evolution of digital dental education also underscores persistent challenges, such as variability in implementation across institutions, the need for faculty development, and gaps in standardized training frameworks.[12][13]

Digital competency is increasingly essential not only for individual dental practitioners but also for enhancing overall patient outcomes and practice efficiency. Proficiency in digital technologies enables improved diagnostic accuracy, more precise treatment planning, and predictable clinical outcomes through tools such as digital imaging, CAD/CAM systems and computer guided workflows.[14] From a patient-care perspective, digital dentistry has been associated with reduced chairside time, fewer clinical errors, improved communication, and enhanced patient satisfaction. At the practice level, digital integration streamlines clinical workflows, optimizes resource utilization and supports evidence-based decision making, ultimately contributing to higher quality, efficient and patient centered dental care. Therefore, embedding digital competency within dental education is critical to preparing graduates for contemporary clinical demands and advancing standards of care.[15][16]

Despite the growing adoption of digital dentistry, several challenges hinder its effective integration into dental education. High initial costs associated with digital equipment, software and maintenance pose significant financial barriers, particularly for resource limited institutions. Additionally, the successful implementation of digital technologies requires adequate faculty training and ongoing technical support, which may be lacking in some educational settings.[17] Resistance to change among faculty and students, often driven by unfamiliarity with digital workflows or concerns regarding increased workload and learning curves, further complicates curriculum reform. These challenges highlight the need for strategic planning, faculty development programs and phased integration models to ensure sustainable and effective adoption of digital dentistry in undergraduate education.[18][19]

The continual refinement of digital dentistry curricula requires active incorporation of feedback from key stakeholders, including dental professionals, educators and students. Input from practicing clinicians ensures that curricular content remains clinically relevant and aligned with evolving technological demands in real world practice. Educator feedback is essential for identifying pedagogical challenges, resource requirements, and effective teaching strategies, while student perspective provide valuable insights into learning experiences, skill acquisition and perceived competency gaps. Integrating multisource feedback supports evidence-based curriculum, promotes learner centered education and facilitates the sustainable and effective implementation of digital technologies in dental education.[20][19]

The broader implications of digital dentistry extend beyond education, signalling a fundamental transformation in the future of the dental profession. Continued advancements in digital imaging, CAD/CAM systems, artificial intelligence, and additive manufacturing are expected to further enhance diagnostic precision, treatment personalization, and clinical predictability. Digital workflows are likely to promote more efficient, minimally invasive, and patient-centered care, while facilitating interdisciplinary collaboration and remote consultation through tele dentistry platforms.[21][22] Additionally, automation and data-driven decisionmaking may redefine traditional clinical roles, emphasizing the importance of digital literacy, adaptability, and lifelong learning among dental professionals. As digital technologies become increasingly embedded in routine practice, they are poised to reshape clinical workflows, practice management models, and professional competencies, underscoring the need for proactive curricular and regulatory adaptation.[23][24]

5 CONCLUSION

In light of the accelerating digital transformation of dental practice, it is imperative that stakeholders in dental education—including academic institutions, curriculum developers, accreditation bodies, and policymakers—prioritize the systematic integration of digital dentistry into undergraduate training. Doing so will ensure the development of digitally competent graduates, enhance the quality and efficiency of patient care, and prepare the dental workforce to meet the evolving demands of contemporary and future clinical practice.

REFERENCES

[1] Ishida Y, Kuwajima Y, Kobayashi T, Yonezawa Y, Asack D, Nagai M, *et al.* (2022). Current implementation of digital dentistry for removable prosthodontics in US dental schools. *Int J Dent.*

[2] Zitzmann NU, Matthisson L, Ohla H, Joda T. (2020). Digital undergraduate education in dentistry: A systematic review. Vol. 17, *International Journal of Environmental Research and Public Health.* MDPI.

[3] Kabra L, Santhosh VN, Sequeira RN, Ankola A V., Coutinho D. (2022). Dental curriculum reform in India: Undergraduate students' awareness and perception on the newly proposed choice based credit system. *J Oral Biol Craniofac Res.* 13(5):630–5.

[4] Ohyama H, Duong ML, Yancoskie AE, Smiley AB, Syed AZ, Reddy MS, *et al.* (2025). Challenges and opportunities in implementing digital technology in dental curriculum: A review and perspective. *Cureus.*

[5] Patil PG. (2020). Digital dentistry in undergraduate curriculum and the fourth industrial revolution. Vol. 10, *International Journal of Prosthodontics and Restorative Dentistry. Jaypee Brothers Medical Publishers (P) Ltd.* p. 46–7.

[6] Schlenz MA, Michel K, Wegner K, Schmidt A, Rehmann P, Wöstmann B. (2022). Undergraduate dental students' perspective on the implementation of digital dentistry in the preclinical curriculum: a questionnaire survey. *BMC Oral Health.* 20(1).

[7] Kavadella A, Tsiklakis K, Vougiouklakis G, Lionarakis A. (2012). Evaluation of a blended learning course for teaching oral radiology to undergraduate dental students. *European Journal of Dental Education.* 16(1).

[8] Nicola U. Zitzmann Rldvbbcssmbja. (2023). Effectiveness of a manual test at the beginning of dental school. *European Journal of Dental Education.*

[9] Alfallaj HA, Afrashtehfar KI, Asiri AK, Almasoud FS, Alnaqa GH, Al-Angari NS. (2023). The status of digital dental technology implementation in the saudi dental schools' curriculum: A national cross-sectional survey for healthcare digitization. *Int J Environ Res Public Health.* 20(1).

[10] Das S, Jha K, Menon I, Kumar G, Singh A, Barman D. (2024). Application of digitalization in dental education - a systematic review. Vol. 35, *Indian Journal of Dental Research.* Wolters Kluwer Medknow Publications; p. 470–7.

[11] Tripathi S, Manoharan PS, Nagda S. (2024). Developing an instructional module of 'digital dentistry' for undergraduate prosthodontics curriculum. *J Oral Biol Craniofac Res.* 14(1):44–8.

[12] Mwogosi A, Mambile C, Simba R, Haruna H. (2025). Integrating digital technologies in clinical dentistry training: a framework for competency-based education. *BMC Med Educ.* 25(1).

[13] Jurado CA, Tsujimoto A, Punj A, Aida N, Miyazaki M, Watanabe H. (2021). Successful development and implementation of a digital dentistry curriculum at a US dental school. *J Oral Sci.* 63(4):358–60.

[14] Revilla-León M, Özcan M. (2019). Additive manufacturing technologies used for processing polymers: Current status and potential application in prosthetic dentistry. Vol. 28, *Journal of Prosthodontics. Blackwell Publishing Inc.*; p. 146–58.

[15] Ho JCY, Chai HH, Huang MZ, Lo ECM, Chu CH. (2025). Impact of Modern Communication in Transforming Dental Care. Vol. 13, *Dentistry Journal. Multidisciplinary Digital Publishing Institute (MDPI).*

[16] Haleem A, Javaid M, Qadri MA, Suman R. (2022). Understanding the role of digital technologies in education: A review. *Sustainable Operations and Computers.* 3:275–85.

[17] Liu CM, Hsu MH, Ng MY, Yu CH. (2025). Digital integration in dental education: A novel self-directed learning model using intraoral scanners for tooth preparation training. *J Dent Sci.* 20(1):639–45.

[18] Tahat DN, Habes M, Tahat K, Pasha SA, Attar RW, Al-Rahmi WM, *et al.* (2023). Technology enhanced learning in undergraduate level education: A case study of students of mass communication. *Sustainability (Switzerland).* 15(21).

[19] Nassani LM, Bencharit S, Schumacher F, Lu WE, Resende R, Fernandes GVO. (2024). The impact of technology teaching in the dental predoctoral curriculum on students' perception of digital dentistry. *Dent J (Basel)*12(3).

[20] Khurshid Z. (2023). Digital dentistry: Transformation of oral health and dental education with technology. Vol. 17, *European Journal of Dentistry. Georg Thieme Verlag*; p. 943–4.

[21] Thurzo A, Strunga M, Urban R, Surovková J, Afrashtehfar KI. (2023). Impact of artificial intelligence on dental education: A review and guide for curriculum update. Vol. 13, *Education Sciences.* MDPI.

[22] Anas M, Ullah I, Usman Sultan M. (2024). Embracing the future: Integrating digital dentistry into undergraduate dental curriculum. Vol. 52, *Journal of the California Dental Association. Taylor and Francis Ltd.*.

[23] Kim CS, Samaniego CS, Sousa Melo SL, Brachvogel WA, Baskaran K, Rulli D. (2023). Artificial intelligence (A.I.) in dental curricula: Ethics and responsible integration. *J Dent Educ.* 87(11):1570–3.

[24] Murbay S, Neelakantan P, Chang JWW, Yeung S. (2020). 'Evaluation of the introduction of a dental virtual simulator on the performance of undergraduate dental students in the pre-clinical operative dentistry course.' *European Journal of Dental Education.* 24(1):5–16.

 ISBN: 978-1-041-32674-8

3D Printing: A New Era of Hands-On Learning in Conservative Dentistry and Endodontics: A Narrative Review

Heta Vaghasia and Kundabala M
Department of Conservative Dentistry and Endodontics, Manipal College of Dental Sciences, Mangalore, Affiliated to Manipal Academy of Higher Education, Manipal, Mangalore, Karnataka

ABSTRACT: The purpose of this review is to explore the transformative impact of 3D printing technology on hands-on learning in conservative dentistry and endodontics. This article reviews various 3D printing technologies and their applications in dental education. The method involved a comprehensive search of literature of recent studies and review of the utilized technologies to create realistic dental models for training and assessment. The 3D printed models are made from printers such as stereolithography (SLA), digital light processing (DLP), and polyjet technology which significantly enhances the training experience by providing detailed accurate replicas of dental structures, which improve students' practical skills and confidence. Positive feedback from students and educators highlights the effectiveness of these models in reducing stress and improving clinical skills. Conclusions drawn from the review suggest that 3D printing is revolutionizing dental education in conservative dentistry and endodontics by providing realistic, customizable models for training and simulation without ethical issues. This technology enhances students' understanding of complex dental anatomy which improves procedural accuracy in restoring teeth and root canal treatment, thereby offering unlimited practice opportunities. Consequently, it significantly increases the quality of dental education and prepares students for real-world clinical challenges. Additionally, 3D printing can provide customized solutions tailored to individual patient anatomy, leading to better treatment results and increased efficiency.

Keywords: 3D Printing, Conservative dentistry, Dental Education, Endodontics, Hands-on learning

1 INTRODUCTION

Technological advancements are fostering a new era of interactive, skill-based learning that is transforming traditional methods of dental education.[1, 2]The integration of digital technology, specially artificial intelligence and 3D printing technology, has revolutionized various industries, including healthcare and dentistry. In the fields of conservative dentistry and endodontics, 3D printing has emerged as a powerful tool that enhances hands-on learning and clinical practice.[3] By enabling the creation of precise anatomical models, it allows students and practitioners to gain valuable practical experience without the need for living patients, thereby improving skills leading to better patient care. [4]

The objective of this review is to explore the role of 3D printing in hands-on learning within conservative dentistry and endodontics. This includes examining how 3D-printed models are used for teaching dental procedures, evaluating their effectiveness compared with conventional learning methods, and identifying the potential of this technology to shape future educational frameworks. The scope covers educational applications, technological advancements, and their impact on clinical training and skill development in these dental specialties.

The significance of this topic lies in its growing relevance in dental education and the expanding body of literature highlighting its benefits. Research suggests that 3D printing offers unmatched precision and flexibility in creating realistic dental models, providing students with opportunities to practice complex procedures in a risk-free environment. As more institutions incorporate this technology into their curriculum, understanding its full potential and limitations becomes crucial for advancing dental education.

The present narrative review describes the types of 3D printers used, the author's name, the publication year, the type of study, the subject, key trends, and its impact of its outcomes on hands-on learning in conservative dentistry and endodontics.

2 METHODOLOGY

A literature search was conducted focused on peer-reviewed articles, reviews, clinical trials, and case studies from the last 10 years and used keywords such as "3D printing," "conservative dentistry," "endodontics," "dental education," and "hands-on learning." Boolean operators (AND, OR, NOT) refined the search results. The relevant

 DOI: 10.1201/9781042016075-63

databases used to capture comprehensive research included PubMed, Scopus, the Cochrane Library, Google Scholar, and ScienceDirect. Studies published in English between 2014 and September 2024 discussing 3D printing in dental education and practice were included. Nondental applications, editorials, and studies whose full texts were unavailable were excluded.

Fifty-one articles were selected by two reviewers to screen titles and abstracts, and any discrepancies were resolved by consensus. Twenty-five full-text articles were reviewed for final selection, and 17 articles were selected for the study as seen in Figure 1 below. The author's name, publication year, type of study, type of printer used, subject, key trends and outcomes were extracted from 17 selected articles for analysis.

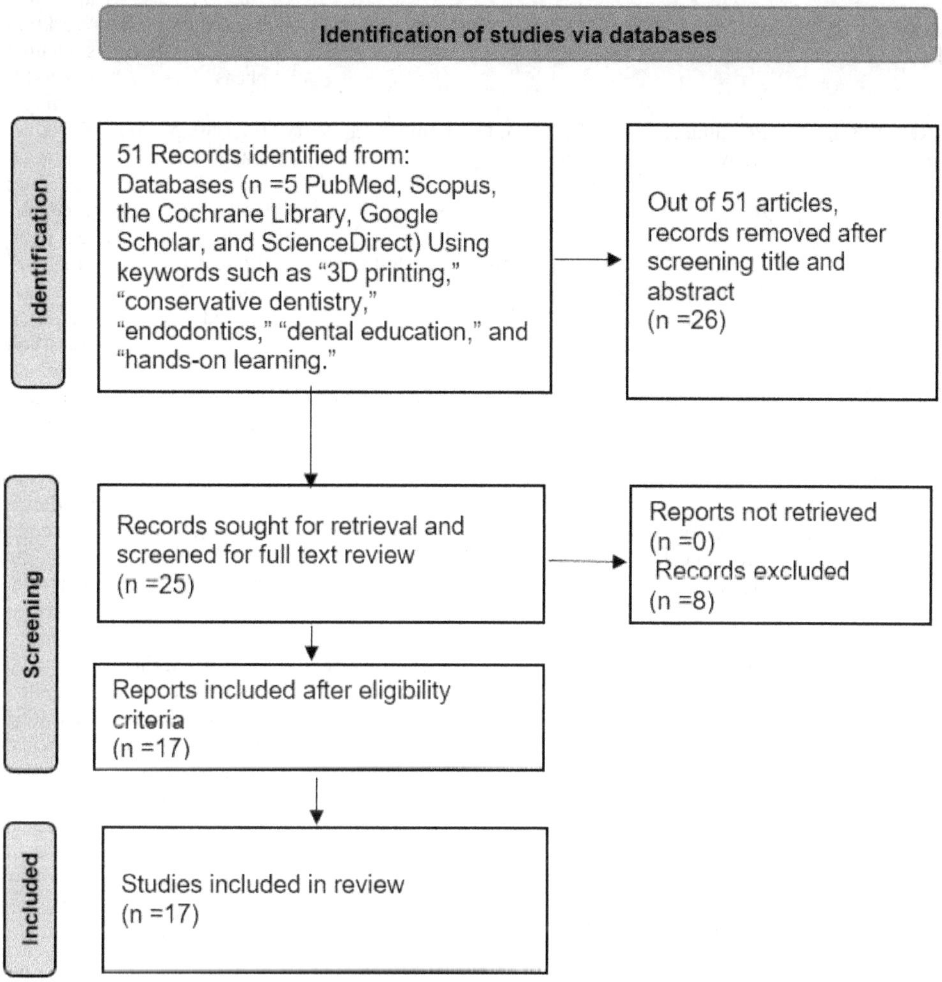

Figure 1. Flow Diagram of Methodology.

3 RESULT

The key findings from the reviewed literature are summarized below in the table. Commonly used 3D printers include Stereolithography, Digital light processing, PolyJet technology etc. According to subject distribution endodontics showed highest no. of articles. Stereolithography was most commonly used printer in endodontics whereas PolyJet technology was commonly used printer in conservative dentistry.

SR NO	AUTHOR NAME	PUBLI-CATION YEAR	TYPE OF STUDY	TYPE OF PRINTER USED	SUBJECT	KEY TRENDS	OUTCOMES
1	Yanglin Zeng *et al.* [5]	2024	Pre-clinical, self – assessment study	PolyJet technology	Conservative Dentistry	3D-printed colored tooth model	Enhanced training experience; improved average scores for in-

(*continued*)

Continued

SR NO	AUTHOR NAME	PUBLICATION YEAR	TYPE OF STUDY	TYPE OF PRINTER USED	SUBJECT	KEY TRENDS	OUTCOMES
							lay preparation.
2	A. Hanafi *et al.*[6]	2020	Pre-clinical study	SLA (Stereolithography)	Endodontics	Modular 3D print model for endodontics	Positive feedback from students; reduced stress during clinical skills application.
3	M. Reymus *et al.*[7]	2018	Undergraduate study	SLA	Endodontics	Feasibility of 3D printed tooth replicas	Workflow feasible; students reported significant benefits in training.
4	Marcel Reymus *et al.*[8]	2021	Pre-clinical study	DLP(Digital Light Processing)	Interdisciplinary	Interdisciplinary teaching model	Effective across endodontics, prosthodontics, and implantology; good comparison to real patient scenarios.
5	Markus Kolling *et al.*[9]	2021	Pre-clinical Training- Questionnaire	Multijet Modeling technology	Endodontics	Student perception of 3D-printed teeth	Students preferred human teeth for tactile realism; acknowledged educational benefits of 3D models.
6	Marco Farronato *et al.* [10]	2023	Invitro Patient Study	PolyJet technology	Endodontics	AR in endodontics	Promising potential for clinical guidance; requires further development for in vivo validation.
7	Matteo Meglioli *et al.* [11]	2023	Self-assessment Pre-clinical study	VAT Photopolymerization 3D printer	Endodontics	Self-assessment on 3D printed models	3D models address availability and variability issues; enhance self-assessment in training.
8	Christian Höhne *et al.* [12]	2023	Pre-Clinical Training Study	SLA	Conservative Dentistry	Modular training model in restorative dentistry	Created affordable, customizable model exceeding traditional tooth features.
9	Przemysław Kustra *et al.* [13]	2020	Teaching Study	SLA	Endodontics	3D models in teaching endodontics	Significant improvement in quality of training; holds potential for better student outcomes with complex scenarios.
10	Sung-Ting Tsai *et al.*[2]	2022	Preclinical Self-Assessment Study	DLP	Endodontics	Self-assessment performance in endodontics	3D model and scoring rubrics were effective for evaluating self-assessment abilities.
11	Oye Peters *et al.*[14]	2021	Pre-clinical Study	NOT MENTIONED	Endodontics	Skills acquisition in endodontics	No significant improvement in obturation skills with 3D-printed models over practice.
12	Mohamed Fakhr *et al.* [4]	2023	Post- Graduate Student Study	SLA	Endodontics	3D models for teaching and treatment outcomes	More accurate results in managing complex tooth morphology; emphasizes time commitment.
13	Sareh Said Yekta-Michael *et al.*[1]	2021	Student Study	NOT MENTIONED	Endodontics	New endodontic tooth models evaluation	DRSK-RCT models shown to improve education quality; potential alternative to extracted teeth.
14	Diva Lugassy *et al.*	2020	Student Study	PolyJet technology	Conservative Dentistry	Augmented feedback from 3D	Positive feedback; both model generations

(*continued*)

Continued

SR NO	AUTHOR NAME	PUBLI-CATION YEAR	TYPE OF STUDY	TYPE OF PRINTER USED	SUBJECT	KEY TRENDS	OUTCOMES
	[15]					models	yielded similar clinical results despite material hardness complaints.
15	Jorge A. Tricio *et al.* [16, 17]	2024	Self-assessment Preclinical study	NOT MENTIONED	Conservative Dentistry	Quality of crown preparations	Practicing on 3D-printed models improved preparation quality; minimized unnecessary tooth reduction.
16	Yiseul Choi *et al.*[17]	2021	Pre-doctoral students	SLA	Endodontics	Access opening guide in dental training	AOG-3DP significantly reduced access opening time; additional imaging and printing time needed.
17	Katarzyna Dobroś *et al.*[3]	2023	Scoping Review	NOT MENTIONED	Conservative Dentistry, Endodontics	Application of 3D models in teaching	3D models provide an effective alternative to traditional teaching models; concerns over soft tissue reproduction.

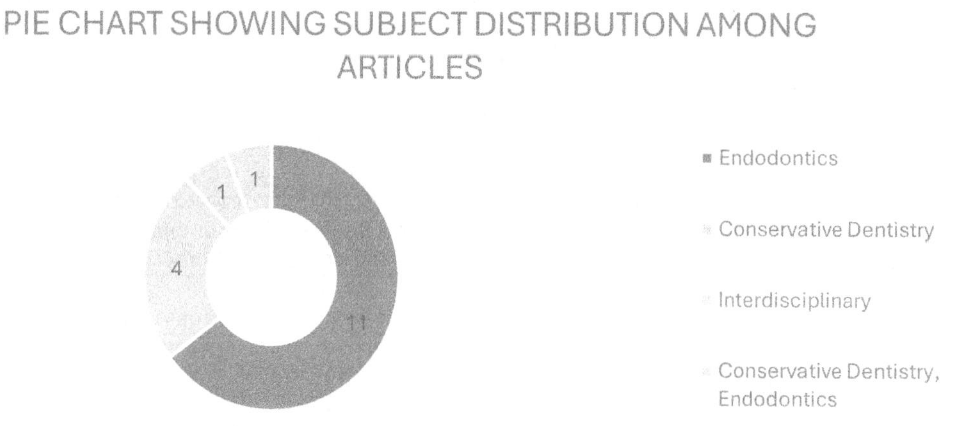

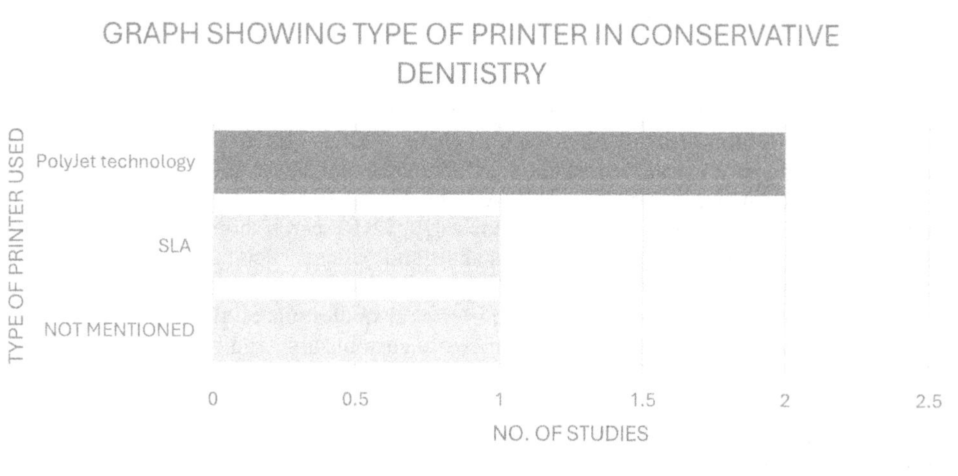

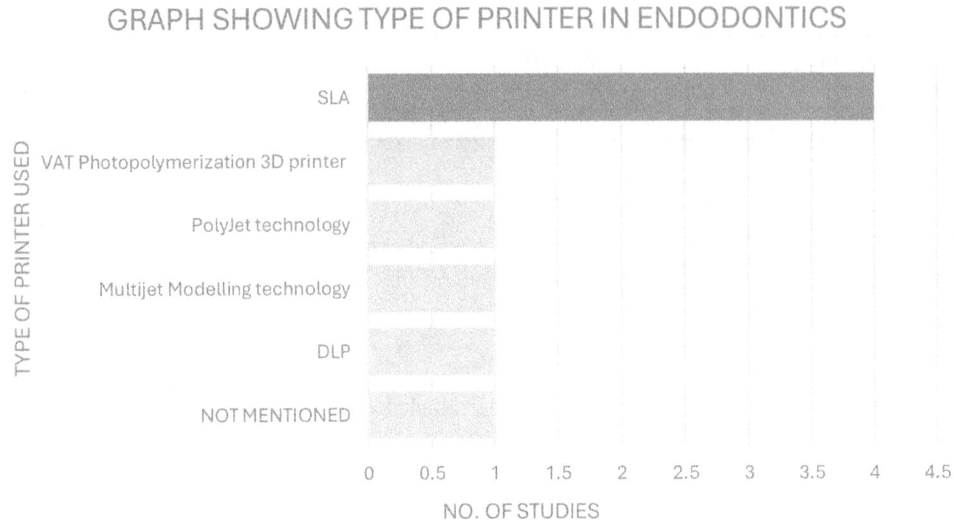

4 DISCUSSION

3D printing technology was introduced in the early 1980s that involves creation of a digital copy of an object and printing it layer by layer using suitable materials. It was initially used for medical applications such as tissues, organoids, surgical tools, models, and custom prosthetics. It relies on medical imaging techniques such as X-rays, CT scans, MRI, and ultrasounds to generate a digital model for printing.[18] Advancements in CBCT and software in dentistry have enabled the creation of life-sized 3D printed tooth models, significantly enhancing diagnosis and treatment planning. In endodontics, this technology allows clinicians to simulate treatments, ensuring a precise access cavity and instrumentation with preservation of dentin.[3, 18]

Most studies in endodontics have utilized SLA printers to create 3D models, as they aid in visualizing and understanding complex root canal anatomy. For example, Mohamed Fakhr et al. concluded that using SLA printers in endodontics resulted in more accurate management of complex tooth morphology, although it requires a significant time commitment[4]. Similarly, Sareh Said Yekta-Michael et al. reported that DRSK RCT models improved education quality, offering a viable alternative to extracted teeth.[1] Additionally, the use of 3D printed guides in presurgical planning can be beneficial, as they allow for the simulation of procedures beforehand, thereby minimizing the risk of iatrogenic injury.[10]

Yanglin Zeng et al. highlighted the benefits of using PolyJet technology in conservative dentistry,to create colored tooth models that enhance training experiences and improve average scores for inlay preparation.[5] Similarly, A. Hanafi and M. Reymus reported positive feedback from students using various types of printers across different dental disciplines. It was also noted that it reduced stress and gave significant training benefits. These studies underscore the potential of 3D printing to revolutionize dental education by providing realistic and customizable training models[6, 8].

However, it was also found in literature that there are several limitations of 3D printing. Markus Kolling et al. reported that while students acknowledged the educational advantages of 3D models in endodontics, they preferred human teeth for tactile realism.[9] This sentiment was echoed by Oye Peters, who reported no significant improvement in obturation skills when practicing with 3D-printed models compared with traditional methods. These findings suggest that while 3D printing offers many benefits, it may not fully replicate the tactile experience of working with real human teeth, which is crucial for developing certain clinical skills.[14]

Exploring multimaterial printing technologies, such as those used by Marco Farronato and Christian Höhne, showed promise in creating more realistic simulations for clinical guidance and restorative dentistry training. Additionally, innovations such as augmented reality (AR) by Marco Farronato require further development but hold potential for enhancing clinical practice in endodontics. [10, 12] Research should also investigate the long-term impact of using 3D-printed models on students' clinical skills and patient outcomes.[10, 12]

The implications of these findings for the field of dental education are profound. The positive feedback from students and the enhanced training experiences reported in several studies suggest that 3D printing can significantly improve the quality of dental education. The ability to create customizable and realistic models allows for more effective training and better preparation for clinical practice. Future research should focus on improving material properties, addressing the limitations related to the hardness and radiopacity of 3D-printed models to make them more comparable to natural teeth. Additionally, exploring the use of augmented reality (AR) and other digital guides can further enhance the training experience. Longitudinal studies are needed to assess the impact of 3D-printed models on students' clinical performance and patient care quality. The development of patient-specific 3D-printed models to provide more tailored training experiences is also crucial. By addressing these areas, dental education can continue to evolve, leveraging 3D printing technology to produce highly skilled and competent dental professionals.

5 CONCLUSION

3D printing is revolutionizing dental education in conservative dentistry and endodontics by providing realistic, customizable models for training and simulation without any ethical issues. This technology enhances students' understanding of complex dental anatomy, improves procedural accuracy in restoring teeth and root canal treatment, and offers unlimited practice opportunities. As a result, it significantly elevates the quality of dental education and prepares students for real-world clinical challenges.3D printing can provide customized solutions tailored to individual patient anatomy, which can lead to better treatment results and increased efficiency. In the area of dental education and research,3D printing can mimic real-life patient scenarios to yield favorable outcomes.

REFERENCES

[1] Yekta-Michael SS, Färber CM, Heinzel A. (2021). Evaluation of new endodontic tooth models in clinical education from the perspective of students and demonstrators. *BMC Med Educ*. 21(1).

[2] Tsai ST, Ho YC, Tsai CL, Yang SF, Lai YL, Lee SY. (2022). Evaluation of students' self-assessment performance in preclinical endodontic training by means of rubrics and a 3D printed model. *Journal of the Formosan Medical Association*. 121(11):2203–10.

[3] Dobroś K, Hajto-Bryk J, Zarzecka J. (2023). Application of 3D-printed teeth models in teaching dentistry students: A scoping review. *European Journal of Dental Education*. 27(1):126–34.

[4] Fakhr M, Nagy MM. (2023). Three-Dimensional tooth models for better teaching and treatment outcomes. *European Journal of Dental Education*. 27(3):695–9.

[5] Zeng Y, Ji X, Dong B, Zhang L, Zheng Q, Wang Y, Han X, Ye L, Huang D, Wang S. (2024). 3D-printed coloured tooth model for inlay preparation in pre-clinical dental education. *European Journal of Dental Education*. 28(2):481–9.

[6] Hanafi A, Donnermeyer D, Schäfer E, Bürklein S. (2022). Perception of a modular 3D print model in undergraduate endodontic education. *Int Endod J*. 53(7):1007–16.

[7] Reymus M, Fotiadou C, Kessler A, Heck K, Hickel R, Diegritz C. (2019). 3D printed replicas for endodontic education. *Int Endod J*. 52(1):123–30.

[8] Reymus M, Liebermann A, Diegritz C, Keßler A. (2021). Development and evaluation of an interdisciplinary teaching model via 3D printing. *Clin Exp Dent Res*. 7(1):3–10.

[9] Kolling M, Backhaus J, Hofmann N, Keß S, Krastl G, Soliman S, *et al.* (2022). Students' perception of three-dimensionally printed teeth in endodontic training. *European Journal of Dental Education*. 26(4):653–61.

[10] Farronato M, Torres A, Pedano MS, Jacobs R. (2023). Novel method for augmented reality guided endodontics: An in vitro study. *J Dent*. 132.

[11] Meglioli M, Mergoni G, Artioli F, Ghezzi B, Manfredi M, Macaluso GM, *et al.* (2023). A novel self-assessment method for training access cavity on 3D printed endodontic models. *Dent J (Basel)*. 11(6).

[12] Höhne C, del Hougne M, Gärtner L, Winter A, Schmitter M. (2024). Modular training model for education of students in restorative and prosthodontic dentistry. *European Journal of Dental Education*. 28(1):347–57.

[13] Kustra P, Dobroś K, Zarzecka J. (2021). Making use of three-dimensional models of teeth, manufactured by stereolithographic technology, in practical teaching of endodontics. *European Journal of Dental Education*. 25(2):299–304.

[14] Peters O, Scott R, Arias A, Lim E, Paqué F, Almassi S, *et al.* (2021). Evaluation of dental students' skills acquisition in endodontics using a 3D printed tooth model. *Eur Endod J*. 6(3):290–4.

[15] Lugassy D, Levanon Y, Rosen G, Livne S, Fridenberg N, Pilo R, *et al.* (2021). Does augmented visual feedback from novel, multicolored, three-dimensional-printed teeth affect dental students' acquisition of manual skills? *Anat Sci Educ*. 14(5):629–40.

[16] Tricio JA, Braithwaite C, Herrera CM, Vicuña DP, Cacciuttolo FR, Jorquera GA, *et al.* (2024). Comparison of digitally assessed quality of posterior crown preparations performed with and without previous practice on patient-specific three-dimensional-printed teeth models. *J Dent Educ*.

[17] Choi Y, Jeon WS, Cho JM, Jeong HG, Shin Y, Park W. (2021). Access opening guide produced using a 3D printer (AOG-3DP) as an effective tool in difficult cases for dental students. *J Dent Educ*. 85(10):1640–5.

[18] Genovese P, Giambò P, Abramo F, Mancini M, Pastore M, D'Amico C. (2024). Advancements and Applications in Digital Dentistry: A Scoping Review. In: *IFMBE Proceedings*. p. 702–9.

Navigating Dental Education Trends and Transforming Dental Pedagogy – Abas and Srikant N (Eds)
© 2027 The Author(s), ISBN: 978-1-041-32674-8

Digital Directions: Using Guided Endodontics as a Tool for Dental Education

Ishan Bhatla and Roma M
Department of Conservative Dentistry and Endodontics, Manipal College of Dental Sciences Mangalore, Manipal Academy of Higher Education, Manipal, India

ABSTRACT: Introduction
Guided endodontics is a straightforward and meticulous technique that can eliminate the extensive experience of the operator performing the endodontic treatment while combining 3-dimensional imaging modalities with analytical software and can serve as a tool for nurturing visualization and improving the skills of a novice dentist. Simulations of dental procedures help achieve optimum results and minimize failure,; this has traditionally been done on typhodont models or extracted teeth, and the incorporation of guided techniques atop this has become a great asset for enhancing the knowledge of dental students. Guided endodontics can be of two types: static navigation with the use of guides and templates, and dynamic navigation with the use of a camera marker system.
Methodology
Biomedical databases like Google scholar, PubMed, Science Direct and Scopus for available literature, the following keywords were used: "guided AND endodontics", "simulation AND dental training".
Results
The present study proves that it is a more precise method of access cavity preparation; it also achieves excellent navigation in teeth with pulpal obliteration and suggests that it is an approach that eliminates the user experience as an influencing factor in comparison with freehand endodontics. The literature also suggests that guided endodontics can be considered a treatment option for managing dens invaginatus cases, involving the removal of glass fiber posts and mineral trioxide aggregates.
Conclusion
Overall, guided endodontics, when combined with simulation technologies, offers substantial benefits for dental education, enhancing both practical skills and theoretical understanding. This innovative approach holds promise for improving the quality of dental training and ultimately leading to better patient outcomes.
Discussion
The improvement of teaching methods to suit modern clinical situations is crucial and integral to improving the clinical judgment, decision -making and practical skills of dental students. Thus, the use of guided techniques as learning tools could shape the future of dental learning.

Keywords: guided endodontics, dynamic navigation, static navigation

1 INTRODUCTION

Guided endodontics is a future of endodontic treatments and is representative of leaping strides in endodontics.[1] Compared with conventional treatments, this approach enhances the precision of root canal treatments and potentially eliminates operator experience as a factor affecting treatment outcomes.[2] This review aims to explore guided endodontics and its potential use as a tool for dental education and how it can improve the proficiency of both students and dental professionals in endodontics.[2]

The primary objective of this study is to understand and analyze the current available literature and explore whether it can be used to improve the existing modalities of education for students, particularly in endodontics.

Guided endodontics can be of two types: static navigation systems and dynamic navigation systems[3]. Static navigation uses a CBCT image of the patient's arch and registers the arch via an intraoral scanner or impression. The images are superimposed via software to design a guide with a drill hole to access the calcified canal directly. Cylindrical sleeves are designed to ensure stable drill access. The design is then exported in STL format for 3D printing. The guide is fitted to the teeth of the patient, and the internal metal or acrylic based cylinder guides the drill to remove calcified tissue, after which the root canal treatment continues conventionally. On the other hand, Dynamic navigation uses CBCT images with reference marks placed in the patient's mouth. A camera attached to a dynamic navigation system coordinates the drill's trajectory in real time, allowing the operator to monitor and alter the angulation of the instruments as needed. This real-time navigation enhances precision and adaptability during the procedure.[4]

The traditional endodontic model work exercises include the use of extracted teeth, which are often found to have pulpal obliteration, thus making practice difficult and incomplete for a learner, since guided endodontics have been

 DOI: 10.1201/9781042016075-64

shown to yield statistically better results with pulpal obliteration. This technique can be used as a great tool to optimize learning skills, optimizing resources, such as the limited number of extracted teeth, while also keeping learners in touch with the upcoming treatment modalities.

As an educational tool, simulation has the potential to be used in conjunction with guided endodontics, with the former using virtual reality and haptic feedback systems and the latter using 3D imaging and printing guides[5][6]. Students can learn treatment in a risk-free environment with the utmost precision, creating an interactive and effective learning experience leading to improved patient treatment outcomes.

2 METHODS

PubMed, Scopus and Science Direc were used to search for available literature via the keywords: "guided AND endodontics", "simulation AND dental training". Duplicate reviews and studies were discarded via Mendeley Desktop reference manager software (Elsevier, AMS, Asterweg, The Netherlands). Manual review was performed, and studies that did not meet the inclusion criteria were excluded. The literature left was read in full, and those that dealt with a topic other than that of interest to this literature review were excluded.

The inclusion criteria of the articles were as follows:

- Keywords: guided AND endodontics, simulation and dental training
- Time period: 2019–2024
- Articles on guided endodontics: its types, uses, advantages, disadvantages, and/or outcomes

Exclusion criteria articles were excluded if they met the following criteria:

- Articles in languages other than English.
- Animal studies.
- Articles that, after their title and abstract were read, did not fit with the subject of interest of this paper.

3 RESULTS

3.1 *Enhanced safety and precision*

A systematic review demonstrated that guided endodontics significantly enhances the accuracy and safety of endodontic procedures, and the combination of 3-dimensional imaging and guided models reduces operator skill-related errors and provides the benefits of easier predictability of root canals, and higher success rates, thus assisting inexperienced operators such as dental students.[7]

3.2 *Improved success rates*

Due to the use of surgical template, the exact direction of the of the access drill can be ensured, whilst also minimizing the dental hard tissue loss and thus contributing to a precise root canal preparation. [8]

3.3 *Conservative access cavity designs*

The combination of the 3-D imaging modality like CBCT with the surgical guide fabrication, the access cavity can be placed directly over the canal orifice, and results in access which is void of operator errors, like gouging or perforations, since the guide will only allow the movement of the drill in the correct direction. [9]

3.4 *Endodontic post removal*

Glass fibre post removal has also been suggested to be a potential approach requiring guided endodontics, and the authors have suggested that it can be of help to novice operators, helping with lesser chairside time, lesser dentine loss and lesser risk of perforations and other iatrogenic errors. [10]

3.5 *Calcific metamorphosis cases*

In cases with calcifications of the pulpal canals, it was found to be more effective in locating and navigating them and required less chairside time. [11][12]

3.6 *Educational benefits*

A literature review that highlights the educational advantages of guided endodontics. indicating that digital visualization and preprocedural planning facilitated by GE help students bridge the gap between theoretical knowledge and clinical practice. This approach was shown to enhance students' understanding and execution of endodontic procedures.[13,14]

3.7 *Canal location accessibility*

An in- vitro study concluded that canal location was more accurate with guided endodontics than with conventional techniques with less substance loss but longer operating times, which can aid in improving canal location, especially in maxillary 1st molars with MB2, and in cases of mid -distal or middle mesial canals, increasing the appreciation and understanding of the anatomy of canal orifices.[15]

3.8 *Clinical applications and limitations*

A systematic review evaluated clinical applications, accuracy, and limitations. The review concluded that while the evidence base is still evolving, guided endodontics are highly accurate and successful in clinical settings, despite some limitations related to the cost and accessibility of advanced technologies.[16,17]

Author	Year	Journal	Title	Result
Connert T *et al.*	2022	International Endodontic Journal	Present status and future directions – Guided endodontics	-
Kulinkovych-Levchuk K *et al.*	2022	International Journal of Environmental Research and Public Health	Guided Endodontics: A Literature Review	• GE has use in accesscavity preparations and locating root canals, especially in pulp canal obliteration cases, microsurgical endodontics, and removing glass fiber posts in endodontic retreatments • In addition, it is independent of an operator's experience • Less time for treatment • higher accuracy and safer than conventional endodontics.
Li Y *et al.*	2021	Journal of Medical Internet Research.	The Current Situation and Future Prospects of Simulators in Dental Education	-
Moreno-Rabié C *et al.*	2020	International Endodontic Journal	Clinical applications, accuracy and limitations of guided endodontics: a systematic review	Guided endodontic procedures offer a highly predictable outcome and lower risk of iatrogenic damage
Ribeiro D, Reis E *et al.*	2022	Journal of Personalized Medicine	Guided Endodontics: Static vs. Dynamic Computer-Aided Techniques	Guided endodontics presented lower risk of iatrogenic damage, especially on use by less experienced operators.
Connert T *et al.*	2019	Journal of Endodontics	Guided Endodontics versus Conventional Access Cavity Preparation: A Comparative Study on Substance Loss Using 3-dimensional–printed Teeth	• Canal location had 91.7% success with the guided approach • There was less substance loss with guided approach • Treatment time was also lower than conventional technique
Honda R	2024	Australian Endodontic Journal	Fibre post removal using ultrasonic tips: A comparative in vitro study using different protocols	Guided endodontics can be used for removal of glass fiber posts
Rane S	2024	Journal of Pharmacy and Bioallied Sciences.	Minimally Invasive Access Cavity Designs: A Review	Virtually fabricated sleeves can help guide the drill with the most conservative path to the root canal
Shah P	2018	Clinical Oral Investigations	3D imaging, 3D printing and 3D virtual planning in endodontics	3D printed models and guides, and haptic simulators have utility in teaching and management of endodontic procedures
Tang WL	2024	Journal of Dental Research	The Use of Dynamic Navigation Systems as a Component of Digital Dentistry	• Enhanced direct visualization, treatment precision, efficiency, safety, and procedural adaptability. • Substantial upfront costs, requires comprehensive training, additional preparatory time, and increased radiation exposure.

(*continued*)

Continued

Author	Year	Journal	Title	Result
Chaniotis A	2024	Journal of Clinical Medicine.	Negotiation of Calcified Canals.	Almost 90% of the calcified canals can be negotiated to the apical third with the help of conventional techniques and microscope. The success rate with follow-up period of 3 years was 80 %.
La Rosa GRM	2024	Australian Endodontic Journal	Advancements in guided surgical endodontics: A scoping review of case report and case series and research implications	Longer follow-up periods, radiographic verifications of bone healing are required to assess the benefit of guided endodontics, which are sparse in currently existing literature
Abdelhafeez MM	2024	Journal of Pharmacy and Bioallied Sciences	Applications of Finite Element Analysis in Endodontics: A Systematic Review and Meta-Analysis	FEA guided endodontics help improve stress distribution and fatigue resistance than conventional techniques
Puri A	2024	cureus	Impact of Guided Endodontics on the Success of Endodontic Treatment: An Umbrella Review of Systematic Reviews and Meta-Analyses	Guided endodntics had improved ,precision, better clinical success rates and lesser procedural errors
Banka A	2024	Journal of Conservative Dentistry and Endodontics	Comparative evaluation between guided endodontics and conventional techniques for calcific metamorphosis – A systematic review and meta-analysis	• Predictable outcomes • Access cavity accuracy • Easier location of root canals in apical third • Reduced chairside time
Dioguardi M	2024		Exploring the Impact of Access Cavity Designs on Canal Orifice Localization and Debris Presence: A Scoping Review	Conventional techniques cause more debris generation whilst guided techniques are more precise

4 DISCUSSION

Guided endodontics is emeging as a transformative tool in dental education, offering significant advantages in both teaching and clinical practice. This technology-driven approach utilizes cone-beam computed tomography (CBCT) and 3D printing to create precise guides for endodontic procedures, enhancing accuracy and predictability.

One of the primary benefits of guided endodontics in dental education is its ability to provide students with a clear, visual understanding of complex anatomical structures. The use of CBCT scans and 3D-printed guides allows for detailed preoperative planning, which can be particularly beneficial in cases involving calcified canals or atypical root anatomies. This detailed visualization helps students grasp the intricacies of root canal systems, which can be challenging to understand through traditional methods.

Moreover, guided endodontics facilitates a minimally invasive approach, preserving more tooth structure and reducing the risk of iatrogenic damage. This is especially important for less experienced operators, such as dental students, who may struggle with the precision required for traditional endodontic techniques. By using static or dynamic navigation systems, students can perform procedures with greater confidence and accuracy, leading to improved clinical outcomes.

One in vitro study in which 3D-printed teeth, were used was conducted by Connert *et al.*. (2019), who compared a guided endodontic procedure with conventional access preparation via three operators of varying experience. The mean substance loss was 9.8 mm3 (SD ± 3.0) for the guided technique and 49.9 mm3 (SD ± 7.7) for the conventional approach by all operators. The guided treatment allowed the operators to find canals, irrespective of experience, 92% of the canals, a statistically greater proportion than the traditional technique did, of 42%,, confirming what was previously indicated in preclinical studies.

Moreover, the combination of GE with simulation tools such as virtual reality (VR) and haptic feedback systems provides a comprehensive, risk-free training environment. This integration improves students' technical skills and prepares them for real-world clinical scenarios.

The integration of guided endodontics into dental curricula also aligns with the trend toward digital dentistry. As dental education increasingly incorporates digital tools and techniques, guided endodontics serves as an excellent example of how technology can enhance learning and clinical practice. Students trained in these advanced techniques are better prepared for modern dental practice, where digital workflows are becoming the norm.

Guided endodontics with advanced simulation technologies represents a significant advancement in dental education. The results from various studies underscore the enhanced precision and safety that GE offers, particularly benefiting dental students by reducing the risk of iatrogenic damage and improving the predictability of root canal treatments. The educational benefits are evident, with digital visualization and preprocedural planning helping students bridge the gap between theoretical knowledge and clinical practice.

While guided endodontics offers numerous benefits, there are several drawbacks to consider. The cost and accessibility of advanced technologies such as CBCT and 3D printing can be prohibitive for some educational institutions. Additionally, the learning curve associated with these technologies may require additional training and resources. Despite these challenges, the long-term benefits for dental education and patient care make the investment worthwhile.

5 CONCLUSION

Guided endodontics (GE) with advanced simulation technologies enhances dental education by improving precision, safety, and predictability in root canal treatments. It bridges theoretical knowledge and clinical practice, especially with tools like VR and haptic feedback, providing a comprehensive, risk-free training environment. Despite high success rates, proper training is crucial to avoid failures due to incorrect use or data limitations. While costs and the learning curve are challenges, the long-term benefits for dental education and patient care justify the investment.

REFERENCES

[1] Connert T, Weiger R, Krastl G. (2022). Present status and future directions – Guided endodontics. *Int Endod J.* 55(S4):995–1002.

[2] Kulinkovych-Levchuk K, Pecci-Lloret MP, Castelo-Baz P, Pecci-Lloret MR, Oñate-Sánchez RE. (2022). Guided endodontics: A literature review. *Int J Environ Res Public Health.* 19(21):13900.

[3] Ribeiro D, Reis E, Marques JA, Falacho RI, Palma PJ. (2022). Guided endodontics: Static vs. dynamic Computer-aided techniques—a literature review. *J Pers Med.* 12(9):1516.

[4] Tang WL, Chao XY, Ye Z, Liu MW, Jiang H. (2024). The use of dynamic navigation systems as a component of digital dentistry. *J Dent Res.* 103(2):119–28.

[5] Shah P, Chong BS. (2018). 3D imaging, 3D printing and 3D virtual planning in endodontics. *Clin Oral Investig.* 22(2):641–54.

[6] Current applications of three-dimensional (3D) printing in pediatric dentistry: a literature review. *Journal of Clinical Pediatric Dentistry.* 48(5):4.

[7] Connert T, Krug R, Eggmann F, Emsermann I, ElAyouti A, Weiger R, *et al.* (2019). Guided endodontics versus conventional access cavity preparation: A comparative study on substance loss using 3-dimensional–printed *Teeth. J Endod.* 45(3):327–31.

[8] Puri A, Abraham D, Gupta A. (2024). Impact of guided endodontics on the success of endodontic treatment: An umbrella review of systematic reviews and meta-analyses. *Cureus.*

[9] Dioguardi M, La Notte D, Sovereto D, Quarta C, Ballini A, Crincoli V, *et al.* (2024). Exploring the impact of access cavity designs on canal orifice localization and debris presence: A scoping review. *Clin Exp Dent Res.* 10(6).

[10] Honda R, Pelepenko LE, Monteiro MF, Marciano MA, Gomes BPFA, de Jesus Soares A, *et al.* (2024). Fibre post removal using ultrasonic tips: A comparative in vitro study using different protocols. *Australian Endodontic Journal.*

[11] Banka A, Patri G, Pradhan PK, Lath H. (2024). Comparative evaluation between guided endodontics and conventional techniques for calcific metamorphosis – A systematic review and meta-analysis. *Journal of Conservative Dentistry and Endodontics.* 27(9):891–6.

[12] Chaniotis A, Sousa Dias H, Chanioti A. (2024). Negotiation of calcified canals. *J Clin Med.* 13(9):2703.

[13] Leung ALS, Yeung C, Chu S, Wong AWY, Yu OY, Chu CH. (2021). Use of computer simulation in dental training with special reference to simodont. *Dent J (Basel).* 9(11):125.

[14] Li Y, Ye H, Ye F, Liu Y, Lv L, Zhang P, *et al.* (2021). The current situation and future prospects of simulators in dental education. *J Med Internet Res.* 23(4):e23635.

[15] Rane S, Pandit V, Gaikwad A, Chavan S, Patil R, Shinde M. (2024). Minimally invasive access cavity designs: A Review. *J pharm bioallied sci.* 16(Suppl 3):S1971–3.

[16] Moreno-Rabié C, Torres A, Lambrechts P, Jacobs R. (2020). Clinical applications, accuracy and limitations of guided endodontics: a systematic review. *Int Endod J.* 53(2):214–31.

[17] La Rosa GRM, Peditto M, Venticinque A, Marcianò A, Bianchi A, Pedullà E. (2024). Advancements in guided surgical endodontics: A scoping review of case report and case series and research implications. *Australian Endodontic Journal.* 50(2):397–408.

Navigating Dental Education Trends and Transforming Dental Pedagogy – Abas and Srikant N (Eds)
© 2027 The Author(s), ISBN: 978-1-041-32674-8

Traditional to Transformative: Innovations in Endodontic Training

Nikki Vasani, Manuel S Thomas, Janina Loren D'Souza, and Sharol Annie Lobo
Department of Conservative Dentistry and Endodontics, Manipal College of Dental Sciences Mangalore, Manipal Academy of Higher Education, Manipal, Karnataka, India

ABSTRACT: The evolution of tooth models for root canal treatment has advanced from simple 2D illustrations and extracted teeth to detailed 3D models and digital simulations. These modern models enhance training, clinical precision, and patient care by providing accurate anatomical detail and realistic textures.

Extracted human teeth have long been the standard for simulating clinical settings, offering a good understanding of internal anatomy and the tactile experience of working on dentine. However, they have several drawbacks: difficulty collecting, ethical considerations, cross-infection risks, and storage issues.

To overcome the drawbacks faced by using natural teeth, resin endodontic blocks with built-in conduits resembling natural root canals are made. However, they lack representation of the crown and root's external anatomy, limiting their educational value.

3D printed models of highly detailed customizable replicas of natural teeth by using micro-CT. These models provide realistic training experiences, can represent various clinical scenarios, and eliminate ethical and logistical issues of using extracted human teeth.

Modern phantom heads feature adjustable jaws, occlusion, and interchangeable teeth to simulate various patient anatomies. These heads can be equipped with integrated root canal models or replaceable sections, offering realistic training while maintaining the full oral context.

Virtual reality (VR) with haptic feedback for teaching root canal treatment offers an advanced, immersive training tool that combines visual simulation with tactile sensations. The haptic feedback mimics the resistance and texture of real teeth, enhancing the learning experience by providing a true-to-life sense of touch.

Keywords: Root canal models, Virtual Reality, Extracted teeth, 3D models

1 INTRODUCTION

Learning and practicing root canals is challenging because of their complex procedural steps, a thorough understanding of tooth anatomy, precise instrumentation skills, and a strong sense of tactile feedback is essential. Historically, training for this procedure relied heavily on extracted human teeth and simple visual aids, which provided students with foundational knowledge but lacked the ability to simulate the full range of clinical scenarios. With modern technologies, the landscape of endodontic training has evolved significantly, offering more realistic and diverse simulation models. The process of learning root canal treatment has evolved from extracted teeth to sophisticated 3D models, virtual simulations, and phantom heads. These advancements enhance training, clinical precision, and patient care by providing accurate anatomical details and realistic textures.[1] This review explores the progression of these models, from traditional approaches to the latest innovations in dental education.

2 TRADITIONAL TRAINING MODELS: EXTRACTED HUMAN TEETH

Extracted human teeth have long been the gold standard for simulating clinical settings in root canal treatment. These teeth provide invaluable insight into the internal anatomy and offer a realistic tactile experience when working on dentine. Practicing on extracted teeth allows students to develop their skills in navigating the root canal system, managing curved canals, and understanding the complexities of tooth morphology.

However, the use of extracted teeth comes with notable limitations. The collection of extracted teeth is often challenging due to ethical concerns, the risk of cross-infection, and the need for stringent storage and sterilization protocols.[2] Additionally, the variability in the anatomy of these teeth can make it challenging to provide standardized training experiences for students.[3] Furthermore, the supply of extracted teeth is inconsistent, making it hard to ensure all students have equal access to quality training specimens. These issues have prompted the need for alternative models that offer a safer, more controlled, and reproducible training environment.

3 SYNTHETIC MODELS: RESIN ENDODONTIC BLOCKS

Resin endodontic blocks were developed as an alternative training tool to address the limitations associated with extracted teeth. These blocks typically contain built-in conduits that mimic the natural root canals of teeth, providing students with a basic understanding of canal navigation and instrumentation techniques. Resin blocks are widely used in preclinical training due to their accessibility, low cost, and consistent anatomical features[4]

However, resin blocks provide a standardized training environment but lacks anatomical complexity and tactile feedback of natural teeth.[5] The artificial nature of the material limits the realism of the training experience, as it does not accurately replicate the feel of working on human dentine. This has driven further innovation in developing more advanced models to simulate the clinical environment better.

4 ADVANCED 3D PRINTED MODELS

3D printing technology has revolutionized the field of dental education by enabling the creation of highly detailed, customizable replicas of natural teeth. These models are often based on micro-CT scans of actual teeth, allowing for precise replication of complex internal structures, including the root canal system.[6] The use of 3D printed models offers several significant advantages over traditional extracted teeth. They can be produced on demand, eliminating ethical and logistical issues, and can be designed to represent a wide range of clinical scenarios, such as teeth with curved canals, calcifications, or resorptive defects.

Moreover, 3D-printed models are made from materials that closely mimic the mechanical properties of natural dentine, providing a more realistic tactile experience. This realism is crucial for developing the manual skills required in root canal treatment, such as the force applied during instrumentation and negotiation of complex canal anatomy. Customizing these models for specific training needs allows educators to tailor their teaching methods, enhancing the overall learning experience before facing similar clinical scenarios.

5 PHANTOM HEADS WITH INTERCHANGEABLE TEETH

Modern phantom heads have become integral to endodontic training, simulating a more comprehensive clinical environment by including adjustable jaws, occlusion, and interchangeable teeth. These heads mimic the oral cavity, allowing students to practice positioning, access, and canal instrumentation within a full oral context. Phantom heads can be equipped with integrated root canal models or replaceable sections, offering versatility and the ability to simulate diverse patient anatomies and clinical conditions.

The use of phantom heads in training provides a bridge between preclinical exercises and real-world patient care. They help students develop a sense of spatial awareness, ergonomic positioning, and the practical application of clinical skills.[7] The realistic setting fosters the development of muscle memory, enhancing the transition from simulation to clinical practice.

6 VIRTUAL REALITY (VR) WITH HAPTIC FEEDBACK

Virtual reality (VR) technology represents the forefront of innovation in endodontic training, offering an immersive learning experience that combines visual simulation with tactile sensations. VR systems equipped with haptic feedback can mimic the resistance and texture of natural teeth, allowing students to feel the sensation of drilling, filing, and obturating a root canal. This technology provides unparalleled realism, enabling users to experience a wide range of clinical scenarios, including complex anatomies and unexpected complications.

The integration of VR in dental education offers numerous benefits, including the ability to practice repeatedly without the need for physical models, instant feedback on performance, and the opportunity to refine techniques in a risk-free environment. VR systems can be programmed to simulate rare or difficult cases, helping students build confidence and competence in managing challenging clinical situations. Combining visual and haptic feedback enhances fine motor skills and decision-making abilities, making VR a powerful tool for teaching root canal treatment. In a study the integration of VR was greatly accepted by students in endodontic training.[8]

The limitations of VR include limited familiarity with the technology among users, the high cost of maintenance, and challenges faced by individuals who wear spectacles, which may hinder the comfortable use of VR headsets.[9,10]

7 DISCUSSION AND CONCLUSION

The evolution of tooth models for root canal treatment reflects the ongoing pursuit of improving dental education and clinical training. Each model type, from traditional extracted teeth to cutting-edge VR simulations, offers unique advantages and contributes to the comprehensive development of endodontic skills. Extracted teeth provide a direct experience of natural anatomy, while resin blocks offer a standardized, cost-effective training tool. Advanced 3D printed models bring unprecedented anatomical accuracy and customization, and phantom heads add a realistic oral context to the learning process. VR with haptic feedback represents the pinnacle of simulation technology, offering an immersive and highly interactive training experience.

The continuous advancement of these models enhances the skill development of students and practitioners, ultimately leading to better clinical outcomes and improved patient care. As technology continues to evolve, the integration of innovative training tools will play a crucial role in shaping the future of endodontic education, ensuring that practitioners are well-equipped to meet the demands of modern dentistry.

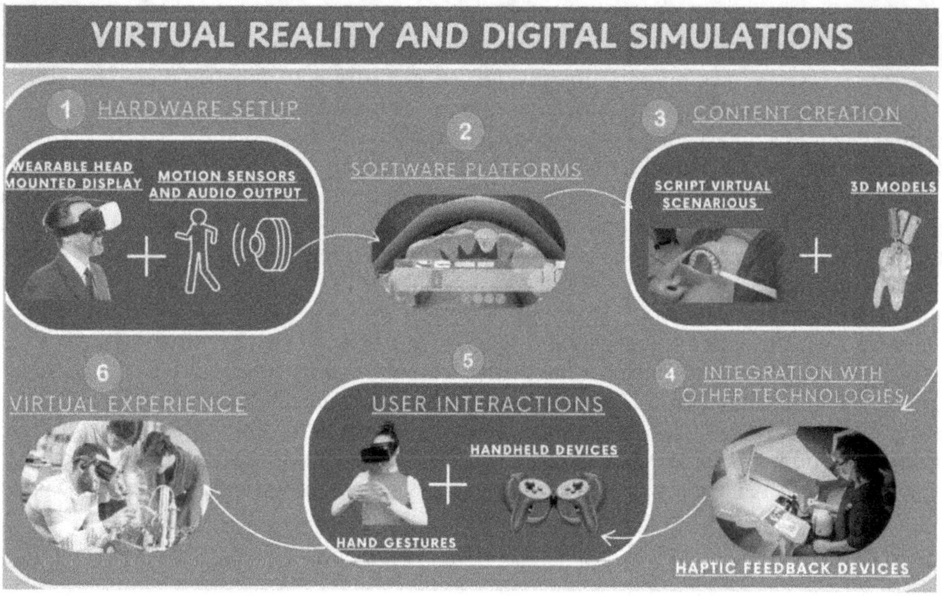

Figure 1. Workflow of Virtual reality integration in endodontic training.

REFERENCES

[1] Fayyaz Y, Ali M, Ullah R, Shaikh MS. (2024). Applications of 3D-printed teeth in dental education: A narrative review. *Journal of Taibah University Medical Sciences*. 19(4):816–22.

[2] Deogade SC, Mantri SS, Saxena S, Sumathi K. (2016). Awareness and knowledge of undergraduate dental students about sterilization/disinfection methods of extracted human teeth. *Ann Med Health Sci Res*. 6(6):348–355. doi:10.4103/amhsr.amhsr_85_16

[3] Decurcio DA, Lim E, Nagendrababu V, Estrela C, Rossi-Fedele G. (2020). Difficulty levels of extracted human teeth used for pre-clinical training in endodontics in an Australian dental school. *Aust Endod J*. 46(1):47–51. doi:10.1111/aej.12355

[4] Soo WK, Thong YL. (2002). Construction of standardised simulated root canals in resin blocks for pre-clinical teaching. *Annals of Dentistry University of Malaya*. 9(1):7–10

[5] Luz DD, de S. Ourique F, Scarparo RK, Vier-Pelisser FV, Morgental RD, Waltrick SB, de Figueiredo JA. (2015). Preparation time and perceptions of Brazilian specialists and dental students regarding simulated root canals for endodontic teaching: a preliminary study. *Journal of Dental Education*. 79(1):56–63.

[6] Cresswell-Boyes AJ, Barber AH, Mills D, Tatla A, Davis GR. (2018). Approaches to 3D printing teeth from X-ray micro tomography. *J Microsc*. 272(3):207–212. doi:10.1111/jmi.12725

[7] Klink A, Engelskirchen F, Kaucher-Fernandez P, Huettig F, Roehler A. (2024). Implementation of patient-individualized 3D-printed models in undergraduate students' education for various prosthetic treatments: A cross-sectional survey study. *Dent J (Basel)*. 12(7):199.

[8] Reymus M, Liebermann A, Diegritz C. (2020). Virtual reality: An effective tool for teaching root canal anatomy to undergraduate dental students–a preliminary study. *International Endodontic Journal*, 53(11):1581–7.

[9] Mansoory MS, Azizi SM, Mirhosseini F, Yousefi D, Moradpoor H. (2022). A study to investigate the effectiveness of the application of virtual reality technology in dental education. *BMC Medical Education*. 22(1):457.

[10] Dzyuba N, Jandu J, Yates J, Kushnerev E. (2022). Virtual and augmented reality in dental education: The good, the bad and the better. *European Journal of Dental Education*

Navigating Dental Education Trends and Transforming Dental Pedagogy – Abas and Srikant N (Eds)
© 2027 The Author(s), ISBN: 978-1-041-32674-8

Virtual Innovations: Enhancing Dental Education Through Teledentistry

Vaishali and Annapoorna Shenoy
Department of Conservative Dentistry and Endodontics, Manipal College of Dental Science Mangalore, Manipal Academy of Higher Education, Manipal, India

ABSTRACT: OBJECTIVE: The primary objective of tele dentistry is to enhance the accessibility, quality and efficiency of learning experience by leveraging digital communication technologies. It supports a more flexible and inclusive learning environment, accommodating diverse learning styles and schedules.

SIGNIFICANCE and CONTRIBUTION TO THE FIELD: Today, it is utilized in academic medical centres, community hospitals, and rural hospitals, and it also facilitates international connections between healthcare providers in developing countries and hospitals in developed nations. Advances in digital communication, telecommunication, and the Internet have created unprecedented opportunities for remote access to medical care.

CONCLUSION: Dentistry mainly involves one to one interaction with the patients, which wasn't possible during the COVID-19 times. Tele dentistry came to the rescue and gained popularity in the dental field. It has a potential to eliminate the disparities in oral health care between urban and rural communities. Also, the integration of teledentistry into dental curricula enhances interactive learning, fosters collaborative education, and facilitates continuous professional development. Additionally, it supports a more flexible and inclusive learning environment, accommodating diverse learning styles and schedules. The implementation of teledentistry tools, such as digital imaging, virtual simulations, and online case discussions, enriches the educational experience. Overall, teledentistry represents a pivotal advancement in oral health care, offering increased accessibility, convenience, and continuity of care, especially in challenging times and undeserved regions.

1 INTRODUCTION

In 1997, Cook et al. defined teledentistry as as "the process of diagnosing patients and offering treatment recommendations via video conferencing technology." This approach utilizes information technology using communication networks to provide healthcare and education in different geographical areas. Teledentistry significantly enhances both dental education and healthcare by leveraging technology for improved learning, training, and patient management.

For dental education, it offers platforms for virtual lectures, remote demonstrations, and interactive simulations, enabling students to learn from experts regardless of their location. It also supports online case discussions and virtual clinics, providing students with access to a wider range of clinical scenarios and patient cases.

In terms of dental healthcare, teledentistry facilitates remote consultations, diagnoses, and treatment planning, enhancing access for patients in underserved areas and reducing the necessity for in-person visits. This technology also aids in ongoing patient monitoring, education on preventive care, and timely interventions, thereby improving overall dental health outcomes. By incorporating teledentistry into both educational and clinical environments, the dental field can advance its practices and broaden access to quality care.

Additionally, today's students are tech-savvy and favor virtual learning resources oveconventional in-person lectures. Farooq and Al-Jandan have noted that lectures that incorporate modern tools, such as videos to illustrate concepts, can enhance student learning. Following the global cessation of educational activities due to the COVID-19 pandemic, teledentistry has emerged as a crucial resource for ongoing instruction and training in dentistry until normalcy returns and physical distancing is no longer necessary.

2 METHODS

Teleconsultation in teledentistry can occur in two primary formats: "Real-Time Consultation" and the "Store-and-Forward Method."

2.1 *Real-time consultation*

This method uses a video conference to enable dental professionals and patients, regardless of their locations, to see, hear, and communicate with one another directly.

 DOI: 10.1201/9781042016075-66

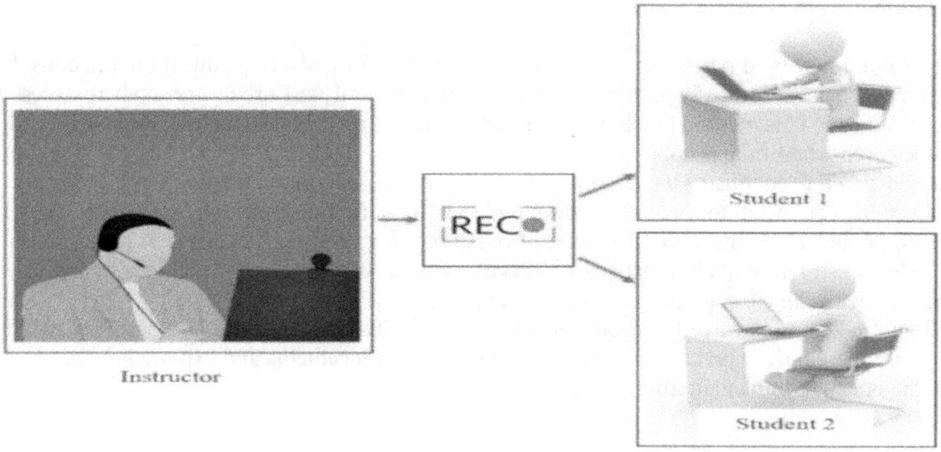

Figure 1. Showing pre-recorded lecture technique to cover didactic component of dental education.

2.2 *Store-and-forward method*

This method involves the dental practitioner gathering and storing clinical information and static images, which are then sent for consultation and treatment planning without the patient's presence. Dentists can share a range of patient information, such as radiographs of periodontal and hard tissues, details of treatments conducted, lab results, tests, notes, photographs, and other pertinent data among multiple providers. This form of data sharing is especially advantageous for patients needing specialist consultations.

3 APPLICATION OF TELEDENTISTRY

1) **Consultations and Screenings:** Patients can have initial consultations via video calls, allowing dentists to assess conditions without an in-person visit.
2) **Follow-Up Care:** After procedures, dentists can check in with patients virtually to monitor healing and address concerns.
3) **Orthodontic Monitoring:** Patients using clear aligners can send progress photos for remote assessment, reducing the need for frequent office visits.
4) **Emergency Assessments:** In urgent situations, patients can receive immediate advice and triage from their dentist without needing to visit the office.
5) **Education and Prevention:** Teledentistry can facilitate virtual education sessions on oral hygiene practices, nutrition, and preventive care.
6) **Access for Underserved Populations:** Remote consultations can improve access to dental care for people in rural or underserved areas.
7) **Integration with Health Records:** Teledentistry platforms can connect with electronic health records, making it easier for dentists to track patient history and treatments.
8) **Collaboration with Specialists:** Dentists can consult with specialists via telecommunication to discuss complex cases, enhancing patient care

4 RESULTS

Advantages of Teledentistry: Teledentistry has below mentioned pros,

1) Improved access to care.
2) Convenience and flexibility
3) Early detection and preventive care
4) Educational benefits
5) Crisis response
6) Reduced wait times

Limitations of Teledentistry: Teledentistry has certain limitations which include,

1) A strong internet connection is necessary.
2) The teacher must be suitably prepared to offer online educational activities.
3) The role of the instructor in clinical training is limited because dentistry is primarily a hands-on field.

5 DISCUSSION

Teledentistry is not a new field but rather an alternative approach for delivering education and consultations using internet resources. Its importance is particularly pronounced in rural and urban areas where access to specialist consultations is limited. This method facilitates timely communication between doctors and patients, allowing them to discuss issues even when time is constrained.

While internet-based teledentistry has become a preferred means of communication, it does come with potential drawbacks, such as the need for adequate training, the pressure for immediate responses, the risk of misunderstandings, privacy concerns, and the chance of overlooking messages. It is essential for practitioners wishing to integrate teledentistry into their practices to educate themselves about the legal, technological, and ethical aspects associated with this new aspect of educating medium.

Dentists should take an initiative to become acquainted with this new future technology. This will help them to understand it's impact on their practices with the use of digital advancements and explore how both the parties can benefit from the effective implementation of this advancement.

6 CONCLUSION

One important development in dental education and treatment is teledentistry. It has made remote learning possible, made specialist information more accessible, and promoted international professional collaboration in the field of dentistry education. Through online mentoring, teleconsultations, and virtual simulations, it enables interactive learning experiences. Additionally, this technology has been crucial in maintaining educational continuity during crises like the COVID-19 epidemic.

It presents encouraging opportunities to advance dental treatment and education, broaden accessibility, and enhance patient results. It signifies a fundamental change toward an integrated and more digital future for oral health services.

REFERENCES

[1] Readul islam, Rafiqul islam, (2022). Sultana fardus teledentistry as an effective tool for the communication improvement between dentists and patients. *Healthcare*. 2022. 10(8):1586 [PubMed]

[2] Bhambal A., Saxena S., Balsaraf S.V. (2010). Teledentistry: Potentials unexplored. *J. Int. Oral. Health*. 2010;2:1–6. [Google Scholar]

[3] Khan S.A., Omar H. (2013). Teledentistry in practice: Literature review. *Telemed. E-Health*. 2013;19:565–567. [PubMed] [CrossRef] [Google Scholar]

[4] Talla P.K., Levin L., Glogauer M., Cable C., Allison P.J. (2020). Delivering dental care as we emerge from the initial phase of the COVID-19 pandemic: Teledentistry and face-to-face consultations in a new clinical world. *Quintessence Int*. 2020;51:672–677. [PubMed] [Google Scholar]

[5] N.D. Jampani, R. Nutalapati, B.S.K Dontula. (2011). Applications of teledentistry: A literature review and update. *J Int Soc Prev Community Dent*. 2011. 1(2): 37–44 [PubMed]

[6] Kirshner M. (2003). The Role of Information Technology and Informatics Research in the Dentist-Patient Relationship. *Adv Dent Res*. 2003;17:77–81. [PubMed] [Google Scholar]

[7] Chang S.U., Plotkin D.R., Mulligan R., Polido J.C., Mah J.K., Meara J.G. (2003). Teledentistry in rural California: A USC initiative. *J. Calif. Dent. Assoc*. 2003;31:601–608. [PubMed] [Google Scholar]

[8] Golder D.T., Brennan K.A. (2000). Practicing dentistry in the age of telemedicine. *J. Am. Dent. Assoc*. 2000;131:734–74. [PubMed] [Google Scholar]

[9] Suetenkov D.E., Popkova O.V., Kiselev A.R. (2020). Possibilities and limitations of teledentistry. *Rev. Cuba. Estomatol*. 2020;57:1–8. [Google Scholar]

[10] Ghai S. (2020). Teledentistry during COVID-19 pandemic. Diabetes Metab. *Syndr. Clin. Res. Rev*. 2020;14:933–935. [PubMed] [Google Scholar]

[11] Farooq I, Al-Jandan BA. (2015) Effect of video triggering during conventional lectures on final grades of dental students in an oral biology course: A two-year retrospective study. *J Dent Educ*. 2015;79(12):1467–1470 [PubMed] [Google Scholar]

[12] Dasgupta A, Deb S. (2008). Telemedicine: A New Horizon in Public Health in India. *Indian J Community Med*. 2008;33:3–8. [PMC free article] [PubMed] [Google Scholar]

[13] Yoshinaga L. (2001). The use of teledentistry for remote learning applications. *Pract Proced Aesthet Dent*. 2001;13:327–8. [PubMed] [Google Scholar]

[14] li S, Noreen S, Farooq I, Bugshan A, Vohra F. (2020). Risk assessment of healthcare workers at the frontline against COVID-19. *Pak J Med Sci*. 2020;36(COVID19-S4):COVID19-S99–S103. [PubMed] [Google Scholar]

[15] Arora P.C., Kaur J., Kaur J., Arora A. (2019). Teledentistry: An innovative tool for the underserved population. *Digit. Med*. 2019;5:6–12. [Google Scholar]

 ISBN: 978-1-041-32674-8

Enhancing Dental Education: Leveraging YouTube for Effective Learning

Meenu Goyat and Ankita Singh
Department of Conservative dentistry and Endodontics, Manipal College of Dental Sciences, Mangalore, Manipal Academy of Higher Education, Manipal

1 INTRODUCTION

YouTube has become one of the most popular and accessible platforms globally, offering a vast range of media content to anyone with internet access. In education, particularly medical and dental education, YouTube has emerged as a significant resource for self-directed learning.

The ability to access educational videos at any time allows students to enhance their theoretical knowledge and practical skills, especially in areas like oral surgery, where hands-on clinical experience is often limited to specific times. This flexibility is particularly advantageous for students who need to balance academic demands with clinical work, offering them the opportunity to revisit procedures and concepts outside of the traditional classroom or clinic setting [2]

Multimedia learning—where information is delivered through a combination of visual and auditory means—has gained substantial attention over the past two decades for its effectiveness in enhancing understanding and retention [3]. YouTube's core value as an educational resource lies in its ability to deliver both visual and verbal information through videos, making it an engaging and versatile tool for learners. Educational videos on YouTube often present real-life clinical examples and well-explained content, which can be difficult to replicate in standard educational environments [3]. As such, it has become an increasingly common tool for supplementing traditional medical education, especially in the e-learning and blended course formats.

However, despite these advantages, the unregulated nature of content on YouTube raises concerns about the quality and accuracy of the information being presented. Unlike peer reviewed educational resources, YouTube content is created and uploaded by individuals or organizations without a formal vetting process. This can result in the dissemination of unscientific, misleading, or even incorrect information, which poses a risk to students who may not have the experience or knowledge to critically evaluate the accuracy of material [4]

For dental students, who rely on accurate and evidence-based knowledge for safe and effective clinical practice, this is a particularly pressing issue.

This review aims to explore the use of YouTube as a self-directed learning resource for dental students, focusing on its role in the education of dental subjects [4]. We will assess the platform's benefits, such as accessibility and multimedia learning potential, while also addressing the limitations and risks associated with unverified content [5]. The goal is to evaluate YouTube's effectiveness and accuracy in supporting the learning needs of dental students and to provide insights into how it can be integrated responsibly into medical education. [6]

2 METHODOLOGY

This review evaluates YouTube as a resource for self-directed learning in dental education using the following steps:

3 LITERATURE REVIEW

(a) Conduct a review of peer-reviewed articles and case studies on YouTube's use in dental and medical education.
(b) Focus on effectiveness, student perceptions, and the quality of content related to clinical procedures and dental theory.

3.1 *Content analysis*

(a) Analyze a sample of popular dental videos (1,000+ views) focusing on clinical procedures (e.g., fillings, root canals).
(b) Evaluate video for:

DOI: 10.1201/9781042016075-67

(i) educational quality (clarity, accuracy, depth)
(ii) Clinical accuracy (alignment with evidence-based practices)
(iii) Visual and auditory quality iv. Engagement (comments, ratings)

3.2 *Data Synthesis and Recommendations*

(a) Synthesize findings from literature, content analysis
(b) Provide recommendations for integrating YouTube into dental education, ensuring content quality, and equipping students with skills to assess content reliability.

3.3 *Expected outcomes*

This methodology will provide a comprehensive assessment of YouTube's educational value in dental education, offering practical insights on improving its effectiveness while addressing concerns about content quality. Recommendations will help educators and institutions guide students in using YouTube as a reliable learning resource.

4 DISCUSSION

YouTube as a learning tool has transformed dental education by providing students with easy access to a wealth of resources, but it comes with both significant advantages and notable challenges. Below is a discussion of the key benefits and drawbacks associated with its use in dental education.

Advantages of Using YouTube in Dental Education

- Accessibility: Available anytime, anywhere, on any device, making it easy to fit learning into students' schedules.
- Visual Learning: Combines visual and auditory elements to enhance understanding of complex procedures.
- Engagement: Interactive content with real-life demonstrations keeps students engaged and improves retention.
- Diverse Perspectives: Exposure to various techniques and approaches from global practitioners and institutions.
- Self-Directed Learning: Allows students to select content based on individual needs and revisit videos for reinforcement.
- Global Content Access: Access to a wide range of updated resources from around the world.

Disadvantages of Using YouTube in Dental Education

- Lack of Peer Review: No formal vetting of content, increasing the risk of errors and misinformation.
- Commercial Bias: Many videos promote commercial products, leading to biased recommendations.
- Non-Professional Content: Non-experts may demonstrate unsafe practices, risking students learning incorrect techniques.
- Content Quality: Difficulty in identifying reliable, evidence-based videos due to YouTube's algorithm favoring popularity over quality.
- Unstructured Learning: Without a formal curriculum, students may struggle to build a cohesive understanding of dental procedures.
- Overreliance on Self-Directed Learning: Students may lack the skills to critically assess the accuracy of content without guidance.
- Global Content Access: Access to a wide range of updated resources from around the world.

  Ethical Guidelines for Using YouTube in Dental Education

  When using YouTube as a resource for dental education, both students and educators must adhere to ethical principles to ensure the content is used responsibly and safely. The following ethical guidelines should be followed:

  Accuracy and Reliability

- Prioritize content from credible sources (e.g., licensed professionals, academic institutions).
- Verify clinical techniques against evidence-based practices to avoid misinformation.

  Avoiding Harmful Practices

- Do not use videos that promote unsafe or unproven dental procedures.
- Report misleading content to YouTube to prevent its spread.

  Student Safety

- Students should not perform complex procedures based solely on YouTube videos. Proper supervision is essential.
- YouTube should supplement, not replace, formal training.

Commercial Bias and Conflicts of Interest

- Ensure videos disclose any commercial relationships or sponsorships.
- Avoid videos with commercial bias; prioritize educational content.

Intellectual Property • Respect copyright laws and give credit to content creators. • Use only licensed or fair-use content for educational purposes.

Privacy and Confidentiality

- Ensure patient data is anonymized and complies with privacy regulations (e.g., HIPAA, GDPR).
- Avoid sharing content that violates patient confidentiality.

Transparency in Content Sharing

- Share videos with clear educational intent aligned with the curriculum.
- Evaluate content before recommending it to students.

Equity and Inclusivity

- Ensure diverse and culturally sensitive content that reflects a range of dental practices.
- Avoid marginalizing or stereotyping any group.

Respecting Student Autonomy

- Encourage students to use YouTube as a supplemental tool, not a replacement for formal education.
- Empower students to critically evaluate content for quality and reliability.

Significance: The integration of YouTube in dental and medical education can address many current challenges associated with traditional educational methods.

- Bridges theory and practice
- Re-playable video content
- Easy integration into busy schedules
- Real-life clinical demonstrations
- Exposure to multiple perspectives
- Engages students visually and audibly
- Promotes hands-on learning visualization
- Accessible on any device
- Supports clinical skill development
- Global content access
- Lack of content regulation
- Encourages interactive discussions
- Instant access to vast resources
- Helps review complex procedures
- Potential for misinformation.

For example, while lectures and textbooks offer foundational knowledge, they often fail to provide the real-life context or visual representation necessary to fully comprehend practical skills [7]. YouTube fills this gap by offering learners a more interactive and engaging way to absorb information. One of the most significant benefits of using YouTube in medical and dental education is its accessibility [7]. Students can access videos from anywhere, at any time, making it easier for them to fit learning into their busy schedules. This flexibility is especially important in clinical education, where students must balance classroom learning with hands-on practice [7]. YouTube also enables students to explore a variety of techniques and approaches from different practitioners around the world, giving them exposure to a diversity of perspectives they might not encounter in their local educational environment. In addition to accessibility, YouTube fosters a sense of community and collaboration among learners [7]. However, despite these advantages, there are significant concerns about the quality and reliability of the content available on YouTube [8]. Dental professionals need to develop critical skills to assess online content, ensuring they rely on accurate and up-to-date information in their learning [8].

Scope:

Educational Potential:

- Complements traditional learning methods
- Bridges gap between theory and practical application
- Visual learning crucial for mastering dental techniques
- Real-time demonstrations of procedures enhance engagement
- Multimedia learning combines visual and verbal elements
- Helps develop cognitive understanding and manual dexterity
- Demonstrates intricate procedures (e.g., dental fillings, root canals)
- Personalization of learning based on individual needs
- Supports self-directed learning for skill enhancement.

The educational potential of YouTube lies in its ability to complement traditional learning methods and bridge the gap between theoretical knowledge and practical application. For dental students, visual learning is especially important, as much of their education revolves around mastering specific techniques and procedures.

In fields like dentistry, where students must develop both cognitive understanding and manual dexterity, video tutorials can be especially helpful in demonstrating the intricate details of procedures such as dental fillings, root canals, and surgeries.

Students can choose videos that align with their specific learning needs, selecting content based on their knowledge gaps or areas of interest. This self-directed learning is becoming increasingly important in modern education, as students seek to take control of their learning journeys and engage with material in a way that suits their personal learning style [8].

Challenges and Limitations:

- Lack of quality control on uploaded videos
- No guarantee of accuracy or up-to-date information
- Risk of incorrect techniques affecting clinical practice
- Search algorithms prioritize popularity over accuracy
- Difficulty differentiating between high- and low-quality content
- Absence of peer-reviewed content on YouTube
- No formal review process to ensure educational value.

Despite its potential, YouTube as an educational resource is not without its challenges. One of the primary concerns is the lack of quality control. This is particularly problematic in medical and dental education, where incorrect information can have serious consequences8. Students may unknowingly rely on videos that present outdated or incorrect techniques, leading to misunderstandings that could affect their clinical practice. Students, especially those who are not yet familiar with advanced topics, may struggle to differentiate between high- and low-quality content.

However, YouTube lacks such a system for educational videos. While some institutions or professionals may upload high-quality content, the absence of a formal review process means that there is no standard by which to measure the educational value of the videos available8.

Role of Peer Review and Quality Control: To maximize the educational value of YouTube in dental education, there needs to be a more structured approach to content review and quality control. One potential solution is the development of a peer-review system for educational videos, like the process used in academic publishing9. Such a system could involve dental professionals reviewing and rating videos based on their accuracy, relevance, and educational value. Another approach could involve collaboration between dental schools and YouTube to create specialized channels or playlists featuring curated content10.

5 CONCLUSION

- YouTube has educational potential
- Lacks quality control
- Students use without guidance
- Content reliability concerns
- Faculty should curate and recommend
- Faculty can create tutorials
- Bridge gap between student use and school endorsement
- Implement video review systems
- Encourage faculty content production
- Research student video search habits
- Focus on content evaluation skills
- Educators need to support better use
- Collaboration between students, educators, institutions
- Enhance YouTube as an effective tool
- Equip students with necessary skills and knowledge

YouTube has the potential to be a valuable educational tool in dental education, but its effectiveness is currently limited by a lack of quality control and faculty involvement. While many dental students use the platform to supplement their learning, they often do so without guidance, leading to concerns about the reliability of the content they find. Faculty members, with their expertise, could play a crucial role in curating content, recommending high-quality videos, and even producing their own tutorials. By doing so, they can help bridge the gap between student use and institutional endorsement of YouTube as a legitimate educational resource. To fully harness the potential of YouTube, dental schools should consider implementing a standardized review system for educational videos, as well as encouraging faculty to take an active role in producing and recommending content. Additionally, future research should focus on understanding how students search for educational videos, how they evaluate the quality of content, and how educators can better support their learning through platforms like YouTube.

By working together, educators, students, and institutions can make YouTube a more effective and reliable tool for dental education, ensuring that future professionals are equipped with the skills and knowledge they need to succeed in their clinical practice.

REFERENCES

[1] Scott J. (1993). Publishing in dental education: a history and systematic analysis. *Eur J Dent Educ* 3(Suppl 1):31–8

[2] Kavadella A, Tsiklakis K, Vougiouklakis G, Lionarakis A. (2012). Evaluation of a blended learning course for teaching oral radiology to undergraduate dental students. *Eur J Dent Educ.* 16(1) doi:10.1111/j.1600-0579.2011.00682.x

[3] R.E. Mayer, (2002). "Multimedia learning," ser. *Psychology of Learning and Motivation.* Academic Press, vol. 41, pp. 85–139.

[4] O'Neill PA. (2008). The role of e-learning in medical education. *Med Teach.* 30(6):555–73. doi:10.1080/01421590802108323

[5] Mayer RE. (2009). *Multimedia learning.* 2nd ed. Cambridge University Press.

[6] Jaffar AA. (2012). YouTube: An emerging tool in anatomy education. *Anat Sci Educ.* 5(3):158–64. doi:10.1002/ase.1268.

[7] Knösel M, Jung K, Bleckmann A. (2011). YouTube, dentistry, and dental education. *J Dent Educ.* 75(12):1558–68. doi:10.1002/j.0022-0337.2011.75.12.tb05139.x.

[8] O'Neill PA. (2008). The role of e-learning in medical education. *Med Teach.* 30(6):555–73. doi:10.1080/01421590802108323

[9] Berman, L.H., and Pomerantz, A. (2016). The impact of YouTube on dental education. *Journal of Dental Education*, 80(10), 1210–1216. doi:10.1002/j.0022 0337.2016.80.

[10] tb06256.x.Azer SA. (2012). Can YouTube help students in learning surface anatomy? *Surg Radiol Anat.* 34(5):465–8. doi:10.1007/s00276-012-0935-x.

[11] Drozd B, Couvillon E, Suarez A. (2018). Medical YouTube videos and methods of evaluation: Literature review. *JMIR Med Educ.* 4(1)doi:10.2196/mededu.8527.

 ISBN: 978-1-041-32674-8

Evolution of Dental Education: From Tradition to Innovation: A Qualitative Review

Ikusdeep Singh and Janina Loren D'Souza
Department of Conservative Dentistry and Endodontics, Manipal College of Dental Sciences Mangalore, Manipal Academy of Higher Education, Manipal, Karnataka, India

ABSTRACT: This paper explores the historical development and current trends in dental education, offering a forward-looking analysis of how these changes are expected to shape the future of the profession.Understanding the evolution and contemporary shifts in dental education is essential for fostering continuous improvement and innovation. This review provides crucial insights that can guide the development of effective educational practices, which will enable us to adapt to emerging trends, and prepare for future advancements. This knowledge is instrumental in advancing dental care and ensuring professional excellence. Innovative teaching methods can significantly impact various aspects of dental education, including curriculum development, educational effectiveness, policy and standards, workforce preparedness, lifelong learning, and equity. Addressing these areas enhances the overall quality and impact of dental education and practice.The transformation in dental education mirrors broader trends in technology, cost management, and instructional delivery. The shift toward decentralized, hybrid, and technology-enhanced educational models offers opportunities for increased efficiency and accessibility. Addressing challenges related to cost, technology integration, and educational structure will be crucial in shaping the future of dental education and practice.The future of dental education is expected to embrace individualized, competency-based, asynchronous, hybrid, and both face-to-face and virtual learning modalities. Virtual education will likely become predominant in didactic and preclinical components, offering flexibility and efficiency through asynchronous learning.

Keywords: Dental, dentists, education, future, evolution, oral health, trend

1 INTRODUCTION

The evolution of dental education has been remarkable since its inception. Over the past 150 years, the reliance on apprenticeships and self-taught skills has shifted toward a comprehensive system of formal lectures. Independent institutions have largely been replaced by university-affiliated dental schools, and postgraduate training in both general and specialized fields has become widely established. The advancement of dental education is fundamentally connected to its ability to increase the quality and efficiency of oral health services through teaching, research, and patient care. To effectively address the upcoming challenges in dental education, active collaboration and support from practitioners, researchers, and policymakers will be crucial.This paper primarily examines the evolution of dental education, covering the shift from apprenticeships to formal schools, changes in financial aspects such as tuition and student debt, and the impact of COVID-19 on curricula. It also explores the incorporation of innovative technologies such as VR(Virtual Reality), AR(Augmented Reality), and AI(Artificial Intelligence), while addressing current challenges and future opportunities for advancement in the field.

2 METHODOLOGY

A research was performed in the biomedical databases PubMed, Scopus and Science Direct for available literature via the following keywords " Dental AND Education", "Evolution AND trends". Duplicates were discarded via Mendly Desktop reference manager software (Elsevier, AMS,Asterweg, The Netherlands), the titles and abstracts were then manually reviewed and those articles that didn't meet the inclusion criteria were excluded. The remaining articles were subsequently read in full and those that dealt with the topic other than that of interest to this literature review were excluded.

The inclusion criteria of the articles were as follows :

- Keywords : Dental AND Education, Evolution AND trends
- Timeline : 1995 - 2024
- Articles on Evolution of dental education : its history, current trends, covid-19 impact , challenges and future.

 DOI: 10.1201/9781042016075-68

Exclusion criteria articles were excluded if they met the following criteria :

- Articles in languages other than English
- Articles that, after their title and abstract were read, did not fit with the subject of interest of this paper.

3 RESULTS

- History of Dental Education :
  - The origins of dental education trace back to an informal apprenticeship-based system in which skilled practitioners teach one another their craft. This practice evolved into a more organized, institutional framework with the establishment of the first dental school in Baltimore,USA in 1840. Today, university-affiliated nonprofit institutions have taken the place of private trade schools as the main providers of dental education.[1]
  - The official beginning of dental education in India occurred with the establishment of the nation's first dental college in Kolkata by Dr. Rafiuddin Ahmed in 1920. Following this, the first private dental school opened in 1966, while all previous institutions were government-run. Since then, the rise of private dental colleges has dramatically reshaped the educational landscape, leaving the government with only 14% of the institutions, while the majority are now privately owned.[2]
  - The elements of dental education have become more intricate. It was sufficient to have a patient, a teacher, a pupil, and a physical location at first. Over the last 183 years, there have been significant advancements in the curriculum and educational environments, including preclinical, classroom, and simulation settings. To increase the quality of the educational experience, institutions have integrated formal assessment methods, comprehensive regulatory frameworks, and diverse, highly qualified faculty.[1]
  - There have been notable changes in the costs associated with dental education, which have increased the burden of student debt. Historically, before becoming independent practitioners, students were required to undergo formal apprenticeships with established dentists for one to two years. In the mid-19th century, these apprenticeships averaged approximately $100. The first dental school was established in 1840, and shortly thereafter, tuition fees ranging from $100 - $200 became standard.[1]
  - From 1880 - 2020, average tuition at private dental schools for DDS(Doctor of Dental Surgery) in the U.S. increased by 555 times, outpacing inflation by 25 times. By 2023, the average debt for graduating dental students reached $280,700
  - BDS(Bachelor of Dental Surgery) fees in India vary by region and institution, typically ranging from INR 80,000 to 5 lakhs annually. Private colleges charge between INR 1.75 lakhs and 5.9 lakhs, whereas government universities offer lower fees, from INR 50,000 to 1.2 lakhs. MDS(Master of Dental Surgery) course fees generally fall between INR 5 and 15 lakhs.

- Profound consequences of COVID - 19 : Dental education was profoundly affected by the COVID - 19 pandemic at all levels ,from admission to graduation and licensure. After lockdown measures were enacted, dental schools had to rapidly evaluate their resources and explore various options to adapt their curricula effectively. Both educators and students faced the challenge of transitioning to new policies, which often involved fully online teaching. Many institutions have replaced traditional classroom instruction with online training via synchronous (live) and asynchronous (on-demand) methods. Consequently, faculty utilized various technology platforms that included teleconferencing and file-sharing capabilities to facilitate online lectures, conduct group discussions, and enhance student engagement.[1] [5]
- Future of Dental Education :
  - The shift in dental education is moving from a centralized model to one that is more decentralized and driven by technology. There is increasing recognition that certain courses can be taught asynchronously and online effectively, utilizing AI-powered feedback and simulators. While face to face interactions remain essential for clinical training, a rigid cohort system is no longer needed. Asynchronous learning and virtual education are expected to play a key role in didactic and preclinical instruction, whereas the clinical aspect will adopt a hybrid model combining virtual and in-person learning.[1][8]
  - The following technological innovations have been incorporated into the current curriculum and hold significant potential for the future :
    - The integration of virtual and augmented reality (VR/AR) into preclinical dental education marks represents transformative development in the field. A study in the Journal of Dental Education revealed that students using VR for tooth preparation demonstrated superior performance and greater confidence in clinical procedures. These technologies provide a controlled, highly realistic environment for practicing dental techniques, reducing risks associated with living patients while enhancing competence and the overall learning experience. Traditional training, where only a few students can observe a surgeon during procedures, limits learning opportunities. However, VR cameras now enable surgeons to stream operations globally, allowing students to virtually "step into"

the operating room using VR goggles, revolutionizing the way clinical skills are taught. In India, dental institutions have begun adopting VR and AR technologies, with their usage expected to grow rapidly.[1][8]

  - The integration of 3D printing technology in dental education is rapidly emerging as a significant trend. This innovative approach enables students to produce realistic models of teeth and gums for hands-on training and practice.Additionally, 3D printing facilitates the creation of customized orthodontic devices and dental implants tailored to each patient's unique requirements. By revolutionizing the way in which dental education is delivered, 3D printing is set to play an increasingly prominent role in the field in the years ahead.[1][8]
  - Another technology that has the potential to completely transform dental education is artificial intelligence (AI). According to an American Dental Association survey, 60% of dentists believe that artificial intelligence will play an essential role in the future of dentistry. AI systems are able to evaluate vast volumes of data and offer insightful analyses that can improve the decision-making of dentists. Artificial intelligence (AI) in dentistry education may be utilized to design individualised learning programs that meet the needs of each learner. Additionally, it may be utilised to build prediction models that can assist in identifying individuals who may be at risk of oral health issues. Although its use in dentistry education is still in its infancy, artificial intelligence has immense promise.[1][8]

- Challenges
  - Financial Barriers :
    - Dental education is costly, with universities facing substantial fixed expenses despite low enrollment.
    - High student debt influences graduates to prioritize high-paying private practices over public health roles, limiting access for low-income families (Nicholson et al., 2015). [6]
  - Loan - Driven Behaviors :
    - Debt repayment pressures may lead to rushed patient visits, negatively affecting care quality and the profession (Mercer, 2018). [6]
  - COVID-19 Impacts :
    - Transition to virtual learning posed challenges, especially for students with limited resources, caregiving responsibilities, or time zone conflicts.
    - Practical training struggled to replicate hands-on experiences due to supervision needs and costly simulation tools. [1][5]
  - Technology Integration :
    - Implementing advanced tools like VR/AR (Virtual/Augmented Reality), 3D printing, and AI (Artificial Intelligence) is expensive and resource-intensive.
    - Faculty training and adapting to new technologies add further complexity, particularly in resource-limited settings like India. [1][8]
  - Practical Training Challenges :
    - The shift to online platforms has yet to overcome barriers in hands-on and clinical training, crucial for skill development. [1][8]

4 DISCUSSION

Institutions should fund costly technologies in dental education through tuition, state appropriations, private donations, and university support. To overcome limited virtual tools, students can leverage existing resources, pursue collaborations, engage in self-directed learning, and participate in hands-on practice through volunteering and peer collaboration. Globally, dental education is shifting toward competency-based learning, technological integration, and harmonized standards, with Europe and Asia leading advancements and Africa addressing unique challenges through international collaboration. While implementing AI(Aritficial intelligence) and VR(Virtual reality) in dental education requires significant time and resources, students are generally supportive, though educators may express concerns about costs, training needs, and ethical considerations like data privacy and professional integrity.

5 CONCLUSION

Predicting the future is inherently uncertain, but several factors will likely shape dental education in the coming years. Dental education will be transformed by rising costs, technological advancements, and the growing demand for accessible and efficient care. In India, these factors, coupled with an increasing population, will drive the adoption of modern technologies and innovative teaching models, ensuring students receive high-quality education.

Hybrid education enhances clinical skills by blending online and offline methods. To maximize technology's potential for cost-efficiency and productivity, careful planning, equitable access, and thorough evaluation are critical.

REFERENCES

[1] Spielman AI. (2024). Dental education and practice: past, present, and future trends. *Frontiers in Oral Health.* 5:1368121

[2] Field MJ, editor. Dental education at the crossroads: challenges and change.

[3] Spielman, AI. (2023). Title of the chapter. In: *Illustrated Encyclopedia of the History of Dentistry*, https://historyofdentistryandmedicine.com/

[4] Jaiswal AK, Srinivas P, Suresh S. (2014). Dental manpower in India: changing trends since 1920. *International Dental Journal.* 64 (4):213–8

[5] Alkadi L. (2021). Dental education in the COVID-19 era: challenges, solutions and opportunities. *The Open Dentistry Journal.* 16;15(1)

[6] Nicholson S, Vujicic M, Wanchek T, Ziebert A, Menezes A. (2015). The effect of education debt on dentists' career decisions. *The Journal of the American Dental Association.* 146(11):800–7

[7] Koshki J, Spielman AI. (2022). The changing life of a dental student-A survey of 140 years.:(Winner of AAHD Student Research Awaed 2022). *Journal of the history of dentistry.*

[8] Thurzo A, Strunga M, Urban R, Surovková J, Afrashtehfar KI. (2023). Impact of artificial intelligence on dental education: A review and guide for curriculum update. *Education Sciences.* 13(2):150

Navigating Dental Education Trends and Transforming Dental Pedagogy – Abas and Srikant N (Eds)
 ISBN: 978-1-041-32674-8

Curriculum Boost for Future Directions to Improve the Scope of Dental Specialty Courses

Saumya Verhwani, Kundabala Mala, and Karthik Shetty
Department of Conservative Dentistry and Endodontics, Manipal College of Dental Sciences, Mangalore, Manipal Academy of Higher Education (MAHE), Manipal, Karnataka

ABSTRACT: Dental education inculcates awareness and imparts practical skills among the budding dental professionals. It caters to produce dental surgeons who are competent enough to address the diverse concerns of the patients. In India, the basis of MDS (Master of Dental Surgery) is patient centered learning; although there are several soft skills that can be included in the curriculum to enhance the education system. Hence, the purpose of this poster is to emphasize the areas where the dental education is lacking. The curriculum barely highlights the handling of patients with physical disabilities and the management of medical emergencies in dental practice, when encountered in a clinic setup during and after dental treatment. The ideas about how to setup a multidisciplinary dental clinic, how to select a location for the setup, marketing of the dental practice and health tourism; that may help a dental setup to grow and flourish; are not discussed in the entire duration of the course. The course also lacks the applied knowledge on digital dentistry, dental ethics and legal intricacies, finance management and technical handling of dental chairs; that are essential for the smooth running of a dental clinic.

Since dental profession has been taking a downward trend in India in comparison to other countries; it is essential for Dental Council of India and dental institutes to include the vistas and skills based on these challenges in the dental curriculum. This would create awareness and improvement of professionalism of the dental specialist.

Keywords: Dental curriculum, multidisciplinary dental clinic, health tourism, dental chairs, Dental Council of India

1 INTRODUCTION

In India, the basis of MDS (Master of Dental Surgery) is patient centered learning; although there are several soft skills that can be included in the curriculum to enhance the education system. A probable solution would be to upgrade the dental education in all perspectives. This gap can be attributed to various factors, such as outdated curriculum, inadequate exposure to clinical practice, and a lack of emphasis on research and critical thinking skills. There are lack of courses on advanced technologies such as digital dentistry, communication skills and training on ethical and legal issues are also inadequate.

2 METHODS

2.1 *Study design and setting*

The present study utilized a cross-sectional observational design and adhered to the STROBE reporting guidelines. Ethical clearance was taken and questionnaire was developed through a six-stage process. Initially, a conceptual framework was developed by drawing on existing literature and expert insights. Subsequently, an item pool was generated, consisting of 20 items for the awareness construct and 22 items for the perception construct. In the third stage, a focus group discussion was conducted with subject experts, followed by cognitive interviews with five representative samples. Throughout these stages, items were subject to continuous evaluation, leading to the addition and removal of specific items based on their relevance.

2.2 *Validity and reliability assessments*

Face validity was assessed by determining the percentage agreement among a panel of five subject experts and it was found to be 84%. Additionally, content validity ratio was determined for the question- naire, and the results indicated that it was a valid tool, with a content validity ratio of 0.78. This was followed by assessment of reliability using Cronbach's alpha coefficient, which was estimated to be 0.85. This indicates that the questionnaire has high internal consistency. Collec- tively, these assessments indicate that the questionnaire is robust and suitable for capturing the intended data in the study.

DOI: 10.1201/9781042016075-69

2.3 *Sample size estimation and sample distribution*

The sample size for the study was estimated based on the findings of the pilot study. The pilot study found that 76.69% of female and 58.85% of male participants had low awareness. The allocation ratio for females to males was 3:1. These proportions were used to calculate the required sample size. Considering Type-I (α) error of 0.05 and Power (1-β) of 0.95, a minimum sample size of 460 participants was determined for the study using G*Power statistical software (Ver. 3.1.9.4.). The final sample size was set as 480 and the list of undergraduate students from two dental colleges in Belagavi was obtained, and it was used as the sampling frame. The participants were selected from this list using a simple random sampling technique by random number table method.

2.4 *Questionnaire characteristics*

The questionnaire used for the study was self-administered and comprised of 23 close-ended questions in English.

2.5 *Data collection*

A single investigator administered the physical questionnaire during working hours at the two dental colleges. The questionnaire was distributed year-wise in a classroom setting on a specified date and time. To ensure unbiased completion in the classroom, volunteers closely supervised the process. Participants were instructed to complete all questions within 15 min.

2.6 *Statistical analysis*

Collected data were entered in Microsoft Excel 2019 and analysed using IBM-SPSS® Statistics-Version 21 (IBM Corp., Armonk, NY, USA). Descriptive statistics were computed, which included percentages, means and standard deviations. The normality of the data distribution was determined using the Kolmogorov–Smirnov test and it was found that the data was normally distributed. Chi-square test was used to check for the association between awareness and perception with the year of study. Analysis Of Variance (ANOVA) test were performed to check for any significant differences among the study groups. Pearson correlation coefficient was used between awareness and perception scores. For all the tests, confidence level and level of significance were set at 95% and 5%, respectively.

3 CONCLUSION

The findings of the study reveal that a significant proportion of dental undergraduate students lacked awareness in the BDS curriculum by DCI.

ACKNOWLEDGMENTS

Reference from article

REFERENCE

Kabra L, Santhosh VN, Sequeira RN, Ankola AV, Coutinho D. (2023), Dental curriculum reform in India: Undergraduate students' awareness and perception on the newly proposed choice based credit system. *J Oral Biol Craniofac Res.* 13(5):630–635. doi: 10.1016/j.jobcr.2023.08.003. Epub 2023 Aug 11. PMID: 37637854; PMCID: PMC10448454 ;was taken.

Navigating Dental Education Trends and Transforming Dental Pedagogy – Abas and Srikant N (Eds)
© 2027 The Author(s), ISBN: 978-1-041-32674-8

Effectiveness of Flipped Classrooms (FCR) in Dental Education: A Literature Review

Krishnapriya and Shivangi Vats
Department of Conservative Dentistry and Endodontics, Manipal College of Dental Sciences Mangalore, Manipal Academy of Higher Education, Manipal, India

1 INTRODUCTION

In traditional classrooms, teachers typically spend most of their time lecturing, with students passively absorbing information. However, educational models are evolving, and one innovative approach gaining traction is the flipped classroom. A flipped classroom (FCR) is a teaching approach that reverses the typical learning model by having students view lectures at home before using class time for interactive activities. Specialized disciplines such as dentistry and innovative teaching methods such as FCR are being adopted to enhance student learning.

This classroom teaching technique aims to prioritize student learning and encourage higher-level learning outcomes on Bloom's taxonomy. Students also placed high value on discussion-based activities in small groups, which enhanced their motivation to learn and boosted their level of engagement and interest in the content being learned. Research has been carried out to understand students' perspectives on flipped classrooms as learning aids and has shown improvements in subject comprehension and retention.1 These innovative methods improve learners' self-confidence, communication skills, creativity, critical thinking, problem-solving, and collaborative learning. Implementing a student-centered, effective teaching strategy is essential for achieving learner engagement in professional courses.2,3 This review aims to understand and summarize the various techniques comprising flipped classrooms for dental undergraduate and postgraduate clinical upskilling.

2 METHODOLOGY

Inclusion and exclusion criteria: All clinical studies, trials and reviews determining the use of flipped classrooms or FCRs in teaching dentistry or dental clinical concepts and topics were included. Studies involving the use of FCR exercises in medical fields other than dentistry were excluded.

The electronic search strategy was developed in Scopus, PubMed, Google Scholar and other databases. The data were synthesized via descriptive statistics. The results were analyzed and discussed.

3 RESULTS

The identified articles were analyzed based on learning resources, students' perspectives, in-class activities, pre-class activities, and the flipped classroom's efficacy in terms of achieving academic success. Abeysekera *et al.* defined FCR as a set of pedagogical approaches that transmit information from classrooms to outside while using class time for social interactive learning activities, thus reducing the cognitive load on the student.3

Table 1. Summary of the identified articles describing the type of study, type of FCR activity and its effects.

Sno.	Authors	Type of Study	Flipped classroom Activity	Effect
1	Park and Howell *et al* [7]	Observational study with intervention	Learning management system, Quiz, Questionnaire	Increased student participation
2	Shapiro *et al* [8]	Observational study with intervention	Online training module	Increase in engagement but cannot replace traditional learning methods.
3	Gallardo *et al* [9]	Questionnaire Survey	Free access to clinical self-explanatory videos	More satisfactory pediatric dentistry learning
4	Quoß M *et al* [10]	Observational study	Inverted Classrooms Peer-assisted teaching and learning	improves students' learning interests and attitudes.
5	Wong G *et al* [11]	Observational study	Instructional videos with background music	Effective in teaching psychomotor skills to dental students

DOI: 10.1201/9781042016075-70

4 DISCUSSION

FCR is a pedagogical approach that employs information and communication technology to replace traditional face-to-face classroom structures. Students essentially engage in activities traditionally termed "homework" in class. Learning management systems (LMS) like Schoology, Moodle, and Blackboard have been employed as platforms for implementing the FC model. LMS grants simple access to content in either downloadable or streaming format, or it could be customized to include a variety of interactive components such as drawing functions and tips, drop-down menus, and drag and drop. [4,5]

Shapiro *et al.* used FCs to assess learners' knowledge in recognizing and reporting cases of neglect and abuse in dentistry. They reported that students enjoy online learning, but it can never substitute for a human teacher. [5]

Students prepared for class by actively participating in discussions and voicing doubts. This strategy is widely used by both trainees and instructors, as evidenced by a growing corpus of literature. Day's study indicated that using the FCR technique in anatomy led to enhanced performance and long-term retention of critical thinking abilities. [9] Students prefer flipped classes, and quizzes, over regular classes, which is an effective teaching method that increases student motivation and engagement. [10,11] Missing classes and attending classes only for the sake of attendance are becoming less important. Gopinath *et al.* assessed the effectiveness of teaching methods in dentistry and reported that video-based education promotes performance in preclinical procedures. Online education is believed to be better retained by students, as mentioned by Varvara *et al.* [13] The drawbacks of flipped classrooms comprise potential challenges in ensuring that all students engage with the material at home, which can lead to gaps in understanding during in-class activities. Additionally, some students may struggle with the self-directed learning aspect, requiring more guidance and support from instructors. [14]

Furthermore, the effectiveness of flipped classrooms can be hindered by varying access to technology, as not all students have reliable internet or devices to participate in online learning. This disparity can exacerbate existing inequalities in education, making it essential for educators to consider these factors when implementing this teaching model. [14]

Preparing interesting video lectures and in-class activities may be difficult for professors who are new to the concept. If a student fails to consistently participate in pre-class activities, they may struggle with classwork. Parents may not understand or agree with the flipped classroom concept, particularly if they see it as a transfer in teaching responsibilities to kids. Traditional assessments may not represent the greater knowledge and engagement it seeks to promote. Students may get overwhelmed and disinterested if the pre-class information is excessively deep or long. Both instructors and students may oppose the flipped paradigm owing to its unfamiliarity or the increased upfront effort required. [14]

5 CONCLUSION

The concept of Flipped Classrooms (FCR) includes a variety of newer modes of learning that include interactive peer sessions moderated by classroom teachers, role reversal, quizzes, course videos, group discussions and peer teaching. Compared with traditional lecture methods, dental clinical upskilling is carried out with FCR more effectively. However, more intervention-based studies with new interactive ideas are needed to clearly define the extent of the flipped class and the activities that can be called as part of FCRs for a better understanding and implementation of this teaching methodology in dental schools worldwide.

CONFLICT OF INTEREST

No conflicts of interest.

FINANCIAL DISCLOSURES

Nil

ACKNOWLEDGMENTS

Nil

REFERENCES

[1] Hew KF, Lo CK. (2018). Flipped classroom improves student learning in health professions education: A metaanalysis. *BMC Med Educ.* 18(1):38. DOI: 10.1186/s12909-018-1144-z PMID: 29544495.

[2] Chen F, Lui AM, Martinelli SM. (2017). A systematic review of the effectiveness of flipped classrooms in medical education. *Med Educ.* 1(6):585–97. DOI:10.1111/medu13272 PMID: 28488303.

[3] Gopinath V, Nallaswamy D. A systematic review on the most effective method for teaching dentistry

[4] Shrestha S, Vikram M, Agrawal N, Ayer A, Shrestha A. (2023). A comparative study of students' performance in flipped classroom and structured interactive session teaching-learning method in Conservative Dentistry and Endodontics. *JGMC Nepal.*16(1): 13–8. DOI: 10.3126/jgmcn.v16i1.51764

[5] Varughese A, M R, S D, *et al.* (2024) Effectiveness of different teaching methods in enhancing dental undergraduate students' knowledge and restorative cement manipulation skills. *Cureus* 16(8): e67999. DOI 10.7759/cureus.67999

[6] Abeysekera L, Dawson P. (2015). Motivation and cognitive load in the flipped classroom: definition, rationale and a call for research. *High Educ Res Dev.* 34(1):1–14.

[7] Park SE, Howell TH. (2015). Implementation of a FC educational model in a predoctoral dental course. *J Dent Educ.* 79(5):563–570.

[8] Shapiro MC, Anderson OR, Lal S. (2014). Assessment of a novel module for training dental students in child abuse recognition and reporting. *J Dent Educ.* 78(8):1167–1175.

[9] Gallardo NE, Caleya AM, Sánchez ME, Feijóo G. (2022). Learning of pediatric dentistry with the flipped classroom model. *Eur J Dent Educ.* 26:302–309. https://doi.org/10.1111/eje.12704

[10] Quoß M, Rüttermann S, Gerhardt-Szep S. (2017). Cross-year peer-assisted learning using the inverted ("flipped") classroom design: a pilot study in dentistry. *Z Evid Fortbild Qual Gesundhwes.* 126:84–93.

[11] Wong G, Apthorpe H, Ruiz K, Nanayakkara S. (2019). An innovative educational approach in using instructional videos to teach dental local anesthetic skills. *Eur J Dent Educ.* 23:28–34.

[12] Day LJ. (2018). A gross anatomy flipped classroom affects performance, retention, and higher-level thinking in lower performing students. *Anat Sci Educ.* 11(6):565–74. DOI: 10.1002/ase.1772 PMID: 29356452

[13] Varvara G, Bernardi S, Bianchi S, Sinjari B, Piattelli M. (2021). Dental education challenges during the COVID 19 pandemic period in Italy: undergraduate student feedback, future perspectives, and the needs of teaching strategies for professional development. *Healthcare (Basel).* 9:454. 10.3390/healthcare9040454

[14] Kraml, Mario. (2024). Advantages and disadvantages of a flipped classroom in adult education using distance learning for learning programming. *EPH-International Journal of Educational Research.*8. 2631. 10.53555/ephijer.v8i1.109.

Navigating Dental Education Trends and Transforming Dental Pedagogy – Abas and Srikant N (Eds)
© 2027 The Author(s), ISBN: 978-1-041-32674-8

Virtual Touch: Enhancing Dental Skills Through Haptic Simulation

N.R Sahitha, Karthik Shetty, and Puttur Laxmish Mallya
Department of Conservative Dentistry and Endodontics, Manipal College of Dental Sciences, Mangalore, Affiliated to Manipal Academy of Higher Education, Manipal

1 INTRODUCTION

Haptic simulation technology has significantly transformed various fields, including healthcare and medical education. Dentistry, a discipline where tactile sensitivity plays a critical role, has greatly benefited from advancements in haptic technologies. Traditionally, dental education has relied heavily on manual skill development using physical models, phantom heads, or live patients. However, as the technology evolves, haptic simulation has gained recognition as an important tool to complement traditional methods in dental training. This review explores the integration of haptic simulation into dentistry and its incorporation into dental curricula, assessing its benefits, challenges, and future prospects.

2 OVERVIEW OF HAPTIC SIMULATION

Haptic simulation refers to the use of technology to create a tactile experience for users in virtual environments. In a medical context, haptics can recreate the sense of touch, force, and texture, providing a more immersive and realistic learning experience. These technologies typically involve force-feedback devices that simulate the physical sensations one would encounter when interacting with real objects. In dentistry, this may include the feel of dental instruments, the hardness of teeth, or the resistance of oral tissues.

In recent years, haptic simulators, such as those developed by companies like Moog Simodont and Virteasy, have been applied to various aspects of dental education, including cavity preparation, endodontics, and other clinical procedures. These tools provide an alternative to traditional methods, enabling students to practice their skills in a risk-free, controlled environment

3 HAPTIC SIMULATION IN DENTAL EDUCATION

3.1 *Enhancing clinical skills training*

Clinical skill development is a critical component of dental education, requiring students to become proficient in fine motor control and tactile feedback. Haptic simulators offer a unique opportunity to simulate clinical scenarios that mirror real-life dental procedures, allowing students to practice these skills before working on actual patients. Simulators can recreate the sensation of drilling teeth, performing root canals, or applying pressure to soft tissues, offering immediate feedback to help students correct mistakes.

A study conducted by Buchanan (2001) emphasized the advantages of virtual reality (VR) and haptic technology in developing psychomotor skills. Buchanan demonstrated that students trained on haptic simulators could perform dental tasks with greater precision compared to those trained solely on traditional methods. Similarly, Laughton *et al.* (2013) reported that students who used haptic feedback devices showed improved accuracy and confidence in their clinical work.

The simulation environment allows for repetitive practice, helping students to refine their skills in areas such as cavity preparation, where accuracy is essential. Unlike real patients or physical models, haptic simulators can be reset easily, and students can repeat tasks as many times as necessary. This ensures that students are well-prepared before performing these procedures in real clinical settings.

3.2 *Reducing risk in clinical training*

A key benefit of haptic simulation is its potential to reduce risk during clinical training. Dental students typically begin practicing on live patients during their final years of study, which can involve some degree of risk, especially if students are not yet confident in their skills. Haptic simulators offer a safe and controlled environment for students to practice procedures without the risk of causing harm to patients.

DOI: 10.1201/9781042016075-71

For instance, in procedures like tooth extractions or cavity preparations, minor errors in force or pressure can result in patient discomfort or damage to tissues. Haptic simulators can train students in the correct application of pressure, the feel of dental tissues, and how to avoid unnecessary damage, thereby minimizing the risk of adverse outcomes when working on real patients.

Additionally, haptic simulation allows instructors to introduce students to more complex cases earlier in their training, which may not be feasible in a clinical setting. These cases might involve rare conditions or complicated procedures that students may not encounter during their limited clinical rotations. Simulating these cases provides a broader scope of experience, ensuring that students are well-prepared for a wider range of clinical situations.

3.3 *Objective evaluation and feedback*

One of the challenges in traditional dental education is the subjective nature of assessment. Instructors rely on visual inspection or patient feedback to evaluate a student's performance, which can sometimes lead to inconsistencies in grading. Haptic simulation offers a solution to this problem by providing objective, quantifiable data on student performance.

Simulators can track a range of metrics, including force applied, angle of entry, and duration of procedures. This data can then be analyzed to provide detailed feedback, allowing students to understand exactly where they made mistakes and how to improve. The objective nature of the feedback also ensures that all students are evaluated based on the same criteria, leading to fairer and more consistent assessments.

Moreover, the instant feedback provided by haptic simulators enables students to learn more efficiently. Instead of waiting for an instructor to assess their work, students can immediately correct their mistakes and continue practicing. This immediate feedback loop enhances the learning experience and helps students to develop their skills more quickly.

4 HAPTIC SIMULATION SYSTEMS IN DENTISTRY

4.1 *Simodont dental trainer*

The Simodont Dental Trainer, developed by Moog Inc., is widely used for dental education. It offers high-precision haptic feedback and simulates various procedures such as cavity preparation, crown placement, and tooth extraction.

Advantages:

- High realism with detailed 3D visuals and tactile sensations.
- Covers a wide range of procedures, from basic to complex.
- Immediate feedback on errors like excessive force or incorrect angulation.
- Can be accessed remotely, allowing flexible learning.

Disadvantages:

- High cost limits accessibility for some institutions.
- Some students find it challenging to transition from virtual simulation to real patients.

4.2 *Virteasy dental simulator*

The Virteasy Dental Simulator offers a user-friendly interface and detailed analytics, making it a popular choice in dental schools.

Advantages:

- Modular system allows for customizability based on educational needs.
- Detailed performance metrics provide objective assessment.
- Cost-effective options compared to other high-end systems.

Disadvantages:

- Less precise haptic feedback compared to Simodont.
- Limited complexity in advanced scenarios.

4.3 *HapTEL (Haptic Technology Enhanced Learning)*

The HapTEL system was developed by King's College London to enhance tactile learning in dental education.

Advantages:

- Strong focus on educational integration, aligning well with traditional curricula.

- Based on pedagogical research, ensuring relevance to dental education.
- More affordable compared to other high-end simulators.

Disadvantages:

- Limited to undergraduate training; lacks depth for postgraduate use.
- Lower haptic fidelity compared to systems like Simodont.

4.4 *DenX Dental Simulator (DentSim)*

The DenX Dental Simulator, also known as DentSim, combines augmented reality (AR) and haptic feedback.

Advantages:

- AR integration allows real instruments to be used with digital feedback.
- Real-time guidance during procedures aids in developing skills.
- More seamless transition from virtual training to patient care.

Disadvantages:

- High cost, particularly for institutions with limited budgets.
- Less sophisticated haptic feedback compared to systems like Simodont.

4.5 *PerioSim*

PerioSim is designed specifically for periodontal training, focusing on tasks like scaling and root planing.

Advantages:

- Highly specialized, making it ideal for periodontal training.
- Interactive feedback helps refine techniques in real time.

Disadvantages:

- Narrow scope limits its use outside of periodontal procedures.
- High cost for a system that covers only a specialized area.

5 CHALLENGES AND LIMITATIONS

Despite the clear advantages of haptic simulation, there are several challenges and limitations to its implementation in dental education.

(1) **Cost:** One of the main barriers to the widespread adoption of haptic simulators is the cost of the equipment. High-end simulators can be expensive to purchase and maintain, making them inaccessible to some dental schools, particularly in developing countries. The financial investment required may deter some institutions from incorporating haptic simulation into their curricula.

(2) **Technology Limitations:** While haptic simulators have advanced significantly in recent years, there are still limitations to the technology. For example, simulating the complexity of soft tissues or replicating the full range of tactile sensations encountered in real-life dental procedures remains a challenge. Current simulators may not fully capture the subtle differences between various types of tissues or the dynamic changes that occur during actual procedures.

(3) **Learning Curve:** Another challenge is the learning curve associated with using haptic devices. Both students and instructors need to become familiar with the technology, which may take time and effort. Some students may initially find it difficult to translate the skills learned on simulators to real-life clinical situations, as the feel of virtual procedures can differ slightly from actual patient interactions.

(4) **Resistance to Change:** The traditional model of dental education has been in place for many years, and some educators may be resistant to adopting new technologies. There is often a reluctance to shift away from tried-and-tested methods, particularly when the long-term benefits of haptic simulation are still being studied. Additionally, integrating haptic simulation into an already packed curriculum may pose logistical challenges.

6 INTEGRATION INTO THE DENTAL CURRICULUM

To fully realize the benefits of haptic simulation, these technologies must be seamlessly integrated into the dental curriculum. This integration involves not only the inclusion of simulation-based learning but also a rethinking of how clinical skills are taught and assessed.

(1) **Preclinical Training:** One of the most effective ways to integrate haptic simulation is in preclinical training, where students are first introduced to clinical procedures. Simulators can be used to teach basic skills such as drilling, cavity preparation, and crown placement. By practicing these skills in a virtual environment, students can develop confidence and proficiency before working on actual patients.
(2) **Blended Learning:** A hybrid approach that combines traditional methods with simulation-based learning is likely to be the most effective. For example, students might use haptic simulators to practice procedures before performing them on physical models or patients. This blended approach allows students to benefit from the strengths of both traditional and simulation-based training.
(3) **Assessment and Competency Testing**: Incorporating haptic simulation into the assessment process can help to standardize competency testing. Simulators can be used to evaluate a student's technical abilities, providing objective data that can be used for grading. This approach can complement traditional assessment methods, offering a more comprehensive evaluation of a student's clinical skills.
(4) **Continuous Development:** As haptic technology continues to evolve, it is essential for dental curricula to remain flexible and adaptable. Regular updates to the curriculum may be necessary to incorporate new technologies and teaching methods. Additionally, ongoing research into the effectiveness of haptic simulation will help to refine its role in dental education.

7 FUTURE PROSPECTS AND RESEARCH DIRECTIONS

The future of haptic simulation in dentistry is promising, with ongoing research and development aimed at addressing the current limitations of the technology. Advances in artificial intelligence, machine learning, and augmented reality could further enhance the capabilities of haptic simulators, making them even more realistic and effective as training tools.

Moreover, as the cost of haptic technology decreases, it is likely that more dental schools will adopt these tools, leading to more widespread use in dental education. Future research should focus on long-term studies to evaluate the impact of haptic simulation on clinical outcomes, as well as the development of more sophisticated simulators that can replicate the full range of tactile sensations encountered in real-life procedures.

8 CONCLUSION

Haptic simulation represents a significant advancement in dental education, offering numerous benefits in terms of skill development, risk reduction, and objective evaluation. Despite challenges such as cost and technology limitations, the integration of haptic simulation into the dental curriculum has the potential to improve the quality of dental training and prepare students for the complexities of clinical practice. As technology continues to evolve, haptic simulation will likely become an increasingly important tool in dental education, helping to shape the next generation of skilled and competent dental professionals.

REFERENCES

Boudokhane S, Collange O, Coronas L, Manderscheid JC, Jacquot B. (2018). Virteasy dental haptic simulator: Evaluation of student learning in oral surgery. *Eur J Dent Educ.* 22(3):e461–5.

Buchanan, J.A. (2001). Use of simulation technology in dental education. *Journal of Dental Education*, 65(11), 1225–1227.

DenX Group. (2024). *DentSim Dental Simulator*. Available from: https://www.dentsim.com/. Accessed August 18.

King's College London. (2024). HapTEL: Haptic technology enhanced learning. Available from: https://www.kcl.ac.uk/haptel. Accessed August 18, 2024.

Laughton, B.D., Vu, H.V., and Goldstein, R.E. (2013). Haptic simulation for competency assessment of crown preparations. *Journal of Prosthetic Dentistry*, 109(6), 361–365.

Lieng MK, Pearson GT. (2010). PerioSim haptic virtual reality periodontal training simulator. *J Dent Educ.* 74(1):126–33.

Lim, K.C., and Neo, B.Y. (2015). Integration of haptic simulators in preclinical dental education: A systematic review. *European Journal of Dental Education*, 19(4), 229–237.

Moog Inc. (2024). *Simodont Dental Trainer*. Available from: https://www.moog.com/products/medical-simulation/simodont-dental-trainer.html. Accessed August 18, 2024.

Suebnukarn S, Haddawy P. (2009). Intelligent dental training simulator with objective skill assessment and feedback. *Artif Intell Med.* 38 (1):25–37.

Navigating Dental Education Trends and Transforming Dental Pedagogy – Abas and Srikant N (Eds)
 ISBN: 978-1-041-32674-8

Guidance in Research and Student Partnership (GRASP): A Novel Training Module for Undergraduate Research

Joanna Baptist
Department of Oral and Maxillofacial Surgery, Manipal College of Dental Sciences Mangalore, Manipal Academy of Higher Education, Manipal, India

Aastha Todi
Consultant Periodontist, Kolkata, India

Swati Pralhad
Department of Periodontology, Manipal College of Dental Sciences Mangalore, Manipal Academy of Higher Education, Manipal, India

Ravikiran Ongole
Department of Oral Medicine and Radiology, Manipal College of Dental Sciences Mangalore, Manipal Academy of Higher Education, Manipal, India

Animesh Jain
Department of Community Medicine, Kasturba Medical College Mangalore, Manipal Academy of Higher Education, Manipal, India

Viral Dave
Department of Orthodontics and Dentofacial Orthopaedics, D Y Patil University School of Dentistry, Navi Mumbai, India

Dilip Naik
Mangalore Campus, Manipal Academy of Higher Education Manipal, India

ABSTRACT: **Objective:** The quality of undergraduate research is enhanced when conducted by a heterogeneous group. Guidance in Student and Research Partnership (GRASP) was one such innovative interdisciplinary research training module that comprised of two faculty from different healthcare disciplines and two students with different levels of academic training (an intern with a third-year student).

Methodology: This program comprised of ten heterogeneous research groups, which was held over a period of seven months. Various topics on steps to research were verbally explained with audiovisual aids. Thorough hands-on training was given to all the participants at every step, to enable them to confidently execute the steps independently on their research studies. Following the training, in each phase, the participants were instructed to implement the same in their research projects.

Results: Data revealed that most of the students were novice in the field of research, as around 85% of students never undertook research before. They were unaware of the various study designs or about the basic research databases like PUBMED or SCOPUS. Also, students were unaware of the format of Manuscript writing. However, with training, all participants satisfactorily completed their research project and 50% of them were able to publish in SCOPUS indexed journals.

Conclusion: Therefore, it is evident that a structured training module in interdisciplinary research leads to good quality research outcomes in short duration. Experiential learning opportunities like these can help students develop research related skills early, and thus, should be formulated and incorporated as a part of the undergraduate curriculum.

Keywords: curriculum, dental undergraduate, research, training module

1 OBJECTIVE

Research is a learning procedure that includes seeking information by a process of building up actualities, pondering about thoughts and proposing hypothesis. An initiative in the field of research at an undergraduate level is a milestone to the idea of learning and thinking out of the box. Stepping into a new stream in dental school, students are enthusiastic with novel ideas, however, the dental and medical education programs and curriculum in India does not give enough emphasis to hands-on learning and critical thinking in terms of research. Improving research

DOI: 10.1201/9781042016075-72

capacity among undergraduates and reflective learning is one of the rising concerns among the health education policy makers. The 4 'I's i.e. Initiative, Impulse, Incentive and Idols have been highlighted as the biggest challenge to research training among undergraduates. [1]

There is a need to provide guidance to students who wish to develop skills in research and foster attributes among dental undergraduates that help develop research. [2] A lot of studies have shown that clinicians are required to pick between performing research and honing in practice, and are finding it progressively hard to incorporate both in their vocations. Research ability is a core competency to achieve in health professionals and it needs to be improved. [3,4] Early introduction of undergraduate dental students to viable research exercises and publication knowledge has evidenced better attitudes towards it. [5]

The quality of undergraduate research is enhanced when conducted by a heterogeneous group.

Guidance in Student and Research Partnership (GRASP) was one such innovative sevenmonth long interdisciplinary research training module that comprised of 10 teams; each with two faculty from different healthcare disciplines and two students with different levels of academic training of Bachelor of Dental Surgery (BDS) undergraduate curriculum (an intern with a third-year student).

This program is recommended to be incorporated in the dental curriculum so that the importance of research is highlighted in the minds of the students and to nurture the research acumen among the young budding researchers.

2 METHODOLOGY

This program was formulated in the form of a short-term training module for a period of seven months. An announcement with the details of the program was made in the dental college where the rules of the modules where clearly listed. As per the circular, twenty students expressed interest and enrolled for the program.

As a part of this module, 10 teams each comprising of a BDS intern was partnered with a third year BDS student who were guided by a faculty from dental college and another faculty from the medical college for carrying out interdisciplinary research. This program also catered to a student centric and student-based research solely performed by the students only guided by the faculty. The module was structured keeping in mind that working together in partnership, the teams would learn the art of teamwork and perform at their best in the given time frame and understand the importance of interdisciplinary research.

This seven-month program was further subdivided into three phases (Figure 1). These phases had sub-sessions according to relevance of each step of research, each of which consisted of didactic lectures using audiovisual tools and was followed by hands-on training to gain confidence to implement them independently by the undergraduate students. These training modules were conducted by experts from the department of Community Medicine.

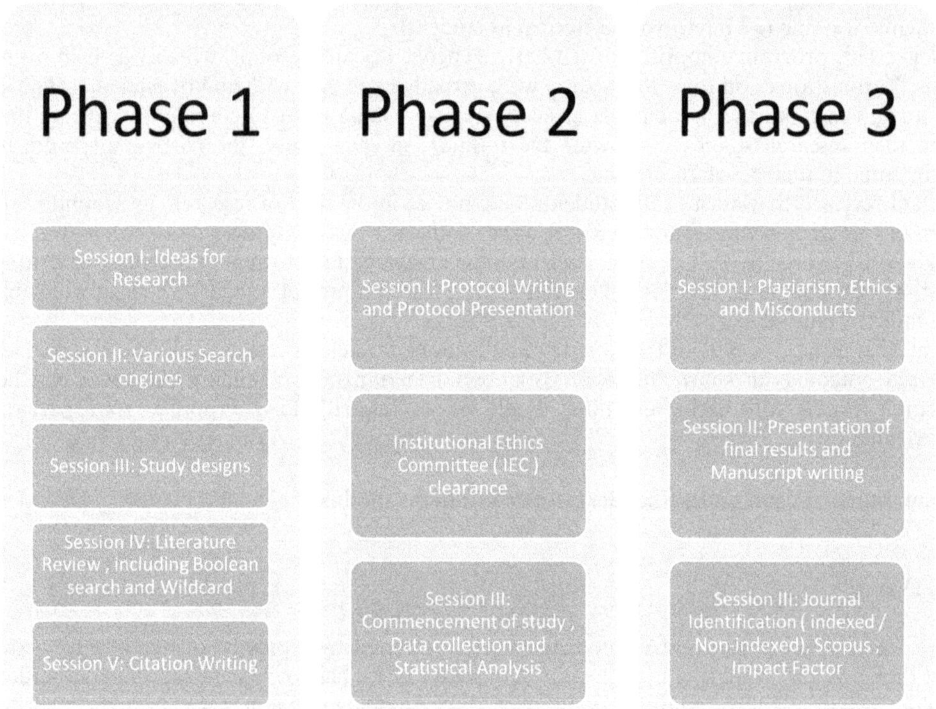

Figure 1. Phases of GRASP.

The phases were as follows:

PHASE 1: Phase 1 was for a period of 2 months where five different steps of research was taught and demonstrated to each pair.

This phase being the first was distributed well so that each participant in the program can grasp as much of information with the basics of research as possible.

PHASE 2: This phase was implemented keeping in mind that the basics were clear to all the participants and there was a need to comprehend them with the knowledge of protocol formulation. This phase consisted of three sessions and was conducted over a period of one month.

PHASE 3: After a gap of three months once the students finished the research project the last phase of this program was crucial as it was utilized to include topics on significance of Publication, selection of journals (indexed and non – indexed journals with high impact factor) and Manuscript writing. Spanning for over a period of one month, this phase marked the end of the various sessions of the program covering all topics relevant to research.

At the end of these sessions, a questionnaire was given to the students to assess their knowledge with a post training evaluation questionnaire. This assessment was combined with a feedback form to all the student participants to assess their experience with this training module and whether such training modules should be incorporated into the existing academic curriculum for the benefit of undergraduate students. The collected data was checked for completeness and consistency and this data was subjected to statistical analysis.

3 RESULTS

A closed ended pre validated questionnaire was given to the participants before commencing and after completion of the training module. Students were asked questions with regards to the importance of research and their knowledge before and after the various training sessions. After obtaining answers to the questions (Table 1) the responses were subjected to statistical analysis.

Table 1. Responses to the questionnaire.

Question	Response	
	Yes (%)	No (%)
Have you conducted any research study (Prior to GRASP)	15	85
Have you presented paper/ poster in a scientific conference previously?	25	75
Do you think research at undergraduate level is important	95	05
Do you think pairing of an Intern with a third year BDS student was useful?	95	05
Do you think you should have a novel idea for starting a research project	85	15
Did you learn any new search engine after the session	85	15
Did you know about the various study designs in research	50	50
Were you aware of how to search for the review of literature before GRASP?	35	65
Did you know the steps of writing protocol before the session?	15	85
Did you know the significance of p value in research (prior to the session)	40	60
Do you believe that you are more confident of presentation skills after the session on presentation of reports	95	05
Did you understand how to write a manuscript after following journals guidelines?	90	10
Were you aware of different indexing agencies before the session?	10	90
Were you aware of the various research misconducts?	40	60

Of the 20 students enrolled for the GRASP, only 3 of them had initiated a research project previously. When asked about the importance of research at the Undergraduate level, 95% of them had a positive opinion. Ninety five percent of students felt that pairing of a third year with an intern for the research project was beneficial. Having a novel idea to begin a research project, was thought to be a necessary factor by 85% of the participants. When questioned about the various search engines before and after the conduction of the session, only 65% of the students were aware of the importance of literature search; but majority of them were unaware of the technique to conduct it before the training session. 85% expressed that they had gained more knowledge and responded correctly that PUBMED and SCOPUS databases were the commonly used search engines for literature search after the training. Half the participants prior to the session were unaware of the types of study designs. Although majority of the participants were able to respond that cross-sectional, case-control, cohort and randomized control trials were the various types of study designs, after the training session. Vancouver style is the most used referencing style and this was known by 16 out of 20 students. There were various sessions related to writing a protocol and only 15% were aware of all the steps before they were trained in these sessions. Fundamentals of statistical analysis relies on the 'p' value and only 40% knew about its significance prior to the session. Sixteen articipants answered on the question regarding various sampling methods, out of which 13 enlisted, simple, random, stratified as the most commonly used sampling methods. Majority of them i.e. 55% were of the opinion that review article need not be reviewed by the Institutional Ethics Committee. 5 out of 8 which accounted for 62% of the participants were of the opinion that, Turnitin is a useful software to check for plagiarism. Manuscript writing according to the various journal guidelines was understood by 90% of students after session education. Only 10% of the participants were conscious of the various indexing agencies before the session. Out of the 20 participants, only sevenf them responded and correctly stated that impact factor is defined by the number of times an article is cited in a journal. Twelve out of the total number of participants were ignorant of the various research misconducts. However, most of them responded that, falsification, fabrication and plagiarism were forms of misconduct after being trained on this topic.

4 DISCUSSION

Research originates with a question or a problem and requires a clear articulation of a goal. Once the correct plan and procedure is drafted, the assumptive answers to certain questions become more assertive and collection and interpretation of data becomes easier. For this knowledge to be disseminated amongst students, research should be incorporated at an early stage in the undergraduate curriculum. [6]

Studies stating the importance of incorporating research at an undergraduate level are very many, however, it still remains a farfetched goal. [7] To reinforce and execute the validity of the fact that research is an integral part of any undergraduate course, the Student Research Forum of Manipal College of Dental Sciences, Mangalore in collaboration with the Department of Community Medicine, Kasturba Medical College, Mangalore initiated this exclusive program called GRASP. This program was organized to enrol 20 undergraduate student participants, who had not completed any research before. These 20 students responded that they were more confident about conducting a research project and presenting it, after they had presented their protocols and final reports in front of the faculty members and experts. When asked about their purpose to join this program, most responded that they were curious and wanted to learn about research under able mentors in a structured program.

The uniqueness of GRASP was the heterogeneous team, where a senior and a junior undergraduate student were paired and, were guided by faculty of two different specialities to conduct an interdisciplinary research project in a structured training module. The students were asked if this concept could be taken forward and most of them agreed supporting it with reasons of teamwork and guidance from mentors at each step in the program was helpful.

This program as already stated was multiphasic and followed a ladder pattern of gradually teaching the research procedures to the participants each step as they moved forwards from basics of research to publication. The phase 1 was subdivided and conducted over 5 sessions namely on the topics of ideas on research, search engines, study designs, literature review, referencing and citation writing. Phase 2 was again split into 3 sessions covering details on protocol writing and its presentation, institutional ethics committee clearance, data collection and statistical analysis. Phase 3 segmented further into three sessions on plagiarism and ethical misconducts, manuscript writing and presentation of final results, steps to publication and identification of indexed and non-indexed journals. A follow up was done after the end of the program and 9 out of 10 studies were ready with their final reports while 5 amongst them were ready in a publishable format and were subsequently published in SCOPUS indexed journals. After the completion of each of these the students were provided with a set of questions assessing their cognitive gain after the session. These results when reviewed clearly produced affirmative data showing that every participant felt that they gained new knowledge through this program. The responses also revealed that the students were appreciative of the didactic lectures and hands on training program imparted to them. They responded that the program had significantly enlightened and motivated them to carry out research projects independently in the future.

As a result, the concept of GRASP needs to be given a serious consideration to be inculcated as a routine in the dental undergraduate curriculum. This research program provides tangible learning objectives that will impact students future professional goals. This program will not only develop and upkeep with the increasing trend of research worldwide but will also be advantageous to the students, mentors and the university.

5 CONCLUSION

Inclusion of research in undergraduate dental curriculum is crucial for developing critical thinking and problem-solving skills in clinical practice. Engaging in research helps students understand the importance of evidence-based medicine that will help them plan treatments effectively. However, the lack of a structured research training in undergraduate curriculum makes it difficult to achieve these goals. Our novel structured training module in interdisciplinary research led to good quality research outcomes in a short duration. Experiential learning opportunities like these can help students develop research related skills early. Training module like GRASP can be offered as an elective in undergraduate curriculum. Credit points for such students can be awarded which can be linked to the formative assessments. However, provision for time within already tight academic schedule and the availability for faculty for training students on a regular basis are some of the challenges.

We firmly believe that our research training module can be easily formulated and incorporated as a part of the undergraduate curriculum in any higher education institute.

REFERENCES

[1] Stephen E. Knight, Jacqueline M. Van Wyk and Saajida Mahomed. (2016). Teaching research: a programme to develop research capacity in undergraduate medical students at the University of KwaZulu-Natal, South Africa. *BMC Medical Education* 16:61.

[2] Laidlaw A, Aiton J, Struthers J, Guild S. (2012). Developing research skills in medical students: *AMEE Guide* No. 69. *Med Teach* 34(9): e754–71.

[3] H Walkington. (2015). Students as researchers: Supporting undergraduate research in the disciplines in higher education. *The higher education academy*. 1: 1–34.

[4] Dolan, E. and Johnson, D. (2009). Towards a Holistic View of Undergraduate Research Experiences: An Exploratory Study of Impact on Graduate/Postdoctoral Mentors. *J Sci Educ Technol* 18: 487.

[5] Walkington, H., & Jenkins, A. (2008). Embedding undergraduate research publication in the student learning experience: Ten suggested strategies. *Brookes E-journal of Learning and Teaching*, 2(3). Retrieved January 2013 from http://bejlt.brookes.ac.uk/article/embedding_undergraduate_research_publication_in_the_student_learning_experi/

[6] Madan CR, Teitge BD. (2013). The benefits of undergraduate research: The student's perspective. *The Mentor: An Academic Advising Journal*. 15:1–3.

[7] Russell SH, Hancock MP, McCullough J. (2007). Benefits of undergraduate research experiences. *Science*. 316 (5824):548–9.

Navigating Dental Education Trends and Transforming Dental Pedagogy – Abas and Srikant N (Eds)
© 2027 The Author(s), ISBN: 978-1-041-32674-8

Complications of Conventional Techniques of IANB and New Learning Curves for Budding Dentists: Review of Literature

Shashank Agarwal, Sandeep K M, and Joanna Baptist
Department of Oral and Maxillofacial Surgery, Manipal College of Dental Sciences Mangalore, Manipal Academy of Higher Education, Manipal, India

Keywords: inferior alveolar nerve block, injection technique, paraesthesia, local anaesthesia

1 INTRODUCTION

In clinical practice, it is essential that patients experience a brief reduction in pain during dental procedures as this can delay the beginning of anxiety. Physicians should be aware that while local anesthetics are dependable and effective medications, problems might nevertheless arise.

Complicated dental procedures including local anesthetics can have systemic to loco-regional effects. According to Haas, the most frequent side effect of local anesthetic injection is anxiety-related adverse events. In addition to a wide range of symptoms (e.g., hyperventilation, nausea, vomiting, and changes in heart rate or blood pressure), the affected patient typically experiences syncope. Furthermore, even though allergies to amide local anesthetics are less common than 1% of the population, allergic reactions can nonetheless occur.

These expressions ought should be included in the differential diagnosis of events that cause worry. Furthermore, a local anesthetic could be hazardous if it enters the bloodstream at a high quantity, particularly if several injections are given or an accidental intravascular injection occurs. Methemoglobinemia is an additional adverse reaction that is mostly linked to certain anesthetic drugs, such as prilocaine, articaine, or the topical anesthetic benzocaine. An overabundance of anesthetic drug metabolites is the source of this occurrence, which leads to systemic cyanosis. There have also been reports of tongue or lip paresthesia or prolonged anesthesia. The lingual nerve is more frequently affected than the inferior alveolar nerve, while it can occasionally become permanent. It is primarily temporary.

Other issues that have been recorded include of: (i) facial nerve paralysis resulting from anesthetic injection into the parotid gland capsule, causing the following symptoms to manifest: (ii) a transient incapacity to close the ipsilateral eye while preserving the integrity of the corneal reflex; (iii) trismus following an injection, which may be caused by hematoma formation, infection, repeated injections, or an overabundance of local anesthetics; (iv) pain resulting from the inoculation of the local anesthetic agent, which may be caused by the anesthetic's quick injection into the tissue or by the shape of the needle; (v) a post-injection infection, potentially due to needle contamination; (vi) needle fracture and additional complications such as edema, hematoma, gingival lesions, soft tissue damage, and taste alteration.

In dentistry, an IAN block is frequently utilized; nonetheless, reports indicate that a significant failure rate of 20–47% has occurred.

Even though these methods yielded varying degrees of success and failure rates, they are nonetheless applied in accordance with clinician comfort levels and clinical circumstances. Additionally, several shortcuts were suggested to increase the success rates of IAN blocks, including creating novel anaesthetics, repositioning the patient, modifying medication dosages and using different methods while teaching the technique to future clinicians.

Some of these methods are: The Glove and Mandible Method, The Mannequin Method, Mobile augmented reality simulator, Visuo-Haptic VR and AR Guidance.

It is not possible to give a precise estimate at this time of the frequency of unfavourable events brought on by IAN anesthetic techniques.

2 DISCUSSION AND REVIEW OF LITERATURE

According to BRIAN WEBBER *et al.* [1] Intentional intravascular injections caused by blockages to the inferior alveolar nerve can lead to frustrating local and systemic effects. It is essential that the dentist identify the issue and provide the necessary care. Occasionally, multiple reactions take place at once. Intra-arterial injections can

 DOI: 10.1201/9781042016075-73

happen during inferior alveolar nerve blocks, even with the greatest of caution on the part of the doctors, who aspirate prior to the injection and record anatomical landmarks. Thankfully, it is uncommon for nerves, mouth and facial tissues, and eyes to sustain permanent damage. To prevent any irreparable repercussions, the practitioner should properly diagnose and treat the issues. The fastest diagnosis and patient reassuring are crucial in controlling a reaction to an intra-arterial injection of local anesthetic. If further symptoms appear, such as syncope or palpitations in the heart, medical professionals should start further suitable care. It is imperative that the dentist explains the situation to the patient and gives him or her the assurance that the prolonged anesthetic is just brief.

According to M. ANTHONY POGREL *et al.* [2] Prospective investigation of patients who were referred to a tertiary care facility and who had permanent changes in their lingual, inferior alveolar, or both nerves' sensation that could only have been caused by an inferior alveolar nerve block. The lingual nerve, inferior alveolar nerve, or both may occasionally become permanently involved after an inferior alveolar nerve block. We still don't know the precise mechanism of participation or its incidence. An inferior alveolar nerve block can very rarely result in permanent nerve damage. There is no known preventive measure, and the precise process is unknown. It's critical to understand the dangers and side effects of local anesthetic.

Wright EF, *et al.* [3] reported a case of myospasm (medial pterygoid trismus) that occurred the day following three inferior alveolar nerve blocks and a standard restoration procedure. An inferior alveolar nerve block may result in a medial pterygoid myospasm. Heat application, muscular stretches, ingestion of analgesics and/or muscle relaxants, and referral to physical therapy are the standard treatments for this disorder. The amount of therapy required usually depends on how severe the disease is.

According to Traeger KA, *et al.* [4] If all or part of the solution is injected intravascularly, the anesthesia for the inferior alveolar nerve may not be acceptable. If a vessel, specifically an artery, is broken or punctured, there's a strong likelihood that blood may seep into the surrounding tissue and develop hematomas. A hematoma is an accumulation of blood that results from a blood vessel rupture into the surrounding tissues. It has long been noted that insufficient inferior alveolar anesthesia may result in the production of hematomas, which can be felt as palpable swelling in the pterygomandibular and retromolar regions. Even though the patient claims that their lip feels numb, partial anesthesia may still be present. In such cases, not getting anesthetic could be the result of dilution of the anaesthetic solution by blood and some of the anesthetic getting deactivated.

According to Doh RM, Shin S, *et al.* [5] Paraesthesia is a change in skin sensation that can include tingling, burning, or partial loss of local sensitivity. The third branch of the trigeminal nerve, the inferior alveolar nerve (IAN), is crucial to dental care. IAN paresthesia has been documented to occur in 0.35% to 8.4% of cases following a variety of dental treatments, including simple anesthetic injections, surgery, and endodontic treatment. There are very few instances of nerve involvement developing later than just after the treatment; instead, the altered feeling usually occurs right away. On the day following surgery, when any local anesthetic effects have worn off, the patient frequently notices the altered sensation. Rarely, nevertheless, individuals report experiencing paraesthesia a few days to months following the surgery. The primary distinction between delayed paraesthesia and classic paresthesia is that the latter happens later and results in restoration to pre-operation, whereas the former starts immediately following the procedure and is not guaranteed to heal.

According to Tzermpos FH, *et al.* [6] Seldom reported side effects of inferior alveolar nerve block anesthesia include facial nerve palsy. Either immediate or delayed paralysis could result from the amount of time that passed between the injection and the beginning of symptoms. Depending on how long passed between the injection and the beginning of symptoms, there could be an immediate or delayed paralysis. In the immediate kind, paralysis sets in minutes after injection, and recovery takes no more than three hours. On the other hand, in the delayed type, healing may take longer than a day and symptoms may manifest between hours to days. This article's goal is to document an instance of delayed facial palsy brought on by an inferior alveolar nerve block that went away eight weeks or so after the anesthesia was administered. This paper presents and discusses the pathophysiology, therapy, and outcomes of an 8-week follow-up for a patient who was sent to a private maxillofacial clinic. The patient was 20 years old.

According to Keskin Yalcin B, *et al.* [7] When the central nervous system and cardiovascular systems are exposed to an adequate (toxic) concentration of anesthetic medication in the blood, local anesthetic systemic toxicity occurs.

Central nervous system symptoms like excitement and convulsions are the first symptoms to manifest, and they are followed by unconsciousness and respiratory arrest. Cardiovascular symptoms like hypertension, tachycardia, and premature ventricular contractions frequently accompany these symptoms. Clinical signs and symptoms typically include objective symptoms including trembling in the extremities, flickering, and rapid talking.

The patient has to be assessed to avoid systemic toxicity. Reduce the amount of local anesthetic used; young or light individuals shouldn't have all four quadrants treated in a single visit with local anesthetic alone; use a precise and gradual injection method; and make adjustments It is advised to use aspiration testing, agents with low toxicity It is advised to use aspiration testing, agents with low toxicity such ropivacaine and levobupivacaine, and dosage split.

According to You JS, *et al.* [8] The most popular technique for providing local anesthetic during intraoral surgery in the posterior mandibular region is the inferior alveolar nerve block. However, as the local anesthetic is being administered, unforeseen issues could arise. The needle fracture is one of these unusual side effects. If the injection needle breaks during the surgery, it should be removed immediately. However, this is one of the most difficult procedures.

According to Jenkins DB, *et al.* [9] A teaching strategy was created to help dental students comprehend and carry out their first inferior alveolar nerve block more easily. Anatomical and clinical information was correlated through lectures, lab sessions, and demonstrations. A key component of this training strategy was the practice and demonstration of injection using cadavers. To preserve the mouth cavity, cadavers were dissected. The superior part of the mandibular ramus was excised, and the skin and masseter muscle were reflected laterally. The inferior alveolar and lingual nerves, as well as the medial pterygoid muscle, were exposed during this surgery, allowing for the monitoring of a syringe needle during inferior alveolar nerve blocks. The mental, infraorbital, and supraorbital nerves were also visible. In addition to offering training and practice sessions prior to the first patient injection, this combined anatomical-clinical experience helped to reduce some of the anxiety that is frequently connected with the initial injection and reinforced the importance of anatomy in clinical practice.

According to Khaled M Mohamed, *et al.* [10] Dental students can learn how to administer local anesthetic (LA) using a variety of techniques. This study sought to determine how two teaching strategies—peer-assisted learning (PAL) and student-to-student learning—affected the proficiency of third-year dentistry students in performing inferior alveolar nerve blocks (IANBs). Peer-assisted learning (PAL) and demonstration using cadavers and dry human skulls are examples of these instructional techniques. Students can also practice on simulation models and real human beings, including as patients or other students. The most popular teaching strategy for the LA administration process and its effective removal during the administration of general or local anesthesia is the student-to-student approach.

Mannequin simulation models have been introduced to avoid possible complications and ethical concerns with student-to-student injections. They consist of an upper head and body mannequin, along with a battery operated electronic typhodont consisting of an upper and lower jaw. The jaws as well as the teeth (32) are fabricated in hard thermosetting material. The gingivae are elastic and removable. This method of teaching is useful as the models give an acoustic signal when the correct region is perforated with a dry syringe. Also, the mannequins are strapped to a dental chair which helps simulate the patients' and the dentist's position to the student. This, however effective it may be, is an expensive method of teaching IANB to students as the models themselves are expensive and might not be affordable by certain educational institutes.

Inferior alveolar nerve block is most used nerve block technique in oral and maxillofacial surgery. It is difficult to master this technique for the undergraduate as it demands knowledge of landmarks and 3-dimensional anatomic knowledge of the vital structures. Various techniques have been employed such as student to student method, mannequin method, student to patient methods to teach students the proper technique of administering IANB.

We have developed This glove and mandible technique , Glove and Mandible Method is a technique devised to give students a chance to gain practical insight into IANB before attempting on patients. A glove was used, mimicking the blind procedure, to cover the ramal and condylar areas of the mandible, and the pterygomandibular raphe (PMR) was marked. A hole is cut into the posterior aspect to visualize the mandibular foramen. Students are then asked to perform a pseudo-nerve block; from the rear end, they could visualize the final position of the needle before depositing the solution. The cause of any discrepancy in the final position of the needle could then be evaluated and rectified easily by simply looking from the rear end, which is not possible on a patient. This method of teaching IANB to budding dentists is economical and is possible in every college.

3 CONCLUSION

Not all complications of inferior alveolar nerve blocks are inevitable, majority can be nullified by knowledge of intricate anatomy of facial skeleton, nerve and blood vessels.

Majority of the complications mentioned above in literature is due to the mishap from the surgeon, such complications can be avoided by utilizing educational tools to master this technique, rather than learning on patients, which possess a threat to patient health.

Newer learning techniques such as, glove and mandible method, mannequin method , cadaver, AI generated models should be employed to teach inferior alveolar nerve block technique to the budding dentists effectively.

REFERENCES

[1] Brian Webber, Herbert Orlansky, Charles Lipton, Mark Stevens, (2001). Complications of an intra-arterial injection from an inferior alveolar nerve block *The Journal of the American Dental Association*, Volume 132, Issue 12, Pages 1702–1704, ISSN 0002-8177

[2] M. Anthony Pogrel, (2000). Sri Thamby, Permanent Nerve Involvement Resulting: From Inferior Alveolar Nerve Blocks, *The Journal of the American Dental Association*, Volume 131, Issue 7,Pages 901–907, ISSN 0002-8177

[3] Wright EF. (2011). Medial pterygoid trismus (myospasm) following inferior alveolar nerve block: case report and literature review. *Gen Dent.* 59(1):64–7. PMID: 21613042.

[4] Traeger KA. (1979). Hematoma following inferior alveolar injection: a possible cause for anesthesia failure. *Anesth Prog.*;26 (5):122–3. PMID: 298458; PMCID: PMC2516859.

[5] Doh RM, Shin S, You TM. (2018). Delayed paresthesia of inferior alveolar nerve after dental surgery: case report and related pathophysiology. *J Dent Anesth Pain Med. 18*(3):177–182. doi: 10.17245/jdapm.2018.18.3.177. Epub 2018 Jun 29. PMID: 29984322; PMCID: PMC6031975.

[6] Tzermpos FH, Cocos A, Kleftogiannis M, Zarakas M, Iatrou I. (2012). Transient delayed facial nerve palsy after inferior alveolar nerve block anesthesia. *Anesth Prog.* 59(1):22–7. doi: 10.2344/11-03.1. PMID: 22428971; PMCID: PMC3309298.

[7] You JS, Kim SG, Oh JS, Choi HI, Jih MK. (2017). Removal of a fractured needle during inferior alveolar nerve block: two case reports. *J Dent Anesth Pain Med.* 17(3):225–229. doi: 10.17245/jdapm.2017.17.3.225. Epub 2017 Sep 25. PMID: 29090254; PMCID: PMC5647823.

[8] Jenkins DB, Spackman GK. (1995). A method for teaching the classical inferior alveolar nerve block. *Clin Anat. 1995*;8(3):231–4. doi: 10.1002/ca.980080310. PMID: 7606599.

[9] Khaled M Mohamed, Fatima M Jadu, Hala M Abdelalim, Amr M Bayoumi, Ahmed M Jan. Impact of Methods for Teaching Inferior Alveolar Nerve Block Anesthesia on Dental Students' Efficiency

Navigating Dental Education Trends and Transforming Dental Pedagogy – Abas and Srikant N (Eds)
© 2027 The Author(s), ISBN: 978-1-041-32674-8

Revitalizing Dental Education: A Review of Advanced Tools and Technology for Future Dentists

Khatheeja Thasneem, M.I. Shanavaz, Nithin Suvarna, Aravind R Kudva, and Prathap M S
Department of Conservative Dentistry and Endodontics, Yenepoya Dental College, Mangalore, Karnataka, India

1 INTRODUCTION

Dental education is essential for equipping professionals to meet diverse patient needs. A well-structured curriculum plays a pivotal role in shaping students clinical skills through defined objectives, methodologies, and assessments [1]Traditional dental curricula in India have been criticized for their rigidity and misalignment with market demands. To address this, the UGC introduced the Choice-Based Credit System (CBCS) in 2015, promoting flexibility, and the DCI aligned it with the NEP 2020 to improve educational quality. [2] The Liaison Committee on Medical Education (LCME) emphasized the need for a "coherent, coordinated, and integrated" curriculum to advance medical education and ensure accreditation and competent healthcare professionals .[3] Adapting these reforms poses challenges but holds transformative potential. As rightly stated by Bland, "successful curricular change only occurs through the dedicated efforts of effective change agents". [4]

Faculty members are key agents of change in implementing new or revised curricula, as they directly influence the process. However, these changes significantly impact faculty, requiring adjustments in teaching philosophy, student assessment, and evaluation processes, alongside intensive faculty development efforts [5,6]. Modern approaches, such as cross-country collaborations, flipped classrooms, flexible lectures, daily quizzes, and online platforms with embedded assessments, are integral to these transitions [7,8]. Advanced technologies, including virtual reality systems, haptic devices, robotic simulators, TEL integration, and 3D imaging and printing, further challenge faculty in adapting to innovative practices [9,10].

Despite the transformative potential of these advancements, challenges persist. Adapting to virtual learning environments, robotics, and nanotechnology requires addressing evolving student needs and treatment trends. Limited infrastructure, unreliable connectivity, and a lack of ergonomic evaluation methods hinder implementation [11,12]. Addressing these barriers is crucial for successfully integrating technology into dental education and healthcare.

1.1 *Objective*

- To examine innovative digital tools and technologies that enhance advanced learning in the dental education curriculum.

1.2 *Scope and limitation*

- The study explored contemporary tools and teaching techniques rather than emphasising traditional methods and challenges.

2 METHODOLOGY

This study employed a qualitative research approach, utilising a random sampling technique. A search of the Web of Science database identified 1,845 articles related to dental education from the past 20 years (2005–2024), including 85 publications from India. Additional data were sourced from databases such as ProQuest Central, Scopus, PubMed, and Google Scholar, yielding 3,590 scholarly works, of which 1,950 were highly relevant. A comprehensive review was conducted on 40 research papers to draw meaningful conclusions. Data collection took place between July and September, supplemented by offline resources, including newspaper articles, e-theses, dissertations, and printed journals.

3 DISCUSSIONS

Integrating advanced tools and technologies (Figure 1) such as AI, robotics, and 3D printing has revolutionised dental education. Historically, dentistry relied heavily on manual image analysis and diagnostic methods, often

 DOI: 10.1201/9781042016075-74

time-intensive and prone to human error. AI now enables the processing of large data sets, resulting in more precise diagnostics and informed decision-making while driving forward research and innovation. [13,14]

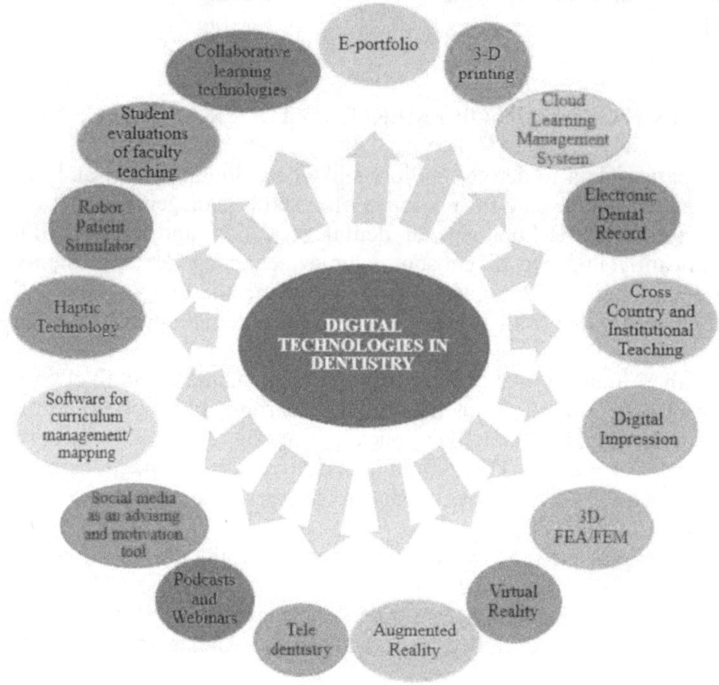

Figure 1. Emerging tools and techniques in dental education.

Virtual and augmented reality (VR and AR) have revolutionized dental pre-clinical training through simulations, enabling students to develop skills and practice procedures in a risk-free, simulated environment before treating real patients. [15] Romane Touati *et al.* presented a case report demonstrating the use of AR in managing complex full-mouth rehabilitation procedures.

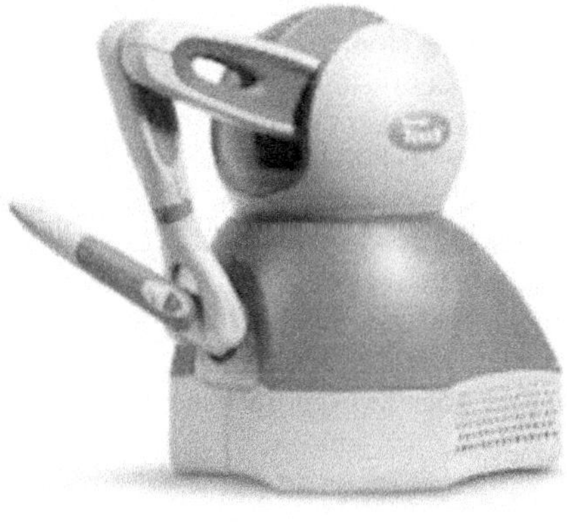

Figure 2. Typical haptic interface device.

Libraries serve as learning content management systems, while lecture theatres and classrooms act as pre-existing virtual learning environments (VLEs). Integrating e-learning with clinical training through mobile technologies and 3D simulations promotes blended learning. Tele-dentistry, an emerging field combining telecommunications with dental care, complements traditional teaching methods and provides innovative learning opportunities for students and practitioners [16]. Robotic patients play a crucial role in training, aiding students in medical emergency scenarios, differential diagnoses, and critical thinking enhancement [17,18].

Digital portfolios, such as those using platforms like PebblePad, foster reflective practice, self-assessment, and goal-setting, enabling students to refine their skills and understanding [19]. Additionally, 3D printing has revolutionized dental education by creating realistic models for clinical simulation, enhancing hands-on learning [20]. Survey condudted at North American dental schools reveal a mixed pace of e-curriculum adoption, with rapid implementation by some institutions and gradual adaptation by others [21]. In the UK, students embrace e-learning more readily than faculty, with some departments resistant to sharing online content, even though they were password protected [22].

4 THE BENEFITS OF INTEGRATION OF EMERGING TOOLS AND TECHNIQUES

Predictive analytics uses patient data to detect conditions like periodontal disease and oral cancer early, enabling personalized treatment and preventive care for proactive oral health management. [23]

Integrating emerging tools and technologies in dental education and practice offers numerous benefits. These innovations significantly improve diagnostic accuracy, enabling dentists to precisely detect conditions and plan more effective treatments. Additionally, they streamline the analysis and interpretation of intraoral and extraoral images, making routine evaluations more efficient and aiding in disease diagnosis and monitoring. [24]

The schematic web enables limitless connectivity through open standards and network layering, transforming stand-alone educational software into platforms that enhance learning and connectivity. IVIDENT tackles dental academic staff shortages with adaptable, globally applicable learning materials and assessments.[11]

Virtual assistants optimize dental workflows and enhance patient satisfaction, while AI-powered robotics improve precision, reduce errors, and boost treatment effectiveness, ensuring accurate interventions through AI-human collaboration.[25]

Simulation technologies offering effective training methods, especially during the pandemic, while digital tools improve preclinical assessments, ensuring standardized and accurate evaluations.[26]

Applying ergonometrics and IT, including telemedicine, teledentistry, and reliable patient record systems, is crucial for addressing the problem, as concluded by an IBM disease management colloquium.[11]

5 CHALLENGES

Implementing an integrated dental curriculum presents multiple challenges despite its importance. Faculty face increased workloads, acting as educational designers, and struggle to manage time amid interruptions and vast data demands. The adoption of modern tools has limited hands-on clinical training, reducing opportunities for physical observation and patient examination. Over-reliance on technology has further diminished essential clinical skills. Many institutions lack infrastructure to support advanced technologies, while unreliable internet disrupts software access, content uploads, and student supervision. [23, 24, 26]

The absence of clear guidelines for incorporating technology into curricula hinders widespread adoption, and reduced face-to-face interactions impair the development of interpersonal clinical skills. Insufficient guidance, frequent turnover, communication delays, and confusion among stakeholders, with parents questioning its necessity and students struggling to adapt. A Hong Kong curriculum reform case study found that only 28.3% of faculty felt their implementation roles were clearly defined, highlighting a lack of clear guidance on their responsibilities. A study by Syeda Kausar and Lubna Baig's identified poor stakeholder communication as a key factor in delaying innovative curriculum implementation. Faculty development programs are often ineffective and pointed that practical implementation was totally different. As per literature frequent faculty turnover hinders smooth curriculum implementation, highlighting the importance of staff retention for workload balance, stability, and knowledge preservation. Also inconsistent funding, rigid curricula, limited career incentives for technology research, and reluctance to share ideas and resources.leadership's prioritization of medical programs over dental education exacerbates issues. [26, 27,28]

6 CONCLUSION

The integration of emerging technologies in dental education presents significant opportunities to transform the field. Innovations such as AI, virtual and augmented reality, haptics, and teledentistry have enhanced diagnostic accuracy, clinical training, and patient care, providing students with controlled environments to build critical skills. However, several challenges persist. The high costs of simulation technologies, lack of faculty preparedness, unclear roles in curriculum reform, and poor stakeholder communication hinder implementation. Faculty burnout, frequent turnover, and insufficient funding for capacity building further complicate progress. E-learning faces additional barriers, including IT skill shortages, unreliable internet connectivity, outdated teaching practices, and the psychomimetic effects of 3D tools. Addressing these issues requires solutions like blended learning, extended clinical programs, robust infection control measures, and fostering leadership support. By overcoming these challenges and investing in modern technologies, dental education can evolve to meet the demands of contemporary practice and improve patient outcomes.

CONFLICT OF INTEREST

There are no conflicts of interest to declare.

ACKNOWLEDGEMENT

The author did not receive any financial support from any institutions or organisations.

REFERENCES

[1] Kabra L, Santhosh VN, Sequeira RN, Ankola AV, Coutinho D. (2023). Dental curriculum reform in India: Undergraduate students' awareness and perception on the newly proposed choice-based credit system. *Journal of Oral Biology and Craniofacial Research.* 13(5):630–5. Available from: https://doi.org/10.1016/j.jobcr.2023.08.003

[2] Muralidharan K, Shanmugan K, Klochkov Y. (2022). The new education policy 2020, digitalization and quality of Life in India: Some reflections. *Education Sciences.* 12(2):75.

[3] Schneiderhan J, Guetterman TC, Dobson ML. (2019). Curriculum development: a how to primer. *iFam Med Com Health.* 7(2): e000046.

[4] Bland CJ, Starnaman S, Wersal L, Moorhead-Rosenberg L, Zonia S, Henry R. (2000). Curricular change in medical schools: how to succeed. *Academic Medicine.* 75(6):575–94.

[5] Reis S. (2018). Curriculum reform: Why? What? How? And how will we know it works? *Isr. J. Health Policy Res.* 7(1): 7–10. doi: 10.1186/s13584-018-0221-4

[6] Baker SE, Edwards R. (2012). How many qualitative interviews is enough? Expert voices and early career reflections on sampling and cases in qualitative research. *National Center for Research Methods.*

[7] Postma TC, White JG. (2015). Developing integrated clinical reasoning competencies in dental students using scaffolded case-based learning – empirical evidence. *European Journal of Dental Education [Internet].* 20(3):180–8. Available from: https://doi.org/10.1111/eje.12159

[8] Kerthana. (2024). AI Revolutionizes dentistry: 6 Powerful applications [Internet]. *Cochin Dental Institute - Dental Technician Course in Kerala.* Available from: https://cochindentalinstitute.com/artificial-intelligence-in-dentistry/

[9] Thomas, Corne, Postma, John, G., White. (2016). Developing integrated clinical reasoning competencies in dental students using scaffolded case-based learning - empirical evidence. *European Journal of Endocrinology,* 20(3):180 188. doi: 10.1111/EJE.12159

[10] Gali, Sivaranjani and Patil, Archana. (2016). The technology of haptics in dental education. *Journal of Dental & Oro-facial Research,*14(02): 70–75

[11] Eaton KA, Reynolds PA, Grayden SK, Wilson NHF. (2008). A vision of dental education in the third millennium. *Br Dent J.* 205 (5):261–71.

[12] McGraw-Hill. (2002). *Ergonometrics. McGraw-Hill Dictionary of Scientifi c and Technical Terms.* 6th ed. New York: McGraw Hill Professional, ISBN: 007042313X

[13] Alam MK, Alftaikhah SAA, Issrani R, Ronsivalle V, Lo Giudice A, Cicciù M, *et al.* (2024). Applications of artificial intelligence in the utilisation of imaging modalities in dentistry: A systematic review and meta-analysis of in-vitro studies. *Heliyon [Internet].* 10(3):e24221. Available from: https://doi.org/10.1016/j.heliyon.2024.e24221

[14] Mohan KR, Fenn SM. (2023). Artificial intelligence and its theranostic applications in dentistry. *Cureus [Internet].* Available from: https://doi.org/10.7759/cureus.38711

[15] Dzyuba N, Jandu J, Yates J, Kushnerev E. (2022). Virtual and augmented reality in dental education: The good, the bad and the better. *European Journal of Dental Education [Internet].* Available from: https://doi.org/10.1111/eje.12871

[16] Chen JW, Hobdell MH, Dunn K, Johnson KA, Zhang J. (2023). Teledentistry and its use in dental education. *The Journal of the American Dental Association [Internet].* 134(3):342–6. Available from: https://doi.org/10.14219/jada.archive.2003.0164

[17] Tanzawa T, Futaki K, Kurabayashi H, Goto K, Yoshihama Y, Hasegawa T, *et al.* (2012). Medical emergency education using a robot patient in a dental setting. *European Journal of Dental Education [Internet].* 17(1). Available from: https://doi.org/10.1111/j.16000579.2012.00770.x

[18] Tanzawa T, Futaki K, Tani C, Hasegawa T, Yamamoto M, Miyazaki T, *et al.* (2011). Introduction of a robot patient into dental education. *European Journal of Dental Education [Internet].* 16(1). Available from: https://doi.org/10.1111/j.1600-0579.2011.00697.x

[19] Gadbury-Amyot CC, Godley LW, Nelson JW. (2019). Measuring the level of reflective ability of predoctoral dental students: Early Outcomes in an E-Portfolio Reflection. *Journal of Dental Education [Internet].* 83(3):275–80. Available from: https://doi.org/10.21815/jde.019.025

[20] Figueiredo-Pina CG, Serro AP. (2023). 3D printing for dental applications. *Materials [Internet].* 16(14):4972. Available from: https://doi.org/10.3390/ma16144972

[21] Hendricson WD, Panagakos F, Eisenberg E, McDonald J, Guest G, Jones P, *et al.* (2004). Electronic Curriculum Implementation at North American Dental Schools. *Journal of Dental Education.* 68(10):1041–57.

[22] Gupta B, White DA, Walmsley AD. (2004). The attitudes of undergraduate students and staff to the use of electronic learning. *Br Dent J.* 196(8):487–92.

[23] Pang M, Zhao X, Lu D, Dong Y, Jiang L, Li J, *et al.* (2022). Preliminary User Evaluation of a new Dental Technology Virtual Simulation System: Development and Validation study. *JMIR Serious Games.* 10(3):e36079. Available from: https://doi.org/10.2196/36079

[24] Lee JI. (2023). Dental education now and in the future. *Journal of Periodontal & Implant Science [Internet].* 53(3):171. Available from: https://doi.org/10.5051/jpis.235303edi01

[25] Scalese RJ, Obeso VT, Issenberg SB. (2007). Simulation technology for skills training and competency assessment in medical education. *Journal of General Internal Medicine [Internet].* 23(S1):46–9. Available from: https://doi.org/10.1007/s11606-007-0283-4

[26] Lin Y, Zhang S, Chen X, Wang C. (2006). A novel method in the design and fabrication of dental splints based on 3D simulation and rapid prototyping technology. *The International Journal of Advanced Manufacturing Technology [Internet].* 28(9–10):919–22. Available from: https://doi.org/10.1007/s00170-004-2197-1

[27] Aslam K, Khan RA, Aslam MA, Javed K, Kamran R, Raja AA. (2022). Faculty Perspective on the Challenges Faced During Implementation of Integrated Curriculum. *J Shalamar Med Dent Coll.* 3(2):159–66.

[28] Rosenberg H, Grad HA, Matear DW. (2003). The effectiveness of computer-aided, self-instructional programs in dental education: a systematic review of the literature. *J Dent Educ.* 67(5):524–32.

 ISBN: 978-1-041-32674-8

Game on in Dental Education: Unlocking Skills and Engagement Through Gamification

Ashwini Anand Kamat and Karthik Shetty
Department of Conservative Dentistry and Endodontics, Manipal College of Dental Sciences Mangalore, Manipal Academy of Higher Education, Karnataka, Manipal, India

ABSTRACT: In contrast to conventional teaching techniques, this study investigates how gaming mechanics improve student engagement, learning outcomes, and clinical skill acquisition in dentistry education. Key components like points, badges, leaderboards, simulations, and interactive challenges were the subject of a review of the body of research on gamification in dental education. In order to evaluate performance and engagement, observational studies of dentistry students utilizing gamified tools were also examined. Gamification significantly improved student engagement, motivation, and aided in retention of theoretical knowledge. Students demonstrated enhanced clinical performance, with greater caliber in practical skills compared to those in conventional learning environments. Collaborative learning and critical thinking were also enhanced. Integrating gamification into dental education shows promise in improving both knowledge retention and clinical skills. The synergistic, engaging nature of gamified learning offers a great solution to traditional education's limitations. However, further research is needed to assess long-term impacts on student success and professional readiness.

Keywords: Gamification, dental education, student engagement, skill acquisition, serious games, interactive learning

1 INTRODUCTION

Lectures and clinical demonstrations were the mainstays of dentistry education in the past. While they were rather successful, they were neither completely captivating nor helpful for retaining skills. Gamification has surfaced as a viable technique to greatly improve learning experiences and skill acquisition as education changes in tandem with technology.

2 OBJECTIVES

With a careful analysis of its effects on student motivation, engagement, and learning outcomes, this review unequivocally examines the crucial role that gamification plays in dental education. The study clearly shows how gamified learning may be successfully used within dentistry curriculum to improve both theoretical knowledge and practical competence by combining new research with interesting case stories.

3 METHODOLOGY

To find pertinent studies, a thorough search method was created. Keywords and phrases were used to search databases like PubMed, Scopus, Google Scholar, and Web of Science. including "gamification," "dental education," "serious games," "engagement," and "learning outcomes." The search was limited to studies published in peer-reviewed journals from 2010-2024.

Inclusion criteria consisted of:

- Studies focusing on gamification in dental education.
- Empirical research (quantitative, qualitative, or mixed methods).
- Studies published in English.

Exclusion criteria included:

- Non-educational settings (e.g., corporate training).
- Articles that did not specifically address gamification elements.
- Reviews, editorials, or opinion pieces.

DOI: 10.1201/9781042016075-75

3.1 *Study selection*

Titles and abstracts were used to filter the search results for relevancy. After that, full-text publications were assessed using the inclusion and exclusion criteria. Two reviewers independently carried out the selection process, and any disagreements were discussed or sorted out with a third reviewer.

3.2 *Data extraction and synthesis*

Data on study characteristics (authors, year of publication, study design), gamification features (points, badges, leaderboards, simulations), and important findings pertaining to learning outcomes and student engagement were extracted using a standardized form. The results from many investigations were compiled and interpreted using a narrative synthesis approach, which revealed recurring themes and variances.

4 KEY FINDINGS/RESULTS

Gamification in dentistry is an innovative approach that integrates game-like elements into educational and clinical settings to enhance engagement and learning outcomes. Dental education games cover a range of types, including simulation and role-playing for practical skills, quizzes and puzzles for testing knowledge, and collaborative multiplayer games for teamwork. They also include augmented reality, serious games, and mobile apps for immersive learning experiences that enhance clinical competency. Table 1 depicts the key findings of this review.

Table 1. Key conclusions from the author's review, the study design, the study components employed, the subject of the gamified versions, and the game description.

Authors	Study design	Study element	Study topic	Description
Yang *et al.* [11]	Prototype	Computer(quiz,training)	Dental casting procedure	The Dental Casting Game and the Dental Casting Question Game are the two modes available in this game. While the second mode uses a question game to broaden the learner's foundational understanding of dental casting, the first mode uses game play to help develop the learner's operating skills in dental lost-wax casting.
Amer *et al.* [12]	RCT	Computer(quiz,training)	Clinical training (dentine bonding)	The three-step resin bonding procedure utilized in the operative dentistry curriculum is taught through an interactive dental videogame that uses Adobe Flash CS3 software.
Paiva *et al.* [13]	Prototype	Computer (Quiz, rewards, levels)	Biosecurity in dentistry	The player's goal is to demonstrate his expertise by accurately completing each challenge and gathering PPE items in the scenario, elevating or lowering the level of biosafety that will determine whether or not the player succeeds. Therefore, the biosafety level will rise as the challenges are correctly answered, and it will fall if the player fails to reach the same level, increasing the spread of viruses.
de Vasconcelos *et al.* [14]	Qualitative	Mobile (Quiz, levels)	Dental prosthesis	The athlete is applying for a position on a renowned dental clinic's prosthesis squad. The candidate must pass the initial interview, internship, and residence phases in order to be hired. Under the supervision of his supervisors, the user encounters progressively more challenging questions at each step. These questions consist of a scenario, a question, and answer possibilities.
Vahed *et al.* [15]	Qualitative	Computer web-based (Quiz, levels)	Teeth morphology	Five sub-games that correspond to varying levels of difficulty about questions pertaining to the discipline content of oral anatomy and tooth morphology make up this web-based game.
Ribeiro *et al.* [16]	Qualitative	Haptic device (Training simulation quiz, rewards, levels, points)	Anaesthesia	The player is in the right position, with the right injection depth and sufficient angulation. Scores are given in accordance with how the anesthetic action is executed. A ranking system is in place to motivate participants to improve their results.

(continued)

Table 1. Continued

Authors	Study design	Study element	Study topic	Description
Rodríguez Andrésetal [17]	Quasi experimental	MicrosoftKinect[a] (Autostereoscopy)	Teeth morphology	Placing each tooth in its proper position is the user's primary objective. Students may see small features that help them identify each tooth and position it correctly by thoroughly examining the 3D models from all sides. There are two main stages to the game: the learning stage and the placement stage.
Sipiyaruk *et al.* [18]	Quasi experimental	Computer Moodle environment (Quiz, feedback)	Dental public health.	The learning scenario is presented to the users in a virtual village. The student was presented with a range of health promotion initiatives to select from.
Feitosa *et al.* [19]	Qualitative	Computer and mobile (Quiz, rewards, levels, points,audio, ranking)	Biosecurity in Dentistry	Based on an educational quiz game, the educational game offers a biosafety learning environment with a 2D UI. Each question's answer time varies according to its degree of difficulty and is shown gradually.

5 DISCUSSION

Gamification has shown promise in various aspects of dental education, including improving academic writing skills among dental students. For instance, a study demonstrated that first-year dental students who participated in a gamified course reported significant improvements in their writing abilities, with satisfaction levels linked to their engagement with the gamified activities. [1]. Additionally, gamification can make complex topics more accessible and enjoyable; a study involving crossword puzzles on bruxism revealed that over 82% of participating students found the activity motivating and stimulating, indicating a positive shift in their learning experience. [2] Simulation games have become an integral part of dental training, providing students with interactive and immersive learning experiences that enhance their clinical skills and knowledge retention. A recent study developed an online serious game specifically for oral diagnosis and treatment planning,[3] which demonstrated significant improvements in students' knowledge acquisition and retention after gameplay, highlighting its effectiveness as a learning tool in dental education. Another review of serious games in dentistry found that these interactive platforms not only matched traditional educational methods in effectiveness but also resulted in higher student satisfaction.[4] Additionally, simulation-based learning environments allow students to practice procedures repeatedly without the constraints of real-world clinical settings, fostering muscle memory and improving fine motor skills. Furthermore, dental simulators utilizing virtual reality (VR) technology provide realistic scenarios for students to engage with, enhancing their understanding of complex procedures while offering immediate feedback on their performance[5]. Quizzes and puzzles play a significant role in dental education by enhancing engagement and reinforcing learning among students. A study highlighted the effectiveness of quizzing as an innovative teaching technique, particularly in complex subjects like cephalometrics, where interactive quizzes helped students retain crucial concepts better than traditional methods. [6] Another review indicated that quizzes not only assess knowledge but also encourage critical thinking and application skills, which are essential in clinical settings. [4] Mobile applications are revolutionizing dental education by providing immersive learning experiences for students. These apps leverage interactive features and engaging content to enhance knowledge retention and practical skills. A study found that dental students who used a mobile app for learning about dental trauma showed significant improvements in their knowledge, with the app being as effective as traditional classroom lectures. [7] Mobile apps are not only beneficial for dental students but also for patient education and communication. The DDS GP app, for example, visually represents over 200 demonstrations of various dental conditions and treatments, helping patients better understand their oral health. [4] Apps like FoodForTeeth and My Dental-Care provide patients with educational resources on dental health, enabling them to take an active role in their oral care. A study investigated the impact of dual-player versus single-player modes in a serious game on dental students' factual knowledge. The study found that dual-player mode significantly enhanced students' learning outcomes compared to single-player mode, [10] suggesting collaborative gameplay fosters better engagement, knowledge retention, and learning efficiency in dental education. The integration of gamification in dental education presents a compelling opportunity to enhance student engagement and skill acquisition, but it also comes with certain limitations that warrant discussion. One significant concern is the variability in the design and implementation of gamified tools, which can affect their effectiveness. Many studies highlight the need for rigorous evaluation of game design elements, including usability and educational impact [4]. Poorly designed games may fail to engage students or may not align well with educational objectives, leading to a superficial understanding of critical concepts rather than deep learning. Additionally, while gamification can enhance motivation, it may also distract from essential foundational knowledge if not integrated thoughtfully into the curriculum [8]. There is also a risk of over-reliance on gamified methods at the expense of traditional learning approaches that provide essential theoretical grounding. Lastly, the effectiveness of gamification may vary among different populations due to cultural differences or individual learning preferences, necessitating further research to identify best practices for diverse student groups [9][4].

6 CONCLUSION

Gamification holds immense potential to transform dental education by enhancing engagement, motivation, and learning outcomes. However, successful integration requires careful planning, support from educators, and ongoing evaluation to ensure its efficacy. As dental curricula continue to adapt to modern educational trends, gamification can play a key role in preparing future dental professionals with both the knowledge and skills necessary for clinical practice. Balancing innovative approaches with established pedagogical principles will be crucial for maximizing the benefits of gamification in dental training.

ACKNOWLEDGEMENTS

None

REFERENCES

[1] Roche CC, Wingo NP, Westfall AO, Azuero A, Dempsey DM, Willig JH. (2018). Educational analytics: a new frontier for gamification?. *CIN: Computers, Informatics, Nursing*. 36(9):458–65.

[2] Schimunda N, de Souza Silva FJ, Fregoneze AP, Petraukas A, Doetzer AD, Spada PC, Torres MF, Brancher JA. (2023). Gamification as a learning resource for dentistry students–experience report. *Revista Contemporânea*. 3(12):29802–14.

[3] Buajeeb W, Chokpipatkun J, Achalanan N, Kriwattanawong N, Sipiyaruk K. (2023). The development of an online serious game for oral diagnosis and treatment planning: evaluation of knowledge acquisition and retention. *BMC Medical Education*. 23(1):830.

[4] Zaror C, Mariño R, Atala-Acevedo C. (2021). Current state of serious games in dentistry: a scoping review. *Games for Health Journal*. 10(2):95–108.

[5] Higgins D, Hayes M, Taylor J, Wallace J. (2020). A scoping review of simulation-based dental education. *MedEdPublish*. 9.

[6] Khan S, Maheshwari S, Ghani S, Hakim S, Gaur A. (2017). Quizzing as an innovative Teaching-Learning technique for undergraduate dental students. *Indian Journal of Orthodontics and Dentofacial Research*. 3(4):235–7.

[7] Dashash M, Alkhadragy R, Scanlan GM. (2024). A phenomenological exploration of experience of Syrian dentists with online Course "Traumatic dental injuries". *Heliyon*. 10(13).

[8] Teerawongpairoj C, Tantipoj C, Sipiyaruk K. (2024). The design and evaluation of gamified online role-play as a telehealth training strategy in dental education: an explanatory sequential mixed-methods study. *Scientific Reports*. 14(1):9216.

[9] Moreira R, Silveira A, Sequeira T, Durão N, Lourenço J, Cascais I, Cabral RM, Gomes TT. (2024). Gamification and Oral Health in Children and Adolescents: Scoping Review. *Interactive Journal of Medical Research* 13(1):e35132.

[10] Krause F, Horn B, Braun A, Fedrowitz S, Bell L, Lemos M. (2024). Who learns more: the impact of dual-player and single-player modes in a serious game on dental students' factual knowledge. *BMC Medical Education*. 24(1):902.

[11] Yang CY, Lo YS, Liu CT. (2010). Developing an interactive dental casting educational game. *Proceedings 2010 3rd IEEE In ternational Conference on Computer Science and Information Technology*, ICCSIT; Chengdu, China; 4, pp. 437–440.

[12] Amer RS, Denehy GE, Cobb DS, *et al.* (2011). Development and evaluation of an interactive dental video game to teach dentin bonding. *J Dent Educ* 75:823–831

[13] Paiva PVF, Machado LS, Valenc,a AMG, *et al.* (2013). Uma pro posta de serious game para o ensino de biosseguranc,a em odontologia. *Pesqui Bras Odontopediatria cli´n Integr* 13:135–139.

[14] de Vasconcelos JE, Salomao J, Madeira B, *et al.* (2014). Odonto Quiz: Um Jogo Se ´rio de Apoio ao estudo da disciplina de pro´ teses denta´rias. *Proceedings of the SBGames*. https://www.sbgames.org/sbgames2014/papers/computing/ short/5_allcomputing-shortpages.pdf (accessed October 1, 2020).

[15] Vahed A. (2016). From dental bite to dental bytes: Students' ex periences of a game-based project. *European Conference on Games Based Learning*; Paisley, United Kingdom; pp. 713–721.

[16] Ribeiro MAO, Corre^a CG, Nunes FLS. (2017). Gamification as a Learning Strategy in a Simulation of Dental Anesthesia, *2017 19th Symposium on Virtual and Augmented Reality (SVR)*, Curitiba, pp. 271–278.

[17] Rodrı´guez-Andre´s D, Carmen J, Molla´ R, Mendez-Lopez M. (2017). A 3D serious game for dental learning in higher education. *IEEE 17th International Conference on Ad vanced Learning Technologies*. http://personales.upv.es/mjuanli/docs/2017_ICALT_Dental.pdf (accessed October 1, 2020).

[18] Sipiyaruk K, Gallagher JE, Hatzipanagos S, Reynolds PA. (2017). Acquiring critical thinking and decision-making skills: An evaluation of a serious game used by Undergraduate Dental Students in Dental Public Health. *Tech Know Learn* 22:209.

[19] Feitosa MLB, Rendeiro MMP, de Oliveira AEF. (2018). Serious Games for good practices in dentistry. [Serious game—paraboas pra´ticas em odontologia]. *Vigil sanit debate* 6: 71–78.

Tooth Tech: The Impact of Augmented Reality on Dental Education: A Literature Review

Adithya Kashyap K
Department of Conservative Dentistry & Endodontics, KVG Dental College & Hospital, Sullia, Karnataka, India

Thesnymol T M
Consultant Endodontist, Thrissur, Kerala, India

K Harish Shetty, Nishi Jayasheelan P, and Prathap M S
Department of Conservative Dentistry & Endodontics, Yenepoya Dental College, Mangalore, Karnataka, India

ABSTRACT: The field of dental education has experienced a remarkable transformation in recent years, thanks to the advent of innovative technologies. Among these, Augmented Reality (AR) stands out as a game-changer, offering unprecedented opportunities for enhancing both the teaching and learning processes. AR overlays digital information onto the physical world, allowing users to interact with both real and virtual elements in real-time. In dental education, AR is revolutionizing how students and professionals alike train and simulate patient scenarios, ultimately leading to improved clinical outcomes. This review aims to provide information about the currently available use of AR in dental education.

Keywords: Augmented Reality, Dental Education, Systematic Review, Learning Outcomes, Educational Technology

1 INTRODUCTION

Dental education has traditionally relied on textbooks, lectures, and hands-on practice in clinical settings to teach students the skills required for diagnosis, treatment, and patient care. However, recent technological advancements, particularly **Augmented Reality (AR)**, are revolutionizing how dental education is delivered.

Augmented reality (AR) refers to the real-time integration of digital information into a user's environment. AR technology overlays content onto the real world, enriching a user's perception of reality rather than replacing it.This immersive technology enhances learning experiences by bridging the gap between theoretical knowledge and practical application.

2 IMPORTANCE OF AR IN EDUCATION

Augmented reality is part of the broader spectrum of immersive technologies, which also includes Virtual Reality (VR) and Mixed Reality (MR). While VR provides a fully immersive digital environment, AR allows users to maintain a connection with the physical world while interacting with virtual enhancements. This feature makes AR particularly suited for medical and dental education, where real-world context and spatial awareness are critical.

In dental education, AR can be utilized to create lifelike simulations of dental procedures, anatomy visualization, and interactive learning modules. The advantages include improved engagement, the ability to practice in a low-risk environment, and an enhanced understanding of complex dental structures. AR can simulate scenarios that are difficult or costly to recreate in traditional training environments, such as rare dental pathologies or emergency situations.

2.1 *Scope of AR in dental education*

(1) AR provides a deeper understanding of complex dental structures and procedures by allowing students to interact with and manipulate 3D models in real-time.
(2) AR enables students to practice procedures in a risk-free environment before working on live patients, reducing the likelihood of mistakes and improving overall confidence.
(3) AR systems can offer real-time feedback on students' performance, allowing them to correct mistakes on the spot and learn more efficiently.

DOI: 10.1201/9781042016075-76

(4) The interactive nature of AR keeps students more engaged than traditional methods, promoting active learning and retention of knowledge.
(5) AR-based learning tools can be implemented in both small and large educational institutions, making it accessible to a wider audience of learners.

2.2 *Objective*

This review paper aims to highlight the effectiveness of AR in dental education, focusing on its impact on student learning outcomes, retention of knowledge, and skill acquisition.

2.3 *Methodology*

An extensive review of peer-reviewed published articles was conducted. Databases such as PubMed, Scopus, and Google Scholar were searched using keywords related to AR in dental education. Studies were analysed for their methodologies, findings, and implications for teaching practices.

2.4 *Inclusion and Exclusion criteria*

Articles addressing the potential application of AR in dental education and published in English language were included in the study. Studies which were not published in English, inability to access the full text were excluded from the review.

3 RESULTS

The review identified several key applications of AR in dental education:

(1) **Applications in Teaching Dental Morphology:**

Traditionally, anatomy has been studied using cadavers, synthetic models, and static 2-dimensional (2D) images like flashcards. However, because anatomical structures are inherently 3D, these methods often fall short, making it difficult for students to fully grasp the subject.

AR based algorithms can be used to learn anatomical structures, making the learning experience easier and more immersive. Moreover, these 3D AR based models can enhance spatial knowledge, helping to bridge the gap between students with varying levels of spatial visualization skills.

Augmented Reality (AR) algorithms offer an improved way to learn anatomical structures, making the experience more engaging and immersive. These 3D AR models can significantly enhance spatial understanding, helping to bridge the gap between students with different levels of spatial visualization skills. A study by Küçük *et al.* highlighted that dental students appear more interested in learning anatomical structures through a 3D model than through traditional 2D methods [1].

(2) **Applications in pre-clinical education:**

A significant proportion of dental education is dedicated to teaching clinical psychomotor skills to students via various pre-clinical activities before trying them directly on the patients. Rather than using synthetic models for these, various dental schools use realistic patient simulators with dental models incorporated to simulate a dental treatment.

Various AR based simulators & their advantages are mentioned in the below table: [22]

S. NO	Simulator name	Application
1.	Moog Simodont dental trainer	Efficient performance in the practice of cavity preparation
2.	Virteasy dental trainer	Caries removal practice for efficient drilling skills improvement
3.	SensAble OMNI and SensAble PHANToM OMNI haptic device	Visuo-tactile caries identification and its removal following minimally invasive techniques
4.	DentSim dental trainer	Visualization of the typhodont teeth and view their work from multiple angles to see their work compared to the ideal.
5.	SimEx-Plus	3D digital interactive real-time training provides real-time feedback of angle, depth, and flatness of the preparation
6.	Mobile- application based	Using a mobile device in a headset and specially designed patterned models for IANB training

These simulators enable instructors to demonstrate techniques that improve students' hand-eye coordination and manual dexterity. This approach ensures a comprehensive learning experience and enhances skill development.

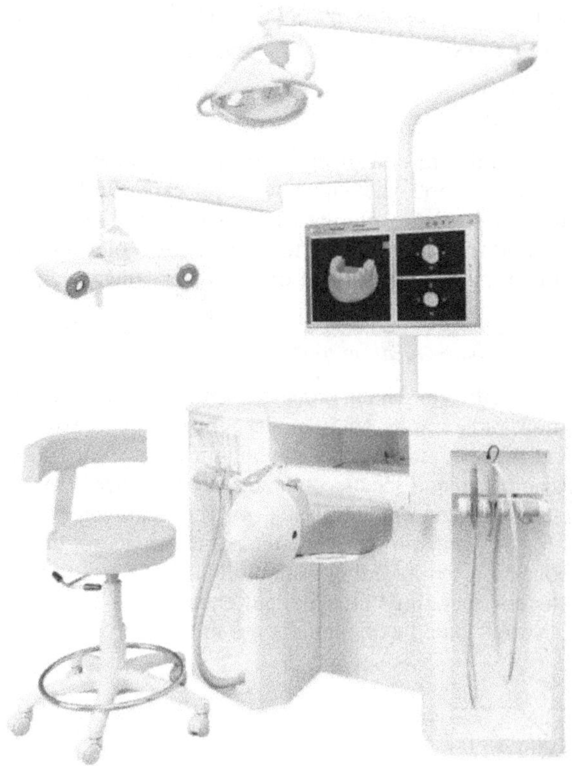

SimEx – Plus based simulator [14].

A study by Dwisaptarini *et al.* found an improvement in performance score in undergraduate dental students when AR based simulator was used in training for caries removal, leading minimal tooth structure damage and higher efficiency [2].

Another advantage of AR technology was during the COVID 19 pandemic, when limitations in pre-clinical education was seen, as many students could not be trained at their institution and lacked a proper guidance and tutoring form their mentor. AR helped in achieving the balance between the training of dental students and limiting the spread of infected cases [3].

3.1 *Applications in clinical practice*

The medical applications of AR are currently concentrated on different surgery types, including neurosurgery, laparoscopic surgery, and plastic surgery. In dentistry, AR is primary used in oral and maxillofacial surgery, dental implant placement and orthognathic surgery [4]. The development of Augmented Reality (AR) devices allows users to overlay medical information, data, and images onto real-world environments. Unlike conventional image-guided surgery, where surgeons have to look away from the operative field to view information, AR guidance systems project real-time intraoperative data directly onto the surgical field [5].

Also, AR based models aid in practising the administration of various local anaesthetic techniques in terms of landmark understanding, time and success rate. A study by Mladenovic *et al.* reported that with the use of AR supported device, undergraduate students were able to perform Inferior alveolar nerve block (IANB) faster, specifically shorter time between uncapping of needle to receiving a negative aspiration test [6].

3.2 *Applications in dental phobia*

An estimated 50–60% of people experience dental anxiety or phobia, making fear-related behaviours one of the toughest challenges in dental patient management. This anxiety often leads individuals to seek dental care only when their condition becomes severe, complicating effective treatment. Clinically, techniques such as cognitive–behavioural treatments, nitrous oxide, and intravenous sedatives administered during dental treatments have been found to minimize patient pain and discomfort during dental care. Following the same concept as distraction, AR based models can serve as an effective non-pharmacologic method managing patients' dental pain.

A recent study by Alabduljabbar R *et al* suggested that an AR-based system is both feasible and effective in managing dental anxiety in young patients [7]. Other studies have also reported that incorporating AR into clinical practice as a distraction technique can be a promising tool for complex procedures and can help to deliver safe and atraumatic experience in paediatric patients [8].

3.3 *Applications in patient education*

Educational and motivational methods are crucial in informing individuals about their oral health and related pathologies, thereby enhancing their compliance with home oral care. Oral health education improves patients' attitudes and practices regarding oral hygiene, offering useful devices and techniques for dental plaque control.

AR can be considered an important and effective tool to educate old and young patients, by teaching the importance of oral health, motivating the prevention of oral diseases, and making oral health practices attractive.

3.4 *Application as Dentist- Patient communication tool*

Clinicians use several tools to collect different data in order to formulate the correct functional and aesthetic treatment plan such as: physical examination, radiographs, study models, intraoral and extraoral photographs. Once the diagnosis has been made, the patient must be informed of the chosen therapeutic modalities, based on his/her clinical situation and on evaluating psychological and socio-economic aspects. Nevertheless, many patients may not have the necessary knowledge to understand the concepts illustrated for the treatment plan and the condition of their oral cavity; thus, it may be difficult for the dentist to persuade the patient to accept the proposed therapeutic option.

AR also enhances patient education by providing visual aids that help patients understand their dental conditions and treatment options, thereby fostering better patient engagement and informed decision-making. Studies indicate that patients who receive AR-based explanations are more likely to adhere to treatment plans and have higher satisfaction levels [9].

4 CHALLENGES AND LIMITATIONS OF AR

(1) Technological and financial barriers
(2) Learning curve and training requirements
(3) Data privacy and security
(4) Technical limitations and integration issues

5 DISCUSSION

As healthcare continues to evolve, dentistry is at the forefront of innovation, emerging as a leader in adopting innovative technologies. Augmented Reality (AR), once primarily used in gaming and entertainment, has now found significant applications in dentistry. This transformative technology is reshaping the field by enhancing precision, improving patient interaction and education, and also advancing diagnostic capabilities, marking a new era of dental care.

Augmented Reality (AR) integrates digital information into the physical environment, thereby offering enhanced visual guidance through wearable devices like smart glasses or headsets. This technology enables dentists, and patients to access real-time visual overlays [10].

The primary function of AR in dentistry is to improve understanding and enhance decision-making by projecting critical information directly into the clinician's view. This may include 3D representations of teeth, radiographic scans, treatment plans, and patient details [11].

With an AR headset, dentists can offer patients a dynamic and visually enriched explanation of their dental health. The headset can project 3D visuals of the patient's teeth, highlighting issues such as decay, misalignment, or gum problems. This allows patients to see and better understand their condition instantly [12,13].

Also the dentists can utilize these visual tools to break down intricate procedures, illustrating how treatments like fillings, crowns, or orthodontics will address specific concerns. They can also provide guided demonstrations of proper oral care techniques, such as brushing and flossing, using interactive overlays, thereby improving communication and awareness, encourages patient involvement, and supports well-informed treatment decisions [12].

AR enables the dental students and practitioners to use virtual simulations to practice procedures in a controlled and risk-free environment. These simulations allow them to experience different clinical scenarios, replicating real-life challenges without the need for a live patient. This approach enables them to refine their techniques, explore complex cases, and learn from mistakes without causing harm. The hands-on experience provided by virtual scenarios build confidence in their abilities and also bridges the gap between theoretical knowledge and practical application, preparing them for real-world patient care [10].

During dental surgeries, this can offer a real-time guidance by enabling dentists to see critical anatomical features, such as nerves, blood vessels, and bone structures, overlaid onto the operative area, thereby enhancing accuracy and safety [10].

AR also monitors the location and movement of surgical tools, allowing dentists to maintain precision throughout the procedure. This level of technology-based feedback ensures accurate execution, particularly in complex tasks like implant placement or extractions, ultimately improving surgical efficiency and outcomes [12].

This particular technology fosters collaborative learning by allowing multiple students to interact with the same virtual model in a shared environment, thereby enhancing the overall learning experience, as it provides an opportunity for the learners to work together on complex cases, share insights, and discuss solutions in real time. Instructors can also leverage AR to provide real-time guidance and feedback, whether they are physically present or teaching remotely. This capability makes dental education more flexible and accessible, especially for institutions in regions with limited resources or for students unable to attend in-person classes. The benefits of AR became particularly evident during the COVID-19 pandemic, as it allowed education to continue despite restrictions on physical interactions, ensuring that students could maintain their learning progress without compromising safety [12,14,15].

These advanced technologies can also enhance communication among dental practitioners, dental technicians, patients, especially when it comes to complex cases requiring a multi-disciplinary approach for problem solving [12,15].

Rhienmora *et al.* (2010) introduced an AR-based dental training simulator incorporating a haptic feedback device, which enabled the students to practice various procedures, such as crown preparation and pulp access, using different dental drill shapes. [16]

Qu *et al.* (2015) developed an AR-assisted navigation technique to enhance surgical precision. Their system displays 3D mandible images with pre-designed cutting planes, providing a visual guide for transferring osteotomy lines and screw positions during procedures [17].

Espejo-Trung *et al.* (2015) created an AR learning tool to teach gold onlay preparation techniques at a dental school in Brazil. The tool garnered strong support from students, demonstrating its effectiveness in improving dental education [18].

One of the primary advantages of AR is its lower development cost compared to VR. AR development can be performed on a standard computer or laptop with a 2 GB off-board video card and 8 GB of RAM or more, using free software. Additionally, AR models can be viewed and interacted with easily on most mobile devices with default settings [19].

When creating 3D models for AR, existing patient data such as CBCT, CT, MRI scans, or digital dental models ordered by the dentist or physician can be utilized. These images are processed similarly across different 3D imaging methods, although digital dental models and digitized plaster models are typically saved in .stl format, while other imaging data is stored in DICOM format. DICOM files are compatible with most 3D image analysis software for viewing and manipulation [19].

Although the potential of AR has a number of advantages, its key limitations include high costs and the complexity of system operation. The expensive hardware and software required for AR applications can be a significant barrier to widespread adoption. Additionally, the systems often have a steep learning curve, making them challenging for users, including dental professionals and students, to operate efficiently. These factors hinder the broader implementation of AR in clinical and educational settings [12].

Other challenges include its time consumption, issues in rendering quality, and cloud storage limitations. The AR creation process is time-consuming due to the need to remove artifacts from 3D models, especially when using CBCT images, which have more noise and metal-induced artifacts. Rendering times can be long, and the quality may not always be optimal, depending on the software and computer specifications. Once created, however, models can be shared globally [19].

Rendering issues arise from thresholding techniques, which can create artifacts, especially in thin bones or areas with metal, like dental fillings or implants. This leads to inaccuracies in 3D reconstructions. Additionally, factors like scan field size and voxel resolution impact the quality of the 3D models.

A significant challenge is cloud storage. Open-source software offers limited space (100 MB), which restricts the creation of more detailed models. Partnerships with commercial AR software can improve model quality and add features like colour adjustments and animations [19].

Although this review outlines the potential applications of AR-assisted learning in various fields of dentistry, more specific information is required regarding its use in different dental specialties. Additionally, there is a lack of research on how AR devices affect the cognitive load of users. A recent systematic review indicated that these devices may result in either lower or comparable cognitive load compared to traditional methods like paper or screen-based instructions. However, further studies are needed to assess cognitive load in real-world clinical and educational settings. To maximize the benefits of AR, future research should focus on ethical issues, learning theories, and cognitive load [12].

6 CONCLUSION

Augmented Reality (AR) has great potential to revolutionize dental education, making it more interactive and effective. To fully harness this potential, ongoing research and investment are crucial. Future advancements may integrate Artificial Intelligence (AI) to create adaptive learning environments, tailoring training programs to individual learning styles. Additionally, haptic feedback technology could further enhance the realism of AR training by simulating tactile sensations of dental procedures.

REFERENCES

[1] Küçük S, Kapakin S, Göktaş Y. (2016). Learning anatomy via mobile augmented reality: Effects on achievement and cognitive load. *Anatomical Sciences Education*. 9(5):411–21.

[2] Dwisaptarini AP, Suebnukarn S, Rhienmora P, Haddawy P, Koontongkaew S. (2018). Effectiveness of the multilayered caries model and visuo-tactile virtual reality simulator for minimally invasive caries removal: A randomized controlled trial. *Operative Dentistry*. 43(3):E110–8.

[3] Ball C, Huang KT, Francis J. (2021). Virtual reality adoption during the COVID-19 pandemic: A uses and gratifications perspective. *Telematics and Informatics*. 65:101728.

[4] Kwon HB, Park YS, Han JS. (2018). Augmented reality in dentistry: a current perspective. *Acta Odontologica Scandinavica*. 76 (7):497–503.

[5] Vávra P, Roman J, Zonča P, Ihnát P, N⊠mec M, Kumar J, Habib N, El-Gendi A. (2017). Recent development of augmented reality in surgery: a review. *Journal of Healthcare Engineering*. 2017(1):4574172.

[6] Mladenovic R, Pereira LA, Mladenovic K, Videnovic N, Bukumiric Z, Mladenovic J. (2019). Effectiveness of augmented reality mobile simulator in teaching local anesthesia of inferior alveolar nerve block. *Journal of Dental Education*. 83(4):423–8.

[7] Alabduljabbar R, Almutawa M, Alkathiri R, Alqahtani A, Alshamlan H. (2023). An interactive augmented and virtual reality system for managing Dental anxiety among young patients: a pilot study. *Applied Sciences*. 13(9):5603.

[8] Yucel G, DemIr B, SmalI FS, YaYIm PS. (2023). Use of Augmented Reality in Alleviating Dental Anxiety among Paediatric Patients: A Randomised Control Study. *Journal of Clinical & Diagnostic Research*. 17(7).

[9] Davis L *et al.* (2022). *J Dent Educ. 86*:487. [PMID: 89012345].

[10] Farronato M, Maspero C, Lanteri V, Fama A, Ferrati F, Pettenuzzo A, Farronato D. (2019). Current state of the art in the use of augmented reality in dentistry: a systematic review of the literature. *BMC oral health*. 19:1–5.

[11] Blanchard J, Koshal S. (2024). Augmented reality: a new perspective in dental education. *Faculty Dental Journal*. 15(2):68–72.

[12] Monterubbianesi R, Tosco V, Vitiello F, Orilisi G, Fraccastoro F, Putignano A, Orsini G. (2022). Augmented, virtual and mixed reality in dentistry: a narrative review on the existing platforms and future challenges. *Applied Sciences*. 12(2):877.

[13] Haji Z, Arif A, Jamal S, Ghafoor R. (2021). Augmented reality in clinical dental training and education. *JPMA. The Journal of the Pakistan Medical Association*. 71(1 (Suppl 1)):S42.

[14] Lai PL, Liu CT, Fu PS, Chen JH, Lan TH, Wang JC, Hung CC. (2024). Achieving new excellence in an augmented reality dental education system. *Journal of Dental Sciences*.

[15] Erdilek D, Gümüştaş B, Güray Efes B. (2023). Digitalization era of dental education: A systematic review. *Dental and Medical Problems*. 60(3):513–25.

[16] Rhienmora P, Gajananan K, Haddawy P, Dailey MN, Suebnukarn S. (2010). Augmented reality haptics system for dental surgical skills training. In *Proceedings of the 17th ACM Symposium on Virtual Reality Software and Technology* (pp. 97–98).

[17] Qu M, Hou Y, Xu Y, Shen C, Zhu M, Xie L, Wang H, Zhang Y, Chai G. (2015). Precise positioning of an intraoral distractor using augmented reality in patients with hemifacial microsomia. *Journal of Cranio-Maxillofacial Surgery*. 43(1):106–12.

[18] Espejo-Trung LC, Elian SN, De Cerqueira Luz MA. (2015). Development and application of a new learning object for teaching operative dentistry using augmented reality. *Journal of Dental Education*. 79(11):1356–62.

[19] Santos GN, da Rosa EL, Leite AF, de Souza Figueiredo PT, de Melo NS. (2016). Augmented reality as a new perspective in dentistry: development of a complementary tool. *Revista da ABENO*. 16(3):19–27.

[20] Mladenovic R. (2020). The usage of augmented reality in dental education. *Augmented Reality in Education: A New Technology for Teaching and Learning*. 139–57.

[21] Li Y, Ye H, Ye F, Liu Y, Lv L, Zhang P, Zhang X, Zhou Y. (2021). The current situation and future prospects of simulators in dental education. *Journal of Medical Internet Research*. 23(4):e23635.

[22] Dzyuba N, Jandu J, Yates J, Kushnerev E. (2022). Virtual and augmented reality in dental education: the good, the bad and the better. *European Journal of Dental Education*.

 ISBN: 978-1-041-32674-8

Comparative Efficacy of Virtual YouTube Instruction, Traditional Chalk-and-Talk, and PowerPoint Presentation Methods in Teaching First-Year BDS Students: A Randomized Controlled Trial in a Kerala

Abdul Saheer P
Department of Public Health Dentistry, Malabar Dental College and Research Centre, Manoor, Edappal, Kerala

Megha J Nair
Department of Pediatric and Preventive Dentistry, Malabar Dental College and Research Centre, Manoor, Edappal, Kerala

ABSTRACT: This study aims to evaluate and compare the effectiveness of three distinct teaching modalities—chalk and talk, PowerPoint presentation, and video learning—in delivering educational content on Root Canal Treatment, Tooth Preparation, and CBCT to first-year BDS students. 60 participants were randomly allocated into three groups. After conducting pre-assessment using objective test on RCT, tooth preparation and CBCT, each group will be exposed to all the three teaching modalities on one of the three topics. The study materials were standardized, and interactions between groups were avoided. Post- assessment were conducted to assess performance using same objective tests. One way ANOVA and post-hoc test, used for comparative analysis of teaching methods revealed that the video-based learning approach, utilizing online videos, was significantly more effective in enhancing student understanding of the topics compared to traditional chalk and talk and PowerPoint presentation methods. Students who engaged with the video content demonstrated superior performance on a standardized test, with notably higher scores and improved comprehension of key concepts. This suggests that video-based instruction offers a more impactful learning experience for first-year BDS students in this context. However, future studies should be done to explore long-term retention and application of knowledge to better understand the sustained impact of each teaching method.

Keywords: Virtual learning, Teaching

1 INTRODUCTION

For many decades the traditional didactic lectures have been the most popular mode of teaching, where a teacher delivers a well prepared lecture orally using black board and chalk to draw the diagram and important points and tries to explain the complex concepts. It has been a universally accepted way of teaching, and adopted in almost all universities. [1,2] However, there has been a shift in the teaching modality from a conventional lecture based method to a more technology oriented, clinical based and student centred approach attributed to advances in information technology as well as time constraints. [3]

PowerPoint (PPT)-based lectures are common in dental schools, similar to other higher education institutions. Nevertheless, there is ongoing debate among educators about whether PPT presentations offer advantages over the traditional chalk-and-board method. Various studies have compared the effectiveness of PPT or overhead projector (OHP) presentations with chalk-and-board lectures, but the results are mixed and inconclusive regarding the superiority of one method over the other. Furthermore, most of these studies have been conducted in developed countries, leaving a gap in research for developing countries. [4]

Video serves as a powerful educational tool that can complement both didactic and Socratic teaching methods. Visual imagery often proves more effective than verbal communication for capturing and maintaining audience attention. Within a limited timeframe, videos can offer detailed explanations, simplifying complex concepts. Incorporating images into the curriculum has been shown to enhance learning retention. Videos can be tailored specifically with voluntary participants, such as students, faculty, and interns, or even actors, and can also be animated to illustrate concepts. Additionally, pre-existing videos can be repurposed for educational use. [5–8]

It is important to understand the effectiveness of these different teaching modalities on students in dental education so that their preferred lecture delivery method could be adopted to make the lectures more useful. There are no studies comparing the effectiveness of online YouTube video learning to other teaching modalities. Thus, this study aimed to evaluate and compare the effectiveness of three distinct teaching modalities—chalk and talk, PowerPoint presentation, and video learning—in delivering educational content on Root Canal Treatment, Tooth Preparation, and CBCT to first-year BDS students.

DOI: 10.1201/9781042016075-77

2 METHODOLOGY

The study aimed to compare the effectiveness of three different teaching modalities—traditional "chalk and talk," PowerPoint presentations, and YouTube videos—on first-year BDS students' learning outcomes in a dental college in Kerala. A total of sixty female students, aged 17-19, who had scored above 80% in their higher secondary examinations and had no prior exposure to the subject matter, were randomly selected for participation. Students with comprehension difficulties in routine classes were excluded from the study. Informed consent was obtained from all participants prior to the study, ensuring that they understood the purpose of the research and the use of their assessment data.

The participants were divided into three groups, each exposed to one of the three teaching modalities. The content focused on Root Canal Treatment (RCT), tooth preparation, and Cone Beam Computed Tomography (CBCT). Each modality was delivered by subject experts with at least 10 years of professional experience in the respective fields. The teaching sessions, whether delivered as a chalk-and-talk lecture, PowerPoint presentation, or YouTube video, were standardized in duration, each lasting 10 minutes to ensure consistency across all groups. Pre- and post-assessments, consisting of objective tests, were conducted offline to evaluate the participants' understanding of the topics. The tests included multiple-choice and short-answer questions, and were designed to measure any improvement in knowledge following the intervention.

The data were analyzed using One-Way ANOVA to compare the effectiveness of the three teaching methods, with post-hoc tests conducted to explore significant differences between the groups. Standardized study materials were used for all groups, and interactions between the groups were prevented to avoid any cross-contamination of learning.

3 RESULTS

Data was analysed using the statistical package SPSS 26.0 (SPSS Inc., Chicago, IL) and level of significance was set at $p<0.05$. Descriptive statistics was performed to assess the mean and standard deviation of the respective groups. Normality of the data was assessed using Shapiro Wilk test. Inferential statistics to find out the difference between the group was done using One-Way ANOVA followed by Bonferroni Post-hoc Test. Within group analysis was done using Paired T test.

		PRE	POST	Mean difference	P Value(t test)
CHALK N BOARD (C)		**3.67±0.40**	**4.66±0.28**	**0.99**	**0.0001***
PPT LECTURE (P)		**3.29±0.54**	**4.93±0.87**	**1.63**	**0.0001***
YOUTUBE (Y)		**3.44±0.72**	**5.38±0.68**	**1.94**	**0.0001***
P value (One way ANOVA)		**0.11**	**0.003***		
POSTHOC TEST	**C vs P**	**0.09**	**0.40**		
	C vs Y	**0.41**	**0.002***		
	P vs Y	**0.68**	**0.08**		

The study assessed the effectiveness of three teaching modalities—chalk and board, PowerPoint presentations, and YouTube videos—on student performance. Pre-assessment scores were 3.67 ± 0.40 for the chalk and board group, 3.29 ± 0.54 for the PowerPoint group, and 3.44 ± 0.72 for the YouTube group. Post-assessment scores showed improvements to 4.66 ± 0.28, 4.93 ± 0.87, and 5.38 ± 0.68, respectively. The mean difference in scores was 0.99 (p = 0.0001) for chalk and board, 1.63 (p = 0.0001) for PowerPoint, and 1.94 (p = 0.0001) for YouTube. One-way ANOVA revealed a significant overall difference between the modalities (p = 0.003). Post-hoc tests showed that while the difference between chalk and board and PowerPoint as well as PowerPoint and YouTube was not significant (p = 0.40, p=0.08), YouTube outperformed the chalk and board (p = 0.002) method.

4 DISCUSSION

The study assessed the effectiveness of three teaching modalities—chalk and board, PowerPoint presentations, and YouTube videos—on student performance. Our study revealed that online YouTube video learning is significantly superior form of lecture delivery as compared to the traditional chalk and talk. Even though not significant, YouTube video learning was found to be more effective than PowerPoint presentation.

The results of our study aligns with another study comparing the chalk and board technique to ppt technique in anatomy subject. In this study ppt based teaching was found to be more effective in teaching students. [9] In another study by Paavizhi *et al.* investigating the effectiveness of Video assisted learning module , it was found that video based learning module outperformed conventional methods which endorses the findings of this study. [10]

5 CONCLUSION

Students who engaged with the video content demonstrated superior performance on a standardized test, with notably higher scores and improved comprehension of key concepts. This suggests that video-based instruction offers a more impactful learning experience for first-year BDS students in this context. However, since this study is the first of its kind, future studies should be done to explore long-term retention and application of knowledge to better understand the sustained impact of each teaching method.

6 LIMITATIONS

This study was performed on a small sample size in a single institution which limits the generalizability of the findings and may lead to institutional bias. Moreover, the objective tests used may not capture all aspects of learning and skill acquisition. This study didn't include any qualitative feedback from participants regarding their experiences or preferences.

7 FUTURE SCOPE

Given the limitations of the current study, several avenues for future research emerge. To enhance the generalizability and external validity of the findings, it would be beneficial to expand the sample size and include a multi-institutional cohort, ensuring a more diverse and representative participant pool. This approach would mitigate institutional bias and provide a broader perspective on the effectiveness of various teaching modalities. Furthermore, while objective assessments offer valuable insights into students' knowledge acquisition, they may not fully capture the development of clinical skills or the long-term retention of concepts. Future studies could incorporate more robust evaluation methods, such as practical exams, clinical assessments, or longitudinal follow-ups, to better assess the application of theoretical knowledge in real-world scenarios. Additionally, qualitative data obtained through participant interviews, surveys, or focus groups could provide deeper insights into students' perceptions of each teaching modality, their preferences, and the perceived effectiveness of the methods. Such qualitative feedback would complement the quantitative data and offer a more comprehensive understanding of how different teaching methods impact students' learning experiences. Finally, as digital education continues to evolve, exploring emerging technologies—such as interactive simulations, virtual reality (VR), and augmented reality (AR)—could offer valuable comparisons to traditional teaching approaches, potentially revolutionizing dental education by providing more engaging, immersive, and effective learning environments. Collectively, these directions for future research have the potential to refine teaching strategies in dental education, leading to more effective, evidence-based pedagogical practices that better prepare students for clinical practice.

ACKNOWLEDGEMENT

We would like to extend our sincere gratitude to all those who supported me throughout the course of this self-funded study.

REFERENCES

[1] Student Affairs Learning Domains. Emporia State University. [Last accessed on 2024 Sept 10]. Available from: https://www.emporia.edu/about-emporiastate-university/leadership-faculty-staff/student-affairs/dean-students/learning-and-assessment/co-curricular-learningdevelopment-model/learning-outcomes-assessment-guide/cocurricular-learning-process/learning-domains/

[2] Jabeen, N., Ghani, A. (2015). Comparison of the Traditional Chalk and Board Lecture System Versus PowerPoint Presentation as a Teaching Technique for Teaching Gross Anatomy to the First Professional Medical Students. *Journal of Evolution of Medical and Dental Sciences*, 4(11): 1811–1817.

[3] Szabo, A., Hastings, N. (2000). Using IT in the Undergraduate Classroom: Should We Replace the Blackboard with PowerPoint? *Computers & Education*, 35(3): 175–187.

[4] Susskind, J.E. (2005). PowerPoint's power in the classroom: Enhancing students' self-efficacy and attitudes. *Computers & Education*, 45(2): 203–215.

[5] Hurtubise, L., Martin, B., Gilliland, A., Mahan, J. (2013). To play or not to play: Leveraging video in medical education. *Journal of Graduate Medical Education*, 5(1): 13.

[6] Fox, G. (2003). Teaching normal development using stimulus videotapes in psychiatric education. *Academic Psychiatry*, 27: 283–288.

[7] Orientale, E.J., Kosowicz, L., Alerte, A., Pfeiffer, C., Harrington, K., Palley, J., *et al.* (2008). Using web-based video to enhance physical examination skills in medical students. *Family Medicine*, 40: 471–476.

[8] Pinsky, L.E., Wipf, J.E. (2000). A picture is worth a thousand words: Practical use of videotape in teaching. *Journal of General Internal Medicine*, 15: 805.

[9] Jabeen, N., Ghani, A. (2015). Comparison of the traditional chalk and blackboard lecture system versus powerpoint presentation as a teaching technique for teaching gross anatomy to the first professional Medical Students. *Journal of Evolution of Medical and Dental Sciences*, 4: 1811–1817.

[10] Paavizhi, K., Palanisamy, P., Saravanakumar, P. (2019). Effectiveness of video assisted learning module. *International Journal of Control and Automation*, 12: 268–275.

 ISBN: 978-1-041-32674-8

Enriching Student's Learning Process Through Project-Based Learning

Ashita Kalaskar and Shailesh Gondivkar
Department Oral Medicine and Radiology, Government Dental College and Hospital, Government Medical College Campus, Medical Square Nagpur, Maharashtra

ABSTRACT: To enhance the understanding of the basics of the subject (Oral Medicine and Radiology) and their clinical applicability, innovative teaching learning method of project based learning (PtBL) was tried with undergraduate students. The methodology included third year undergraduate students who were explained about the steps involved in PtBL. In a batch of 60 students, 55 were eligible and were divided into eleven groups of 5 each. They were allotted team-based PtBL topics which were mainly related to radiographic techniques and clinical examination. Students were expected to complete the projects in 7-10 days and present a final product of their project work either in the form of poster, video or power point presentation. Students maintained a logbook which was evaluated periodically by the allotted faculties. Student's perceptions were obtained by a pre-validated survey questionnaire. Data obtained was tabulated and statistically analysed. The results obtained revealed that a total of 50 students completed the projects and presented the final product as poster, video and power point presentation. Majority of the students perceived that the topics for PtBL were relevant. Satisfactory report was commented by the allotted faculties for the overall project work. Students perceptions regarding the integration of the basics of the provided topics with that of clinical skills development was appreciated as a positive impact on knowledge and overall skill development by most of the students. Thus it can be concluded that the innovative, team-based PtBL modules were well-perceived by most of the students.

Keywords: clinical applicability, project based learning, team based topics

1 INTRODUCTION

The aim behind providing dental education is to train the graduates so that they become efficient enough to take care of the oral health needs of the society at large. But the present dental curriculum which is mostly teacher centred, provides limited period and emphasises more on summative assessment, so achieving the above goal might seem to be difficult. Competency based medical education (CBME) seems to provide solutions in this aspect, which focuses on student centred learning and formative assessments which helps in developing the desired competencies in the students [1]. Problem-based learning, case-based learning, early clinical exposure, project based learning are few examples of CBME [1].

Project based learning (PtBL) is an instructional, active teaching learning method [2]. Its early proponents include John Dewey whose ideas of "learning by doing" were further popularized by his pupil William Heard Kilpatric [3]. In this method students utilize their previous knowledge and experience to systematically solve the given challenge or problem. While doing this they learn many new things which further helps in enhancing their knowledge and skills [4]. Although PtBL sounds similar to problem based learning, but the key differences are noteworthy. PjBL focuses on constructing the outcome of the given challenge, with the facilitators role being only advisory, giving the learners more control of their learning and thus making the process more flexible. On the contrary problem based learning focuses on making the learners study, with the facilitator role being present throughout the session and certain steps are needed to be followed scrupulously [5]. Also it is different from case based learning in which certain case scenarios are discussed mimicking the real world exposure, whereas in PjBL the learner goes a step ahead to perform in the real world [6].

PtBL has been utilized earlier as teaching learning method in higher education and initial years of medical education, providing beneficial results [7–9]. In dentistry, few PjBL models have been tried especially concerning Public Health Dentistry with regards to community services [10]. But as stated by Shah H.N et.al "PtBL is context-specific, its design varies according to the setting and purpose of its use" [2], its utilization and usefulness in Oral Medicine and Radiology (OMR) needs to be explored further.

OMR speciality includes dual subjects dealing with detailed clinical examination and radiographic investigations so as to provide diagnosis and medicinal treatment. Thus the undergraduates are required to understand and learn the technical aspects as well as the clinical skills efficiently to reach to a diagnosis to plan appropriate treatment. Therefore to enhance the understanding of the basics of the subject and their clinical applicability, PtBL was tried in undergraduate students.

 DOI: 10.1201/9781042016075-78

2 MATERIALS AND METHODS

After receiving the institutional ethical clearance, an interventional educational research was planned for the third year students undergoing Bachelor in Dental Surgery (BDS). The study was conducted from March 2022 to January 2023. Third year students were selected for the PtBL as OMR subject is introduced theoretically and practically in this year. Following the convenience sampling method, third year BDS students, who had attended the relevant lectures and practical demonstrations and consented to participate were included in the study.

The third year students batch consisted of 60 students, out of which 55 students fulfilled the inclusion criteria. The students were briefed about the PtBL. They were made aware about the projects they would be allotted and what they are expected to do. PtBL is a team based teaching learning method therefore eleven teams of 5 students each were made for the projects. The project was done by the students during their clinical posting in department, as this time they could devote solely to the project work. The time allotted for completion and submission of project was 7- 10 days. Students were asked to maintain a logbook in which they entered their daily activities, their experiences, knowledge gained, skill learned and solutions they could come across to solve the given challenge or problem. Each group was allotted a faculty who kept the track of all the activities the students were performing from initial step to the last, which also included checking their log book. Students followed the seven step process of PtBL as shown in Figure 1 [9]. These steps ensured that the students work in team, interact, discuss, explore the literature to find answers and gain relevant clinical exposure whenever possible (as the project work was done during clinical posting timing), thus fostering communication skills, critical thinking, clinical reasoning and skills while completing the project.

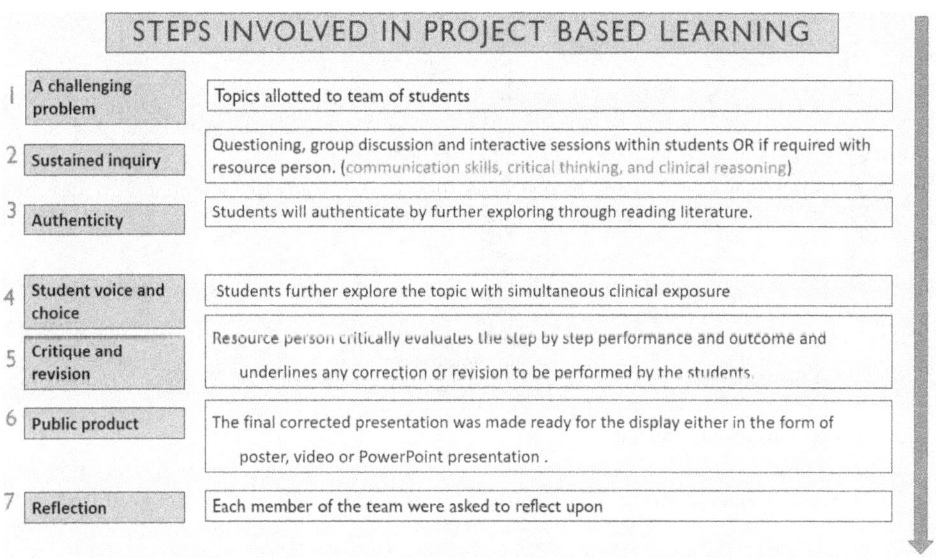

Figure 1. Seven steps involved in project based learning.

The concerned faculty worked as a silent observer, providing assistance whenever required and gave feedback at the end regarding any modifications or corrections to be done prior to submission of the final project work. The final corrected project was made ready for the display either in the form of poster, video or Power Point presentation, which the students presented in front of the entire class. The overall project work performed in teams was evaluated by a questionnaire containing 10 questions (questions related to communication, collaboration, active participation, responsibilities, accountability, timeline followed, information gathered, clinical applicability, corrections performed and final displaly of project work). The facilitators ticked the most appropriate response out of the four responses of slightly dissatisfactory, dissatisfactory, slightly satisfactory and satisfactory. The scoring for the responses was as follows: slightly dissatisfactory= 1, dissatisfactory= 2, slightly satisfactory= 3 and satisfactory= 4. For reporting convenience, slightly dissatisfactory and dissatisfactory were combined and reported as dissatisfactory (score=1 to 20), and slightly satisfactory and satisfactory were combined and reported as satisfactory (score= 21 to 40). The concerned faculty reported on the overall work of the teams as satisfactory or dissatisfactory.

Students perceptions were evaluated by a validated self-structured survey containing 20 item questionnaire (17 questions had responses on 5-point Lickert scale, 2 had responses as yes / no and one was an open ended questions) [12].

3 RESULTS

Students were in the age range of 20-21 years, with more females (41) than males (14). All 11 teams completed the projects satisfactorily with few students (5) unable to continue due to health related issues. Log book was maintained by most of the students (47). The survey questionnaire was completed by 50 students. For reporting purpose, the responses related to agree and strongly agree were combined to agree and responses related to disagree and strongly disagree were combined to disagree. Majority students agreed that the provided topics for PtBL were relevant to the subject (50) and PtBL could be expanded to other subject topics as well (45). Regarding the perceptions related to students understanding and overall improvement, majority students agreed that the steps involved in PtBL emphasized the technical as well as academic aspects(43), enhanced the understanding of the topic (47) and had a positive impact on academic growth (43) and clinical skill improvement (48). Regarding perceptions related to overall PtBL, all students agreed that there was fair assessment of their work and PtBL enhanced positive interaction between teachers and students. Presenting the project in front of all the students helped to expand the benefits to others. Forty one students agreed to this. 40 students agreed that they would like to do PtBL activities in future and also would like to try in other subjects of dentistry also (44). Almost all agreed that they preferd to do the PtBL activity in team rather than individually. Good learning experience, fun-filled interactive activities and good opportunity to improve communication and clinical skills were few of the suggestions provided by the students (Graphs 1,2,3).

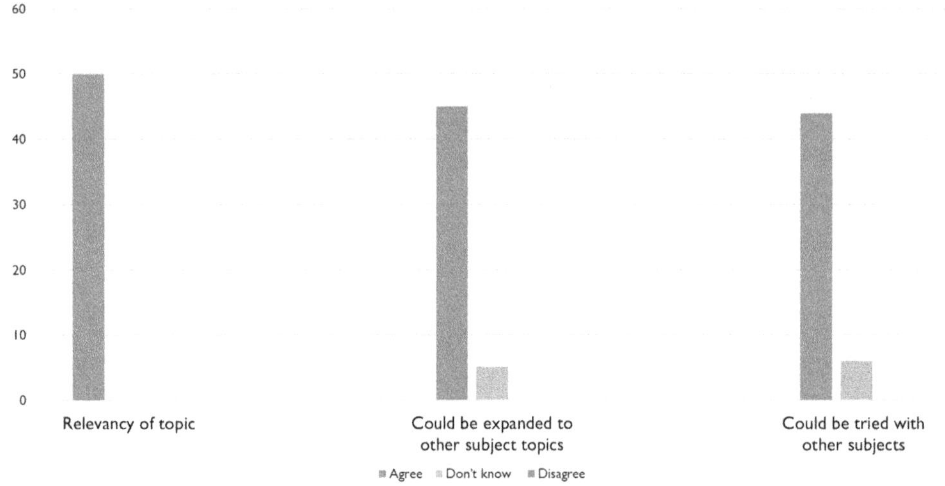

Graph 1. Students Perceptions related to topic.

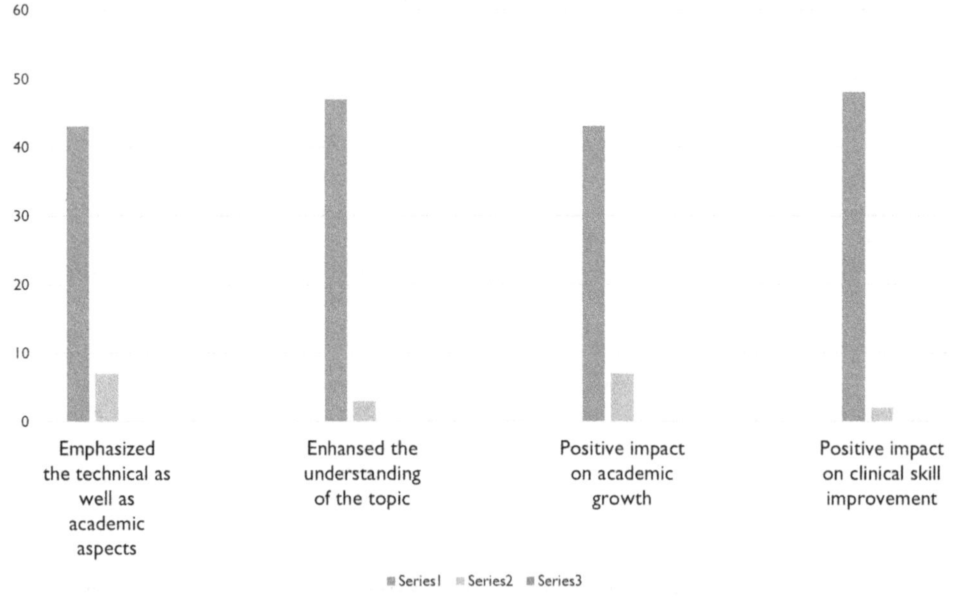

Graph 2. Students perceptions related to topic understanding and overall improvement.

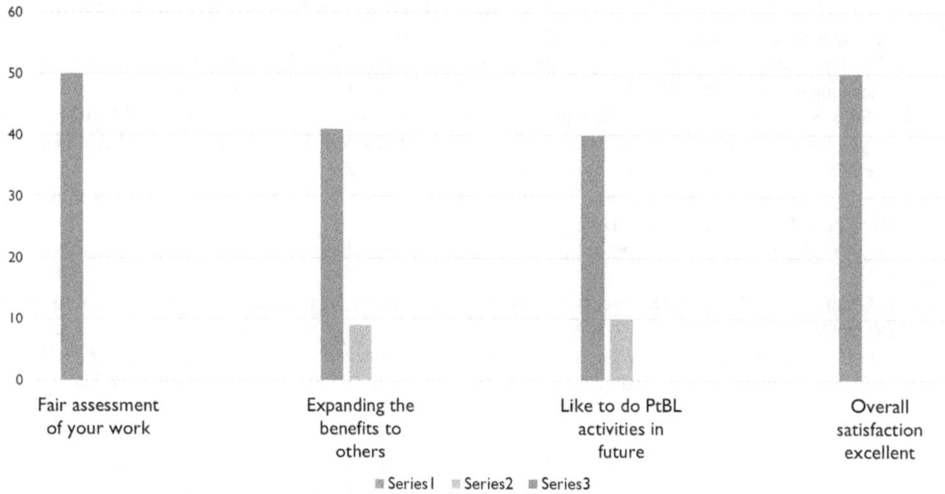

Graph 3. Students perceptions related to overall PtBL.

4 DISCUSSION

PtBL is a team based, student centred, self directed teaching learning method. It is based on the theory of constructivism which says that "learners construct knowledge rather than just passively take in information. As people experience the world and reflect upon those experiences, they build their own representations and incorporate new information into their pre-existing knowledge (schemas)" [13]. In the present study as the students went on performing the seven steps of PtBL they explored the possibilities of improving their communication skills through interactive sessions, improve their critical thinking through group discussions and improve their clinical reasoning skills by connecting basics of theory to clinical exposure. This ensures in-depth understanding which helps to improve quick recall of those topics and increase academic performance. The agreeing of most of the students in the present study regarding positive impact on academic growth and clinical skill improvement helps to justify this. Also most of the students preferred team work over individual work which highlights the possibilities of improving communication skills amongst the peers. Their willingness to perform more such activities in the future also shows their inclination toward student centred self-directed learning.

Presenting the completed project work in front of the class was well appreciated by most of the students. This helped in expanding the knowledge and experiences of the teams with other students.

Similar reports of PtBL were also reported by Shah H.N. et.al and Elkhamisy F.A.A. *et al.* who tried PtBL in MBBS students [2,12]. In dentistry, Costa-Silva *et al.* reported that PjBL model enhanced understanding of cell biology additionally with respect to its clinical application [14]. In yet another PjBL model by Yoo S H et.al. oral hygiene issues could be better identified from the society, enabling the learners to execute early and quick solutions to address them [15]. All these examples offer promising results with respect to PjBL.

There are few limitations in the present study. Objective based formative assessments of the students could give us the outcome related to effectiveness of PtBL, but as each group of students was given a different topic, formative assessment outcome could have varied in-between teams. Also control group could not be included owing to less number of students in class.

5 CONCLUSION

Within the limitations of the present study it can be concluded that PtBL can be used as an active teaching learning method in Oral Medicine and Radiology subject. Future studies involving vertical and horizontal integration of subjects involving larger sample of students, multicentre involvement and longitudinal study to evaluate PtBL's impact on summative assessment are required.

ACKNOWLEDGEMENT

We acknowledge all the students and faculties for conducting this research.

REFERENCES

[1] Shah N, Desai C, Jorwekar G, Badyal D, Singh T. (2016). Competency-based medical education: An overview and application in pharmacology. *Indian J Pharmacol.* 48(1):S5–S9.

[2] Shah H.N., Patel D.S, Chhatriwala M.N. (2021). Project-Based Learning, an Effective Tool for the Active Teaching-learning Method for First-year Medical Students. *Int J Cur Res Rev.* 13 (10):41–46

[3] Perry, S.B (2020). The students' guide to learning design and research, Project Based learning https://edtechbooks.org/studentguide/project-based_learning as taken on 17/09/24

[4] Indrawan E, Jalinus N, Syahril S. (2019). Review project based learning. *Int J Sci Res (IJSR)*. 8: 1014–1018.

[5] Bédard D, Lison C, Dalle D, *et al.* (2012). Problem-based and project-based learning in engineering and medicine: Determinants of students' engagement and persistence. *Interdisciplinary Journal of Problem-Based Learning*. 6:2.

[6] McLean SF. (2016). Case-Based Learning and its Application in Medical and Health-Care Fields: A Review of Worldwide Literature. *J Med Educ Curric Dev.* 3:JMECD.S20377.

[7] Guo P, Saab N, Post LS, *et al.* (2020). A review of project-based learning in higher education: Student outcomes and measures. *Int J Educ Res.* 102.

[8] Nerurkar AB, Dhanani JV. (2016). Effectiveness of project based learning in teaching microbiology to undergraduate medical students. *IOSR-JRME.* 6(5):19–22.

[9] Kim K-J. (2020). Project-based learning approach to increase medical student empathy. *Medical Education Online*. 25(1):1742965.

[10] Lee, Jihyun. (2015). Designing a Project-based Service-Learning Course for Pre-dental Education: A Theoretical Exploration. *Educational Technology International.* 16. 249–272.

[11] https://www.pblworks.org/what-is-pbl as assessed on 15/9/23

[12] Elkhamisy, F.A.A., Zidan, A.H., and Fathelbab, M.F. (2022). Using project-based learning to enhance curricular integration and relevance of basic medical sciences in pre-clerkship years. *Alexandria Journal of Medicine*, *58*(1), 1–7.

[13] Kokotsaki D, Menzies V, Wiggins A. (2016). Project-based learning: A review of the literature. *Improv School.* 19(3):267–277.

[14] Costa-Silva D, Cortes J, Bachinski R, Spiegel C, Alves G. (2018). Teaching cell biology to dental students with a project-based learning approach. *J Dent Educ* 82(3):322e31.

[15] Yoo S-H, Bae S-M, Shin B-M, Shin S-J. (2020). The effect of project based learning modules on a community dental hygiene practicum in South Korea. *J Dent Educ* 84(4):418e28.

Navigating Dental Education Trends and Transforming Dental Pedagogy – Abas and Srikant N (Eds)
© 2027 The Author(s), ISBN: 978-1-041-32674-8

Redefining Dental Curriculum: The Impact of Digital Innovations and Emerging Educational Trends

Suviksha Suresh Naik
Manipal College of Dental Sciences Mangalore, Manipal Academy of Higher Education, Manipal, India

Sharon J.R. Saldanha
Department of Prosthodontics and Crown & Bridge, Manipal College of Dental Sciences Mangalore, Manipal Academy of Higher Education, Manipal, India

ABSTRACT: The objective of this review article is to explore how digital innovations and emerging educational trends are reshaping dental curricula. This examination is crucial for understanding how technological advancements, such as virtual reality (VR), augmented reality (AR), and artificial intelligence (AI), are revolutionizing dental education by enhancing simulation-based learning and providing personalized feedback.The significance of this review lies in its contribution to identify how these digital tools are bridging gaps in traditional dental training, thus improving clinical competence and adaptability among students. Key trends highlighted include the increased integration of immersive technologies that offer realistic training environments and the shift towards competency-based and interprofessional education models that emphasize collaborative skills. Patterns in the literature indicate a growing recognition of the need for curricula that incorporate these innovations to stay relevant in a rapidly evolving field. However, gaps remain in understanding the long-term impacts of these technologies on educational outcomes and their practical implementation across diverse educational settings.In conclusion, this review underscores the transformative potential of digital innovations in dental education and suggests future research directions to evaluate their effectiveness and guide the development of curricula that fully leverage these advancements.

Keywords: dental education, digital innovations, AI in dental curricula, competency based education

1 INTRODUCTION

Technology continues to impact the way education is provided at unprecedented speed and the field of dentistry education is not left behind. The traditional paradigm is based on scientific understanding of discipline and was influenced by the Gies Report of 1926. Traditional dentistry courses have undergone radical and progressive change. [1]

What is significant about this is that it is now accepted that conventional dental education, though basic, may be inadequate in equipping students for the contemporary changing face of dentistry.Therefore, this review seeks to integrate existing literature on how dental education has been incorporated with information and communication technologies, explore important themes and patterns, and fill in the vacuums created in the literature. [2]

Artificial intelligence (AI) focuses on solving complex problems and performing natural tasks like vision or language understanding, which traditional algorithms cannot address. It emphasizes knowledge acquisition, representation, and application, with knowledge-based systems being a key area of development. [3]

The significance of this analysis is to highlight transforming aspects in digital innovations and novel trends in education with regard to dental teaching curricula. More specifically, this paper aims to study the use of new technology in education like virtual reality (VR), augmented reality (AR), and artificial intelligence (AI) and the turn to competency-based or interprofessional education approaches. The review will also look into how these trends can enhance clinical competence, flexibility, and collaboration skills in dental students. In addition it wishes to further the existing debate on how reforming dental education would enhance the students' preparedness towards the impending demands of the profession. [4]

2 METHODS

For the purposes of this review, a systematic search of peer reviewed journals, academic sources and industry sources was carried out. The overview lasted for the past decade since there have been many developments in technology lately. Several keywords were searched in various data bases such as PubMed, Scopus, and Google Scholar including "Dental education", "Digital innovations", "Virtual reality in dentistry", "Augmented reality in dental training", "AI in dental curricula", "Competency based education", "Interprofessional education in

DOI: 10.1201/9781042016075-79

dentistry" and many more. Articles that featured innovative technologies to enhance dental education and articles that focused on developments in dentistry education were included.

A criteria to include articles that were published in the English language between 2013 and 2023 and focused on dental education digitally and through new pedagogical. There were article type limitations, only studies that involved empirical work, case studies and other literature reviews indicating how these technologies changed learning outcomes were allowed. Articles that were excluded are the papers not directly related to dental curricula and papers that discussed technologies without clear application to dental training.

3 RESULTS

3.1 *Integration of digital technologies in dental education*

The particular literature shows a self-reinforcement toward the incorporation of VR, AR and AI technologies in dental education curriculum. Considering specifically VR and AR technologies, these are primarily used in offering simulation based teaching learning strategies that assist in mastering dentistry skills. Such VR platforms as Simodont, for instance, are utilized in few dental schools to replace clinical attachments in enabling procedure investigation of the patients by the students in a safe environment before undertaking the real clinical duties. AI on the other hand has increasingly been engaged to give specific students feedback or assessments. As an example, if a student is currently in a simulation and is not performing well in the specific tasks simulating a particular procedure, AI can identify this problem and suggest that the student practice certain procedures or learn about them. It is likely that most learning will improve in this case, rather than in traditional teaching mechanisms. [5]

3.2 *AR and VR in dentistry: Revolutionizing dental education*

Augmented Reality (AR) and Virtual Reality (VR) are transforming dental education by providing immersive learning experiences that enhance traditional teaching methods. These technologies help students visualize and practice complex processes in a risk-free environment and redefine learning and teaching.

3.3 *Augmented reality (AR) in dentistry*

AR overlays digital images on real-world objects. Improved anatomy visualization, guided replication and interactive learning. It allows students to view 3D dental structures in real time. Perform a virtual surgery and follow real-time step instructions.

3.4 *Virtual reality (VR) in dentistry*

VR immerses students in a simulated medical environment. By giving training on virtual patients. It includes a haptic feedback system to simulate the sensation of touch. Helps students practice skills and decision-making in a realistic, risk-free environment.

AR and VR improve dental education by increasing engagement, helps keep procedures risk-free and provide a personalized learning experience. But challenges include high operating costs, limited haptic feedback on some systems. Learning curve for students and educators despite these obstacles, the benefits of interactive and immersive learning make AR and VR critical in modernizing dental curricula and bridging the gap between theoretical knowledge and clinical practice. [6]

3.5 *Shift towards competency-based education*

Another broad trend noted in the literature is time-based to competency-based education (CBE) trend. The emerging environment demands the development of new approaches of learning, to enable learners to meet the new challenges in the workplace. Conventional model of dental education has entailed practices where certain specified periods are assigned for instance for the completion of courses as well as clinical training. However, there is increasing concern that students do not learn at a similar speed and therefore they need to be taught in another flexible manner that addresses the outcomes. Competency-based models are learning systems whereby the learners are promoted depending on their learning progress and not the time taken in learning. This brings the probability that students are well trained before they advance, which might result in better levels of clinical skills when they complete their programs. Education literature still recognizes the importance of informing CBE with the use of digital tools such as AI that would help monitor a student's progress and, at the same time, advise the learner on his/her competencies' status. [7]

3.6 *Incline in interprofessional education*

Another trend in modern dental education is interprofessional education (IPE), focusing on students' interaction between representatives of different branches of healthcare. As dentistry is becoming essential with the general healthcare systems, the dentist should have closer interaction with the physician, nurse, pharmacist, etc. The authors found out that by including IPE in dental curricula the students' collaborative competencies are enhanced hence making them a great asset to any inter professional health practice team. [8]

3.7 *Gaps in the literature*

Although there are lots of publications about the use of digital innovations in dental education, the literature lacks detailed insights about the effectiveness of using digital tools in the course of dental education in the long run. Very few investigations have examined the impacts of such technologies on student performance within a long-term basis. Moreover, there are still numerous debates regarding VR and AR even though they are included as a major element of modern technologies; however, the use of these technologies varies between the different educational contexts. There is no proper study on the real-life trouble that the institutions are encountered while implementing these technologies into current usually structured programs. [9]

Table 1. Summary of key findings from the literature.

Key Trends	Description
Merging of VR & AR	Use of virtual and augmented reality in role-based learning procedures of dentistry.
AI for Personalized Learning	Interaction of artificial application in respect of giving specific feedback and assessments.
Competency based Education	Change from Traditional Credit Hour System into outcomes approach that has been boosted by technological interventions.
Interprofessional Education	More focus on interaction between students of various faculties and using various methods which presupposes teamwork.
Complications in research	Lack of more longitudinal studies into the effects of the technology and skills, and of the application of the tools.

4 DISCUSSION

As was demonstrated in the course of this review, it is possible to enhance the impact of innovations in the sphere of digital technologies in dental education significantly. The major advantage of using VR and AR in education is that, given a simulation, students can practice a subject in a manner that was unrealistic before. These technologies can enhance the knowledge to clinical application, guaranteeing that the learners become combat ready when handling real live patients. While conventional learning structures can prove to be beneficial, they can barrier or hinder learning, AI can offer an effective solution through providing learners with feedback which can help them to increase the pace of learning.

But, at the same time, it is evident that the possibilities of these technologies are great and their application entails several issues. Incorporating VR, AR, and AI in dental curricula also demands some types of funding, and training for professors in the use of these technologies. There is also the need to ensure that these technologies are available to students from different backgrounds and as well as institutions especially for developing countries where the resources are limited. [6]

Competency-based education takes the wheel of dental education and therefore is a significant change in the system of education. Since CBE outcome based this helps in achieving positive results of students since the college does not compromise the quality of training by providing the students with adequate time for practice before they leave college. Another advantage of this model which can be achieved with the help of digital tools is the potential ability to generate more competent and adaptable graduates. However further research has to be carried out to refine on how CBE can be incorporated within current learning and teaching frameworks and how technology can play a pivotal role towards this end. [7]

IPE is slowly gaining popularity especially because different health care sectors are overlapping more than before. This is one area that dental education should change so that students are in a position to care about dental patients as part of a team. The integration of IPE into dental curricula enhances team-building skills and prepares learners for todays' health systems. But more research is still required in order to understand how IPE is to be incorporated into dental programs effectively and also to identify how these digital technologies can support this development. [8]

5 CONCLUSION

This review focuses on revealing the trends and new educational improvements that affect the dental curricula to a great extent due to the digital innovations. The incorporation of the novel displays like VR, AR, as well as the artificial intelligence is exponentially changing how dental education is provided and enhanced with a more engaging, flexible, as well as individualized learning environment for the students. At the same time, education based on competencies and developed in an interprofessional manner can be characterized as the trend toward outcomes-based, integrated education. [9]

However, whereas these trends are promising they have a number of issues that need to be resolved. More studies are required to assess the sustained effects of such innovations on the learning achievements of students and to study the optimal ways utilizing the technologies as part of learning environments. [8]

All in all, one can speak about the changes that digital innovations and trends in the sphere of education bring to dental curricula as the perspectives, which can cause great changes in the way students learn and affect educational results positively. In this way, by further examining these trends, even the educators and institutions can come up with better and innovative forms of dental education. Besides, there is a need to accompany the technological activities with practicable implementation approaches that allow all the learners to access those technologies. Meeting these changes in a progressive and sensitive manner will be another integral factor important in the social construction of tomorrow's dentists to practice in the dynamic and complex dental care environment.

Nevertheless, even as there have been arguments that these innovations will cause a revolution in education, there are still some gaps in their effects on learners' performance and how these have been actualized across different types of schools.

This study and such similar studies will continue being conducted to help in striving for the development of dental curricula as well as help in improving the quality of dental education. [10]

REFERENCES

[1] Donoff RB. (2002). The Gies Report and research. *J Am Coll Dent.* 69(2):22–5.

[2] Pyle M. New models of dental education and curricular change: their potential impact on dental education. *J Dent Educ.* 76:89–97. doi:10.1002/j.0022-0337.2012.76.1.tb05237.x.

[3] Haton JP. (2006). A brief introduction to artificial intelligence. *IFAC Proc Vol.* 39(4):8–16. doi:10.3182/20060522-3-FR-2904.00003.

[4] Gandedkar N, Wong M, Prasad S, Darendeliler MA. (2023). Augmented/virtual reality and artificial intelligence in dental education and research. In: *Augmented and Virtual Reality for Dental and Medical Applications.* Springer; doi:10.1007/978-3-031-27166-3_9.

[5] Zitzmann NU, Matthisson L, Ohla H, Joda T. (2020). Digital undergraduate education in dentistry: a systematic review. *Int J Environ Res Public Health.* 17(9):3269. doi:10.3390/ijerph17093269.

[6] Fahim S, Maqsood A, Das G, Ahmed N, Saquib S, Lal A, *et al.* (2022). Augmented reality and virtual reality in dentistry: highlights from the current research. *Appl Sci.* 12(8):3719. doi:10.3390/app12083719.

[7] Rashwan N, Mahmoud MR. (2021). Application of competency-based education in dentistry: a review article. *Int J Dent Sci Res.* 9 (2):23–6. doi:10.12691/ijdsr-9-2-1.

[8] Tabrizi M, Lee WC. (2020). A pilot study of an interprofessional program involving dental, medical, nursing, and pharmacy students. *Front Public Health.* 8:602957. doi:10.3389/fpubh.2020.602957.

[9] Huang TK, Yang CH, Hsieh YH, Wang JC, Hung CC. (2018). Augmented reality (AR) and virtual reality (VR) applied in dentistry. *Kaohsiung J Med Sci.* 34(1):36–43. doi:10.1016/j.kjms.2018.01.009.

[10] Khurshid Z. (2023). Digital dentistry: transformation of oral health and dental education with technology. *Eur J Dent.* 17(4):943–4. doi:10.1055/s-0043-1772674.

[11] Artificial intelligence in dentistry: Current state and future directions. *Bull R Coll Surg Engl.* 105:380-3. doi:10.1308/rcsbull.2023.132.

Navigating Dental Education Trends and Transforming Dental Pedagogy – Abas and Srikant N (Eds)
 ISBN: 978-1-041-32674-8

Artificial Intelligence (Fuzzy Logic) in Shade Selection: A Review

Aashna D
Department of Conservative Dentistry and Endodontics, Yenepoya Dental College

1 INTRODUCTION

Dentistry is a rapidly evolving field that continuously seeks to align with modern technological and intellectual advancements. To meet the latest demands within the dental community, integrating technology with dental practices is essential review.

This integration has led to the development of innovative tools, particularly in aesthetic dentistry and color research, highlighting the role of artificial intelligence (AI).

The concept of "artificial intelligence" (AI), refers to the simulation of human cognitive processes by computer systems. Since its inception, AI has witnessed remarkable growth and has become integral to numerous fields in dentistry [1]. Machine learning (ML), deep learning (DL), and fuzzy logic aid in minimizing the gap between human perception of color and computational representation of colors in digital devices [2]. Color information plays a crucial role in achieving accurate color matching, with hue (H) and saturation (S) being particularly effective for enhancing precision. To enhance accuracy, dental shade matching is done using machine learning-derived coefficients such as the fuzzy logic, to obtain a highly accurate result [3][4][5]. The perception of a color tone can be influenced by various factors, including the lighting conditions on the object's surface, the technique applied, and the visual acuity and experience of the professional. Thus, Computer vision can aid in this task, minimizing the subjectivity of measurements [6].

1.1 *Aim*

This poster aims to present a scoping review of the current applications of AI in shade selection within aesthetic dentistry.

1.2 *Objective*

To perform a review of the use of artificial intelligence (AI) in dentistry, providing broader insights on various applications and advances in artificial intelligence in the field of esthetic dentistry.

2 METHODOLOGY

An extensive electronic search was conducted across databases such as Google Scholar, PubMed, and Scopus to gather relevant studies and insights. This review has no meta – analysis as no difficult estimation to be calculated. All titles and abstracts were subject to the inclusion criteria of the studies. Open access, free access articles, studies published in English language were included. Studies that were not AI based, studies that were not related to dentistry and related to other disciplines in dentistry other than restorative dentistry, closed access articles, studies in any other language other than English and without evidence-based reviews were excluded.

3 RESULTS

The systematic review reveals significant AI applications in shade selection for dentistry. AI-driven algorithms are capable of creating sophisticated models that predict optimal tooth shades based on various factors, including lighting conditions, patient characteristics, and existing dental materials. Moreover, AI tools can analyze images of patients' teeth to provide real-time shade recommendations, ensuring enhanced accuracy and consistency in shade matching.

4 DISCUSSION

Over the past two decades, artificial intelligence (AI) has undergone significant advancements, driven by innovations in digitized data acquisition, machine learning (ML), and improvements in computing power. These developments have

DOI: 10.1201/9781042016075-80

expanded AI applications into fields that were once heavily reliant on human expertise, including healthcare and dentistry. AI's integration into various professional sectors is transforming how tasks are performed, enhancing both efficiency and accuracy.

In the realm of aesthetic dentistry, AI holds great promise, particularly in areas such as diagnostic precision, treatment planning, and patient care. Machine learning (ML), deep learning (DL), and federated learning (FL) are some of the key AI methodologies being employed to address complex challenges in dental practices. ML algorithms enable systems to analyze vast amounts of data, learning from patterns and improving over time. Deep learning techniques, which mimic the human brain's neural networks, offer even greater potential by enabling the system to recognize intricate details in images or patient records, allowing for highly accurate diagnoses and personalized treatment recommendations. Meanwhile, federated learning, which enables data training without the need for centralized data storage, provides an added layer of privacy and security, which is particularly beneficial in healthcare settings.

One area where AI is making a significant impact is in the shade selection process in aesthetic dentistry. Traditionally, selecting the correct shade of dental materials to match a patient's natural teeth has been a subjective and challenging task, requiring the expertise of trained professionals. However, with AI, this process can be enhanced through the use of advanced image analysis, pattern recognition, and color matching algorithms. AI tools can analyze images of a patient's teeth and compare them to a database of shades, providing more consistent and accurate results than traditional methods. This advancement not only improves the aesthetic outcomes but also helps in making faster and more reliable decisions during treatment planning.

This review aims to provide a comprehensive overview of the current and future applications of AI in the field of shade selection in aesthetic dentistry. By examining the advancements in AI technologies and their potential to revolutionize the way dental professionals approach shade matching, the review highlights the growing role of AI in improving patient outcomes, optimizing treatment procedures, and reshaping the future of dental practice.

5 CONCLUSION

The impact of artificial intelligence (AI) and machine learning (ML) on the dental profession is rapidly growing, playing a crucial role in advancing digital technologies within treatment planning and aesthetic procedures. AI is revolutionizing how dental professionals approach diagnosis, treatment decisions, and patient care by leveraging data-driven insights and automating complex tasks. One of the primary benefits of integrating AI into dental practices is its ability to enhance precision in procedures that require meticulous attention to detail, such as in aesthetic dentistry. AI tools can analyze images, patient records, and other clinical data to provide more accurate assessments, reducing human error and allowing for tailored treatments based on individual patient needs.

In addition to improving diagnostic accuracy, AI is transforming treatment planning and execution. AI's capacity to analyze and process large amounts of data also enables dentists to make more informed decisions about treatment options, considering factors such as a patient's medical history, genetic predisposition, and lifestyle. In aesthetic procedures, such as smile design and shade matching, AI plays a vital role in ensuring that dental treatments achieve the desired cosmetic results. AI-powered systems can assess a patient's facial features, skin tone, and other aesthetic factors, offering suggestions for optimal dental work that enhances natural beauty. Additionally, machine learning algorithms help match dental restorations, such as crowns and veneers, to the patient's natural tooth color with greater accuracy, reducing the risk of color mismatch and ensuring a more harmonious result. As AI continues to evolve, its integration into dental practices will undoubtedly continue to enhance the overall quality of care. It not only increases the precision and effectiveness of treatments but also streamlines workflows, reduces the likelihood of errors, and provides dentists with more advanced tools to enhance patient experiences. Ultimately, the growing influence of AI and ML in dentistry promises to improve both the clinical and aesthetic aspects of dental practice, leading to better outcomes for patients and greater efficiency in the delivery of care.

REFERENCES

[1] Where Is the Artificial Intelligence Applied in Dentistry? Systematic Review and Literature Analysis Andrej Thurzo,1,2,* Wanda Urbanová,3 Bohuslav Novák,1 Ladislav Czako,4 Tomáš Siebert. (n.d.)

[2] Carrillo-Perez F, Pecho OE, Morales JC, Paravina RD, Della Bona A, Ghinea R, *et al.* (2022). Applications of artificial intelligence in dentistry: A comprehensive review. *J Esthet Restor Dent* 34:259–80. https://doi.org/10.1111/jerd.12844.

[3] Chen S-L, Zhou H-S, Chen T-Y, Lee T-H, Chen C-A, Lin T-L, *et al.* (2020). Dental shade matching method based on hue, saturation, value color model with machine learning and fuzzy decision. *Sens Mater* 32:3185. https://doi.org/10.18494/sam.2020.2848.

[4] Lin T-L, Chuang C-H, Chen S-L, Lin N-H, Miaou S-G, Lin S-Y, *et al.* (2019). An efficient image processing methodology based on fuzzy decision for dental shade matching. *J Intell Fuzzy Syst* 36:1133–42. https://doi.org/10.3233/jifs-169887.

[5] Shetty S, Gali S, Augustine D, Sv S. (2024). Artificial intelligence systems in dental shade-matching: A systematic review. *J Prosthodont* 33:519–32. https://doi.org/10.1111/jopr.13805.

[6] Helio Pedrini; (n.d.) Dental shade matching assisted by computer vision techniques Willian Pulido Beneducci, Marcelo Lucchesi Teixeira.

Navigating Dental Education Trends and Transforming Dental Pedagogy – Abas and Srikant N (Eds)

Need for Updating Dental Surgery Curricula for Contemporary Practice, Innovations and Assessment: A Review

Anupama Prasad D.
Department of Prosthodontics and Crown & Bridge, AB Shetty Memorial Institute of Dental Sciences, NITTE (Deemed to be University), Deralakatte, Mangaluru, Karnataka, India

ABSTRACT: The Bachelor of Dental Surgery (BDS) curriculum must constantly progress to stride with innovations in dental technology and the needs of the community in. This paper highlights the necessity of regular curriculum assessment and modification in dental education, emphasizing the integration of modern innovations and responsiveness to community requirements. Traditional curricula have undergone minimal changes over the years, relying on established learning methods. However, the need to update these curricula to reflect the current and future demands of dental practice is pressing.

Modern dental education should encompass aspects that foster empathy, social responsibility, and a commitment to lifelong learning. The curriculum must adapt to include emerging technologies in the dental field and breakdown courses to manage the increasing complexity of the discipline. A successful dental program not only teaches students technical skills but also allows them to navigate rapid changes in the field and engage in self-directed learning.

This paper suggests that curriculum development should strike a balance between theoretical knowledge and practical application, guided by systematic, evidence-based assessments. The ultimate aim is to produce skilled, adaptable professionals who are prepared to meet the changing demands of global oral health care.

Keywords: Dental education, Dental curriculum, National education policy, Problem-based learning, Choice-based credit system

1 INTRODUCTION

"Education is not just about filling a bucket; it is more like sparking a fire." – William Butler Yeats. Education in dentistry is highly important for making skilful dental specialists who can meet the many essentials of patients. The dental curriculum of India is outdated and lacks flexibility. This has made it difficult for graduates to meet what employers expect. Students in dental schools face a great deal of stress in trying to fit into this rigid curriculum, which seems disconnected from their needs. A major issue is that "Tomorrow's doctors are taught by today's teachers using yesterday's lessons," as Sethuraman noted. [1,2]

The conventional dental curriculum is designed with theoretical instructions, preclinical exposure, and training in clinical subjects, all aimed at shaping future practitioners. Each educational establishment is tasked with providing a curriculum that is clinically pertinent, scientifically grounded, medically up to date, and socially accountable. This approach enables patient tailored care by students and also to adds to disease deterrence and health promotion, ultimately benefiting the healthcare system and the wider population. [3] The provision of suitable educational programs aligned with clear objectives, along with principled evaluation and assessment, are fundamental principles of curriculum development. [4] In present context, the curriculum of dental education in India must constantly progress to stride with innovations in dental technology, the needs of the community and the shifting healthcare landscape. [5]

2 METHODOLOGY

A total of 24 articles were collected from journals published from 2009–2023 in the English language. Only 9 articles that matched the objective of the review were considered (Figure 1). The keywords used were dental curriculum, curriculum revision, problem-based learning, and national education policy.

Kern has given a six-step approach (Figure 2) for developing a curriculum that, when followed, leads to an effective method of preparing dental graduates to face the world more efficiently.

DOI: 10.1201/9781042016075-81

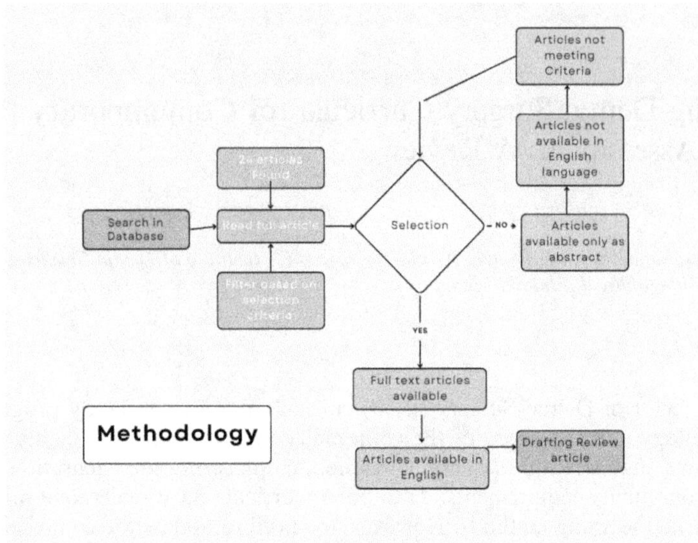

Figure 1. Methodology.

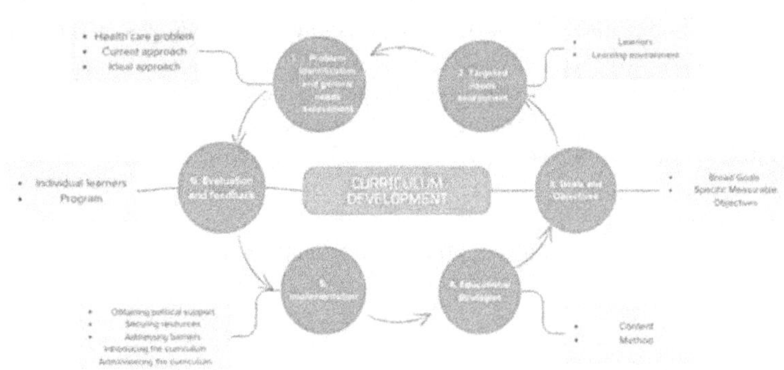

Figure 2. Kern's six-step approach to curriculum development [2].

Step 1: Identifying problem and assessment of needs

The primary step involves identifying and critically analysing a healthcare need or issue. This could be related to a specific health problem or the skills and qualities required of healthcare providers, such as the requirement of physicians to become autonomous continuous learners capable of adapting to evolving medical knowledge. It might also concern societal health care needs, such as whether the current number and the physicians currently being trained meet the necessary requirements. A comprehensive assessment of the issue includes analysis of the acceptance of the needs by patients, doctors, the education system, and society. Afterwards, an ideal approach is outlined, comparing what is currently done to what should be done. The gap between these two forms the basis for a broad need analysis. [2]

Step 2: Targeted Needs Analysis

Second step focuses on understanding the specific requirements of the aimed cluster of knowledge seekers and their learning institution or environment that can differ from those of the general learner population. It helps customize a curriculum for a particular context, fosters communication with stakeholders, and ensures that curriculum development aligns with available resources and institutional goals. [2]

Step 3: Aims and Purposes

Once the requirements of the learners in focus are identified, general goals and specific purposes can be developed. These purposes can cover cognitive (intellectual), affective (emotional), or psychomotor (skills and behavior) domains. Objectives could also pertain to the curriculum's processes or desired outcomes in terms of healthcare delivery or patient health. [2]

Step 4: Educational Strategies

After the objectives are defined, the next step is to select appropriate content of curriculum and teaching methods that are most likely to attain these aims. [2]

Step 5: Implementation

This step involves the actual deployment of the curriculum and includes obtaining political and institutional support, securing necessary resources, addressing barriers to implementation, administering the curriculum, and continuously refining it through iterative cycles. Effective implementation is key to bringing the curriculum from concept to realism. [2]

Step 6: Assessment and Response

Evaluation has two main components: assessing individual performance (individual assessment) and evaluating the curriculum as a whole (program evaluation). Evaluations can be formative (providing ongoing feedback to improve learning or curriculum) or summative (offering a final assessment or grade). Evaluation serves multiple purposes, from improving the curriculum and securing support to answering research questions about the effectiveness of different educational strategies. [2]

3 ALIGNED TEACHING METHODS

Baseline knowledge is often best attained through books, classes, or asynchronous virtual modules. Diagnostic tasks and critical-thinking activities, which engage learners, seem to be effective than lectures at improving clinical reasoning.

Effective teamwork is best cultivated through participation in interprofessional learning and collaborative work experiences rather than through reading. Skills such as discussions, diagnosis, and clinical techniques are best learned in simulated environments, where learners can practice, receive feedback, and reflect on their performance. Curriculum development is an ongoing process. It continuously evolves on the basis of evaluation outcomes, resource changes, shifts in learner needs, and updates to the subject matter. [2]

Emphasis of National Education Policy (NEP) 2020 in India lays the importance of recognizing and promoting the unique capabilities of every learner. In alignment with this, the Dental Council of India (DCI) has proposed a choice-based credit system (CBCS) model for dental curriculum. Originally introduced by the University Grants Commission (UGC) in 2015, CBCS aims to improve the excellence of training by offering learners with flexibility in course selection, credit allocation, and assessment methods. This student-centered approach allows for personalized learning tailored to individual interests, capacities, and professional aims, thus CBC is more beneficial than the orthodox system of education. [1]

Dental curricula require regular updates to remain aligned with advancements in both scientific knowledge and societal needs. Senior students of dentistry, as key stakeholders, hold a decisive role in shaping these revisions. There is a need to incorporate modern educational strategies into dental programs. These strategies include methods such as problem-based learning, flipped classrooms, simulation, simulated reality, tech-driven education, online education, and gamification. The proficiencies with the minimum sufficiency, in both hypothetical and applied areas, fall into three main categories: 1. Evidence-based dentistry and research: There is an identified gap in skills such as "implementation of evidence-based dentistry principles" and "conducting medical research". "2. Procedure-based aptitudes: Skills such as "performing intraoral surgeries (beyond tooth extraction), "endodontic retreatment of multirooted teeth," "surgical extraction of wisdom teeth," "performing periodontal surgeries," and "fabricating space maintainers" were found to be lacking. This may be due to the complex nature of these procedures. Soft skills and practice management: abilities such as "maintaining dental equipment," "practice management," "handling medical emergencies," "professional conduct with colleagues," and "prescribing necessary medications" are not sufficiently addressed in the curriculum. [6]

Age old hypothetical education dominates, that is not conducive to participatory learning. Moreover, there exists a noticeable limited availability of courses on next generation technologies such as multimedia learning, along with insufficient resources in communication skills, ethics, and legal issues. [1] The Dental Council of India does not currently offer specific guidelines for incorporating communication skills into the undergraduate dental curriculum. Extending the existing dental program by an additional year presents an opportunity to introduce training in professionalism, communication, social skills, and computer information technologies (CITs). The development of proficiency in communication, team building, and global awareness is gradually becoming a crucial aspect of dental education in India. [7] Electives can be categorized into two main groups: a) General: Athletics, soft skills, music, dance, and yoga; and b) Wellness related: Investigative sciences, biochemistry, technology of nanomaterials, science of neurology, and management courses in health service. [8]

To address gaps in traditional methods, many universities have integrated problem-based learning (PBL), which shifts the concentration from a instructor-led approach to a inquiry-based learning. Main goals in PBL include enhancing information retention, promoting independent and collaborative work, fostering problem-solving and interdisciplinary thinking, and engaging students more actively in their learning. A hybrid system, which combines information-focused learning of preclinical classes with PBL of clinical teaching and maintains simulation labs for practical preparation, is a recommended model for maximizing both theoretical understanding and practical skill development. [3]

Interestingly, undergraduate education has changed substantially recently. Initiatives began with the Eleventh Five Year Plan (2007–2012) aimed at improving teaching following suggestions from the National Knowledge Commission and Yashpal Committee (2008–2009). One change was the introduction of the choice-based credit system (CBCS) by the University Grants Commission (UGC) in 2015. This system was designed to increase the quality of education while giving students more choices in what they study.

More excitingly, CBCS creates a student-focused environment where learning can be tailored to what each student enjoys and wants to do in their careers. It's much better than the old ways of learning. The National Educational Policy (NEP) of India in 2020 also supports this focus on individual student talent. The DCI aims to make these changes with the CBCS model in dental education. In this CBCS model, students do not just obtain percentages for each course; they receive grade points on the basis of their performance and attendance throughout their studies. These points are determined by multiplying grade values by credit numbers—students can even choose electives that spark their interest. Studying things such as forensics or basic life support (BLS) adds important skills beyond regular dentistry topics. Many believe that advanced therapies such as implantology should also be included in courses. The new curriculum does emphasize better communication skills and soft skills instead of just memorizing facts as previous versions did.

One benefit of this model is that it can help students study abroad and transfer credits easily. Having credit systems also helps compare courses across different countries. transferring credits between institutions will be ideal—especially if someone wants to pursue higher education or specializes elsewhere. This system opens doors for those needing flexibility for personal reasons. The CBCS model fits well with NEP 2020 scheme of India ,since it aims at a versatile educational set-up that encourages creativity and critical thinking. It allows future dentists to select courses that resonate with them while enhancing lifelong learning. However, rolling it out nationwide won't be easy; it's a big job for everyone involved. Authorities must work together closely, offering special training to teachers at various institutions while also keeping students informed about these changes. In short, this approach is definitely a step forward for educators and policymakers seeking to improve dental education in India. [1]

4 CONCLUSION

Curriculum development must consider several factors, including advanced academic qualifications, national authorisation body guidelines, and internationally accepted standards. Teachers and Learners, as internal participants, play crucial roles in ensuring the quality of the curriculum, and their contentment and opinion must be regularly analysed to inform modifications and reforms. Intuitions of Dentistry must thoughtfully plan their courses to align with the expected graduate competencies while also considering available resources. In traditional curricula, students often play a passive role in lectures, which can become repetitive and focused on memorization, leading to decreased motivation.

In contrast, active curriculum models such as PBL and case-based learning (CBL) promote interactive learning through small group tutorials between students and faculty and mutual evaluation. However, implementing such methods requires multidisciplinary coordination. [9]

REFERENCES

[1] Kabra L, Santhosh VN, Sequeira RN, Ankola AV, Coutinho D. (2023). Dental curriculum reform in India: Undergraduate students' awareness and perception on the newly proposed choice based credit system. *J Oral Biol Craniofac Res*. 2023;13(5):630–635.

[2] Kern DE. (2009). A six-step approach to curriculum development. In *Curriculum Development for Medical Education a Six-Step Approach* (pp. 5–9). Baltimore: The Johns Hopkins University Press.

[3] Won J, Guan G, Mei L, *et al*. (2021). A multicenter study of dental curricula in Asia/Pacific nations: The views and experiences of final-year dental students. *J Dent Educ*. 85:660–668.

[4] Dabaghi-Tabriz F, Rahbar M, Somi MH, Taghizadieh A, Hanaee J, Ghaffari R, Dehghani AH, Partovi P. (2019). *Comparing the Curriculum of Five Specialized Fields of Dentistry in Iran and 10 Top Faculties of the World. Maedica (Bucur)*. 2019 Mar;14 (1):30–37.

[5] Deshmukh SV. (2023). Change in dental curriculum in India a need of an hour. *J Int Clin Dent Res Organ* 15:65–6.

[6] Salmani A, Keshavarz H, Akbari M, Kharrazifard MJ, Varmazyari S, Khami MR. (2023). Evaluation of national dental curriculum in Iran using senior dental students' feedback. *BMC Oral Health*. 26;23(1):45.

[7] Sangappa SB, Tekian A.(2013). Communication skills course in an Indian undergraduate dental curriculum:a randomized controlled trial. *J Dent Educ*. 77(8):1092–8.

[8] Rao LN, Hegde M, P Shetty C. (2014). Comparison of dental curriculum in India versus developed countries. *Nitte Univ J Health Sci* 2014;4:121–4.

[9] Abdelsalam M, Rodriguez TE, Brallier L. (2020). Student and Faculty Satisfaction with Their Dental Curriculum in a Dental College in Saudi Arabia. *Int J Dent*. 2020 8;2020:6839717.

Navigating Dental Education Trends and Transforming Dental Pedagogy – Abas and Srikant N (Eds)
© 2027 The Author(s), ISBN: 978-1-041-32674-8

Online e-Group Discussions Through Collaborative Learning for Faculty Development of Medical Educators

Shwetha KM
Public Health Dentistry, Faculty of Dental Sciences, M.S. Ramaiah University of Applied Sciences, Bengaluru, Karnataka

Nagesh KR
Forensic Medicine, Father Muller Medical College, Mangalore, Karnataka

Thomas V. Chacko
Medical Education & Community Medicine, Believers Church Medical College & Hospital, St Thomas Nagar, Kuttapuzha, Thiruvalla, Kerala State, India

ABSTRACT: **Background:** Continuing professional development (CPD) is essential for health professional educators (HPEs) to stay updated with the latest knowledge and effectively train the next generation of students. **Objectives: 1)** To design and describe an online e-group discussion on a specific topic for HPEs. 2) To measure the effectiveness of the online E-group discussion via the Kirkpatrick model. **Methodology:** The FAIMER listserv discussion model and the mentor-learning (ML) web platform were used for online e-group discussions. The topics and a moderating team for the ML web discussion were selected during the onsite session. Professionalism in healthcare was one of the topics chosen for the CPD. The weekly objectives, content, and activities for the one-month ML web discussion were developed. A presurvey assessed the need for professionalism and prioritized discussion content. At the end of the month, effectiveness was evaluated via Kirkpatrick's model (levels one and two). **Results:** A total of 32 HPEs from medical, dental, nursing, and physiotherapy disciplines, representing Indian, Nepali, and Malaysian nationalities, participated. The presurvey indicated that 69% of the respondents felt that professionalism was missing in their curriculum. During the month-long discussion, 477 emails were exchanged. The results revealed a greater than 50% improvement in participants' knowledge about the topic, and 70% reported that they would apply the knowledge gained in their academic and work environments. **Conclusion:** Online platforms are effective for facilitating CPD, enhancing HPEs' knowledge of relevant topics and extending reach across broader geographic regions within available resources.

Keywords: Continuing professional development, health educators, online learning

1 INTRODUCTION

Lifelong learning is essential for healthcare professionals to provide evidence-based, high-quality care to patients. The main goal of medical education is to improve the health of community members, which can be achieved at the organizational level by aligning the curriculum with local health needs, creating a community-centred learning atmosphere, training basic healthcare workers, and participating in national policy development and implementation. [1]

For the past few years, there has been a demand for evidence-based health care for patients. The self-determination of healthcare professionals taking initiative in their own learning needs to update their knowledge and skills by attending conferences, workshops, and seminars for continuing education/professional development. [2,3] Additionally, online education has gained significant popularity among healthcare professionals because of its flexibility in terms of scheduling, cost-effectiveness, and ability to participate without taking time off from work. Despite these logistical benefits, the primary objective remains the same: to acquire knowledge and improve patient care. [4–8]

The contents of online discussions are prepared on the basis of the principles of education, adult learning, and pedagogy. [5,6] Adult learning is self-directed learning with an appropriate platform where the participants are self-motivated and take ownership of their learning. Collaborative learning is a form of group learning in which some meaningful learning interactions occur between learners. This approach is increasingly valued in education for enabling learning through shared ideas and resources, with moderators or mentors facilitating meaningful activities. [9]

The Foundation for Advancement of International Medical Education and Research (FAIMER) fellowship program uses an online platform for the implementation phase. [1,10,11] The FAIMER fellowship program at PSG FAIMER Regional Institute (PSG-FRI), Coimbatore, India, provides a capacity-building platform for health professional educators (HPEs). [10] The present article discusses the findings observed during the Mentor–Learner web (M-L web) discussion on professionalism in health care workers, with the following objectives: 1) To design and describe an online e-group discussion on a professionalism in healthcare for HPEs. 2) To measure the effectiveness of the online e-group discussion using the Kirkpatrick model.

2 METHODOLOGY

The online focussed e-group discussion (ML web) was conducted in February 2016. The planning for the same was started two months prior. The participants were year one, year two fellows, and alumni of the FAIMER regional institute under the observation of faculty members. This process facilitates collaborative learning, where each learner learns from the discussion under the supervision of faculty moderators and the director of the regional institute.

This process of self-determined learning during the mentor-learner (M-L) Web starts with the identification of the topics by year one Fellows (the mentees) that they want to learn more during the implementation phase. [1,10,11] Usually, they list those topics that would be useful for them (needed) for project implementation as well as for those areas that they would need to build expertise on for them to transfer knowledge to the workplace as much sought after Facilitators of Learning and Change managers in their home institution. They then vote for the topics that need to be shortlisted and included in the seven monthly learning slots available and sequence them so that this focused learning should take place while keeping in mind where they would need it to help them with activities for which capacity building is needed through the month-long discussion.

The year two Fellows (Mentors) then choose which topics and month they would like to be the moderator-Mentors of the month. The choice of their month and topic for which they would be actively participating and facilitating the learning is also self-determined according to their own needs for further professional development. Our topic for the ML web discussion was *professionalism in health care*. Medical education focuses more on the cognitive and psychomotor domains, which are taught in professional schools through a structured curriculum. [12–14] Professionalism is considered a secondary competency skill that includes noncognitive skills that are presently learned through a hidden curriculum. In recent years, there has been growing interest among healthcare professional educators in teaching professionalism during the training period; hence, this topic was selected. [15–18]

The scope for interacting with the team was also provided for two afternoon sessions during the onsite session. Once the offsite session started, the list of topics was shared on the listserv (the common mail group for fellows) with the alumni to choose the topic. Finally, the ML web team was formed with year one and year two fellows as moderators and the faculty as mentors.

The resources were collected from various search engines, such as MEDLINE, EBSCO, Google Scholar, and textbooks. These materials were shared by the team members via group mail and approved by the mentor. A preliminary survey (via SurveyMonkey) was conducted to gauge participants' expectations on the topic and maintain engagement throughout the month. On the basis of the participants' responses and resource materials, weekly objectives, content, and activities were designed for month-long sessions.

Each week, the moderator posted discussion topics to a designated Listserv group email, where participants responded within the same thread. The moderator guided discussions by acknowledging the contributions, encouraging participation, and highlighting key points. This format continued weekly, with each week focusing on a specific objective and including planned activities and shared resources sent via email attachments. The participants contributed by sharing their insights, experiences, and additional resources. The activities involved critical thinking questions, culminating in curriculum suggestions with examples by the month's end.

~~Midway through the discussions, a survey was conducted to assess the participants' knowledge and engagement with challenging aspects of the topic, such as the unprofessional behaviors observed.~~ Nonparticipants were regularly reminded via mobile messages and emails to encourage involvement.

The effectiveness of the ML web discussion was evaluated via the Kirkpatrick model. [19] The first level was assessed through participants' feedback via an open-ended questionnaire, whereas the second level measured knowledge improvement through a retrospective questionnaire for self-assessment. This type of questionnaire allows participants to compare their level of understanding before and after the discussion simultaneously. Additionally, questions concerning facilitating and hindering factors were also included. All notifications were sent via email, with reminders additionally sent through mobile messages.

3 RESULTS

The participants were HPEs from medical, dental, nursing and physiotherapy specialties with Indian, Nepali and Malaysian nationalities. They are assistant professors with a minimum of three years of experience. Some of the participants were heads of the department.

There were 477 mails posted for the entire month by the participants and the moderators. The maximum number of mails shared for the topic in week 4 was 139, followed by 115 for week 2, 114 for week 1 and 109 for week 3. There were 106 mails exchanged by the moderators, faculty mentors and director during the prediscussion.

In the preliminary survey, 69% of the participants ranked professionalism as a missing component in the present curriculum as the reason for unprofessional behaviour among some of the health professionals. The participants opined that the faculty is not well equipped to teach and assess professionalism to students, as it was not part of student assessment.

The participants were given options to rank the topics for building their capacity to implement professionalism in the undergraduate curriculum. They ranked first for topics to be included (63.4%), second for teaching learning methods (63.4%), and third for student assessment methods (60%) for professionalism (Figure 1).

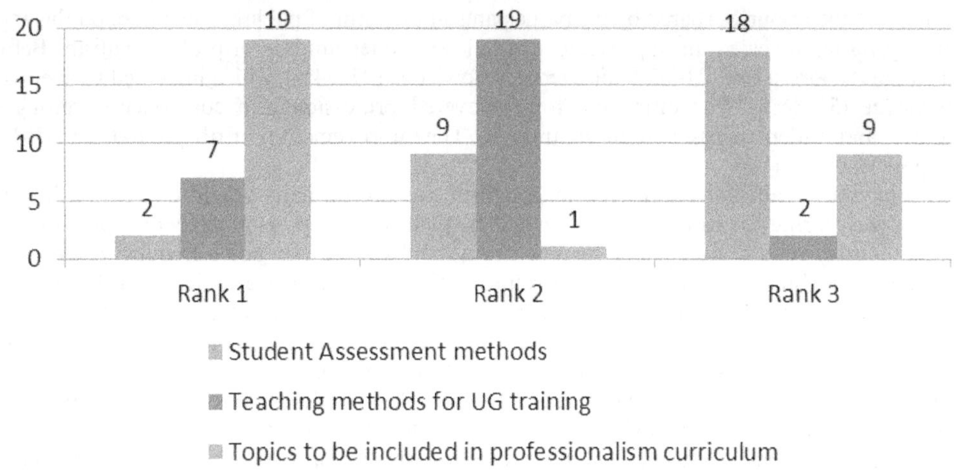

Figure 1. Responses to participants' expectations of professionalism in healthcare ML web discussions.

The responses to the open-ended feedback questions indicated that most participants found the sessions to be resourceful and effective in enhancing their understanding of the topic. They highlighted well-planned discussions, professional moderation, and quality resources as key facilitators of learning. The excerpts of participants' responses are as follows: "*1. The activities were thought provoking and required the participants to read, analyse, and reflect before answering. 2. Responses from the participants were informative, and reading materials shared is a treasure trove of information*". While more than half reported no obstacles, a few noted time constraints and an excess of emails as challenges.

The results of the Retropre questionnaire are given in Table 1. The results show that their level of understanding of the topics of professionalism improved. Before the ML web discussion, most of the participants had either little knowledge or average knowledge about the topics discussed, but the participants graded themselves as having good knowledge to average knowledge after they participated in a one-month discussion.

Table 1. The results of the postsurvey regarding their knowledge of the topic (professionalism) before and after the ML web discussion.

Questions	Before ML web						After ML web					
	No knowledge	Little knowledge	Average knowledge	Good knowledge	Total	Weighted average	No knowledge	Little knowledge	Average knowledge	Good knowledge	Total	Weighted average
Need for professionalism	0.0% (0)	50.0% (10)	45.0% (9)	5.0% (1)	20	2.55	0.0% (0)	0.0% (0)	13.6% (3)	86.4% (19)	22	3.86
Components/attributes of professionalism	0.0% (0)	68.2% (15)	27.23% (6)	4.6% (1)	22	2.36	0.0% (0)	0.0% (0)	18.2% (4)	81.8% (18)	22	3.82
Framing/formulating learning outcomes for each attributes	19.1% (4)	47.6% (10)	33.3% (7)	0.0% (0)	21	2.14	0.0% (0)	0.0% (0)	43.5% (10)	56.5% (13)	23	3.57
Assessment for professionalism among students	19.1% (4)	57.1% (12)	23.8% (5)	0.0% (0)	21	2.05	0.0% (0)	0.0% (0)	34.8% (8)	65.2% (15)	23	3.65
Differentiation between unprofessional and professional behaviours in health care	0.0% (0)	21.1% (4)	73.7% (14)	5.3% (1)	19	2.84	0.0% (0)	0.0% (0)	13.6% (3)	86.4% (19)	22	3.86
How well will you be able to transfer what you learnt in this session to your academic and work environment			To a great extent			To some extent			Not at all			Total
responses			69.6% (16)			30.4% (7)			0.0% (0)			23

Approximately 70% of the participants opined that they would transfer the learning from this session to their academic and work environment to a great extent.

4 DISCUSSION

The ML Web discussion was conducted on the topic of professionalism in healthcare for FAIMER fellows. This platform was utilized as CPD for fellows, as the topics were selected by them during the onsite session at the regional institute.

The moderators planned the discussion involving the participants in the initial stages of preparation by conducting a preliminary survey, resulting in a well-structured program with defined objectives achieved through appropriately designed activities and useful resource materials. This is also evident from the number of responses, i.e., 477 emails for the entire month, and the resources shared by the participants in the form of published literature on this topic.

The postsurvey results revealed an improvement in fellows' understanding of professionalism. Before the discussion, participants reported low (21–68%) or average knowledge (27–74%), which increased to average (14–43%) or good knowledge (56–86%). The discussion topics covered professionalism components, setting objectives, teaching methods, and student assessment during training. The improvement is attributed to the FAIMER system, which fosters peer learning. [1]

The chosen topic was significant because professionalism was not formally taught in our healthcare education system. A mid-survey during the discussion highlighted frequent unprofessional behavior: approximately 60% of the participants reported regular derogatory remarks from faculty, and 57% noted frequent offensive sarcasm in front of their colleagues. Such behaviors are concerning, as they may influence students. Professionalism is often learned through hidden curricula, with role modelling being a key method, as noted in the literature. [15,17,18,20] Therefore, before teaching students, faculty across institutions must be sensitized and trained to teach this topic. However, training faculty nationwide poses significant logistical challenges.

After the discussion, the participating fellows responded that they would transfer the learning from the ML web discussion to their academic and work environment to some extent (30.43%, 69.57%).

An inherent challenge of online learning is nonparticipation or nonresponsiveness, which is encountered during online discussions. However, measures, such as reminders and encouragement through text messages, WhatsApp, and mails, were taken to overcome this problem to some extent. As this was conducted online, the fellows were in their home institutions, and it is known that fellows had other responsibilities and preoccupied activities in their home institution.10 The reminders and encouragement for participating were crucial for the moderators to sustain interest among the group.

There were some hindrances to learning, as reported by 50% of the fellows as too much content to follow for a week; few had time constraints, and some of them had health issues. Otherwise, most of them appreciated encouragement from moderators, shared resources and interesting activities that were planned for the entire month.

Overall, the online platform bridges distances and unites professionals across regions to share knowledge for their professional development. [21] This approach can be utilized for training the basics of the topic, which can cover wide geographic regions, as the participants were from different parts of India, Nepal and Malaysia. Further advanced courses can be conducted in the form of workshops to hone skills to teach and assess the students for professionalism. Since the beginning of the COVID-19 pandemic, online platforms have been extensively utilized for meetings, training sessions, and certification courses. These platforms offer a cost-effective, blended approach to learning that transcends geographical boundaries. [22]

5 CONCLUSION

The topic of the online discussion was tailored to the needs of the participants and effectively enhanced their understanding of professionalism in healthcare. This approach successfully reached a broader geographic audience and improved the level of comprehension among HPEs.

ACKNOWLEDGEMENTS

We acknowledge the moderating team Dr. Archana Prabhu K, Dr. Zayapragasarazan, Dr. Rus, Dr. Savitha, faculty and alumni of the PSG FAIMER regional institute Dr. Animesh Jain, Dr. Sudha Ramlingam, Dr. Jayalakshmi, Dr. Rashmi Jain, Dr. Rams, Dr. Vivek Saoji, for their support during the ML web discussion.

REFERENCES

[1] Burdick WP, Morahan PS, Norcini JJ. (2007). Capacity building in medical education and health outcomes in developing countries: the missing link. *Educ Heal.* 20:65.

[2] Gonzalez P. (2010). Conceptualizing Capacity Building. *Cent to Improv Proj Perform (CIPP), Westat US.* 33(1):153–160.

[3] Hawe P, King L, Noort M, Jordens C LB. (2000). *Indicators to Help with Capacity Buildings in Health Promotion.* NSW Health Department, Sydney.

[4] Belfield CR, Morris ZS, Bullock a D, Frame JW. (2001). The benefits and costs of continuing professional development (CPD) for general dental practice: A discussion. *Eur J Dent Educ.* 2001;5(2):47–52.

[5] Kennedy A. (2005). Models of continuing professional development: a framework for analysis. *J in-service Educ.* 2005;31(2):235–250.

[6] Chacko TV. (2018). Emerging pedagogies for effective adult learning: From andragogy to heutagogy. *Archives of Medicine and Health Sciences.* 6(2):278–83.

[7] Johnson LA, Lohman MC, Sharp JD, Krenz TS. (2000). Continuing dental education via an interactive video network: course development, implementation and evaluation. *J Educ Media.* 2000;25(2):129–140.

[8] Laister J, Kober S. (2002). Social aspects of collaborative learning in virtual learning environments. In: *In Proceedings of the Networked Learning Conference Sheffield, Marc.*

[9] Schönwetter DJ, Hamilton J, Sawatzky JA. (2015). Exploring professional development needs of educators in the health sciences professions. *Journal of dental education.* 79(2):113–23.

[10] Anshu, Bansal P, Mennin SG, Burdick WP, Singh T. (2008). Online faculty development for medical educators: Experience of a South Asian program. *Educ Health (Abingdon).* 21(3):175.

[11] Dongre AR, Chacko T V., Banu S, et al. (2010). On-line capacity-building program on "analysis of data" for medical educators in the South Asia region: a qualitative exploration of our experience. *Educ Health (Abingdon).* 23(3):425.

[12] Kusumawati W, Prihatiningsih TS, Rahayu GR, Sastrowijoto S. (2015). Identification of professional Behavior Attributes for Indonesian Medical Educaton. *South Asian J Med Educ.* 9(1):19–25.

[13] Zijlstra-Shaw S, Robinson PG, Roberts T. (2016). Assessing professionalism within dental education; the need for a definition. *Eur J Dent Educ.* 16(1).

[14] Tim WJ, Winnie WB, Doug KL. (2009). A blueprint to assess professionalism: Results of a systematic review. *Acad Med.* 2009;84 (5):551–58.

[15] Adkoli B V., Al-Umran KU, Al-Sheikh M, Deepak KK, Al-Rubaish AM. (2011). Medical students' perception of professionalism: A qualitative study from Saudi Arabia. *Med Teach.* 2011;33(10):840–845.

[16] Kirk LM. (2007). Professionalism in medicine: definitions and considerations for teaching. *Proc (Bayl Univ Med Cent).* 2007;20 (1):13–16.

[17] Passi V, Doug M, Peile E, Thistlethwaite J, Johnson N. (2010). Developing medical professionalism in future doctors : a systematic review. *Int J Med Educ.* 2010;(1):19–29.

[18] Birden H, Glass N, Wilson I, Harrison M, Usherwood T, Nass D. (2013). BEME Guide: Teaching professionalism in medical education: a Best Evidence Medical Education (BEME) systematic review. BEME Guide No. 25. *Med Teach.* 2013;35(7):e1252–66.

[19] Bates R. (2004). A critical analysis of evaluation practice: the Kirkpatrick model and the principle of beneficence. *Eval Program Plann.* 2004;27(3):341–347.

[20] Wearn A, Wilson H, Hawken SJ, Child S, Mitchell CJ. (2010). In search of professionalism: implications for medical education. *N Z Med J.* 123(1314):123–132.

[21] Ferreira D, Paterson R, Hakone K. (2018). The Growth of e-Learning in Higher Education: Preparing an Agenda for a Professional Development Workshop. *Language Research Bulletin.* 32:20–31.

[22] Ghobrini M, Ghobrini RE, Benaicha F. (2024). A Digital Leap in the Evolution of Continuous Professional Development for Teachers. *International Journal of Science Annals.* 7(1): 17–25.

Navigating Dental Education Trends and Transforming Dental Pedagogy – Abas and Srikant N (Eds)
 ISBN: 978-1-041-32674-8

Application of "Hand as Foot Teaching Method" in Dental Education: A Comprehensive Literature Review

Shivangi Vats, Manuel S Thomas, and Janina Loren D'Souza
Department of Conservative Dentistry and Endodontics, Manipal College of Dental Sciences Mangalore, Manipal Academy of Higher Education, Manipal, India

1 INTRODUCTION

It is a crucial obligation to provide undergraduate students with the knowledge and skills they need to practice dentistry. Graduates must understand the diagnosis and treatment of pulpal and peri-radicular disorders, as well as the preservation and repair of pulp in damaged teeth. The teaching objectives of endodontic learning depend upon an easy understanding of oral structures, oral and dental anatomy, and oral functions.

The technique called "Hand as Foot Teaching Method" has been used to teach key and difficult problems in medical education. [1] It is an innovative teaching strategy that uses hand gestures to help students understand anatomical structures and functions. It's used in medical education, particularly in human anatomy and surgery classes, comparing the orientation of hands to the orientation of a patient's foot or other anatomical structures. However, the applications of this teaching method extend to few areas of dental education as well. This technique has been and further can be applied in clinical teaching. This is an image teaching method using hand actions to improve the teaching effect, enliven the classroom atmosphere, and enhance the interaction between teachers and students thus, transforming student's learning process from abstract to intuitive, from simple rote memorization to comprehension and memory, achieving satisfactory results.

This article aims to understand the concept and extent of usage, of hand as a foot teaching method in various fields of dental education.

2 METHODOLOGY

Inclusion Criteria: All the literature text, and journal articles discussing hand as foot technique as a teaching method in dentistry or dental schools or dental institutes in the worldwide population were collected using keywords finalized after a brief literature review. Primary studies with any design published in peer-reviewed academic journals were included. Letters to Editors were also included. Hand as foot technique as a teaching method in medical education was also included.

Exclusion Criteria: Articles and text discussing other clinical medical and dental education teaching methods were excluded.

The electronic search strategy was developed in Pubmed, Google Scholar and Scopus databases. A search string was created, and articles were shortlisted according to inclusion criteria using Rayyan software by two independent reviewers. Data was synthesized using descriptive statistics. Results were analyzed and discussed.

3 RESULTS

Most of the articles describe the use of hand as foot technique in imparting clinical knowledge of anatomical structures in dentistry and medicine. It has also been used to describe various muscle movements in the temporomandibular joint, anatomic memorization of visceral structures and general surgical principles. In the field of dental education, it has been used to simplify the memorisation of classifications of root canal anatomy, root apex anatomy, and dental anatomical structure classification e.g CEJ. However, very few dental clinical simulations using hand as foot teaching method has been found. (Table 1)

 DOI: 10.1201/9781042016075-83

Table 1. Summary of included articles reporting the subject area, study type, and educational benefits of the "Hand as Foot" teaching method.

Sno.	Study	Type of study/article	Subject	Application
1.	Song *et al.* [2] Deng *et al.* [3]	Letter to Editor	*Portal vein anatomy Anatomy*	• Anatomy Memorization • Three-dimensional structure building • Accurate implementation of the hepatic portal vein related surgery • Learning efficiency improvement • Strengthening teacher-student interaction • Activating classroom atmosphere
2.	Liu J *et al.* [4]	Letter to Editor	Hepatic Anatomy	• Anatomy memorization • Three-dimensional structure building • Correct decisions on the best course of treatment during surgery • Learning efficiency improvement
3.	L. Zhang *et al.* [5]	Letter to Editor	Classification of C-shaped root canal anatomy	• Illustrative approach • Enhanced dental student understanding and management of unique dental morphology. • Enhanced Photographic memory and better clinical application of knowledge
4.	J. Zhang *et al.* [6]	Letter to Editor	Types of Cementoenamel Junction	• Facilitation of memory retention • deepening conceptual comprehension • Boost in learning management • Enhancement in learning efficiency.
5.	Wang S *et al.* [7]	Letter to Editor	Morphological classification of the tooth root canal	• Easier to remember root canal morphology • More intuitive learning
6.	Shi L *et al.* [8]	Letter to Editor	Tooth apex root anatomy	• Ease of remembering root canal morphology • Better recollection of root apex
7.	Su YN *et al.* [9]	Randomised Control Trial (Clinical Study)	Human Physiology	• Superior effectiveness in engaging students. • Facilitating comprehension • Enabling students to visualize complex physiological mechanisms. • Fostered active student participation with desire for deeper understanding.
8.	He B *et al.* [10]	Cohort Study	Characteristics of the motion system injury course	• Facilitating teachers to optimize the integration of knowledge points • Shortens the teaching time.
9.	Jiang T *et al.* [11]	Letter to Editor	Movements of Temporomandibular Joint	• combines the advantages of figurative analogy method and comparative method. • Simulate the human body structure morphology and joint movement.

4 DISCUSSION

The "Hand as Foot" teaching method demonstrates higher mental engagement of students, improving comprehension skills, and enhancing recollection. The "Hand as Foot teaching method" emphasizes the concept of "similarities in differences and similarities in differences" by using the analogy between upper and lower limb injuries. [10] It uses the analogy between human fingers and root canals. [7] This approach helps teachers integrate knowledge points more effectively and reduces teaching time. Currently, students and teachers recognize this teaching method. However, statistical analysis is required to confirm its feasibility and effectiveness. Therefore, relevant experiments should be designed to further validate its benefits and feasibility. Additionally, the gestural picture teaching method may generate psychological issues for students with physical disabilities.

5 CONCLUSION

In Dentistry, the "Hand as Foot" teaching approach combines "teach and learn" for teachers, "hand and brain" for learners thus, reinforcing learning mechanisms. This technique combined with multimedia teaching aids can potentially animate the learning process of difficult and confusing dental concepts for dental undergraduate students. However further research is needed in this area to further validate this technique as an essential teaching tool in student- teacher interactive environment.

CONFLICT OF INTEREST

The Authors claim that they have no conflict of interest.

FINANCIAL DISCLOSURES

Nil

ACKNOWLEDGEMENTS

Nil

REFERENCES

[1] Sana L, Dhaker T, Rahma Y, Marwa I, Wassim T, Faouzi C. (2023). Applications of "hand as foot" teaching methods in digestive and visceral surgery: A systemic review. *Educational Research (IJMCER)*. 5(3):147–53.

[2] Song XQ, Wang N. (2022). The "Hand as foot" teaching method in the anatomy of portal vein. *Asian J Surg*

[3] Deng L, Liu D, Jia P, Yan L. (2022). The "Hand as Foot" teaching method in hepatic portal vein branch. *Asian J Surg.*

[4] Liu J, Xue D, Wang P. (2022). The "Hand as Foot" teaching method in liver segment anatomy. *Asian J Surg* 45:565e567.

[5] L. Zhang, H. Liu and Y. Shen, (2022). The "Hand as Foot" teaching method in the classification of C-shaped root canal system in mandibular second molars, *Asian Journal of Surgery*, https://doi.org/10.1016/j.asjsur.2023.08.151

[6] J. Zhang, H. Liu and Y. Shen, (2022). The "Hand as Foot" teaching method in the classification of cementoenamel junction, *Asian Journal of Surgery*, https://doi.org/10.1016/j.asjsur.2023.08.176

[7] Wang S, Yu H, Li Z, Feng J. (2023). The "hand as foot" teaching method in morphologic classification of tooth root canal. *Asian J Surg*. 46(8):3077–3079. doi: 10.1016/j.asjsur.2023.02.058. Epub 2023 Mar 23. PMID: 36966109.

[8] Shi L, Liu H. (2024). The "Hand as Foot" teaching method in the tooth apical root anatomy. *Asian J Surg*. 47(2):1131–1132. doi: 10.1016/j.asjsur.2023.10.141. Epub 2023 Nov 25. PMID: 38008620.

[9] Su YN, Zhao DY. (2024). Effectiveness of the "Hand as Foot" teaching method in human physiology: A randomized controlled trial. *Asian J Surg*. 47(2):953–958. doi: 10.1016/j.asjsur.2023.12.178. Epub 2024 Jan 6. PMID: 38185549.

[10] He B, Li Q, Zhao J, Liu R, Li Y, Xu Y. (2021). The innovation and practice of "Hand as Foot teaching method" in the teaching of motion system injury course. *BMC Med Educ*. 21(1):553. doi: 10.1186/s12909-021-02944-w. Erratum in: BMC Med Educ. 23(1):13. doi: 10.1186/s12909-022-03818-5. PMID: 34717612; PMCID: PMC8557065.

[11] Jiang T, Liu R, Zhao J, He B. (2021). Application of "hand as foot" teaching method in temporomandibular joint movement teaching. *Asian J Surg*. 44(3):605–606. doi: 10.1016/j.asjsur.2020.12.023. Epub 2021 Feb 9. PMID: 33579605.

Navigating Dental Education Trends and Transforming Dental Pedagogy – Abas and Srikant N (Eds)
© 2027 The Author(s), ISBN: 978-1-041-32674-8

From the Classroom to the Clinic: Assessing and Improving Empathy in Dental Students by Implementing an Empathy Module

Jaishree Chahande
Department of Prosthodontics, Ranjeet Deshmukh Dental College & Research Centre, Nagpur. (formerly, VSPM's Dental College & Research Centre, Nagpur-Maharashtra)

ABSTRACT: **Purpose:** Empathy is considered one of the cornerstones of healthcare services and plays a vital role in doctor-patient relationships. According to the Association of American Medical Colleges and the American Dental Education Association, one of the most crucial goals of clinical training is empathy. There are gaps in the research on dental students, while there is a plethora of material evaluating medical students' empathy levels. This study aims to assess and compare empathy levels among undergraduate and postgraduate dental students with clinical exposure and to evaluate the impact of an empathy-training module on 2nd year undergraduate dental students. **Methods:** This study was conducted among all clinical undergraduates and postgraduate students. A validated, *'Jefferson Scale of Empathy Health Care Provider Student's Version'* was used for data collection. An empathy module was implemented for second-year dental students before they began their clinical training. The impact of this module was measured by pretest and posttest evaluations. **Results:** Empathy levels increased with increasing years of dental education. Undergraduate students demonstrated higher empathy levels in later years, indicating a potential lack of empathy training in earlier years. Compared with their male peers, female students presented greater empathy scores. The implementation of the empathy module for second-year undergraduate students resulted in a significant increase in empathy scores after training. **Conclusion:** This study observed how different student groups differed in their empathy. The findings suggest that incorporating empathy-training modules into the dental curriculum could enhance empathy among students, thereby improving patient care and doctor-patient relationships.

Keywords: Empathy, Dental, Doctor-patient relationship, Curriculum, Module

1 INTRODUCTION

Empathy is regarded one of the pillars of healthcare services. It plays a vital role in doctor-patient relationships ultimately influencing patient satisfaction and treatment efficacy. [1] Empathy is a crucial component of effective patient care, particularly in fields such as dentistry where patient anxiety and discomfort are common. [2–4] The word empathy came from the *German* word *'Einfulung'* and was derived from the *Greek* words *'em'* and *'pathos'*, which mean *'feeling into'*. 'Sympathy' and 'empathy' are sometimes used interchangeably. Sympathy is 'the experience of another person's emotions and when feel sorry for someone but might not do anything to help'. While, empathy is 'a cognitive attribute that involves an ability to understand the patient's experiences, pain, suffering and perspective combined with a capability to communicate this understanding and intention to help'. As per Pederson in 2009, empathy is considered the 'appropriate understanding of the patient'. [5]

The three domains of empathy are: cognitive, affective and behavioral. The cognitive domain enables us to see the outside world from other people's perspectives and comprehend the inner experiences of others. We can participate or enter another person's experience through the affective domain. [6] The behavioural domain facilitates to take action. Since, both empathy and sympathy entail sharing, they should be distinguished in the context of patient care because they are frequently confused. [7]

Empathy was highlighted as one of the primary goals of clinical training by the *'Association of American Medical Colleges'* (AAMC) [8] and the *'American Dental Education Association'* (ADEA) [9]; however gaps exist in applying these principles to dental education. Dental students deal with their patients in close proximity in clinics, and the dentist-patient relationship strengthens by the empathy. [10]

With this in mind, a longitudinal comparative analytical study was conducted among clinical dental students to assess empathy. [11–13] However, whereas there is a lot of literature assessing medical students' empathy skills, there are gaps in studies on dental students. Only a few studies have been undertaken with regard to the Indian context. Traditional dental curricula often emphasize technical skills over interpersonal skills, potentially leading to a gap in empathetic patient interactions. Therefore, this study aims to fill this research gap by assessing and comparing empathy levels among undergraduate and postgraduate dental students between different years of study with clinical exposure and to evaluate the impact of an empathy training module implemented for second-year BDS (Bachelor of Dental Surgery) students prior to their clinical exposure.

DOI: 10.1201/9781042016075-84

2 MATERIALS AND METHODS

2.1 *Study design and population*

A longitudinal mixed-methods comparative analytical study design was used to evaluate the impact of the empathy module.

After approval was obtained from the Institutional Ethics Committee, the undergraduate students with clinical exposure included third, final year students, interns, and postgraduates, including first-final year students, of Ranjeet Deshmukh Dental College & Research Centre, Nagpur (formerly, *VSPM's Dental College & Research Centre, Nagpur-Maharashtra*) participated in study.

2.2 *Data collection technique*

This study was conducted in two phases.

Phase I: Phase I included data collection from all Undergraduates with clinical exposure and postgraduate students via a pre validated, self-administered questionnaire including demographic details. The questionnaire consisted of two parts: Part I included demographic details of the participants, including age, sex, and year of study. Part II included the '*Jefferson Scale of Empathy Health Care Provider Student's Version*' *(JSE-HPS)*. [5,11,14] In this twenty items instrument, responses are given on a seven-point Likert scale, with 1 denoting 'strongly disagree' and 7 denoting 'strongly agree.' Ten negatively phrased items on the scale were reverse scored out of the 20 questions. [15,16] A higher score denotes a behavioural propensity favouring empathic engagement in patient care; the total score goes from 20 to 140.

The questionnaire was distributed to all the students, and a statistical analysis was performed.

Phase II: Empathy Module:

On the basis of initial assessments, an empathy module was designed and implemented for second-year BDS students as a part of the value-added course on *'Emotional Intelligence'* to inculcate empathy before beginning their clinical postings.

2.3 *The empathy module consisted of the following:*

- **Interactive Workshops**: Focus on understanding patient perspectives and effective communication, including empathetic communication, patient-centred care, using positive gestures and nonverbal clues, like making eye contact, using open body language, taking notes, active listening, and repeating what a patient says to make sure they understand. [17]
- **Group Task on identifying the statements**: Displaying clinical scenarios to differentiate between sympathy and empathy.
- **Role-playing exercises**: Simulated patient scenarios to practice empathy. Practice empathetic and sympathetic responses by pair-up and role-playing different patient scenarios. One person acts as the patient, and the other practices empathetic and sympathetic responses and then switches roles and discusses experiences. [18]
- **Reflections and discussion on the applied aspect of empathy**: Students documented their experiences and reflections on empathy during the clinical practice scenario. Patient history during clinical work and lifelong clinical practice. [19]

Questions for Reflection like-

- How did the role-play exercise feel?
- What challenges did you face in practicing empathy or sympathy?
- How can you incorporate these skills into your daily patient interactions during case history taking, clinical work and lifelong clinical practice?
- **Resources and Further Reading:** Books and articles are shared with students.
- **Follow-up:** Additional follow-up assessments will be conducted before clinical exposure.

2.4 *Data collection of the Empathy Module*

Quantitative: Empathy was measured via the *'Jefferson Scale of Empathy for Healthcare Providers'* (JSE-HCP) before and after the module by Pretest and Posttest to evaluate its impact. [5]

Qualitative: Interviews and reflections using feedback provided insights into students' experiences and perceived changes. Pretests were conducted before the module, and posttests were administered immediately after the module to evaluate its impact.

2.5 *Statistical analysis*

The data were analysed via descriptive statistics and inferential tests. The empathy scores were compared across different groups via t tests where appropriate. A p value of <0.05 was considered to indicate statistical significance.

3 RESULTS

Demographics: The study included 352 students, including 279 undergraduate and 73 postgraduate students. A total of 62 males and 290 female participants with a mean age of 23.42 years were included.

Empathy Levels: Table 1 presents the average empathy scores by student group.

Table 1. Empathy scores by student group and gender.

Year of study	Group	Male Empathy Scores	Female Empathy Scores	Mean Empathy Score	Std. Deviation	p value
Undergraduates	Third-Year	66.28	90.18	78.23	10.183	<0.001
	Final-Year	79.83	101.63	90.73	12.124	
	Interns	86.55	109.23	97.89	14.193	
Postgraduates	First-Year	92.90	120.18	106.54	16.85	<0.005
	Second-Year	109.00	119.54	114.27	18.574	
	Final-Year	120.11	129.47	124.79	20.154	
Mean Empathy Score		92.445	111.705	102.075		

Graph 1-Empathy scores by student group and gender

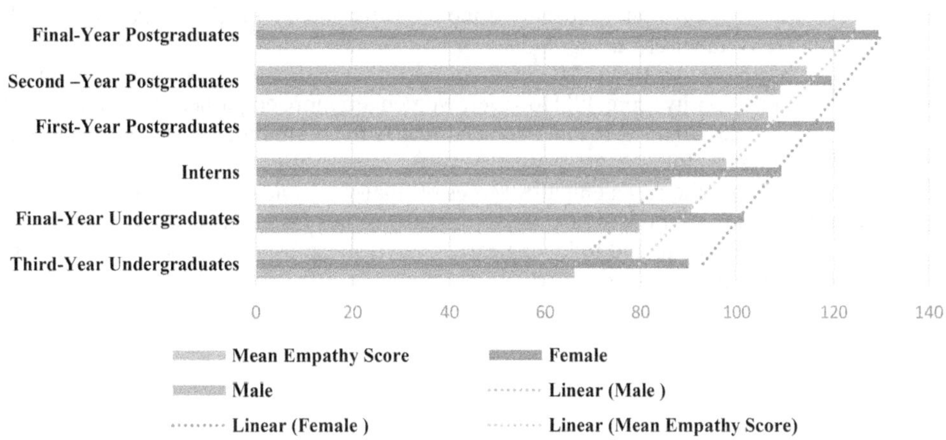

Graph 1. Shows that the trend line increases as the year of study progresses for undergraduates and Postgraduates.

The analysis revealed a significant increase in empathy scores as the students progressed through their dental education ($p < 0.001$).

Undergraduate students: Empathy levels increased significantly from third-year to final-year students and interns ($p < 0.001$). Specifically, empathy scores were higher among interns than among final and third BDS students.

Postgraduate students: There was a noticeable increase in empathy scores from first-year to final-year postgraduates ($p < 0.05$).

Gender differences: Female students consistently scored higher on empathy measures than male students did ($p < 0.05$).

Impact of Empathy Module: For second-year BDS students, there was a statistically significant increase in empathy scores, with a male pretest mean score of 60.28 and a posttest mean score of 103.52 and a t value of 8.65, with $p < 0.001$. The female pretest empathy mean score was 70.56, the posttest empathy mean score was 112.45, and the t value was 8.38, with $p < 0.001$ indicating statistical significance. This finding indicates that the empathy module has a positive impact on the second BDS student's empathy scores, which are further assessed when they join clinical postings.

Feedback: After the empathy module, feedback was collected from second BDS students.

Table 2 shows the statements of the second BDS students regarding empathy module feedback on a five-point Likert scale ranging from strongly disagree (1) to strongly agree (5). The results of the chi-square goodness-of-fit test, indicate that there are statistically significant differences in the level of agreement of the second BDS students regarding the statements.

Table 2. Feedback from Second BDS students about the Empathy Module.

Statement	Chi-Square	df	p value
(1) I am now able to differentiate between sympathy and empathy	39.700	2	.000
(1) I learned empathetic communication skills	51.600	2	.000
(1) I enjoyed role play techniques	33.600	2	.000
(1) Group activities were engaging	63.300	2	.000
(1) I faced challenges while practicing empathy initially during group task	38.700	2	.000
(1) I feel that every dental student should learn empathy for patient care	48.500	2	.000
(1) I will incorporate these skills into my daily patient interactions during case history taking, clinical work and lifelong clinical practice	47.200	2	.000
(1) Shared resource materials to learn empathy are interesting	34.900	2	.000
(1) Can continue Empathy Module in future	35.300	2	.000

4 DISCUSSION

These findings indicate that empathy levels among dental students improve with increasing years of study, likely due to increased clinical experience and exposure. The higher empathy scores observed in female students suggest potential gender-based differences in empathic tendencies. The positive impact of the empathy module highlights its potential as a valuable addition to the dental curriculum, fostering greater empathic engagement from the early stages of clinical training. Research has indicated that empathy enhances therapeutic results, treatment compliance, and patient satisfaction. Feeling heard and understood increases the likelihood that patients will adhere to their treatment plan and take care of themselves.

The findings of a study conducted by Babar MG *et al.* revealed that male students outperformed female students in terms of their overall mean empathy score. [9] However, women are more empathetic than men in this study and the majority of others. [15,20–22] Hojat M *et al.* contended that women are more sensitive to emotional cues and that empathy is a feminine quality. [6]

According to Sherman JJ *et al.*, the mean empathy scores of final-year students were greater than those of other years. This result was similar to that of this study, where empathy scores increased as the year of study progressed. [20] According to Beattie *et al.*, prior to and following early analytical exposure to behavioral sciences and clinical encounters, empathy levels significantly increased. [23]

5 LIMITATIONS

This study is limited to only data collected during the empathy module, and further observations are awaited until second BDS students join their clinical postings. Only empathy scale scores were compared on the basis of the pre validated empathy scale, but clinical observations during clinical work can yield actual empathy scores.

6 CONCLUSION

This study highlights the variability in empathy levels among dental students and underscores the need for structured empathy training within the dental curriculum. The incorporation of empathy modules can significantly enhance empathic skills, contributing to better patient interactions and overall treatment outcomes. Building empathetic relationships with our patients also reduces disagreements and can increase reimbursement due to improved patient experience score. We can establish a deeper human connection with our patients when we take the time to understand them.

7 SUGGESTIONS

Comparative studies between different dental schools and international settings could provide broader insights into empathy training, and further research could explore the integration of empathy training across different stages of dental education and its effects on various competencies in dental practice.

ACKNOWLEDGMENT

I would like to express my gratitude to every student who took part in this study.

REFERENCES

[1] Williams B, Sadasivan S, Kadirvelu A, Olaussen A. (2014). Empathy levels among first year Malaysian medical students: an observational study. *Adv Med Educ Pract.* 5:149–56. doi: 10.2147/AMEP.S58094. PMID: 24876799; PMCID: PMC4035026.

[2] Hojat M, Gonnella JS, Mangione S, Nasca TJ, Veloski JJ, Erdmann JB, Callahan CA, Magee M. (2002). Empathy in medical students as related to academic performance, clinical competence and gender. *Med Educ.* 36(6):522–7. doi: 10.1046/j.1365-2923.2002.01234.x. PMID: 12047665.

[3] Mercer SW, Maxwell M, Heaney D, Watt GC. (2004). The consultation and relational empathy (CARE) measure: development and preliminary validation and reliability of an empathy-based consultation process measure. *Fam Pract.* 21(6):699–705. doi: 10.1093/fampra/cmh621. Epub 2004 Nov 4. PMID: 15528286.

[4] Wiltshire AD, Ross MW, Brimlow DL. (2002). Empathic communication between dental professionals and persons living with HIV and AIDS. *J Dent Educ.* 66(1):86–93. PMID: 12358105.

[5] Hojat M, Mangione S, Nasca TJ, CohenMJM, Gonnella JS, Erdmann JB, and Magee M. (2001). The jefferson scale of physician empathy: Development and preliminary psychometric data. educational and psychological measurement - *EDUC PSYCHOL MEAS.* 61. 349–365. 10.1177/00131640121971158.

[6] Hojat M, Gonnella JS, Nasca TJ, Mangione S, Vergare M, Magee M. (2002). Physician empathy: definition, components, measurement, and relationship to gender and specialty. *Am J Psychiatry.* 159(9):1563–9. doi: 10.1176/appi.ajp.159.9.1563. PMID: 12202278.

[7] Wispe L. (1986). The distinction between sympathy and empathy: To call forth a concept, a word is needed. *J Pers Soc Psychol 1986.* Vol. 50(2):314–321. DOI: 10.1037/0022-3514.50.2.314.

[8] Barbosa P, Raymond G, Zlotnick C, Wilk J, Toomey R 3rd, Mitchell J 3rd. (2013). Mindfulness-based stress reduction training is associated with greater empathy and reduced anxiety for graduate healthcare students. *Educ Health (Abingdon).* 2013 Jan-Apr;26 (1):9–14. doi: 10.4103/1357-6283.112794. PMID: 23823667.

[9] Babar MG, Omar H, Lim LP, Khan SA, Mitha S, Ahmad SFB, Hasan SS. (2013). An assessment of dental students' empathy levels in Malaysia. *Int J Med Educ.* 4:223–9. doi: 10.5116/ijme.5259.4513. PMCID: PMC4205538.

[10] Díaz-Narváez, V.P., Gutierrez-Ventura, F., de Villalba, T.V., Salcedo-Rioja, M., Calzadilla-Núñez, A., Hamdan-Rodríguez, M. and Cervantes, M. (2015) Empathy levels of dentistry students in peru and argentina. *Health,* 7, 1268–1274. http://dx.doi.org/10.4236/health.2015.710141

[11] Prabhu S, Kumar VS, Prasanth SS, Kishore S. (2014). Standing in patients' shoes – Survey on empathy among dental students in India. *J Educ Ethics Dent* 2014;4:69–73 10.4103/0974-7761.148990..

[12] Datta G, Vanishree N, Nayak SS, Bullappa D, Naveen N, Lakshmikantha R, Prasad KS, Anushri M. (2016). Measuring empathy towards patients among dental under graduate students of bangalore city-a cross sectional study. *J. Med. Public Health,* 6(3):113–6.

[13] Aggarwal VP, Garg R, Goyal N, Kaur P, Singhal S, Singla N, Gijwani D, Sharma A. (2016). Exploring the missing link - Empathy among dental students: An institutional cross-sectional survey. *Dent Res J (Isfahan).* 13(5):419–423. doi: 10.4103/1735-3327.192279. PMID: 27857767; PMCID: PMC5091000.

[14] Hojat, Mohammadreza. (2016). *Empathy in Health Professions Education and Patient Care.* 10.1007/978-3-319-27625-0

[15] Boyle MJ, Williams BA, Brown GT, Molloy AM, McKenna LG, Molloy E *et al.* (2010). Levels of empathy in undergraduate health science students. *The Internet Journal of Medical Education.* 1(1):1–14.

[16] Jefferson Scale of Empathy (JSE). Center for research in medical education and health care (CRMEHC). [cited 1 July 2013]; Available from: http://www.jefferson.edu/jmc/crmehc/jse.html.

[17] Baker DP, Day R, Salas E. (2006). Teamwork as an essential component of high-reliability organizations. *Health Serv Res.* 41(4 Pt 2):1576–98. doi: 10.1111/j.1475-6773.2006.00566.x. PMID: 16898980; PMCID: PMC1955345.

[18] Derksen F, Bensing J, Lagro-Janssen A. (2013). Effectiveness of empathy in general practice: a systematic review. *Br J Gen Pract.* 63(606):e76–84. doi: 10.3399/bjgp13X660814. PMID: 23336477; PMCID: PMC3529296.

[19] Schön, D.A. (1983). *The Reflective Practitioner: How Professionals Think in Action.* Basic Books.

[20] Sherman JJ, Cramer A. (2005). A measurement of changes in empathy during dental school. *J Dent Educ.* 69(3):338–45.

[21] Magalhaes E, Salgueira AP, Costa P, Costa MJ. (2011). Empathy in senior year and first year medical students: a cross-sectional study. *BMC Med Educ.* 11:52.

[22] Kataoka HU, Koide N, Ochi K, Hojat MR, Gonnella JS. (2009). Measurement of empathy among Japanese medical students: psychometrics and score differences by gender and level of medical education. *Acad Med.* 84: 1192–7.

[23] Beattie A, Durham J, Harvey J, Steele J, McHanwell S. (2012). Does empathy change in first-year dental students? *Eur J Dent Educ.* 16: e111–e116.

Navigating Dental Education Trends and Transforming Dental Pedagogy – Abas and Srikant N (Eds)
 ISBN: 978-1-041-32674-8

Digitally Advanced Axiographic Tool for New Trends in Teaching and Assessment of Recording Condylar Guidance in Dental Education

Ganaraj Shetty
Department of Prosthodontics, AB Shetty Memorial Institute of Dental, Sciences, NITTE (Deemed to be University), Deralakatte, Mangaluru, Karnataka, India

Manoj Shetty
Department of Oral Implantology, AB Shetty Memorial Institute, of Dental Sciences, NITTE (Deemed to be University), Deralakatte, Mangaluru, Karnataka, India

ABSTRACT: Aim and objective: The study aims to systematically analyse the digitally advanced Axiographic tool in recording condylar guidance that focuses on introducing the innovative technique in teaching dental students, and assessment of recording the condylar guidance to facilitate providing designed occlusion in complete denture prosthesis.

Materials and methods: 50 completely edentulous subjects referred to the Department of Prosthodontics for receiving complete denture prostheses were considered to participate in the study. The condylar guidance was recorded using the conventional technique (Gothic arch tracing technique, interocclusal bite recording technique,) and digitally advanced Axiographic tool to record the condylar guidance following which the programming of the articulator was done to achieve balanced occlusion.

Results: The data on various study parameters were obtained and summarized using appropriate statistical measures. No significant difference was observed in recording condylar guidance amongst the Gothic arch tracing, interocclusal bite record, and axiographic tracings. The mean difference between the Gothic arch tracing and the interocclusal bite record is 1.19°. The mean difference between the Gothic arch tracing and the axiographic tracings is 0.96°. And between the interocclusal bite record tracing and the axiographic tracings is 0.23°.

Conclusion: The digitally advanced Axiographic tool can substitute the use of the conventional techniques which is less time consuming and will ease the procedure in recording condylar guidance, which aids in accurately programming the semi-adjustable articulator to facilitate providing the designed balanced occlusion in complete denture prosthesis and may also help in introducing the technique in teaching and for dental students.

Keywords: Axiographic recording, Condylar guidance, Extraoral tracing intraoral tracing

1 INTRODUCTION

The documentation of the maxillomandibular relationship and recording of the condylar guidance values have to be done with the utmost care, as the values help us set the condylar guidance and program the semi-adjustable articulator following which the balanced complete denture prosthesis is fabricated without any error in occlusion [1–3]. The condylar guidance values obtained from the records of centric and eccentric relation help the operator to program the semiadjustable articulator that indirectly aids in the diagnosis, designing the treatment paln, and contiving the complete denture prosthesis. The intersection of the arcs is produced by the movement of the condyle on right side and left side of the form the head of apex of the arrow, the record obtained which is known as the Gothic arch tracing record [4]. The development in digital technology have made it more feasible to inspect and evaluate the movements of the mandibular jaw with the highest degree of precision and accuracy; in the present study, a contactless-type of mandibular tracking device, which is known as Axioquick recording is used to record condylar guidance. Hence, The study aims to systematically analyse the digitally advanced Axiographic tool in recording condylar guidance that focuses on introducing the innovative technique in teaching dental students, and assessment of recording the condylar guidance to facilitate providing designed occlusion in complete denture prosthesis.

2 MATERIALS AND METHODS

The study was carried out in the Department of Prosthodontics and Crown & Bridge at our institute after obtaining ethical clearance from the institute's Ethical Clearance Committee with the Registration No NU/CEC/2016-2017/0080. A total of 50 completely edentulous subjects with high, well-rounded class I ridges, sufficient interarch space, and good neuromuscular coordination were randomly selected to participate in the study.

 DOI: 10.1201/9781042016075-85

3 RESULTS

Table 1. Comparison of the right and left sides in group I (Gothic arch tracing)

	N	*Mean*	*SD*	*Mean Difference*	*95% Confidence interval (CI) of the difference*		*t*	*Degree of freedom (df)*	*p-value*
					Lower	*Upper*			
Left	53	29.06	2.78	0.19	-0.41	0.79	0.63	52	0.53 (NS)
Right	53	28.87	3.62						

Paired t-test; $*p < 0.05$ statistically significant; $p > 0.05$, not significant; NS, nonsignificant

Table 2. Comparison of the right and left sides in group II (Interocclusal bite record)

	N	*Mean*	*SD*	*Mean Difference*	*95% (CI) of the difference*		*t*	*df*	*p-value*
					Lower	*Upper*			
Left	53	27.74	3.61	0.06	-0.43	0.54	0.24	52	0.82 (NS)
Right	53	27.68	4.03						

Paired t-test; $*p < 0.05$ statistically significant; $p > 0.05$, not significant; nonsignificant, NS

Table 3. Comparison of the right and left sides in group III (axiographic tracing)

	N	*Mean*	*SD*	*Mean Difference*	*95% (CI) of the difference*		*t*	*df*	*p-value*
					Lower	*Upper*			
Left	53	28.08	3.23	0.17	-0.46	0.8	0.54	52	0.59 (NS)
Right	53	27.91	3.44						

Paired t-test; $*p < 0.05$ statistically significant; $p > 0.05$, not significant; NS, nonsignificant

Table 4. Comparison between the study groups (group I: graphic tracing; group II: interocclusal records; group III: axiograph reading) readings using ANOVA

	Study groups	*N*	*Mean*	*SD*	*Min*	*Max*	*ANOVA*	
							F	*p-value*
Left	1	53	29.06	2.78	25	35	2.40	0.09(NS)
	2	53	27.74	3.61	20	35		
	3	53	28.08	3.23	21	34		

$*p < 0.05$, statistically significant; $p > 0.05$, not significant; NS, nonsignificant

Table 5. Comparison between the study groups (group I: graphic tracing; group II: interocclusal records; group III: axiograph reading) readings using ANOVA

	Study groups	*N*	*Mean*	*SD*	*Min*	*Max*	*ANOVA*	
							F	*p-value*
Left	1	53	28.87	3.62	20	35	1.54	0.22 (NS)
	2	53	27.68	4.03	20	35		
	3	53	27.91	3.44	21	35		

$*p < 0.05$, statistically significant; $p > 0.05$, not significant; NS, nonsignificant

Comparison between the study groups (group I: graphic tracing; group II: interocclusal records; group III: axiograph reading)using ANOVA. The condylar guidance value on the left side was maximum in group I with a mean value of 29.06 ± 2.78, followed by 28.08 ± 3.23 for group III and least in group II with a mean value of 27.74 ± 3.61. However, there was no significant difference in the left condylar guidance value between the three groups ($p > 0.05$)

Comparison between the study groups (group I: graphic tracing; group II: interocclusal records; group III: axiograph reading) using ANOVA Similarly, on the right side, the mean condylar guidance value was highest in group I with a mean value of 28.87 ± 3.62 followed by 27.91 ± 3.44 for group III and least in group II with a mean value of 27.68 ± 4.03. Group I showed maximum variation when compared to groups II and III on the right side and left side, with no significant difference in condylar guidance value between the three groups ($p > 0.05$).

In a pairwise comparison between the groups on the left side, when group I was compared with group II, the mean difference obtained was 1.32° with a nonsignificant *p*-value of 0.09. Similarly, when group I was compared with group II, the mean difference obtained was 0.98° with a nonsignificant *p*-value of 0.26. Similarly, when group II was compared with group III, the mean difference obtained was 0.34 with a nonsignificant value *p*-value of 1.82.

Pairwise comparison between the groups on the right side, when the group I was compared with group II the mean difference obtained was 1.19° with a nonsignificant *p*-value of 0.23. Similarly, when group I was compared with group II, the mean difference obtained was 0.96° with a nonsignificant *p*-value of 0.38 which was the value. Similarly, when group II was compared with group III, the mean difference obtained was 0.23 with a nonsignificant *p*-value of 0.95.

4 DISCUSSION

The accomplishment of successful Prosthodontic practice can be strengthened by accurately simulating the direction of the movement of the condylar head over the articular eminence of the completely edentulous patient on a semi-adjustable articulator. It facilitates the operator to record the condylar path that can be traced by the movement of the condyles in centric and all the eccentric mandibular movements and also to design the morphology of the occlusal surfaces, which in turn aids in restoring the occlusion without interferences [5,6]. The "high tracers" are the type of gothic arch tracing device which is specially designed to trace the condylar guidance by eliminating all the inconveniences so often experienced during the recording of the condylar guidance [7]. Christensen proposed the use of a protrusive interocclusal record for programming the semi-adjustable articulator in the year 1902; further, Hanau's formula was introduced in 1930, equating $L = H/8 + 12$ to calculate lateral condylar guidance used to record and obtain the condylar guidance values to program the semi-adjustable articulators [8,9]. In the philosophies published recently and literature reviews attesting to the inaccuracies of interocclusal bite registrations, many clinicians use the average condylar guidance value to program the semi-adjustable articulator obtained from the mean published values. The axiography is a graphical recording technique used to record the path of condylar guidance with high precision and accurately provide numerical data of these movements. In the present study, the axiography was used solely for the objective of digitally recording the path of condylar guidance. The present study can be a step toward evaluating the ability of the conventionally followed Gothic arch tracing technique and finding more reliable techniques to overcome the limitations and shortcomings of all the techniques used earlier. there are presently no studies comparing horizontal condylar guidance obtained by extraoral Gothic arch tracing, interocclusal bite records, and axiographic tracings. The condylar guidance values obtained from above mentioned three techniques shows no statistically significant variations. Thus, the null hypothesis stating no significant difference in the condyle guidance values recorded using the Gothic arch tracing technique, interocclusal bite recording technique, and axiographic tracings is accepted.

5 CONCLUSION

The digitally advanced Axiographic tool can substitute the use of the conventional techniques which is less time consuming and will ease the procedure in recording condylar guidance, which aids in accurately programming the semi-adjustable articulator to facilitate providing the designed balanced occlusion in complete denture prosthesis and may also help in introducing the technique in teaching and for dental students.

REFERENCES

[1] Vikas C. A Critical Evaluation of Different Methods of Recording Centric Jaw Relation of Completely Edentulous Individuals: An in Vivo Study (Doctoral dissertation, Tamil Nadu Government Dental College and Hospital, Chennai).

[2] Bansal S, Palaskar J. (2009). Critical evaluation of methods to record centric jaw relation. *The J Indian Prosthodont Soc* 9(3):120–126. DOI: 10.4103/0972-4052.57080

[3] Hernandez AI, Jasinevicius TR, Kaleinikova Z, *et al.* (2010). Symmetry of horizontal and sagittal condylar path angles: an in vivo study. *Cranio* 28(1):60–66. DOI: 10.1179/crn.2010.008

[4] Patil R, Dubey S, Patil A, *et al.* (2015). Correlation between sagittal condylar guidance obtained by Gothic arch tracing an interocclusal record and by panoramic radiographic tracing in edentulous subjects: A clinicoradiographic analysis. *IOSR J Dent Med Sci* 14(1):57–59. DOI: 10.9790/0853-14155759

[5] Jerath S, Rani S, Kumar M, *et al.* (2019). Clinico-radiographic comparative evaluation of horizontal condylar guidance angle by interocclusal wax record, CBCT and Gothic arch tracing method-an in vivo study. *Int J Recent Sci Res* 10(7):33715–33720. DOI: 10.24327/ijrsr.2019.1007.3732

[6] Sabarigirinathan C, Vinayagavel K, Gunasekar C, *et al.* (2013). A critical evaluation of different methods of recording centric jaw relation of completely edentulous individuals: An in vivo study. *IJOART* 2(12):31–39.

[7] Bhawsar SV, Marathe AS, Ansari SA. (2015). Evaluation of Hanau's formula in determination of lateral condylar guidance: a clinical research study. *J Indian Prosthodont Soc* 15(4):326–330. DOI: 10.4103/0972-4052.161566

[8] Curtis TA, Taylor RC, Rositano SA. (1975). Physical problems in obtaining records of the maxillofacial patient. *J Prosthet Dent* 34 (5):539–554. DOI: 10.1016/0022-3913(75)90042-6

[9] Gilboa I, Cardash HS, Kaffe I, *et al.* (2008). Condylar guidance: correlation between articular morphology and panoramic radiographic images in dry human skulls. *J Prosthet Dent* 99(6):477–482. DOI: 10.1016/ S0022-3913(08)60112-2

 ISBN: 978-1-041-32674-8

Emotional Intelligence: A Critical Aspect of Dental Education in India

Ashwin Rao
Department of Pediatric and Preventive Dentistry, Manipal College of Dental Sciences Mangalore, Manipal Academy of Higher Education, Manipal, India

ABSTRACT: Emotional intelligence (EI) is a broad spectrum with various diverse facets. EI plays a vital role in personal and professional success and easily scales with intelligence quotient or cognition. EI has a major influence on the dental profession considering the nature of its work. Awareness of EI is a very important aspect of a career in dentistry, as the dentist negotiates difficult professional challenges involving hard skills, patients and failures and finances. This awareness of EI, however, cannot be developed overnight and hence needs to be incorporated into the dental curriculum for undergraduates. In India, students from various economic, financial and educational backgrounds join dentistry. Patients also tend to come from diverse economic, cultural and religious backgrounds. An awareness of the concept of EI therefore becomes critically important in the Indian context both during the period of dental education to help patients cope with the stress of education and later to communicate with patients. Dentists who had impressive technical skills but poor communication ability had poor patient satisfaction scores. However, dental schools in India lack a formal curriculum in this area. EI is touched upon only briefly in the curriculum through theories of psychology in the subject of pediatric dentistry as part of child psychology. This review therefore explored the need for a structured format to teach the concept of emotional intelligence to undergraduate dental students in India.

Keywords: emotional intelligence, emotional quotient, dental education and dentistry under graduation, dental curriculum, India

1 INTRODUCTION

Emotional intelligence (EI) is a broad spectrum with various diverse facets. The dental profession, owing to its nature, has been acknowledged to be a very stressful area of work [1,2]. Knowledge of personality development and emotional intelligence are very important aspects for a career in dentistry, as the dentist negotiates challenging professional challenges involving hard skills, patients and failures and finances. The challenges involve raising their heads at the beginning of dental school, starting with a demanding curriculum [3]. However, the student is not formally taught to address mental challenges that lie ahead in the student life and subsequently in their career. The aspect of EI is touched upon only briefly in the curriculum through theories of psychology in the subject of pediatric dentistry as part of child psychology. However, the fact that these theories have implications for budding dentists, which go beyond the realms of child management in dentistry, is lost to the students. The psychoanalytic theory of Sigmund Freud is a key example here. Through its key components of the Psychic triad, the Iceberg phenomenon, psychosexual stages and defense mechanisms teach the development of personality and emotional intelligence. However, it is taught within the circumference of the application of child management only. This paper reviews the need for a structured format to teach the concept of emotional intelligence to undergraduate dental students, especially in India, which is a culturally diverse country [4] in terms of language, religion and income.

2 MATERIALS AND METHODS

A literature search was conducted using the keywords "emotional intelligence", "emotional quotient", "dental education", "dental under graduation", "dental postgraduate", "dental curriculum" and "India". The search was conducted in various databases, including Scopus, Medline via PubMed, CINAHL and Embase. Boolean operators such as 'AND' and 'OR' were employed to refine the search within each database. Original studies and review articles specifically addressing the subject of emotional intelligence and dental education in India after 2000 were included. Articles related to emotional intelligence not related to dental education, the curriculum, or India were excluded.

From the initial search of 102 articles, 7 met our inclusion criteria after screening titles and abstracts. These studies are relevant to emotional intelligence and dental education in India. However, upon full-text review, 2 of these articles were excluded. Ultimately, we included 5 articles that explored emotional intelligence and dentistry under graduation and were relevant to India. (Table 1).

 DOI: 10.1201/9781042016075-86

Table 1. List of included studies with methods and conclusion.

Author	Year	Type	Conclusion
Bhaskar D J *et al.* [6]	2012	Original research	Both male and female Pedodontic postgraduates had a high EI
Ravichandra K S *et al.* [4]	2015	Original Research	Major percentage of students Surveyed not aware of EI
Kumar A *et al.* [7]	2015	Original research	More than half the participants had high EI scores though not in all domains
Yadav V *et al.* [5]	2020	Original research	Significant difference between males and females with respect to handling stress
Saoji SS [8]	2024	Original research	High level of EI in post graduate students

3 RESULTS

In 2015, Ravichandra K S *et al.* [4] conducted a cross-sectional survey among undergraduate dental students to assess their EI in six domains. Only 11.55% of the participants had good EI, with scores above 20 in all domains. They recommended interventions to make undergraduate students aware of the EI concept and its impact on their dental education and careers [4].

Yadv V *et al.*. in 2020 [5] conducted a cross-sectional survey among 323 dental undergraduates across Delhi. They used the Schutte Emotional Intelligence and Perceived Stress scale for this purpose. The results revealed an inverse relationship between EI and perceived stress. They recommended stress prevention and intervention programs within the dental curriculum. Using

Bhaskar J D *et al.* [6]. conducted a survey among 300 Pedodontic postgraduate students evaluating their EI. The results revealed high EI among both male and female Pedodontic postgraduates.

Kumar A *et al.*. [7] in 2015 determined the association between EI and the academic performance of final-year undergraduate dental students across six colleges in Bengaluru. They reported that EI was positively associated with academic performance and recommended that dental students' EI be developed.

Saoji SS *et al.*. [8] in 2024 determined the association between confidence fatigue and EI among postgraduate students in India. They reported a high EI level despite high confidence fatigue (CF) and recommended formal EI awareness to combat the CF.

4 DISCUSSION

4.1 *Understanding emotional intelligence*

EI is defined as *'a form of intelligence that involves the ability to monitor one's own and others' feelings and emotions, to discriminate among them and to use this information to guide one's thinking and actions'* [9]. The first references of EI can be traced back to the roots of emotional intelligence (EI), which can be traced back to the "multiple intelligence theory" by Gardner [10] and the "social intelligence theory" by Thorndike [11]. The concept of EI was proposed by Salovey and Mayer [9]. They explained the importance of being aware of one's own emotions and channelized the balanced use of emotions to guide their actions. Various terms have been used to define emotional intelligence, including emotional quotient, social intelligence and emotional literacy. The EI includes six important facets [12]. These include self-confidence, self-awareness, empathy, self-control, motivation and social competency. Self-confidence is a basic belief that a person can do what is required to produce the desired outcome despite the prevailing situation. Self-awareness is a deep understanding of one's self and one's own strengths and weakness. Empathy is the ability to be kind to other situations and feelings. Self-control broadly addresses being able to control emotional outbursts. The traits of persistence and passion comprise motivation. Social competency comprises a genuine interest in other people and seeing the good in them. It has been argued by Goleman [12] that EI plays a vital role in personal and professional success and easily scales with intelligence quotients or cognition. Its role in healthcare areas in terms of mental health and success in practice are now being increasingly recognized.

4.2 *Emotional intelligence and the dental profession*

The dental profession especially has an intimate association with EI [13]. The surgical aspect of this field in an environment where the patient is conscious and aware of the pain is very unique to dentistry among all healthcare specialties. The dentist also works near the patient very much in the patient's personal space where the patient can also sense his/her vibration and emotions. The dentist must therefore understand the individual patient's behavior and work according to the needs of each patient. This, in EI terms, is called empathy, which is a trait where the individual is aware and considerate of another human being's feelings. These emotional expectations put considerable pressure on the dental surgeon, who has to have strong control over his/her emotional reactions to carry out this sensitive work on a daily basis. This is even more pertinent considering that dentists and other healthcare professionals invariably bring their emotions to the workplace. In addition, considering that the Dentist population ratio, especially in rural India, is 1:20000 [14], dentists are burdened with a heavy workload. This, in the long run, can take a toll on her/his mental health. Pankey demonstrated that dentists with good EI skills tend to have more harmonious practice environments with better conflict resolving skills [15]. Communication is another vital skill required by the dentist because demanding procedures are performed on conscious patients under local anesthesia. Good communication skills can allay patient anxiety, leading to improved treatment outcomes. Sarnat H *et al.* [16] reported that dentists who had impressive technical skills but poor communication abilities had poor patient satisfaction scores.

4.3 *Emotional Intelligence in the dental curriculum*

This awareness of EI, however, cannot be developed overnight and hence needs to be incorporated into the dental curriculum as an undergraduate. In India, students from various economic, financial and educational backgrounds join dentistry. These students are not formally aware of the concept of EI, as they learn to deal with emotions only informally through family and, to an extent, through the society around them [17]. Hence, when they are subjected to the rigors of dental education, many are often not able to cope. This is especially true in the freshman year. It is a life-changing experience in which people leave home, live in a new environment, meet new people and face new academic challenges that can be very overwhelming. Formal EI training can therefore help dental students cope with demanding programs such as dentistry, where the student is expected to develop a wide range of skills and competencies. Studies have consistently shown that students with high EI handle stressful situations much better and excel in academics. Pau and Croucher, in their study of undergraduates in the UK studying dentistry, revealed that students who scored high on EI coped with stress much better [18]. Further studies have shown that students who score low on EI are more stressed by situations and are drawn toward unhealthy addictions such as smoking and being socially withdrawn [19].

Another aspect of dental education in India now concerns the large percentage of females joining the profession. There is a perception among women that dentistry will enhance their stature in society professionally and financially [20]. This raises the question of differences in EI between men and women. Petrides *et al.* [21] reported that EI scores are higher in men than in women. In contrast, Austin *et al.* [22] reported the opposite, citing higher female EI scores. There are also reports based on the "Emotional Quotient Inventory (EQ-i) Bar", which state that there are no differences between men and women in their overall EI scores, but the scores may vary across specific EI domains [23]. These domains include empathy, interpersonal relationships, social responsibility, assertiveness and stress tolerance. These specific differences can be traced back to gender role expectations in childhood and biological differences. However, women consistently scored higher than men did in the empathy domain, which could explain the higher percentage of women opting for the speciality of pediatric dentistry, where the importance of this domain becomes paramount [24]. Ravichandra KS *et al.* [4] conducted a study among undergraduate dental students to assess their EI. They evaluated six aspects of EI, namely, self-awareness, self-confidence, self-control, empathy, motivation, and social competency among the students. The results revealed that only 11.55% of the dental students in India had acceptable EI, and most of them needed definite intervention to improve their EI. India has more than 300 dental colleges with students from diverse backgrounds. They will, in turn, be trained to treat people from diverse backgrounds. This training will be qualitatively incomplete if an important soft skill such as EI is not formally inducted into the curriculum. Pediatric and preventive dentistry is the only subject in the dental curriculum that, to some extent, trains postgraduates in EI. This is because it is an integral part of being able to deal empathetically with the fearful child and their apprehensive parents. Bhaskar *et al.* conducted a study assessing the EI of postgraduate students studying pedodontics and preventive dentistry in India. The results revealed high EI scores for both male and female postgraduate students [5]. However, at the undergraduate level, child psychology continues to remain only a minute part of a large dental curriculum.

5 CONCLUSION

This paper emphasizes the importance of emotional intelligence for the profession of dentistry. It also highlights that this important aspect has not received importance in the literature. The blending of this important life skill into the dental profession requires it to be an integral part of the dental curriculum in India at the undergraduate level.

REFERENCES

[1] Polychronopoulou A, Divaris K. (2009). Dental students' perceived sources of stress: A multicountry study. *J Dent Educ* 73(5):631–9.

[2] Kay EJ, Lowe JC. (2008). A survey of stress levels, self-perceived health and health-related behaviors of UK dental practitioners in 2005. *Br Dent J* 204(11):E19.

[3] Yarascavitch C, Regehr G, Hodges B, Haas DA. (2009). Changes in dental student empathy during training. *J Dent Educ* 73(4):509–7.

[4] Ravichandra KS, Ravi GR, Kandregula CR, Vundavalli S, Srikanth K, Lakhotia D. (2015). Emotional intelligence among dental undergraduate students: An indispensable and ignored aspect in dentistry. *J Int Oral Health.* 7(4):69–72.

[5] Yadav V, Mohanty V, Balappanavar AY, Verma A, Chahar P, Yadav G. (2020). Emotional Intelligence and Perceived Stress among Dental Undergraduates in Delhi. *Int J Clin Pediatr Dent.* 13(4):344–347. doi: 10.5005/jp-journals-10005-1789.

[6] Bhaskar DJ, Aruna DS, Rajesh G, Suganna M, Suvarna M. (2013). Emotional intelligence of pedodontics and preventive dentistry postgraduate students in India. *Eur J Dent Educ.* 17(1):e5–9. doi:10.1111/j.1600-0579.2012.00750.x.

[7] Kumar A, Puranik MP, Sowmya KR. (2016). Association between dental students' emotional intelligence and academic performance: A study at six dental colleges in India. *J Dent Educ.* 80(5):526–32.

[8] Saoji SS, Paul P, Sontakke PD, Reche A, Awghad S. (2024). Determining the emotional intelligence and compassion fatigue among postgraduate dental students using the emotional intelligence scale and the quality of life scale: an observational study. *Cureus.* 16(7):e64060. doi: 10.7759/cureus.64060.

[9] Mayer JD, Salovey P. (1993). The intelligence of emotional intelligence. *Intelligence* 17(4): 433–442.

[10] Gardner H. (1983). Frames of Mind: The theory of multiple intelligences. New York: Basic Books.

[11] Thorndike EL. (1920). Intelligence and its uses. *Harper's Magazine* 140: 227–235.

[12] Goleman D. (1998). *Working with Emotional Intelligence.* New York: Bantam Books.

[13] Yarascavitch C, Regehr G, Hodges B, Haas DA. (2009). Changes in dental student empathy during training. *J Dent Educ* 73(4):509–7.

[14] Aggarwal A, Mehta S, Gupta D, Sheikh S, Pallagatti S, Singh R, *et al.* (2012). Dental students motivations and perceptions of dental professional career in India. *J Dent Educ* 76(11):1532–9.

[15] Becker IM, Ackley D, Green RA. The value of emotional intelligence in dentistry. *Dent Today*, 22(10): 106.

[16] Sarnat H, Arad P, Hanauer D, *et al.* (2001). Communication strategies used during pediatric dental treatment: A pilot study. *Pediatr Dent* 23: 337–342.

[17] Singh D. (2003). *Emotional Intelligence at Work*, 2nd edn. New Delhi: Sage Publications.

[18] Pau AK, Croucher R. (2003). Emotional intelligence and perceived stress in dental undergraduates. *J Dent Educ* 67(9):1023–8.

[19] Brackett MA, Mayer JD, Warner RM. (2004). Emotional intelligence and its relation to everyday behavior. *Pers Indiv Diff* 36:1387–402.

[20] dos Santos BF, Nicolau B, Muller K, Bedos C, Zuanon AC. (2013). Brazilian dental students intentions and motivations towardstheir professional career. *J Dent Educ* 77(3):337–44.

[21] Petrides KV, Furnham A, Martin GN. (2004). Estimates of emotional andpsychometric intelligence: evidence for gender-based stereotypes. *JSoc Psychol* 144(2): 149–162.

[22] Austin EJ, Evans P, Goldwater R, Potter V. (2005). A preliminary study of emotional intelligence, empathy and exam performance in first year medical students. *Personality Individ Differ* 39(8):1395–1405.

[23] Bar-On R. (2000). Emotional and social intelligence: Insights from the Emotional Quotient Inventory. In: Bar-On R, Parker JDA eds *The Handbook of Emotional Intelligence.* San Francisco: Jossey-Bass,363–388.

[24] Benjamin P, Hagit G, Diana R. (2003). Child-management techniques. Are there differences in the way female and male pediatric dentists inIsrael practice?. *Braz Dent J* 14(2): 82–86.

Author Index

For Product Safety Concerns and Information please contact our EU
representative GPSR@taylorandfrancis.com
Taylor & Francis Verlag GmbH, Kaufingerstraße 24, 80331 München, Germany

www.ingramcontent.com/pod-product-compliance
Lightning Source LLC
LaVergne TN
LVHW081210220826
846195LV00029B/313